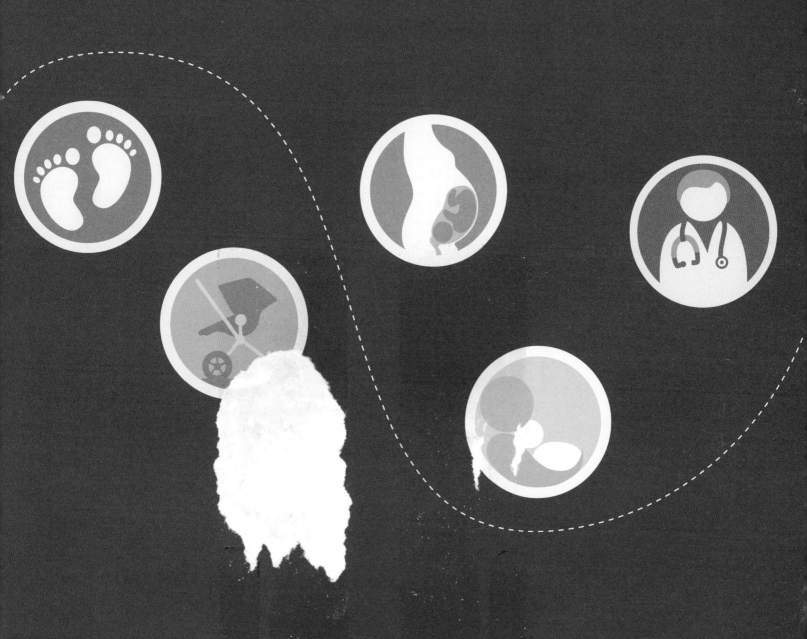

THE Pregnancy
ENCYCLOPEDIA

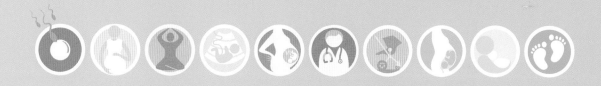

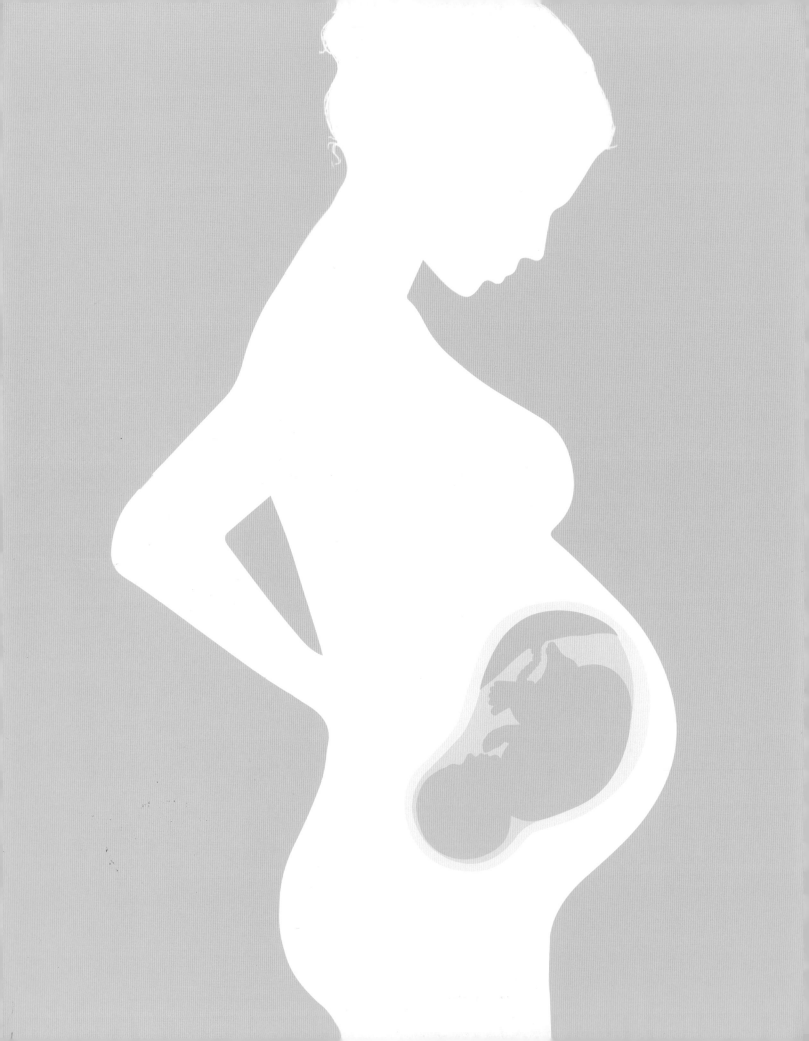

THE
Pregnancy
ENCYCLOPEDIA

All your questions answered

Consultant Editor Paula Amato, M.D.
Editor-in-chief Dr. Chandrima Biswas, Consultant Obstetrician

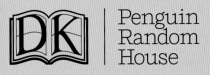

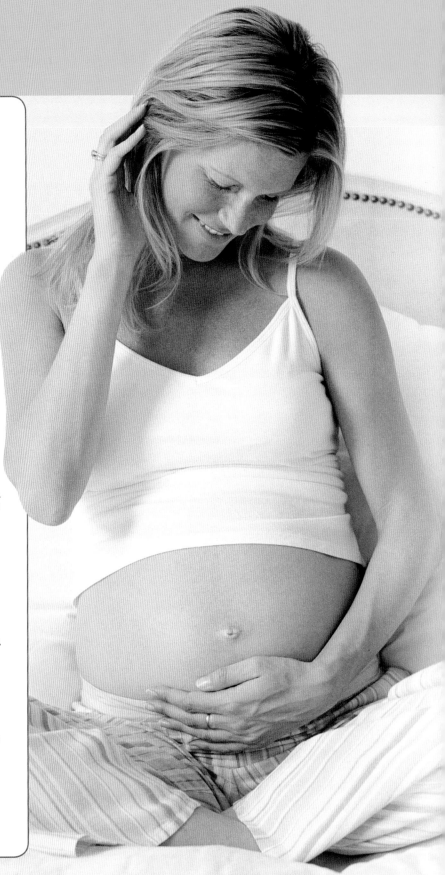

Editor-in-chief Dr. Chandrima Biswas
Consultants Dr. Anastasia Alcock, Dr. Jenny Hall,
Dr. Su Laurent, Professor Lesley Page
US Editorial Consultant Lisa Fields
US Medical Consultant Dr. Paula Amato
Writers Judy Barratt, Claire Cross, Susannah Steel
Senior Editors Carrie Love, Victoria Heyworth-Dunne
US Editor Jane Perlmutter
US Senior Editor Shannon Beatty
Senior Art Editors Nicola Rodway, Alison Gardner, Collette Sadler
Project Editors Shashwati Tia Sarkar, Victoria Marshallsay,
Dawn Bates, Hilary Mandleberg, Ruth O'Rourke
Project Designers Emma Forge, Tom Forge
Jacket Designer Nicola Powling
Jacket Editor Francesca Young
Preproduction Producer Andy Hilliard
Senior Print Producer Stephanie McConnell
Creative Technical Support Sonia Charbonnier
New illustrations Peter Bull
New photography Ruth Jenkinson
Picture Researchers Lucy Claxton, Martin Copeland
Managing Editor Lisa Dyer
Managing Art Editor Marianne Markham
Art Director Maxine Pedliham
Publishing Director Mary-Clare Jerram

First American Edition, 2016
Published in the United States by DK Publishing
345 Hudson Street, New York, New York 10014

Copyright © 2016 Dorling Kindersley Limited
DK, a Division of Penguin Random House LLC
16 17 18 19   10 9 8 7 6 5 4 3 2 1
001–280240–Feb/16

Published in Great Britain by Dorling Kindersley Limited.
A catalog record for this book is available from the Library of Congress.
ISBN: 978-1-4654-4378-6

DK books are available at special discounts when purchased in bulk for sales
promotions, premiums, fund-raising, or educational use. For details, contact:
DK Publishing Special Markets, 345 Hudson Street, New York, New York 10014
SpecialSales@dk.com

Printed and bound in China

All images © Dorling Kindersley Limited
For further information see: www.dkimages.com

A WORLD OF IDEAS:
SEE ALL THERE IS TO KNOW

www.dk.com

Contents

Foreword

Your pregnancy journey, the first time and each time you embark on it, is incredible and unique to you. From my professional working life in obstetrics, and seeing patients from all sorts of backgrounds, I have found there are as many different pregnancies and birth experiences as there are individual women.

Finding out you are pregnant for the first time, or indeed the second, third, or fourth times, can bring on a myriad of emotions—joy, excitement, reticence, fear, awe, curiosity, and, of course, anxiety. These feelings are entirely natural, as is the need for advice. In the past, societies with large families and different social structures created a network of sisterly support to help and inform women about all matters pregnancy related. By contrast, today we may talk about our pregnancy to only a handful of family members and girlfriends; and to our obstetrician or midwife every couple of weeks.

Often, our first step is to perform an Internet search. Here there is an abundance of information (and misinformation), and anecdotes of the pregnancy and childbirth experiences of other parents—including those that are unusually good or unusually disappointing. Sometimes search results are informative but too often they can be confusing and lead to further anxiety about our own experience.

Your questions answered

On the following pages, we have aimed to provide the balanced advice and support you need at one of the most important times of your life. We have covered every stage: pre-conception, the pregnancy, labor, birth, and even the first three monthst of your baby's life. We have arranged the chapters by theme, and question, helping you to find the answers you are seeking, as well as other related subjects you might want to know about. A timetable of prenatal care is outlined and expert advice is given on

Q Who are the consultants?

Editor-in-chief	Consultant	Consultant
Dr. Chandrima Biswas	**Dr. Anastasia Alcock**	**Dr. Jenny Hall**
MRCOG MBBS	MRCPCH MBBS DTM&H DPID DRCOG	EdD RM ADM MSc PGDip(HE)

Dr. Chandrima Biswas is clinical director at the Whittington Hospital in London, and is also the obstetric lead for the North Central London Maternity Network. She is a fellow of the Royal College of Obstetrics and Gynaecology, and a former president of the Maternity and Newborn Forum of the Royal Society of Medicine. She specializes in high-risk obstetrics, in particular the problems associated with maternal obesity.

Dr. Anastasia Alcock is a pediatrician specializing in emergency medicine and infectious diseases. She is currently working at the John Radcliffe Hospital in Oxford, having graduated from Imperial College School of Medicine, London. Anastasia is the founder of The Prenatal Classroom, which provides prenatal and postpartum advice. She is the author of *Your Baby's First Year*, which guides parents through the ups and downs of the first year.

Dr. Jenny Hall has been involved with the British National Health Service for more than 35 years, as a nurse and midwife and then as an educator. She is currently senior lecturer at Bournemouth University and researches particularly spirituality and dignity in care. She was the editor for *The Practising Midwife Journal* for ten years and is currently associate editor for *Women & Birth* journal. She is the author and coauthor of a variety of midwifery articles and books.

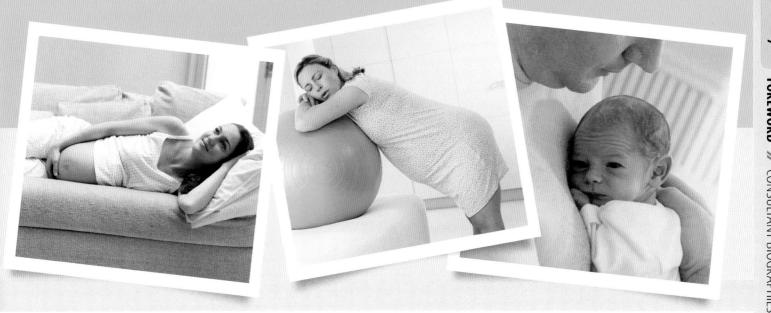

what is likely to occur during your pregnancy, from procedures and ultrasounds to birth plans and labor techniques. You will learn about nutrition and exercise, and how to keep healthy, as well as the biological changes taking place in your body and your baby's. There are also sections on clothes to buy to accommodate your increasingly large belly, and also what to buy to prepare for your new arrival. You'll find guidance on all concerns from common complaints during the first trimester to taking care of your newborn. When the time comes to seek advice from your own obstetrician, we have asked you to do so.

Your journey to birth and beyond
The story of the beginnings of your baby's life is told in a visually beautiful, easy-to-read, and factually

accurate account. Throughout, in-depth medical information and authoritative advice will enable you to feel confident about what to expect before, during, and after the birth, while information on lifestyle, working, and well-being will help you have a balanced and joyful pregnancy, and look forward to meeting the newest member of your family.

To all those contemplating pregnancy, or who are already pregnant, I hope you will find that this fascinating book helps you understand and enjoy the very beginning of your baby's life.

Dr. Chandrima Biswas

Consultant
Dr. Su Laurent
MRCP, FRCPCH

Dr. Su Laurent has been a consulting pediatrician at Barnet Hospital, London since 1993. Her special interests include asthma, and the interaction between the mind and body and how this affects physical health. She has written several books on parenting and child health. She is the medical advisor to the charity Child Bereavement UK and was the expert pediatrician for *Mother and Baby* magazine for many years.

Consultant
Professor Lesley Page CBE
PhD MSc BA RM RN
Honorary DSc HFRCM

Professor Lesley Page is president of the Royal College of Midwives. She was the first professor of midwifery in the UK at Thames Valley University and Queen Charlotte's Hospital. She is a renowned international academic, advocate, and activist for midwives, mothers, and babies. She has contributed to the development of woman centered maternity care. She has practiced midwifery in the community, hospital, and home-birth settings for more than 32 years.

US Consultant Editor
Paula Amato
M.D.

Dr. Paula Amato is a reproductive endocrinologist and is an associate professor at the Oregon Health and Science University (OHSU) in Oregon. She received her degree from the University of Toronto, where she also completed her residency in obstetrics and gynecology. She was subsequently a fellow in reproductive endocrinology and infertility at the University of California. She is board certified in obstetrics, gynecology, reproductive endocrinology, and infertility.

How do I use this book?

The Pregnancy Encyclopedia is a one-stop reference that will guide and inform you throughout these special nine months. Presented in an easy-to-navigate question-and-answer format, the book covers all aspects of pregnancy and labor, and looks ahead to life with your brand-new baby and the first few weeks of family life.

HOW EACH CHAPTER IS ARRANGED

Chapters are arranged thematically, allowing you to find the answers to all your questions on a topic in one place. Whether you want to learn all about the pregnancy tests and ultrasounds, find out exactly what you should and shouldn't eat, explore your baby's development, or check what equipment you will need when your newborn arrives, dedicated chapters provide a complete reference on each topic.

Within each chapter, sections explore particular elements of a topic, beginning with a summary and then an accessible question-and-answer format. Special feature pages examine key questions in depth, and gorgeous visual highlight pages take a closer look at areas of interest.

Navigation A mini contents list tells you where to find the section you're looking for

Introduction An overview gives some background to questions you might have

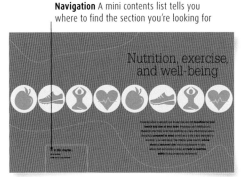

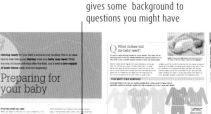
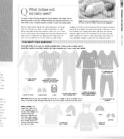

Book chapters Themed chapters make it easy to find what you need to know about a particular area of pregnancy.

Chapter sections Sections take aspects of the chapter's topic and explore them in detail.

Questions Informative answers from trusted professionals are given

Visual explanations Tricky concepts are made easy to understand

Single question Key topics are given a thorough treatment

Side headings At-a-glance guide to the contents of each page

Steps Processes are explained through clearly marked steps

Fun facts Lists of amazing facts will fill you with awe

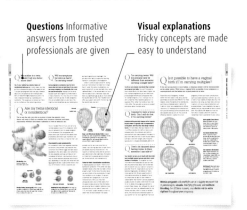
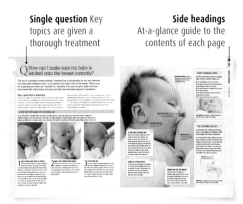
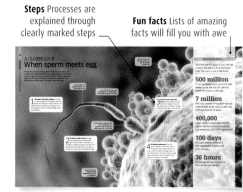

Q&A pages Find answers to your most-asked questions with this easy-to-follow format. Full of clear illustrations to help explain the information.

Special features Feature pages look at the big questions in depth. Detailed answers and visuals give you the full picture on a variety of topics.

Highlight pages Beautiful visuals and fascinating facts celebrate the wonder of pregnancy and having a newborn baby.

THE CHAPTERS IN THIS BOOK

WELCOME TO YOUR PREGNANCY

» pages 10–25

Illustrations See how your baby grows at each week throughout your pregnancy

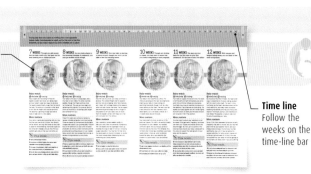

Time line Follow the weeks on the time-line bar

Week-by-week guidance for your pregnancy

is given in the initial chapter of this book. There are weekly digests on the progress of your baby's development in "Baby watch" and you can follow your own pregnancy journey in "Mom matters." Read about the incredible changes that take place within each week of the three trimesters. Helpful hints and reminders are given for each week, such as when to arrange childbirth classes.

Welcome chapter Your baby's size and weight are listed for each week, along with possible symptoms you might be experiencing

CONCEPTION

The first step in your pregnancy journey, this chapter looks at the incredible chain of events that lead to conception, with detailed explanations of how your monthly cycle prepares your body for pregnancy, and on how pregnancy is established with the implantation of the tiny embryo. From optimizing fertility to the early signs of pregnancy, this chapter helps you prepare for and navigate these first important weeks.

NUTRITION, EXERCISE, AND WELL-BEING

Pregnancy comes with a bewildering array of advice on what you should and shouldn't do to keep you and your baby healthy. This chapter provides clear-cut guidelines on which foods to avoid, and explains how healthy eating can optimize your baby's early development. Sensible exercise advice and relaxation techniques help you deal with common pregnancy concerns, and develop stamina and focus for labor.

PRENATAL CARE

The type of care you receive is a primary concern in pregnancy. This chapter details the options for prenatal care and who you can expect to take care of you. It also prompts you to think about where you want to give birth, who you would like to be with you, and what type of birth you would prefer. A section on all the tests and ultrasounds you will be offered in pregnancy helps you to understand why these are done and how they can benefit you and your baby.

ALL ABOUT YOU

The changes to your body in pregnancy impact many aspects of life, from your relationship with your partner to your ability to stay comfortable and sleep, to making travel arrangements. In addition to these practical matters, this chapter also explores the many physical and emotional changes pregnancy brings, and looks at some of the common complaints and complications of pregnancy and how to manage them.

YOUR GROWING BABY

Nothing is more fascinating in pregnancy than the incredible development of your baby in the uterus. This chapter documents each step of your baby's progress, showing how, within a matter of weeks, your baby develops from a tiny bundle of cells to a recognizably human fetus. In addition to her external growth and features, we look at how your baby's vital organs develop and at the unique genetic inheritance your baby holds.

PRACTICAL PREPARATIONS

From maternity and nursing bras, support belts, and pregnancy jeans, through to nursing pillows, strollers, cribs, and sleep suits, there's a whole host of items you will need for your pregnancy and your baby when he arrives. This chapter helps you to make practical choices, gives tips on what to buy when, and ensures that you have all you need to get you through pregnancy and the early weeks and months with your new baby.

LABOR AND BIRTH

A dedicated chapter on labor and birth guides you through each stage of labor, showing you how to recognize when labor is really underway and how to chart its progress. Guidance on pain-relief options will help you consider which techniques and medications you might prefer to use in labor. And you can find out what happens right after the birth: how your baby is taken care of, how you might feel, and how to kick-start the bonding process.

THE POSTPARTUM PERIOD

During pregnancy, you will want to think ahead to life with your new baby. This chapter allows you to do just that, providing a glimpse into what you can expect, and preparing you for the everyday care of your baby. You can read up on essential areas such as feeding, washing, dressing, comforting, transporting your baby, and dealing with first illnesses. You'll also find advice and tips on how to give yourself time to heal and recover gently after the birth.

SPECIAL SITUATIONS

Sometimes pregnancy brings up painful and unexpected situations, whether the actual loss of the pregnancy, a baby that arrives too early and needs special care, or a newborn who has a particular medical concern or long-term condition. This chapter looks at some of the difficult and challenging scenarios families can face and offers advice, information, and guidance to help families understand, come to terms with, and cope with these situations.

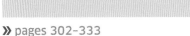

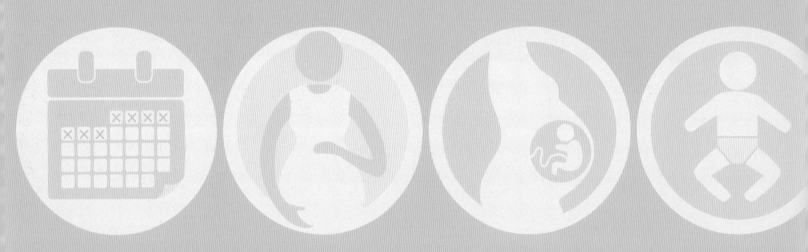

Welcome to your pregnancy

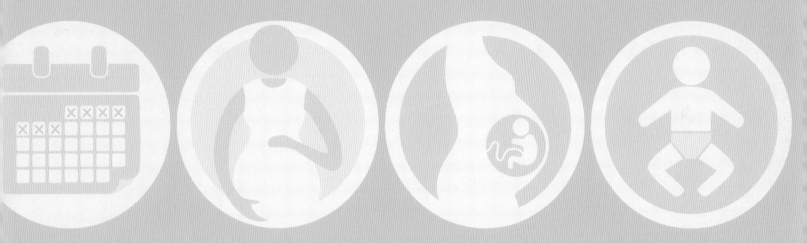

Congratulations—**you're pregnant**, or at least you think
you might be! In this chapter you'll find a summary of **what
to expect during each week** of pregnancy. You can then
turn to the chapters later in the book for more detailed
information on each subject.

Time line

From the moment of conception, you and your growing baby go through a multitude of extraordinary changes. Your pregnancy is dated from the first day of your last period. The average length of pregnancy is 40 weeks and it is divided into three parts, or trimesters, which last approximately three months each. Throughout this book, when a "week" is referred to, it means a completed week of pregnancy. This time line of key events gives you an at-a-glance view of your pregnancy journey.

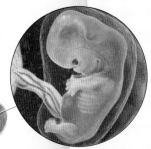

Menstruation Pregnancy is dated from the first day of your last period, so for the first two weeks you are not actually pregnant.

Supplements Take folic acid before you become pregnant, or as soon as you know you are, and continue until 12 weeks pregnant. Take vitamin D throughout your pregnancy, and beyond if you plan to breast-feed.

YOUR DEVELOPING BABY
Although no bigger than a large grape, your baby is developing rapidly. A tiny heart is beating, a little face is taking shape, and limbs are starting to form.

8-WEEK-OLD EMBRYO

THE ANATOMY SCAN
This ultrasound checks your baby's organs, body systems, and limbs. The sonographer may also be able to tell you whether it's a boy or a girl.

First trimester

0	1	2	3	4	5	6	7	8	9	10	11	12

Second trimester

13	14	15	16	17	18	19	20

CONCEPTION
Once a sperm fertilizes an egg, your baby begins life. After several days, it burrows into the lining of the uterus. The place where it implants will develop into the placenta.

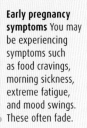

Early pregnancy symptoms You may be experiencing symptoms such as food cravings, morning sickness, extreme fatigue, and mood swings. These often fade.

Prenatal appointments Your first appointment takes place at around 6 to 8 weeks. It will be really thorough and you'll be able to ask the doctor any pregnancy-related questions that you may have.

Telling others After the first trimester, or when you've had your first ultrasound, is a good time to tell the wider world about your pregnancy.

Exercise Keep active and healthy. Your regular exercise may be too strenuous now, so adapt your routine and consider exercise classes especially tailored for pregnant women.

Flu vaccine Potentially harmful to you and your unborn baby, flu can be prevented through vaccination at any point during pregnancy. Ask your doctor for a flu shot.

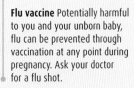

You're pregnant! A pregnancy test will detect the presence of a certain hormone that will confirm that you are expecting a baby.

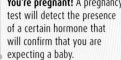

GOOD NEWS!

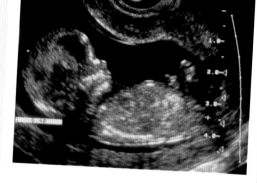

FIRST ULTRASOUND
When you are 8 to 14 weeks pregnant, your baby will be measured from crown to rump and you'll be given an estimated delivery date. Keep in mind, though, that there's a five-week range when birth could happen. You will be offered a nuchal translucency test if you are 11 to 14 weeks.

YOUR BABY'S POSITION

At this late stage, your baby's growth continues to be assessed as well as the efficiency of the placenta. By this point, your baby is nearly at full term and space is tight inside your uterus. Her head may begin to move into the pelvic cavity. Engagement occurs when the widest part of the baby's head has entered the pelvic inlet. This is one of the ways your body prepares itself for labor.

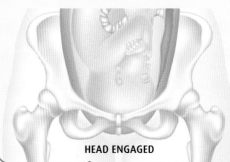

HEAD ENGAGED

Baby equipment Start thinking about the equipment you will need for your baby. You'll want to try out strollers, car seats, front-pack carriers, and slings. Think about whether your baby will sleep in a crib or bassinet.

Your birth plan Now is a good time to decide where you would like to give birth, who you would like to be there, and the labor techniques you might consider.

Telling your employer There's no requirement that dictates you tell your employer about your pregnancy. But you may decide to tell a boss or supervisor, as many women do, by the time you're showing.

Whooping cough vaccine This is offered to you between 28 and 38 weeks. It protects your baby from birth until her first vaccinations.

Childbirth classes Classes may start around now. They are popular, so enroll at least 12 weeks in advance. Your doctor will explain what is available.

Due date It's normal for babies to be born between 37 and 42 weeks, so don't worry if yours hasn't arrived.

Third trimester

| 22 | 23 | 24 | 25 | 26 | 27 | 28 | 29 | 30 | 31 | 32 | 33 | 34 | 35 | 36 | 37 | 38 | 39 | 40+ |

YOUR MOVING BABY

For the last couple of weeks your baby's movements have become more obvious; you may be able to feel her hiccups and she will be growing used to the sound of your voice. Be aware of your baby's pattern of behavior and report unusual changes to your doctor.

The nesting instinct Try to rest as much as you can. If you feel the urge to clean and scrub, be careful not to overdo it.

Prepare your hospital bag Pack your hospital bag well in advance, in case you go into labor early. Add a copy of your birth plan. Make sure your birth partner knows where everything is.

Preparing for labor Practice exercises that might ease labor. Spend time on all fours or sitting on an exercise ball; start relaxation and breathing techniques; try massaging your perineum to make the area more supple.

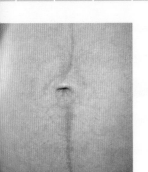

COMMON SIDE EFFECTS OF PREGNANCY

Many women feel full of energy and positive in the second trimester. You may begin to experience common side effects, including swollen hands and feet, bleeding gums, hemorrhoids, cramps, and skin changes. Some women get a dark line called a linea nigra on their abdomen that fades after birth.

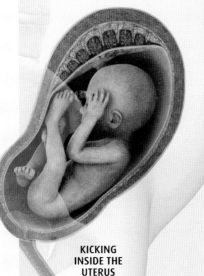

KICKING INSIDE THE UTERUS

ARE YOU READY?

Watch out for early labor signs such as a "bloody show," water breaking, and contractions beginning. If you go over 41 to 42 weeks you'll be overdue. This is very common and you can speak to your doctor about the next course of action.

First trimester

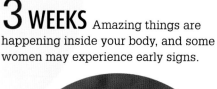

DAYS 1–14 The countdown of your pregnancy begins with your period—the start of the fertility cycle.

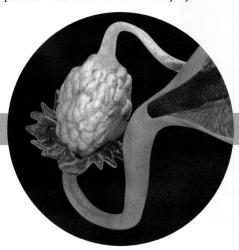

Baby watch

There is no baby yet, but the ovarian follicles are working to ripen the next egg.

Mom matters

Since it is often hard to be sure of the exact date when fertilization takes place, the first day of your last menstrual period (LMP) is used as a marker. In the first two weeks the body is resetting the fertility cycle: in the first week, the previous month's uterine lining sheds; in the second week, the uterine lining has begun to thicken in preparation for the next opportunity to conceive a baby.

 This week...

» Start taking 400 mcg folic acid daily, before conception.

» Both you and your partner should adopt a healthy lifestyle to increase your chances of becoming pregnant and having a trouble-free pregnancy—stop smoking and drinking alcohol, reduce caffeine intake, and get regular exercise.

» It's a good idea to get your health checked by a doctor, making sure your immunizations are up to date, and seeking advice on how to get existing conditions under control.

» Obesity can result in high-risk pregnancies, and should be tackled before you conceive. It can also interfere with your hormones and lower your chances of conceiving.

2 WEEKS A mature egg is released from the ovaries and if a sperm fertilizes it, a baby is conceived.

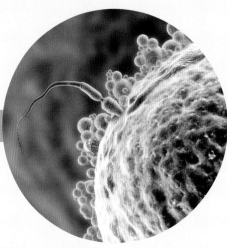

Baby watch

Length: approximately ½₅ in (0.1 mm)

Once released, an egg can survive for up to 24 hours as it waits to be fertilized. Around 200–500 million sperm are ejaculated during orgasm, but only a few hundred will make it all the way to the egg, where one winning sperm will penetrate and fertilize it. Shortly after fertilization, the outer layer of the egg thickens so that no other sperm can enter. The sperm and egg fuse their genetic material to start making your baby, which begins life as a single cell called a zygote.

Mom matters

The zygote will signal its existence to the pituitary gland in your brain. A new hormone is released called human chorionic gonadotrophin (hCG) that overrides your usual monthly cycle.

 This week...

» Enjoy sex frequently to give yourselves the best chance of conceiving. Have sex at least every two to three days throughout the month.

» Make sure you find time to relax and unwind—stress may affect your ability to become pregnant. It's no wonder that many couples seem to conceive while on vacation.

3 WEEKS Amazing things are happening inside your body, and some women may experience early signs.

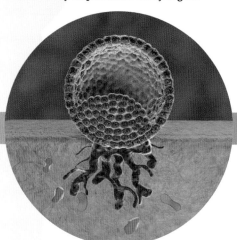

Baby watch

Length: > ½₃₂ in (1 mm)

Your baby-to-be is now a ball of around 100 cells called a blastocyst. It burrows into the lining of the uterus, which has become sticky to help it attach securely. The place where it implants will eventually develop into a placenta; for now a yolk sac is forming to nourish your baby in the earliest stages.

Mom matters

Hormones, including estrogen and progesterone, surge through your body to help the blastocyst settle safely. It's possible to experience very early symptoms such as sore breasts and fatigue. When the egg implants, it can cause some slight bleeding or "spotting," but this bleeding should be light, brief, and not painful.

 This week...

» While you are waiting to find out whether you are pregnant, avoid alcohol, smoking, and caffeine and eat a balanced diet. This will give your baby a great start.

» You may be able to find out whether you are pregnant this week using an extra-sensitive pregnancy test.

» Consult your doctor about whether or not it is safe to continue taking any existing medication.

The first trimester is a crucial time, during which all the major organs are formed. The pregnancy is supported by hormones from the ovary until the placenta takes over at around 10 weeks.

KEY

 Average height:
Up to 20 weeks crown to rump
From 20 weeks crown to heel

Average weight

4 WEEKS If you miss a period this week, it could be the first time you wonder, "Am I pregnant?"

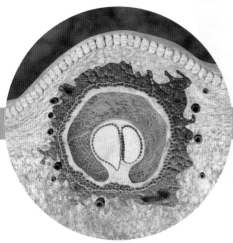

Baby watch

Length: 1/16 in (2 mm)

Your tiny baby has begun life as an embryo and is currently a disc of layered cells that is developing fast. It is floating in a fluid-filled amniotic sac. A basic blood circulation system has been established, and the brain and nervous system have begun to develop.

Mom matters

You might experience a variety of pregnancy symptoms including morning sickness. The levels of human chorionic gonadotrophin (hCG) hormone the fertilized egg is producing are high enough now that a pregnancy test will register positive.

 This week...

» Take a pregnancy test.

» Start taking 400 mcg folic acid and 10 mcg vitamin D daily, if you aren't already.

» Find out about stopping your contraception, if your pregnancy wasn't planned.

» Call your doctor to make an appointment for prenatal care.

» Stop drinking alcohol, smoking, and keep caffeine to no more than 200 mg per day.

5 WEEKS You won't be looking pregnant but as your body adapts to the pregnancy, you might well be feeling it.

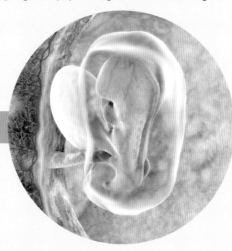

Baby watch

1/8 in (4 mm)

The embryo now resembles a tiny tadpole. The body has lengthened, and a row of dark cells has formed along the back, which is the beginning of the spinal cord. Dark spots on the face are the earliest hints of eyes, and bud like growths will become limbs. The heart is growing fast and by the end of this week it will start beating.

Mom matters

Common first trimester symptoms could be in full swing now. Most of the time they fade after 12 weeks. If you are suffering from morning sickness try eating plain foods and taking ginger. If you can't keep anything down, speak to your doctor.

 This week...

» Learn about what to eat for a healthy pregnancy and avoid foods that can cause food poisoning, such as undercooked egg and meats, pâté and liver, and unpasteurized dairy products and soft cheeses.

» If you have a hazardous or physically strenuous job, tell your employer about your pregnancy so that he or she can make provisions for you.

» Think about what type of prenatal care you would like, and compile questions to ask at your first prenatal appointment.

6 WEEKS Although there is no visible belly bump, it doesn't mean your body isn't changing in other ways.

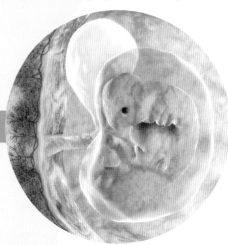

Baby watch

3/8 in (8 mm)

Your baby has doubled in length and resembles a small shrimp. The head and brain are growing at an incredible rate, and dark spots that will develop into eyes have appeared on the sides of the head. Primitive retinas are already forming.

Mom matters

Your metabolism speeds up, your lungs are working harder, and your blood volume is already increasing. Don't be surprised to find a little weight gain already, even though there's no sign of a belly. Your blood pressure drops as your blood vessels relax; this can cause dizziness so try to avoid standing up for long periods. Your nipples and the circles of skin around them (the areolae) may be darker and a mucus plug in the cervix seals off the uterus to protect the baby from infection.

This week...

» Your first prenatal visit can take place between six and eight weeks of pregnancy. At this appointment you will be weighed and your blood pressure checked. You will have your blood drawn for tests and will leave a urine sample to be checked.

» You may be given an early ultrasound to check your pregnancy if you have had any bleeding or a previous miscarriage.

During this time your baby is evolving into a recognizably human baby. Development is rapid, and by the end of the first trimester, all the major organs and body systems are in place.

7 WEEKS
Though you still cannot feel the baby inside you, the heart can be seen beating on an ultrasound now.

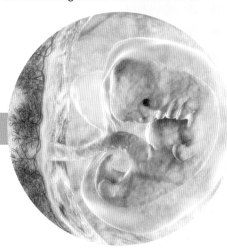

Baby watch
⬥ ⁵⁄₈ in (1.6 cm) ⬥ ¹⁄₃₂ oz (1 g)

Major organs are now being formed; the digestive system and bowel are taking shape and your baby's lungs have begun to develop. The head is proportionally larger than the rest of the body. The embryo is covered in a thin layer of skin and the fingers and toes are primitive. The placenta is growing stronger and will be ready to take over in a few weeks.

Mom matters

Your uterus is gradually expanding, and you may find that your waistline is thicker. Your breasts will be heavier and may feel tender as they start to adapt for breast-feeding. Hormonal surges can also bring skin changes, and you may find you suddenly get acne, or that your skin dries out.

 ## This week...

» Start practicing Kegel exercises.

» Be attentive to kitchen hygiene since you are more vulnerable to food poisoning in pregnancy.

» Be aware of toxoplasmosis, which can be found in cat feces, undercooked meat, and contaminated soil.

» Be safe when using cleaning products—wear protective gloves and open windows so that you don't inhale fumes.

8 WEEKS
As your body adapts to the hormonal changes of pregnancy, you may get sudden mood swings.

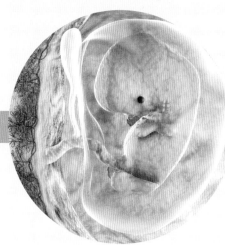

Baby watch
⬥ ⁷⁄₈ in (2.3 cm) ⬥ ¹⁄₁₆ oz (2 g)

Your baby is the size of a large grape, and a tiny nose is now visible. The limbs resemble paddles, though the fingers and toes have not formed yet. The eyes are now larger and darkening with pigment. The yolk sac starts to shrink as the embryo increasingly gets oxygen and nutrients from you.

Mom matters

These first weeks are commonly marked by nausea, complete exhaustion, and mood swings. These are caused by hormonal and physiological changes that support your growing baby. Frequent trips to the bathroom are due to the increased production of urine by certain hormones and the growing uterus putting pressure on your bladder. Many women also have strange food cravings, or develop strong aversions to some foods.

 ## This week...

» Make an appointment with the dentist (you should already be going twice a year) to check your gum health since gums soften and bleed in pregnancy.

» If your breasts feel fuller, get your bust measured by an experienced fitter and buy a supportive maternity bra.

» Get a flu shot at any time to protect your baby and yourself.

9 WEEKS
Your tiny baby is starting to move around, though you won't yet be able to feel this exciting action.

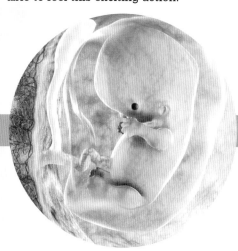

Baby watch
⬥ 1¼ in (3 cm) ⬥ ⅛ oz (4 g)

Now the size of a prune, your baby continues to develop. The webbed fingers start to separate and tiny toes are emerging. Early facial features are in place. Soft cartilage makes up the skeleton, which will later harden into bone. The sex organs and external genitalia begin to form, though it's not possible to tell your baby's sex yet. Buds from the bladder connect with tissue cells that will eventually form the kidneys.

Mom matters

Your respiratory system adapts rapidly to help your body meet the demands of pregnancy. The ribs expand and the diaphragm moves up, enabling the lungs to take in more air, increasing oxygen absorption. You may feel the heat since the blood supply to the skin increases; to counter this, blood vessels dilate, dispersing heat and controlling your blood pressure.

 ## This week...

» Start to budget for when the baby arrives.

» Keep up with or start some gentle exercise—the more fit you keep yourself, the easier labor and delivery will be.

10 WEEKS
Though not obvious to others, you may start to notice that your body is beginning to look pregnant.

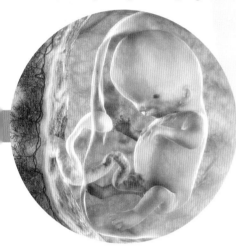

Baby watch
📏 1⅝ in (4.1 cm) ⚖️ ¼ oz (7 g)

Your baby is now classified as a fetus. The limbs are growing and the neck has lengthened, enabling your baby to make kicking and squirming movements, though it will be a few weeks before you feel them. The heart now has a basic structure, with four chambers, and it beats rapidly, up to 160 beats a minute, as it circulates blood around the body.

Mom matters
Your uterus starts to move up and out of the pelvis as it grows. This shift in its position means less pressure on your bladder. Your breasts continue to grow, and you may go up two or three bra sizes by the end of this trimester. It is normal to feel increasingly breathless—your body needs to take in more air, which is directed toward the baby, uterus, and placenta—but mention it to your doctor if you are alarmed.

 ## This week...

» Look at your employee handbook to see whether you'll be offered maternity leave.

» If your breasts are tender, wear a softer bra at night.

» Start looking into childbirth classes to sign up for.

11 WEEKS
You may see your baby for the first time on your first ultrasound. It's the start of your love affair!

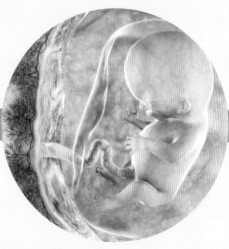

Baby watch
📏 2⅛ in (5.4 cm) ⚖️ ½ oz (14 g)

Your baby is roughly the size of a lime. The brain is forming left and right hemispheres and at the same time, primitive reflexes are developing. Your baby may move in response to pressure on the abdomen. Facial features are developing. The eyelids are fused together and will remain tightly shut until about 26 weeks, but the eyes and ears are not quite in their final position.

Mom matters
You may need to adjust your waistband or opt for looser-fitting garments. Pregnancy hormones can mean your nipples and areolae darken and become bigger. By now, up to a quarter of the blood pumped around your body is being sent to the uterus to support the rapid growth of your baby and the placenta.

 ## This week...

» A first ultrasound is done between 8 and 14 weeks. Various measurements are taken and you are given an estimated delivery date (EDD). The ultrasound also checks whether you are having one baby or more.

» You may have first screening tests to assess your baby's risk of chromosomal and genetic conditions. Your doctor will talk to you about what is available.

12 WEEKS
With nausea and fatigue fading away, you are likely to feel more invigorated.

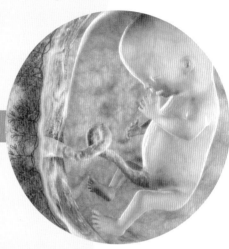

Baby watch
📏 2⅞ in (7.4 cm) ⚖️ ¾ oz (23 g)

By the end of this first trimester, the head is still large in proportion to the body, taking up about half the crown-rump length. The heart is fully functional, but the heart rate slows down. As the chest wall forms, your baby starts to practice breathing movements, and may also hiccup and swallow. The mouth, stomach, and intestines are now linked. The placenta is ready to take over the job of nourishing your baby.

Mom matters
Some of the more unpleasant symptoms of early pregnancy may start to recede, and you may feel great relief as your appetite returns, and your energy levels increase. The hormone hCG falls significantly now, which may be behind the nausea subsiding. For some women, nausea can continue to around week 20. If this is the case, rest assured that your baby will still be getting all the nutrients she needs, even if you are suffering!

 ## This week...

» If you've been waiting until your first ultrasound to tell family and friends, have fun breaking the good news.

» You may be offered the nuchal translucency test around now (often at the same time as your first ultrasound). This is used to help assess your baby's risk of Down syndrome.

Second trimester

13 WEEKS
Changes inside your body mean that you are glowing now. Sit back and enjoy this settled period.

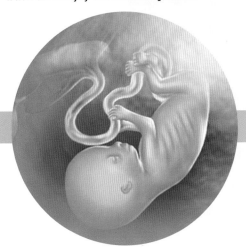

Baby watch
 3⅜ in (8.7 cm) 1½ oz (43 g)

Your baby will begin to look more in proportion as the torso starts to lengthen. The hands and feet are no longer webbed, toenails continue to develop, and the numerous bones of the hands and feet start to form.

Mom matters

The hormone relaxin is softening your joints and ligaments in preparation for birth. The downside is the added strain on your ligaments; you may start to feel some discomfort. As your blood volume continues to increase, your skin may start to take on the characteristic pregnancy "glow;" this, together with your more noticeable belly can start to signal to others that you're pregnant.

This week...

» Now is a great time to take a vacation if you want, while you feel more energetic and are not uncomfortably big. Most airlines don't let women fly in advanced pregnancy, so check their latest dates for flying before you buy a ticket.

» Keep a diary or photo journal of your pregnancy. You can record your growing belly, feelings, and changing symptoms.

» Keep up your regular exercise if it is gentle enough. Walking and swimming are ideal, and moderate jogging is fine if you're used to this.

14 WEEKS
Your pregnancy may be becoming obvious, and you may feel an incredible sense of well-being.

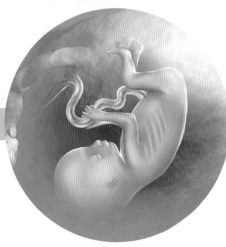

Baby watch
 4 in (10.1 cm) 2½ oz (70 g)

The umbilical cord, your baby's lifeline, is growing thicker and longer as it transports an increasing volume of oxygen-rich blood and nutrients to your baby. In baby girls, the ovaries are forming thousands of eggs, and the ovaries themselves are moving down into the pelvis. The external genitalia are increasingly visible now, and could possibly be seen on an ultrasound.

Mom matters

It's not uncommon to have a permanently stuffy nose, nosebleeds, and sinus headaches. These are caused by the extra blood flow to the mucous membranes. New symptoms may emerge such as constipation and indigestion. These are thought to be side effects of the hormones that make your digestive system sluggish.

This week...

» You may need to shop for some pregnancy clothes since waistbands may be growing too tight.

» If you have been referred for diagnostic tests such as CVS or amniocentesis, they could be done around this time.

» You are not obliged to tell your employer about your pregnancy, but discussing it sooner means you can talk through plans. Approach your boss or human resources.

15 WEEKS
It is normal to have mixed feelings about your changing body shape and curves.

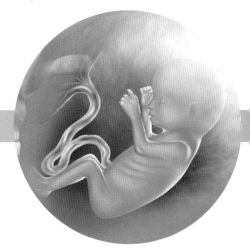

Baby watch
 4⅝ in (11.6 cm) 3½ oz (100 g)

Your baby's kidneys are functioning and can filter blood and eliminate waste from the body. The messages from the baby's brain and the rest of the body travel with more speed, allowing for more coordinated actions, including slow eye movements.

Mom matters

In addition to glowing skin, you may also find that your hair is fuller and more glossy as hormonal conditions prolong the growth phase of hair and less hair falls out on a daily basis than usual. Nails become healthier and stronger too.

This week...

» If you don't already exercise, put a gentle, regular exercise regimen into place. Now is a good time to start a pregnancy yoga class.

» It's not too early to start thinking about your birth plan—where you would like to give birth, who you would like to be with you, and birthing techniques you might consider.

» If you plan to take one enroll in childbirth classes this week, if you haven't done so already. These don't start until later in pregnancy but can fill up quickly. Your doctor can give you details of hospital and private classes.

» Try to set aside time for you and your partner.

Your pregnancy is well-established as the risk of miscarriage drops significantly, and you may enjoy a resurgence of energy now. The fetus grows dramatically, and your abdomen will soon develop a rounded belly.

16 WEEKS You will definitely start to look pregnant now, even if you don't feel that different.

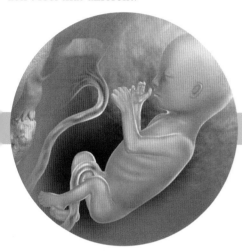

Baby watch

 5⅛ in (13 cm) ⌷ 5 oz (140 g)

The fetus is now larger than the placenta. The torso and limbs are growing quickly, and head growth slows, so the fetus looks more in proportion. You may hear your baby's heartbeat for the first time now as your doctor listens in with a fetal heart monitor that is placed on your abdomen to measure sound waves.

Mom matters

A rise in the production of melanin, the pigment that gives your skin and hair its color, can create temporary skin changes. Dark patches, called "chloasma," may appear on your cheeks, forehead, upper lip, and neck. You may develop a dark vertical line down your abdomen, called a linea nigra. These lighten or disappear after birth.

This week...

» Your doctor will talk to you about the anatomy scan (ultrasound) due soon. If blood tests revealed you were anemic, you may be offered iron supplements.

» If you wear contact lenses, you may find your eyes are drier than usual. Your optician can give you special drops.

» Dieting isn't recommended in pregnancy; try to stick to fresh, healthy foods.

17 WEEKS The bloom of pregnancy may be showing in your skin, and even in your mood.

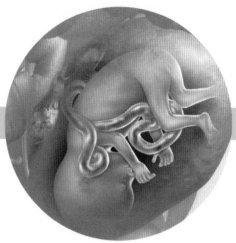

Baby watch

 5⅝ in (14.2 cm) ⌷ 6¾ oz (190 g)

The baby's sexual organs are well-developed now and will be clearly visible. By the end of this week, all your baby's milk teeth buds have formed and are nestled in place under the gums.

Mom matters

Your heart is now working at twice its normal rate to pump the increased blood volume around your body. To deal with this extra volume of blood and stop your blood pressure from rising, your blood vessels become more flexible and dilate. As more blood is diverted to the skin, you may look positively glowing and healthy. You may have a renewed interest in sex, helped by the increased blood flow to the pelvic area.

This week...

» Due to hormonal changes you may feel hotter than usual; dress in breathable fabrics or layers you can adjust.

» Support your baby's developing nervous system by eating foods containing omega-3 fatty acids, such as fish that's low in mercury, flaxseed and olive oil. Don't eat more than 8 to 12 ounces of low-mercury fish each week.

» While your energy levels may have picked up, be careful not to overdo things. Plan plenty of relaxation time.

18 WEEKS You may experience your baby's early, fluttering movements. These are known as "quickening."

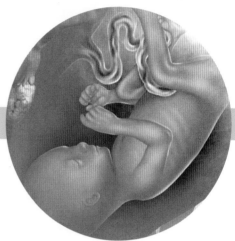

Baby watch

 6 in (15.3 cm) ⌷ 8½ oz (240 g)

Your baby increasingly resembles the little person you will meet. Facial features are well formed and unique fingerprints have begun to develop. Though the eyelids are still shut, the eyeballs can move from side to side.

Mom matters

You may feel your baby move for the very first time from this point. These early movements are known as "quickening" and can feel like a fluttery sensation. Each week your uterus grows around ⅜ in (1 cm), and the top of the uterus (the fundus) is almost level with your belly button. The ligaments that support the pelvic area stretch and thin, which can cause hip and back pain.

This week...

» Your anatomy scan (ultrasound) takes place around this time, so think ahead as to whether or not you want to discover your baby's sex.

» As your belly becomes ever more prominent, you may attract comments on your appearance and people may want to touch your belly. It is fine to ask people not to.

» Your changing shape and size means your center of gravity shifts, and you may feel a little wobbly. It may be time to put your high heels aside.

By the end of this second trimester, your baby has doubled her weight, and the major organs continue to develop apace. You will look obviously pregnant now, and are likely to feel a calm sense of well-being.

19 WEEKS You are almost halfway through your journey. Congratulations!

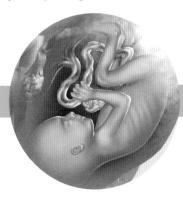

Baby watch

6½ in (16.4 cm) 10½ oz (300 g)

The legs are longer than the arms, and areas of hard bone continue to form. Your baby's senses of sight, sound, taste, touch, and smell are developing in the brain.

Mom matters

Your weight gain accelerates in this trimester. On average, women gain 1–2 lb (0.5–1 kg) per week from now up until delivery. Your baby accounts for only some of this extra weight; the rest is increased blood volume, breast size, amniotic fluid, and fat reserves. As your uterus continues to move upward, pressing into the stomach, and progesterone relaxes the abdominal muscles, digestion can become sluggish. You may suffer from heartburn, indigestion, and constipation, or existing symptoms may worsen.

 This week...

» Include plenty of fiber in your diet and drink plenty of fluids to help keep your stool soft and avoid uncomfortable constipation.

» Start thinking about baby names, and compile a list of your favorites.

20 WEEKS Your ultrasound gives you a glimpse of your well-formed baby.

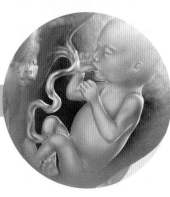

Baby watch

10½ in (26.7 cm) 12¼ oz (360 g)

The skin is covered in fine, downy lanugo hair and fat is beginning to be deposited under the skin. The skin forms two distinct layers: the epidermis and the dermis. Your baby is regularly swallowing more amniotic fluid, the kidneys are processing this, and she is urinating. Your baby's skin begins to release a white, waxy substance called "vernix caseosa," which forms a protective coating on the skin.

Mom matters

Your belly is increasingly rounded; it sits just below your belly button. Your extra blood volume helps supply the organs, which are working harder now to support you and your baby.

 This week...

» You will be given an anatomy scan (ultrasound) between 18 and 22 weeks. This takes various key measurements of your baby and checks her organs and body systems, and you can ask the sonographer to reveal your baby's gender if you want. The position of your placenta will also be checked.

21 WEEKS You are becoming more aware of your lively baby.

Baby watch

10⅞ in (27.8 cm) 15 oz (430 g)

The nerves and tiny bones in your baby's inner ear are developed enough for her to detect sounds. As the nervous system develops, your baby's movements become more deliberate: she kicks and may suck her thumb.

Mom matters

A large proportion of your increased blood volume is sent to your uterus, and this change in the distribution of your blood can make you feel dizzy at times. Your baby's movements become more obvious. Once you become aware of your baby's pattern of movement (rather than the actual number of movements), this becomes a good indicator of fetal well-being. If you don't feel any movement for 24 hours, contact your doctor.

 This week...

» This is an ideal time to go on a "babymoon" vacation, before you're in your third trimester.

» Continue to eat a healthy diet, and avoid fatty, rich foods to counter indigestion.

22 WEEKS You may see some unwanted, though usually temporary, side effects.

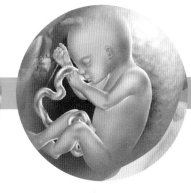

Baby watch

11⅜ in (28.9 cm) 1.1 lb (501 g)

Bathed in amniotic fluid and with just a little subcutaneous fat, your baby looks a little wrinkly. The skin cells start to produce a protective layer of keratin. Tiny nails start to emerge at the base of the nail beds, hair might be appearing on the scalp, and your baby now has eyelashes and eyebrows.

Mom matters

As the uterus expands, thinning the skin's collagen and elastin fibers, stretch marks may appear. These fade from red or dark purple to a shiny, paler color after pregnancy. Your skin may feel very dry and itchy. Keeping hydrated and using an unperfumed moisturizer can help. Painful leg-muscle cramps are a common symptom during this time, with spasms often occurring at night. Flexing the foot and massage can relieve cramps.

 This week...

» Anecdotally, foods containing potassium (such as bananas) or calcium may help to reduce the incidence of cramps. Staying well hydrated also helps prevent them.

23 WEEKS Keeping active means you will be well prepared for the birth, and primed for a rapid recovery.

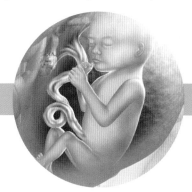

Baby watch

⬇ 12 in (30 cm) ⏱ 1 lb 5 oz (600 g)

Your baby's lungs start to produce a substance called surfactant now, which supports the tiny air sacs (alveoli) in the lungs, strengthening them in preparation for breathing outside of the uterus. In the inner ear, the cochlea is fully developed and allows hearing. Your baby may startle at loud noises and turn her head in response to sounds. She is also becoming familiar with your voice, which she'll recognize at birth.

Mom matters

Regular gentle exercise will help to keep your muscles and ligaments strong and supple. This will also help to relieve pregnancy complaints such as backaches. There's also some evidence that women who exercise have a shorter labor, and that the fetal heartbeat is stronger. Kegel exercises are very important too, helping to strengthen the hammock of muscles that support the pelvic area and organs, including the uterus.

 This week...

≫ If you haven't already done so, think about how to tell an older child about the baby's arrival. A young child may have little concept of timings, though, so keep explanations simple. There are also books you can use to introduce the idea.

≫ Good sources of protein such as lean meat, legumes, eggs, and cheese are essential for the healthy growth of your baby.

24 WEEKS Your baby might be active when you want to sleep— kicking, yawning, and even hiccupping.

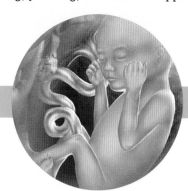

Baby watch

⬇ 13⅝ in (34.6 cm) ⏱ 1 lb 8 oz (660 g)

Your baby is starting to develop a primitive memory as the brain becomes more complex, and brain waves now are similar to those of a newborn's. You may notice your baby's hiccups now, and your baby may yawn as she develops a cycle of sleeping and waking. The nostrils are open, and the adult teeth buds are developing in the gums. By the end of this trimester, the fetal heartbeat has slowed to 140–150 beats a minute.

Mom matters

You will notice your abdomen expanding quickly as it stretches to accommodate your rapidly growing baby. As your belly protrudes outward and rises, it presses on your diaphragm, and you may feel breathless. It also nudges against your stomach, which can lead to heartburn and acid reflux.

 This week...

≫ As your belly gets bigger, you may feel off-balance. Be aware of compensating for this with bad posture that puts an additional strain on your back.

≫ You may have to shift the position that you sleep in as your belly continues to grow larger. If you tend to sleep on your stomach, that may no longer be an option. Sleeping on your back doesn't allow for the best blood flow to your baby; try sleeping on your side. Either is fine, but the left side is recommended.

25 WEEKS At the close of the second trimester, your thoughts might turn to the birth.

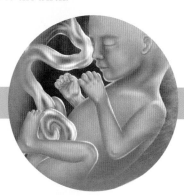

Baby watch

⬇ 14 in (35.6 cm) ⏱ 1 lb 10¼ oz (760 g)

With fully formed hands, your baby can grasp anything she comes into contact with. She may have discovered the pleasure of thumb-sucking. There's still room in the uterus for quite a bit of movement; some babies make a pedaling motion akin to walking. In boys, the testes start to move down from the lower abdomen into the scrotum.

Mom matters

Your uterus continues to move upward. Your organs are compressed by the expanding uterus, and you could feel a bit cramped inside. Blood volume has increased to around 8¾ pints (5 liters), and your heart is working hard to pump it around. The blood vessels have relaxed as much as possible, so your blood pressure may rise a little now. It is normal for your hands, feet, and ankles to swell as a result of fluid retention (edema). Severe swelling will need to be monitored.

 This week...

≫ You may have an prenatal appointment this week. The doctor will measure the height of your uterus (the fundus) to check that your baby is growing as expected.

≫ If you have had a previous late miscarriage, you may be given an ultrasound now to check the length of your cervix.

≫ As your digestive system is squashed, it may be easier to eat smaller, more frequent meals instead of the usual three large meals.

Third trimester

26 WEEKS It's the home stretch. Your belly is a source of pride, and you will marvel as it grows.

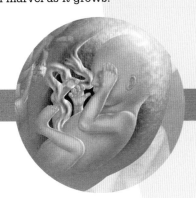

Baby watch

🔲 14⅜ in (36.6 cm) ⏲ 1 lb 14½ oz (875 g)

Your baby's eyelids open for the very first time around now. He is sensitive to light passing through the abdominal wall, though at the moment he can see only in black, white, and grays. As the kidneys mature, more urine is produced and excreted into the amniotic sac. The waxy vernix that is coating your baby helps prevent his skin from being irritated by the urine.

Mom matters

Don't be surprised if your breasts start leaking a little fluid now. This premilk, called colostrum, is produced in pregnancy, ready for your baby right after birth. You may feel a sense of relief as your reach the third trimester.

 This week...

» Talking to your unborn baby now can kick-start the bonding process as your voice becomes familiar to him.

» If you are suffering from hemorrhoids, keep up your fiber intake to keep stool-soft.

» If varicose veins are a problem, wear support hose and put your feet up as much as possible.

» Make a checklist of everything you will need for your baby. Start doing research on which big items to borrow or buy and begin purchasing things if you feel comfortable doing so.

27 WEEKS Reassuringly, babies who are born at this stage in pregnancy have a 90 percent survival rate.

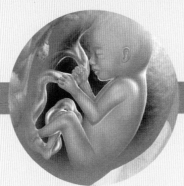

Baby watch

🔲 14⅝ in (37.6 cm) ⏲ 2 lb 4 oz (1 kg)

Your steadily growing baby fits ever more snugly in the uterus, but he can still manage to turn and flex his limbs. Your baby's muscle and organ development is supported by amino acids (the building blocks of protein) passed on from your blood. Baby boys start to outgrow girls now. Creases form on the palms of the hands and in the tooth buds, enamel, and dentine develop.

Mom matters

With the production of amniotic fluid slowing and your baby becoming increasingly active, you're likely to feel plenty of kicks. Note your baby's pattern of activities; if there are changes in his normal behavior (such as slowing down or stopping completely), you should report them to your doctor. Some women develop a pregnancy "waddle" as they grow, caused by their changing shape and the loosening of ligaments and tissues. This might become more exaggerated over the coming weeks. Many women find they become clumsier at this stage. Be careful on slippery surfaces such as the shower or bathtub.

 This week...

» Be careful with your movements to avoid straining your back.

28 WEEKS At this point, you may not remember how you felt without a belly.

Baby watch

🔲 15⅛ in (38.6 cm) ⏲ 2 lb 8 oz (1.2 g)

Vital development is continuing in the lungs, preparing your baby to breathe at birth. The folds of the brain have increased to house millions of new brain cells, and the cerebral cortex can send electrical impulses.

Mom matters

Your breasts are gearing up for feeding your baby. Pregnancy hormones increase the blood flow to the breasts and cause changes to the tissue, the veins become more prominent, and they may increase in size. The nipple area, or areola, also continues to grow and darken. You may notice small bumps known as Montgomery's tubercules forming around your nipples.

This week...

» You may have an prenatal appointment this week. Your doctor may give you bloods tests to check for anemia and pregnancy-induced gestational diabetes.

» If your blood group is Rhesus negative, you will be offered an injection called Rh immunoglobulin (RhIg) to avoid complications in this and future pregnancies.

» If you're suffering from restless leg syndrome, avoid caffeine late in the day, and eat foods containing the amino acid tryptophan, such as pumpkin seeds and yogurt, that triggers the release of the calming brain chemical serotonin, promoting good sleep.

Though your baby could survive in the outside world with assistance if born now, the uterus is still the best place for him as his lungs and digestive system mature and the brain continues to develop.

29 WEEKS You may start to feel sharp kicks from your baby.

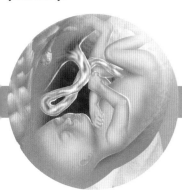

Baby watch

15⅝ in (39.9 cm) · 3 lb (1.3 kg)

Your baby makes practice breathing movements as he swallows amniotic fluid. His nervous system is becoming more complex, refining his movements and developing his sucking reflex. He starts to fill out more as muscle and fat are laid down. Between now and the end of pregnancy, his weight will double.

Mom matters

Your lung capacity has increased and your ribs have spread out sideways to help your lungs work harder. There is pressure on your other organs; you may find symptoms such as heartburn, constipation, and palpitations worsen, and you experience twinges, aches, and pains.

 This week...

» You will be offered the whooping cough vaccine to protect your unborn baby from this virus.

» If it's hard to stay comfortable at night, position pillows to support your belly. V-shaped pillows are helpful.

30 WEEKS Review your birth plan around now. It's not too late to make changes.

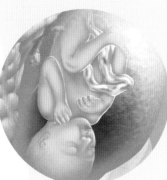

Baby watch

16⅛ in (41.1 cm) · 3 lb 3 oz (1.5 kg)

The skin is developing a pinker hue as fat builds up underneath and your baby will now be able to regulate his own body temperature. Although he is increasingly cramped for space, your baby is very flexible and can easily bring his feet up to his head, and even suck on his toes!

Mom matters

Although labor is a couple of months off, your uterus is preparing for the event by making practice "Braxton Hicks" contractions—you may start to notice tightening sensations around your abdomen around now or in later weeks. These range from being mild to a stronger cramp like feeling, but their irregularity and the fact they aren't very painful means this isn't the real thing.

 This week...

» Childbirth classes start around this time. Encourage your partner to attend so he knows what to expect. It's the perfect chance to start building a support network.

» Monitor swollen hands and feet.

31 WEEKS Your baby may be lying in any number of positions.

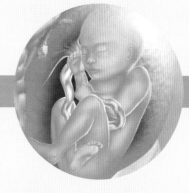

Baby watch

16⅝ in (42.4 cm) · 3 lb 10 oz (1.7 kg)

As your baby exercises his limbs, his muscle mass increases and muscle tone improves, so his movements become stronger and more purposeful. His practice breathing movements are regular and rhythmic, moving his diaphragm and chest wall.

Mom matters

Your blood volume peaks around this time. This extra volume is largely due to an increase in the plasma and fluid content of the blood, while the number of red blood cells remains the same. This means the red blood cells become less concentrated, a common cause of anemia in late pregnancy. There's no need to worry about the baby, though, since he will still receive all the nutrients and oxygen he needs to thrive.

 This week...

» You may have a routine prenatal appointment where your blood pressure and urine are checked, and your uterus will be measured. You will also be checked for signs of preeclampsia.

32 WEEKS Now is a good time to start thinking about practical preparations.

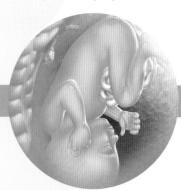

Baby watch

17⅛ in (43.7 cm) · 4 lb 3½ oz (1.9 kg)

Fine tuning is taking place in your baby's nervous system as brain cells are gradually coded into distinct areas that will control specific functions. Your baby will now be looking more substantial and plump as the wrinkles start filling out.

Mom matters

The size of your belly puts pressure on your veins; this can lead to varicose veins. Gentle exercise, rest, and support hose can bring relief, and symptoms should settle down after the birth. Your belly button may pop out around now. If this bothers you, rest assured that it should go back after the birth.

This week...

» Spend time on all fours, sitting on an exercise ball, or leaning over a bean bag or ball to move your baby into the best position.

» Check out the route to the hospital now. Find out how long the trip is at different times of day.

» Talk to your doctor and partner about any anxieties you may have about the approaching labor.

In these final weeks, your baby continues to lay down insulating fat deposits for life outside of the uterus, and the lungs are ready to take their first breath. Your baby will settle into his final position, ready for the birth.

33 WEEKS Each day, your baby is preparing for survival in the outside world.

34 WEEKS Practicing relaxation techniques will help you prepare for labor.

35 WEEKS Your body is well and truly gearing up for the big day.

36 WEEKS Make sure you have a plan ready for when you go into labor.

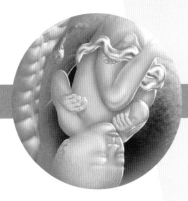
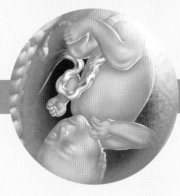
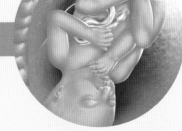
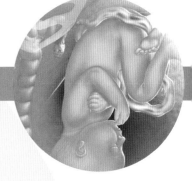

Baby watch

👶 17⅝ in (45 cm)   ⏱ 4 lb 11½ oz (2.1 kg)

Your baby is increasingly awake and active, and is becoming more aware of her surroundings, as she touches her face and pulls on the umbilical cord. Her sucking reflex is strong enough now that if born this early, she should be able to feed independently. Her fingernails are reaching the tips of her nail beds, and may need a trim at birth.

Mom matters

Your heart works extra hard now as you approach the home stretch–your heart rate increases by 10 to 15 beats a minute and the heart works up to 50 percent harder. It's not uncommon to experience fluttery palpitations; these are usually harmless, though mention them to your doctor if accompanied by breathlessness or chest pain.

 ## This week...

>> Regularly massaging your perineum can help make this area more supple and reduces your risk of tearing during the delivery.

>> Start thinking about who will give support once the baby is here, and also in the future.

Baby watch

👶 18⅛ in (46.2 cm)   ⏱ 5 lb 5 oz (2.4 kg)

Your baby looks far more in proportion, and is nicely plump. In the limbs, the bones continue to harden. Waste from the amniotic fluid is building up in the gut, forming a sticky substance called meconium, which will be your baby's first greenish-black poop after the birth.

Mom matters

Your baby is most likely to be lying vertically by this stage of pregnancy, though occasionally, babies are in a diagonal or horizontal position. As your baby gets bigger, her movements are likely to feel stronger, more frequent, and have a recognizable pattern now rather than seeming like isolated kicks.

 ## This week...

>> If you have an older child, have someone lined up to watch her when you go to the hospital.

>> Pack your hospital bag and keep your birth plan on hand. Make sure your partner knows where everything is too.

Baby watch

👶 18⅝ in (47.4 cm)   ⏱ 5 lb 10 oz (2.6 kg)

Your baby may have stationed herself in a head-down position, ready for her exit later this month. She is still busy laying down fat to insulate her after birth. At the same time, she will shed her lanugo hair, and may have just a few patches left over the back and shoulders.

Mom matters

With labor approaching, your baby's head may begin to "engage" (descend into your pelvis), and your belly may sit lower. The release of pressure on the diaphragm makes it easier to breathe. This is known as "lightening." The baby's head now presses on your bladder, which means frequent bathroom stops and interrupted sleep. Aches and pains in the pelvic area may well increase.

 ## This week...

>> Get fitted for a nursing bra now and get equipped for breast-feeding.

>> Prepare instructions for those filling in for you at work if you're starting maternity leave.

>> Keep practicing your Kegel exercises regularly to avoid stress incontinence later.

Baby watch

👶 19⅛ in (48.6 cm)   ⏱ 6 lb 5 oz (2.9 kg)

Your baby is almost full term, and her lungs are fully developed now, which means she could breathe without help if born from this point. She is losing the waxy vernix, though some may linger at birth.

Mom matters

Braxton Hicks contractions may be occurring with increasing regularity, and production of the hormone relaxin increases, helping to relax the pelvic ligaments and to soften the cervix. A combination of hormonal surges, anxiety about labor, lack of sleep, and aches and pains may leave you feeling a little vulnerable. Mood swings are quite common in these final weeks.

 ## This week...

>> Keep an eye on the strength and pattern of your baby's movements and report any changes to your doctor.

>> Learn about the signs of labor so that you know what to expect, and feel confident about when to call your doctor.

>> Finalize your birth plan.

37 WEEKS At this point you are probably as big as you are going to get.

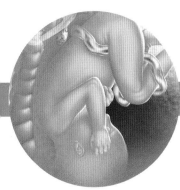

Baby watch

📏 19⅝ in (49.8 cm) ⚖️ 6 lb 10 oz (3.1 kg)

Now at full term, space is at a premium for your baby, and she may draw her legs and arms into her body in the classic fetal pose. The skull bones aren't fused, which allows the bony plates to overlap and elongate to help your baby squeeze through the birth canal.

Mom matters

Your movement may slow since your size makes it difficult to move quickly and maintain balance. Your breasts are ready to feed your baby at birth. The milk ducts have branched off, creating a transportation system to deliver milk to your baby.

 This week...

≫ You will have a prenatal appointment this week. Your blood pressure and the baby's growth and position will be checked. Your doctor will talk to you about your options if you pass your due date, and will discuss the hospital's policy on inducing labor.

≫ Make a few home-cooked dishes to pop in the freezer for after the birth.

≫ Pack your hospital bag or make preparations for a home birth.

38 WEEKS Double-check your birth plan; it's not too late to make changes.

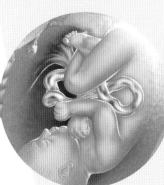

Baby watch

📏 20 in (50.7 cm) ⚖️ 7 lb 3 oz (3.3 kg)

The gray matter of the brain, the cortex, develops in layers of cells. As each layer is complete, more connections are made between cells, which help to fine-tune your baby's movements. Thanks to antibodies from your blood, your baby has some protection from infection, and after birth she can continue to receive antibodies from your breast milk.

Mom matters

You may feel very fatigued in these final stages since you carry all the extra weight of the fetus, uterus, and extra fluid. Your heart is working at full capacity. Taking some time to lie down increases the blood flow to your baby, and helps you rest and recuperate.

 This week...

≫ You may have a late burst of energy now and an urge to clean and scrub. If the "nesting" urge hits you, by all means go with it, but be careful not to overdo it.

≫ Practice breathing and relaxation techniques to help reduce anxiety.

39 WEEKS Make sure you are clear on how to recognize the signs of labor.

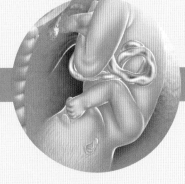

Baby watch

📏 20⅛ in (51.2 cm) ⚖️ 7 lb 11 oz (3.5 kg)

With her arrival imminent, your baby is well-prepared for life on the outside. Eyebrows, eyelashes, and nails are all in place, and her organs and body systems are sufficiently developed, though many of these will continue to develop after the birth.

Mom matters

It's best to take it easy now and conserve your energy for labor. Combine rests with periods of gentle activity. You are likely to feel a mounting pressure in your pubic region and your baby may be partially or fully engaged in your pelvis, although in second and subsequent pregnancies, this often happens later on.

 This week...

≫ You will have a prenatal appointment this week where your doctor can check if the head is engaged and assess your baby's well-being.

≫ Relieve backaches with warm baths and a soothing massage.

40 WEEKS Very soon you will be holding your new baby in your arms.

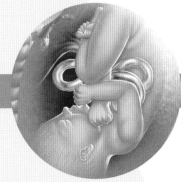

Baby watch

📏 20⅛ in (51.2 cm) ⚖️ 7 lb 11 oz (3.5 kg)

At 40 weeks your baby has little space to move around. You're likely to feel her limbs protruding or her hiccupping. If she is born after 40 weeks she will have some vernix on her skin and may have less amniotic fluid surrounding her.

Mom matters

Approximately 45 percent of women haven't given birth at 40 weeks. However, the majority deliver during the next week and only 15 percent go above 41 weeks. You might be offered a "sweep" to induce labor. This encourages the release of hormones that help to start contractions.

 This week...

≫ Keep your birth plan with you at all times. Your packed hospital bag should also be on hand.

≫ Make sure you have fuel in your car, coins for parking, and a fully charged phone and camera in your bag.

≫ Make sure the birthing center has your birth plan if that's where you will be giving birth.

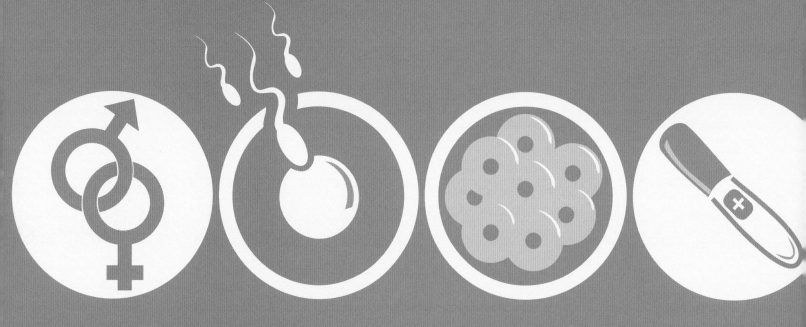

Conception

The moment you conceive a baby is **incredibly special**. You may not even realize conception has taken place, but **life is stirring deep inside you**. If you have only just decided to try for a baby there are steps you can take to improve your fertility and chances of getting pregnant. This chapter includes detailed explanations on how the male and female **reproductive systems** actually work. It also answers questions and concerns surrounding fertility, assisted conception, and unexpected pregnancy.

If you have decided to **try to get pregnant,** you may be excited but unsure of what to do next. There are ways to **maximize your fertility** and prepare for pregnancy, but once you've done those things, relax and **let nature take its course.** If you don't conceive quickly, try not to get disheartened. It is normal for it to take some time.

Trying to conceive

Preparing for pregnancy

Once you've decided to get pregnant, there are some practical steps you need to take—from stopping any birth control and making lifestyle changes to checking your immunity to certain infections. Taking these actions before you conceive will put you in the best possible health for pregnancy.

During pregnancy, the focus is understandably on the woman. However, at this preconception stage it really is about both of you. Men, as well as women, can do much to improve their fertility by making dietary and lifestyle changes, with the added advantage that when the baby arrives he will have two fit and healthy parents.

You can maximize your chances of becoming pregnant by tracking your menstrual cycle and knowing the optimal time to conceive. In addition to using an ovulation prediction kit, you can learn to spot the natural signs that you are ovulating. Be aware, though, of the importance of relaxing and enjoying the process of getting pregnant. Becoming too focused on conceiving and feeling stressed can spoil your enjoyment of this special and exciting time, and actually adversely affect your fertility. It can also negatively affect your relationship if your lovemaking is all about getting pregnant.

Couples who have been trying to get pregnant for some time may want to investigate why they have had no success so far. This is especially true of older couples, who may want to seek advice sooner rather than later. There is a great deal of help available, starting with basic fertility tests, such as blood tests and ultrasounds, to rule out any physical problems. Sometimes knowing that your reproductive organs are in good health can help you relax and actually improve your chances of conceiving.

For couples who are considering having fertility treatment, this chapter outlines the options available, such as in vitro fertilization (IVF). There is a wide range of fertility treatments available and success rates are improving gradually all the time.

Getting pregnant again

If you are trying to have another baby, the preparation is the same. Although it is harder to prioritize yourself once you are a mother, being in good shape will benefit your conception chances and provide the energy to care for more children. If you had any problems conceiving or during previous pregnancies, discuss these with your doctor so you can go into this pregnancy feeling happy and confident.

Q I want to have a baby. Should I just stop using birth control?

It depends on which type of birth control you use. Condoms and spermicides can be stopped immediately. If you are on the pill or minipill, finish the course so you have a bleed. Although it may take a few months for ovulation to return to normal, you can conceive immediately after stopping without any risks to your baby.

If you have an IUD in place, or an implant, make an appointment for it to be removed. If you are on injections, simply stop renewing them and the hormones will gradually decrease. It can, however, take a year for your cycle to return to normal.

Whichever contraception you use, you may want to make diet and lifestyle changes and have medical checkups before you get pregnant. It may be worth doing this preconception preparation before you stop your birth control in case you become pregnant quickly.

Q Why should I have my immunity checked before conceiving?

Some infections are dangerous to catch in pregnancy, so it is wise to get your immunity checked before you conceive. Your doctor can arrange blood tests for this purpose. If you are not immune to certain infectious diseases, you can be vaccinated before you get pregnant, but not afterward. Rubella (German measles) is most dangerous to the fetus in the first 16 weeks, capable of causing miscarriage, stillbirth, or abnormalities such as hearing loss and brain damage. Chicken pox can cause miscarriage and birth defects. Vaccination prevents rubella and lessens the chance of getting chicken pox and makes it milder if you do contract it.

Hepatitis causes liver disease and can be passed to your baby; if you are at high risk of infection you should be immunized. Tests can also be done for group B streptococcus and chlamydia.

Toxoplasmosis is a parasitic infection that can be present in cat feces and undercooked meat. Avoid changing cat litter, and wash your hands thoroughly after gardening or handling raw meat. Wash all vegetables and fruit before eating. If you think you may be at risk of toxoplasmosis (see p.108), ask your doctor to test you.

Q Can we do anything to improve our chances of getting pregnant?

Improving your diet and lifestyle will put you in the best possible position to conceive—and that works for both of you. Sperm and egg cells both take three months to fully mature, so taking action early will produce the healthiest cells.

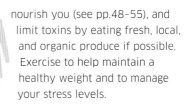

To be in the best shape for fertility and parenthood, remove unhealthy indulgences such as fast-food, refined carbohydrates, alcohol, caffeine, and tobacco from your life. Eat foods that nourish you (see pp.48–55), and limit toxins by eating fresh, local, and organic produce if possible. Exercise to help maintain a healthy weight and to manage your stress levels.

TIPS FOR MALE FERTILITY

Improve the health of your sperm and be in the best shape for parenthood:

 » Take a multivitamin: choose one that includes selenium, zinc, and folate for optimal sperm production and health.

 » Clean up your diet: eat plenty of fruit and vegetables because their antioxidants promote sperm health.

 » Maintain a healthy weight: too much or too little body weight can inhibit the production of reproductive hormones and affect sperm quality.

 » Quit smoking tobacco or marijuana: both substances can affect fertility. Seek help to quit if necessary.

 » Limit alcohol: too much can affect sperm quality.

 » Enjoy a caffeine boost: there's nothing wrong with an occasional coffee.

 » Exercise moderately: bicycling a lot could compress the testes, but bicycling in moderation is fine.

 » Reduce stress: being stressed may affect certain hormones required for sperm production.

TIPS FOR FEMALE FERTILITY

Prevent hormone imbalances and help regulate your menstrual cycle:

 » Take folic acid: take 400 mcg a day, either as a single supplement or as part of a preconception multivitamin.

 » Eat well: make sure your diet is well balanced to maximize essential nutrients.

 » Maintain a healthy weight: being overweight or underweight can affect fertility. Stay at a healthy weight by eating a balanced diet and exercising moderately.

 » Watch what you drink: alcohol and caffeine can affect fertility. Your doctor will tell you to quit drinking alcoholic beverages to protect your baby, but if you don't want to give up coffee, that's okay. Limit your caffeine intake to 200 mg a day (about two cups of coffee). Remember, soft drinks, energy drinks, and tea also contain caffeine. Choose decaffeinated and fruit teas.

 » Quit smoking: the toxins in cigarettes age your ovaries, damage your eggs, and adversely affect fertilization and implantation. Seek help to quit if necessary.

 » Manage stress: find ways to relax. Try your best not to make getting pregnant your main focus.

Being **relaxed** can double your chances of becoming pregnant within a year—so **have fun and enjoy** trying to get pregnant!

Q At what point in my menstrual cycle should we have sex in order to get pregnant?

The best way to maximize your chances is to have sex regularly—every two to three days throughout the month—but if you want you can also try tracking your ovulation.

You are most likely to conceive in the five to six days leading up to and including ovulation (when your body releases an egg). This is called the "fertile window." Aside from charting your monthly cycle, there are a few ways to figure out when you might be ovulating.

Monitor your cervical mucus

Just before the fertile window, a sticky, thick, cloudy white mucus appears. It turns thinner, clearer, and stretchy at ovulation. After ovulation, the mucus decreases and disappears. To check the mucus, wash your hands and insert your fingers into your vagina or wipe yourself with toilet paper. Stretch the mucus between your fingers. Note the color and consistency.

Use an ovulation predictor kit

An ovulation kit helps predict your fertile window by measuring levels of luteinizing hormone (LH), the hormone that releases your egg. You simply test your urine to detect LH surges up to two days before ovulation, which is useful if you have an irregular cycle.

Measure your basal temperature

Your basal body temperature (BBT) changes throughout the month. Before ovulation, your

BBT is usually about 96–98°F (35–37°C). Just after ovulation, the progesterone released into the body raises your body temperature slightly (approximately 0.4°F/0.2°C) until your next period. So you can determine when ovulation has happened, but not predict it, using BBT.

If you chart your temperature changes over a few months, you may see a pattern forming of when ovulation is likely. Buy a special basal body thermometer from a pharmacy. Note your temperature at the same time every morning before you eat or drink.

There are a lot of apps available for monitoring your monthly cycle.

CHANGES DURING THE MENSTRUAL CYCLE

This graph shows a 28-day menstrual cycle and the changes that help predict the fertile window, which is in the middle of the cycle and lasts five to six days. If your menstrual cycle is not 28 days long (most are between 21 and 35 days), the fertile window will still fall roughly in the middle.

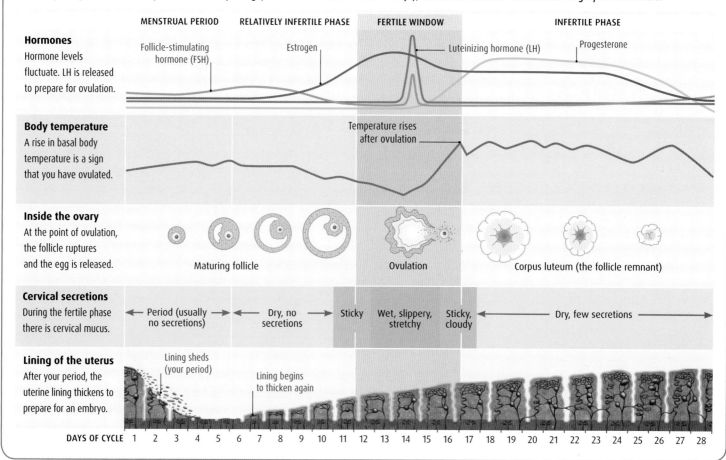

Q Are there any sexual positions that might help us conceive?

No, there is no scientific evidence that having sex in a particular position increases your chances of conception. There are unsupported claims that it helps to have sex in the missionary position so that the man is on top, or in positions that allow deep penetration, and that a female orgasm can help to pull sperm farther into the cervix. You don't need to lie on your back with your legs raised after sex to give the sperm the best chance of success either! However, it certainly doesn't hurt to give any of these methods a try–just having sex, in whatever position you like, will improve your chances of getting pregnant.

Q I've got two sons. How can I improve my chances of conceiving a girl?

It would be nice to think that you can influence the gender of your baby, but unfortunately there is no evidence that you can. Whether your baby is a boy or a girl is dependent on whether the sperm that fertilizes the egg carries an X chromosome (for a girl) or a Y chromosome (for a boy), and this is purely a matter of chance.

Nevertheless, you are not the first to ask this question and there are lots of old wives' tales about it! In the 1960s, a theory called the Shettles Method claimed that X-bearing sperm survive longer in the cervix but move more slowly than faster, smaller, though less healthy, Y-bearing sperm. With this in mind, the theory suggested that you should have sex as close to ovulation as possible for a boy, but two to three days before ovulation for a girl. There are some sex-selection kits available online that utilize this theory, but this method has not been scientifically proven.

Another theory for natural sex selection, also not scientifically proven, is the Whelan Method. This advises having sex two to three days before ovulation for a girl and four to five days before the basal body temperature rises to conceive a boy–which is the opposite advice to the Shettles Method. The Whelan Method also advocates eating a diet that is high in calcium and magnesium for a boy, and eating lots of salty and potassium-rich foods for a girl.

Q How long will it take for us to get pregnant?

The time it takes will depend on many different factors, but be aware that it is normal for even a fertile couple to take a year, or even two, to conceive.

Figures reveal that on average more than 80 percent of couples under the age of 40 get pregnant within a year if they have regular unprotected sex; more than 90 percent achieve pregnancy in two years. Naturally, it is frustrating if conception is taking a long time for you, but the figures show that it is worthwhile to keep going.

Whatever your age, you can both make dietary and lifestyle changes to improve your chances of conceiving (see pp.50–51). You can also monitor when you ovulate to increase your chances of success (see opposite).

However, some experts argue that staying relaxed and not focusing too much on tracking ovulation will help you to conceive.

If you have been having unprotected sex for a year without success, consider seeing your doctor about your fertility health.

If you are a woman over 35 and you haven't conceived after six months of regular unprotected sex, seek medical advice at this point (statistically, fertility rates drop at age 35). You should also seek advice if you have irregular periods or are worried about your fallopian tubes due to your medical history.

Make sure you are having sex on a **regular basis**. Some couples simply don't have sex often enough to get pregnant!

AVERAGE CONCEPTION RATES IN FERTILE COUPLES

After a year of trying, 93 out of 100 couples in a US study achieved a pregnancy, at the rates set out below.

MONTH	1	2	3	4	5	6	7	8	9	10	11	12
PERCENTAGE OF COUPLES PREGNANT	20	36	49	59	67	74	79	83	86	89	91	93

Q We have one child and know we want another. How long should we wait before trying to get pregnant?

This may depend on your experience the first time around. If you had a normal pregnancy with no complications, there is no reason not to conceive again once you feel ready. However, consider factors such as whether you have the energy to care for a young baby while pregnant and whether you want some time to enjoy the child that you have.

If it took a while for you to conceive, you may want to start trying to get pregnant as soon as you feel ready, though be prepared that you could conceive more quickly this time around. Conversely, if you conceived very quickly last time, it is not unusual for it to take longer to get pregnant again.

If you had a cesarean section with your first baby, wait for at least a year before getting pregnant again. This is to give your body enough time to recover–becoming pregnant sooner can double the risk of complications in the next pregnancy. Waiting a year also gives your incision a chance to heal. If you would like a vaginal birth next time and you're not completely healed, there is more chance of rupture during a VBAC (vaginal birth after cesarean section).

Any medical complications experienced in your first pregnancy, such as severe vomiting (hyperemesis gravidarum), preeclampsia, gestational diabetes, or a premature birth, could reoccur. You may want to discuss the likelihood of this with your doctor before you begin trying to get pregnant again.

Becoming pregnant is a complex biological process. First, it requires the release of an egg from the ovary. This egg must then be fertilized by a sperm in the fallopian tube. Once fertilized, the egg becomes a ball of cells that must travel down the fallopian tube and implant in the lining of the uterus. When this occurs, you have conceived and are pregnant.

Creating new life

You will have the best chance of conceiving if your reproductive organs are healthy and functioning well. Sperm are produced in a man's testes. Once matured in the epididymis, the sperm travel into a tube, the vas deferens, which leads to a sac like structure. When a man ejaculates, semen—a fluid containing the sperm—discharges into the urethra inside the penis. In a woman, the ovaries are positioned on either side of the uterus. They contain the eggs, or ova, that are released each month (ovulation).

The egg's journey

All the eggs in an ovary are exposed to follicle-stimulating hormone (FSH) each month in order to mature, but only about 20 develop. Eggs mature within follicles, fluid-filled structures that enlarge in response to FSH. Usually only one follicle matures fully and releases an egg, while the other follicles shrivel and their eggs are lost.

If a woman has a nonidentical twin pregnancy, it means two of her follicles have matured and each one released an egg that month.

Ovulation triggers

The mature egg is surrounded by cells that produce the hormone estrogen. This stimulates the growth of tissue in the breasts, thickens the uterine lining, and nourishes the egg. As the levels of estrogen rise, the hypothalamus in the brain triggers a burst of luteinizing hormone (LH) that works to release the egg from its follicle: ovulation occurs.

The fallopian tube

At the point of ovulation, the newly released egg is wafted into the nearby fallopian tube by delicate frondlike strands called fimbriae. It is encouraged down the tube toward the uterus by tiny hairlike projections, known as cilia, in the lining. This can take five days or more. If a woman has sexual intercourse around this time, the egg may be fertilized by a sperm while it is in the fallopian tube.

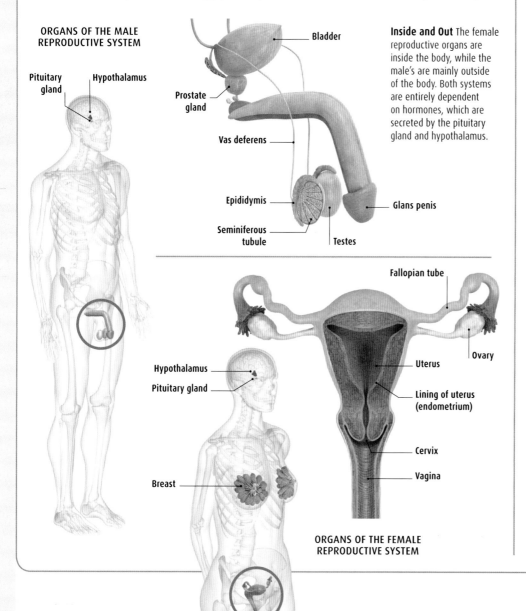

ORGANS OF THE MALE REPRODUCTIVE SYSTEM

Pituitary gland
Hypothalamus

Bladder

Prostate gland

Vas deferens

Epididymis

Glans penis

Seminiferous tubule

Testes

Inside and Out The female reproductive organs are inside the body, while the male's are mainly outside of the body. Both systems are entirely dependent on hormones, which are secreted by the pituitary gland and hypothalamus.

Fallopian tube

Hypothalamus
Pituitary gland

Uterus

Lining of uterus (endometrium)

Ovary

Cervix

Vagina

Breast

ORGANS OF THE FEMALE REPRODUCTIVE SYSTEM

2 FERTILIZATION

A single sperm penetrates the outer layers of the egg to fertilize it, while it is in the fallopian tube. The 23 chromosomes (which contain DNA, the genetic information needed for the development of a cell) in the sperm join with the 23 in the egg. Together these 46 chromosomes create a blueprint that makes your baby unique.

The fertilized egg, now called a zygote, divides into two identical cells. Within hours, the zygote divides multiple times into a microscopic ball of cells (morula) as it heads toward the uterus.

Uterus At this stage the uterus is the size of a plum, but will expand as your developing baby grows

Fallopian tube

Path of egg

Zygote Once fertilized, the egg is known as a zygote

Morula Around three to four days after fertilization, a ball of around 16 cells heads toward the uterus

Fimbriae Fingerlike projections sweep the egg into the fallopian tube

Ovary A mature egg is released from the ovary

Blastocyst By the time it implants in the uterus, about a week after fertilization, what was a single cell is now a ball of up to 100 cells

3 IMPLANTATION

About a week after fertilization, the ball of cells, now known as a blastocyst, implants itself in the lining of the uterus. The blastocyst has an outer layer of cells, which will develop into the placenta, and an inner mass of cells that will become the embryo.

Once implanted, the blastocyst begins to secrete the pregnancy hormone hCG, which helps to maintain the thick lining of the uterus and prevents it from shedding (your monthly period). This is the hormone that can be detected in your urine when you take a pregnancy test.

1 OVULATION

The ovaries typically alternate in releasing an egg during each monthly cycle, so ovulation takes place from just one ovary. One—or occasionally more than one—fully mature egg is released from an ovary and is wafted into a nearby fallopian tube.

Once the egg begins its journey, the ovaries produce the hormone progesterone, which causes the uterine lining to thicken and ripen in anticipation of a possible pregnancy. It also produces the nutrients necessary to support a developing embryo, and causes the breast lobules (milk glands) to swell.

FROM OVULATION TO IMPLANTATION

Q I had an abortion when I was younger. Can I still get pregnant?

If your abortion was conducted before 14 weeks of pregnancy, and as long as your fallopian tubes were not damaged for any reason, you should still be able to get pregnant. If your abortion was between 14 and 24 weeks, there may be a slight risk of premature delivery if you become pregnant again. If you have been trying to conceive for a year or more, or for six months if you are over 35, you may want to see your doctor to have some basic fertility tests.

Q I'm on long-term medication. Will this affect my fertility?

Some medication prescribed for long-term medical conditions may affect your ability to conceive. If you have an existing medical condition, it's important to talk to your doctor before you try to get pregnant.

Such conditions include asthma, diabetes, heart disease, inflammatory bowel disease (IBD) lupus, epilepsy, migraine, mental health problems, acne, high blood pressure, anemia, obesity, and being underweight. The type or dose of prescription drugs, vitamins, herbal medicine, or other supplements you take may need to be adjusted before and during pregnancy. Don't stop taking any medication you've been prescribed until advised to do so by your doctor. Don't forget to mention any allergies and over-the-counter medications too.

You may need to take a higher dose of folic acid if you are at risk of having a pregnancy affected by a neural tube defect (see p.49). This may be the case if you take medication for epilepsy, you are diabetic, if you had a neural tube defect in a previous pregnancy, or there is a history of neural tube defects in your family.

Q I think my partner and I have fertility issues. What should we do?

The first thing to do is make an appointment with your doctor, especially if the female partner has irregular or painful periods, feels pain during intercourse, has previously had a pelvic infection or surgery, or if there's any reason the male partner might have abnormal

Q What is genetic screening and should we have it before we conceive?

Genetic screening may be done to find out if couples who are planning to conceive are carrying a particular altered gene that could lead to their baby inheriting a specific medical condition. It helps couples to prepare for the likelihood of their child having the condition.

Some genetic disorders are more common in particular ethnic groups. Sickle-cell disease is most common in those of African descent, while most cases of Tay-Sachs disease and cystic fibrosis affect Ashkenazi Jews and northern white Europeans respectively. Contact your doctor to be referred for

screening. The test usually involves giving a blood or sample tissue so that your DNA can be analyzed. It may take weeks, or sometimes months, to get the results. It is vital to remember that screening is not foolproof or conclusive. Genetic counseling is often provided to inform and support parents.

Sickle-cell anemia In this example both parents are carriers—they each have one sickle-cell gene. If the baby inherits a sickle-cell gene from each parent, he will have sickle-cell anemia. If he inherits only one, he will be a carrier. He may inherit neither of the sickle-cell genes.

Both genes A child who inherits both sickle-cell genes will have the condition

ONE SICKLE-CELL GENE (CARRIER)

ONE SICKLE-CELL GENE (CARRIER)

NO SICKLE-CELL GENES

ONE SICKLE-CELL GENE (CARRIER)

ONE SICKLE-CELL GENE (CARRIER)

PAIR OF SICKLE-CELL GENES (SICKLE-CELL ANEMIA)

semen. Your doctor will ask you how long you have been trying to conceive, the current state of your health, and about any past health issues. If appropriate, he or she will suggest a range of tests that may establish the cause.

For women, the possible causes include damaged or blocked fallopian tubes, failure to ovulate, endometriosis, fibroids, cysts on the ovaries, and pelvic inflammatory disease. The most common tests are blood tests to check levels of hormones linked to ovulation, ultrasound scans to look at the reproductive organs, and X-rays of the uterus and fallopian tubes. For men, the causes include poor sperm count, blockage of the tubes, and infections.

Tests will assess sperm quality, hormones, the reproductive organs, and chromosomes.

Depending on the situation, there are various treatment options such as medicines and drugs to assist fertility, surgical procedures, and assisted conception. Although the tests may discover the root of the problem there are occasions where fertility can be unexplained.

Going through these tests can be extremely stressful and frustrating. During this time, it is vital to learn everything you can about your medical situation, so ask your doctor or specialist if you have any questions or concerns and communicate with your partner about your feelings.

Q Is it still possible to have a baby in our forties, or have we waited too long?

Women are increasingly having babies in their forties, particularly if they have assisted conception. Statistically, the odds aren't in your favor, but it depends on your individual circumstances and health.

Talk to your doctor if you haven't conceived after having unprotected sex for six months. He or she will begin initial tests (see opposite) to check whether you have any problems that could be affecting your fertility.

Do all that you can to maximize your fertility by making diet and lifestyle changes (see p.29). In addition to improving your chances of conceiving naturally, these changes will also ensure you are in the best possible health for pregnancy and parenthood.

You may be advised that your best option of conceiving is to have fertility treatment. Using donated eggs is often an effective treatment for women who are in their forties. This is combined with in vitro fertilization (IVF) to try to achieve a pregnancy. Be aware that IVF can cost thousands of dollars, and the procedure may not be covered by your health insurance. Even if it is covered, you may be limited on how many cycles of IVF you can try before you pay out of pocket, so keep your budget in mind.

> The number of babies born to women who are 40 and over has **more than quadrupled** over the last three decades.

AVERAGE RATES OF INFERTILITY IN WOMEN

Women are most fertile in their 20s, with only a 3 percent likelihood of being infertile. By age 35 this has risen to 15 percent and by age 40, a woman has a 32 percent chance of infertility. Women in their late forties have a 69 percent likelihood of infertility.

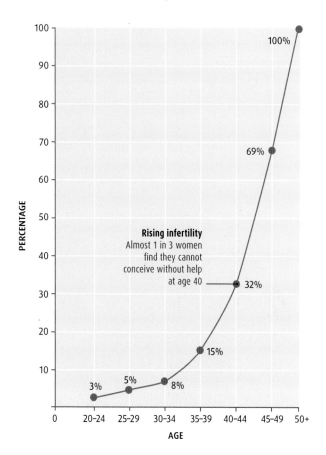

Rising infertility
Almost 1 in 3 women find they cannot conceive without help at age 40

Biological clock As this graph shows, a woman is nearly twice as likely to have fertility issues at age 35 as she did at age 30. That likelihood doubles again by 40.

KEY
● Likelihood of infertility

Q Is it true that it's more common to have twins when you are older?

Since women over the age of 35 are more likely to release more than one egg per cycle, yes, they do have a higher chance of conceiving a multiple pregnancy. Another reason is the number of older women who are taking advantage of assisted conception, which carries with it the possibility of a multiple pregnancy because the treatments sometimes use more than one embryo at a time. Multiple pregnancy is the biggest risk factor to an unborn baby, due to the high chance of premature birth.

Q My partner is a few years older than I am. Will this affect how long it takes us to conceive?

Male fertility begins to decline after the age of 40, when the quality of the sperm deteriorates. This can affect the health of the children born to the man as well as having an impact on his rate of fertility. Statistically, the average time for a man to conceive with his partner if he is under 25 is just four-and-a-half months; if the female partner is under 25 and the man is 40, it is likely to take nearly two years—five times as long—to conceive.

Q We've been trying to get pregnant for six months. Do we need to see a doctor?

If you are under 35, the recommended time to wait before consulting your doctor is one year. In the meantime, try not to worry, maintain a healthy lifestyle, and keep having sex regularly.

If you are over 35, or have a history of gynecological issues, you are more likely to have problems conceiving. See your doctor if you've been unsuccessful after six months of trying to get pregnant so that the necessary tests and investigations can be done

Q We are considering IVF. How successful is it and what does it involve?

The live birth rate from IVF is increasing gradually. In 2012, US success rates were 32.8 percent for women under 35; 27.3 percent for 35–37 years; 20.7 percent for 38–39 years; 13.1 percent for 40–42 years; and 4.4 percent for 43 years plus.

1 in 50
babies **in the US** are **born as a result of IVF treatment** (2014).

IVF is the process by which an egg and sperm are mixed together in a petri dish outside the body. Following fertilization, an embryo (possibly more than one) is transferred to the uterus. The process is extremely time-consuming and involves many appointments. You are also required to take medication by injection and undergo a minor surgical procedure. Before beginning IVF, it is crucial to prepare yourself for the fact that it can be an extremely fraught and draining experience. It can put an enormous amount of pressure on a couple and it is vital, therefore, that both partners are in complete agreement about the course of action.

Before embarking on the treatment, speak to your doctor and consider doing your own research into hospitals, clinics, and the procedure. IVF is appropriate in some medical situations, but not in others. There are also some couples for whom IVF is likely to be of little help, so a full understanding of what it involves is essential.

WHAT HAPPENS WHEN?

A number of eggs are usually required to increase the likelihood of conceiving a viable embryo. IVF treatment involves injections to encourage the ovaries to ripen more than one egg. Your progress is monitored with scans and a specialist will choose an optimum point to collect the eggs for fertilization.

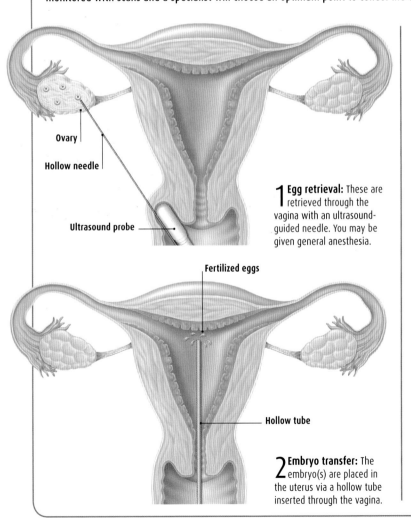

Ovary

Hollow needle

Ultrasound probe

1 Egg retrieval: These are retrieved through the vagina with an ultrasound-guided needle. You may be given general anesthesia.

Fertilized eggs

Hollow tube

2 Embryo transfer: The embryo(s) are placed in the uterus via a hollow tube inserted through the vagina.

THE STAGES OF IVF

Stage 1–Suppression

In some treatments, the ovaries are suppressed before stimulating them to produce multiple eggs. This stage can begin one week before your period is due or the day after it begins. You take a nasal spray or inject a drug for one to two weeks to suppress your natural cycle. This prevents the pituitary gland from producing follicle-stimulating hormones (FSH). Other treatments go straight to stimulation (see below) and suppress the release of mature eggs afterward.

Stage 2–Stimulation

An ultrasound scan is done to confirm that the ovaries are not active. Following this, you take FSH as a daily injection for 10 to 12 days. This increases the number of eggs your ovaries produce. During this time regular hormone tests are done to indicate how well the follicles are responding to the FSH. A last injection given approximately 36 hours before egg collection helps the eggs to mature.

Stage 3–Egg retrieval

This is usually done using a vaginal ultrasound that shows an image of each ovary. The eggs are sucked into a test tube and given to an embryologist who places them in special fluid to be examined.

Stage 4–Embryo selection

The male partner produces semen and his sperm are mixed with the eggs and placed in an incubator. The embryos are assessed 48 hours later and checked to ensure they look normal. The ideal time to transfer the embryo(s) is after about five days when it has developed into a blastocyst. This gives a higher chance of pregnancy.

Stage 5–Embryo transfer

An embryo (or embryos) is put into a fine plastic tube and this is inserted through the cervix into the uterus.

Q My doctor said we might want to consider having ICSI rather than normal IVF treatment. What is it?

This is only different from IVF at the point of fertilization. Instead of the egg and sperm being left to fertilize naturally in a petri dish, one healthy sperm is selected and injected directly into a mature egg.

ICSI (intra-cytoplasmic sperm injection) is recommended to couples if the man has a very low sperm count, for example, or other sperm problems that mean the egg is unlikely to be fertilized naturally. This treatment may be recommended if you have had low—or even zero—fertilization rates in a previous IVF cycle—the eggs that have been collected have failed to turn into embryos in the first 24 hours.

The process of stimulating the ovaries to produce more eggs and egg collection is the same as for IVF. Following the ICSI fertilization procedure, the IVF treatment continues as normal in that the embryo (or embryos) is placed into the uterus (see opposite). Be aware that if you are paying for your IVF treatment, there is an additional expense for ICSI.

ICSI

In the ICSI procedure, the sperm and egg are brought together instead of being left to fertilize naturally.

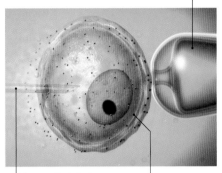

Pipette This holds the egg still

Fine needle A single sperm is injected directly

Egg

Q I know someone who got pregnant by having IUI. What exactly is it?

IUI stands for intrauterine insemination and is a procedure where sperm is placed directly into the uterus. Before being considered for IUI, your fallopian tubes are tested to ensure that they are open. You are given a blood or urine test to detect ovulation. As soon as the egg is mature, a hormone injection is given to release it. Then 36-40 hours after this your partner provides a sperm sample. The fastest-moving, least-sluggish sperm are selected and inserted into your uterus using a catheter. It is a quick and painless procedure.

The rest is left to nature in the hope that one sperm fertilizes the egg. You may be advised to have up to six cycles of IUI. You may be recommended to opt for IUI if you have ovulation problems, your partner is impotent, or you are trying to get pregnant using donated sperm. IUI may or may not be covered by your health insurance company.

Q We're using donor eggs. Will my body naturally accept them?

If you are not ovulating (an inability to produce eggs is not rare) and require a donated egg, the lining of your uterus probably won't be thick enough for an embryo to implant in it. You will

need a cycle of hormone replacement prior to the egg being implanted to ensure the uterine lining can nourish the embryo. This is the main key to a successful pregnancy from a donated egg. The principle risk for you is a multiple birth if you have more than one fertilized egg transferred.

Q I've heard that some women freeze their eggs. Is this something I should consider doing?

Freezing and storing your eggs may enable you to use them for treatment in the future. Since many women are leaving childbearing to later in life, egg freezing is becoming more common. Aside from preserving fertility, it is something that is recommended for women under 40 who need cancer treatment that may make them infertile or for those who cannot wait for another IVF attempt (due to age or illness) if the first one fails. The procedure for collecting eggs is the same as the first stages of a cycle of IVF treatment where drugs are used to stimulate the ovaries to produce follicles (which contain the eggs). When the follicles are large enough, the eggs are retrieved and placed in storage in liquid nitrogen. Until relatively recently, using eggs that had been frozen carried certain risks and the success rate had been poor. Due to improved freezing methods (vitrification), this is now changing.

Women undergoing IVF or ICSI often have a number of unused embryos. Some people choose

to have these frozen for use in another treatment cycle if the first fails, to attempt another pregnancy with a sibling embryo, or to donate to others. The chances of a successful pregnancy using a thawed frozen embryo are not affected by the amount of time the embryo is stored and frozen. However, not all embryos survive the thawing process. The clinic will advise you on the best procedure for using your frozen embryos. There are options depending on your personal and medical circumstances.

There have been lawsuits in the US recently regarding the fate of frozen embryos after a couple splits up, since both partners contributed to the embryo. If you are considering freezing embryos with your partner, you may want to sign a contract or consent form to spell out what would happen to the embryos in the event that the relationship ended.

Q Did you know...

Eating oysters is good for male fertility. They are high in zinc, which helps sperm count, sperm motility (the way sperm moves), and increases testosterone levels. If you can't stomach oysters, other good sources of zinc are legumes, nuts, spinach, and lean beef and lamb, or you could take a daily zinc supplement.

Discovering that you are pregnant will be one of the most **transformative and memorable** experiences of your life. Even if the pregnancy is planned, you are likely to feel a range of **emotions** from joy to trepidation. Take time to adjust and then start to learn about the many miraculous changes taking place **inside your body**.

Pregnant!

Finding out that you are pregnant

Congratulations! You are now on an amazing, life-changing journey. Perhaps you have missed your period, or noticed symptoms such as sore breasts, nausea, and extreme fatigue. Maybe you know just how far along you must be, or it has taken weeks to realize you could be pregnant. Whether you have been actively trying to get pregnant, have been undergoing fertility treatment, or your pregnancy was unplanned, enjoy the moment of discovery—there is no more exciting and momentous news.

Most women find out they are pregnant by doing a home pregnancy test since these are so accurate and reliable. In some circumstances, a blood test or ultrasound may be needed to confirm a pregnancy.

One or both of you may feel overwhelmed that you are going to be parents. It is quite normal to have a number of questions and concerns—about your stage of pregnancy and when your baby is due, and whether your baby is healthy. You may look to the future and wonder about how much life will change, but try not to get too anxious—you have plenty of time until your baby is born.

If you are a single parent, whether you have an unexpected or a planned pregnancy, you may be experiencing some anxiety, as well as shock or delight.

There is no right or wrong time to tell people that you are having a baby. You may want to confide only in immediate family members until you are into your second trimester and the likelihood of miscarriage is minimal. Otherwise, trust your instincts and tell those close friends and family members whom you know will actively support you through the first weeks of pregnancy.

If you work, you may want to wait until you have had your first ultrasound before you tell your boss. However, if you are experiencing symptoms such as nausea and vomiting it can be more difficult to hide your pregnancy. Also, if your job involves chemicals or heavy lifting then you will definitely need to tell your manager.

What to expect

It is worth familiarizing yourself with the common symptoms of early pregnancy, such as fatigue and nausea, and finding ways to cope with them. Equally, be reassured that you may not have any symptoms and this is normal for some women.

Many of the more difficult symptoms, such as vomiting and fatigue lessen by early in the second trimester and you may find at that time you begin to relax and enjoy your pregnancy a bit more.

Q I think I may be pregnant. How do I find out for sure?

A urine test is the quickest and simplest way to measure whether you have high levels of the pregnancy hormone human chorionic gonadotrophin (hCG) in your body, which starts rising several days after conception.

You can buy a pregnancy testing kit from a pharmacy or a supermarket to use at home, or you can go to your doctor's office to have them perform an in-office lab test.

Most home testing kits can be used on the first day of your missed period; any earlier, and the test is less reliable (see graph, below). However, some brands claim to provide an accurate result up to four days before your period is due.

If you have irregular periods and you aren't sure when the first day of your missed period will be, do a test three weeks after you last had unprotected sex.

How to test

It is advisable, but not essential, to do the test soon after you wake in the morning since your urine has the highest concentration of hormones at that time. You simply urinate on the test stick for a few seconds and wait for the positive or negative symbol or the words "Pregnant" or "Not Pregnant" to appear on the screen. The result should show on the screen within a couple of minutes. If you follow the instructions correctly, a positive result means you are almost certainly pregnant. If you have a negative result and your period still hasn't

arrived, you may have tested too early. Although any delay can feel incredibly frustrating, it's worthwhile to wait a few days before testing again.

Doctors accept pregnancy home testing kits as accurate. If there is any doubt, a blood test may be done to detect the exact levels of hCG in your body, even if those levels are still low. This may be recommended if you are undergoing fertility treatment.

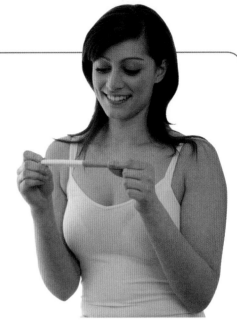

Testing at home Pregnancy testing kits are usually easy-to-use sticks that test the hormone levels in your urine.

HCG LEVELS IN PREGNANCY

The hormone that signals you are pregnant is called hCG. As the graph shows, hCG levels start rising a week after conception—a little at first and then steadily until your baby is well-established in the uterus. The other main pregnancy hormones, estrogen and progesterone, surge later on.

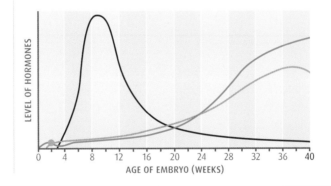

KEY

— Human chorionic gonadotrophin (hCG)

— Estrogen

— Progesterone

● Conception

Increased hormones Note the huge surge in hCG (the purple line) following conception.

Q My home pregnancy test result is positive. Can I be sure it's right? What happens next?

A positive pregnancy test result means you have raised levels of the pregnancy hormone hCG in your body. Even if the positive symbol or words on the test screen are faint, you are still likely to be pregnant. Many women often do another test just to make sure (many home pregnancy tests come in a double pack), though this isn't necessary.

Make an appointment with your doctor as soon as you can to let him or her know you are pregnant. At the appointment you will find out about your prenatal care and have the chance to

ask questions. Many women schedule this first appointment so they see the doctor when they are about 6 or 8 weeks pregnant.

Your doctor will want to discuss nutrition and lifestyle with you and ensure you know about taking folic acid (see p.49). He or she will also discuss your medical history in case you need additional prenatal screenings or need to adapt any current medication.

Your doctor will give you an estimated delivery date (EDD). You can use a due-date calendar to figure out your EDD yourself (see p.42). They are most useful if you have a regular menstrual cycle: simply look up the first date of your last menstrual period to find your EDD. However, it's an estimate and only 4 percent of women give birth on their EDD. Some doctors do

an ultrasound at the initial appointment (between 7 and 9 weeks). Others wait until 11–14 weeks. If you've had a miscarriage, have a suspected ectopic pregnancy, or you're experiencing bleeding, an earlier scan may be recommended.

> The accuracy of **home pregnancy tests is more than 99 percent.** So if it says "pregnant" on that little screen, you can be fairly certain that you are!

A CLOSER LOOK
When sperm meets egg

This is the moment of the miracle: when a single sperm from the 200–500 million contenders in a single ejaculate penetrates a mature egg that only survives for 24 hours. The journey has taken the tiny sperm around 5–20 minutes, and most of its brothers have fallen by the wayside in the vital race.

A long, whip-like tail propels the sperm on its swim toward the egg.

The midsection houses a spiral mitochondrion—it's the powerhouse that provides the sperm with energy.

1 **This sperm has beaten millions** of others to reach the egg in the fallopian tube. Only about 200–300 sperm made it this far. The others bind to the surface of the egg, but this winning sperm pushes through the egg's layers to penetrate it.

The sperm head contains the male DNA—including the X or Y chromosome that will determine whether your baby is a girl or boy.

2 **The sperm is able to enter** the egg's corona radiata and zona pellucida layers with the help of enzymes in its acrosome—a caplike structure on its head. The acrosome will shed when the job is done, so the sperm can fuse with and fertilize the egg.

The egg is encased by a thick transparent double membrane called a zona pellucida.

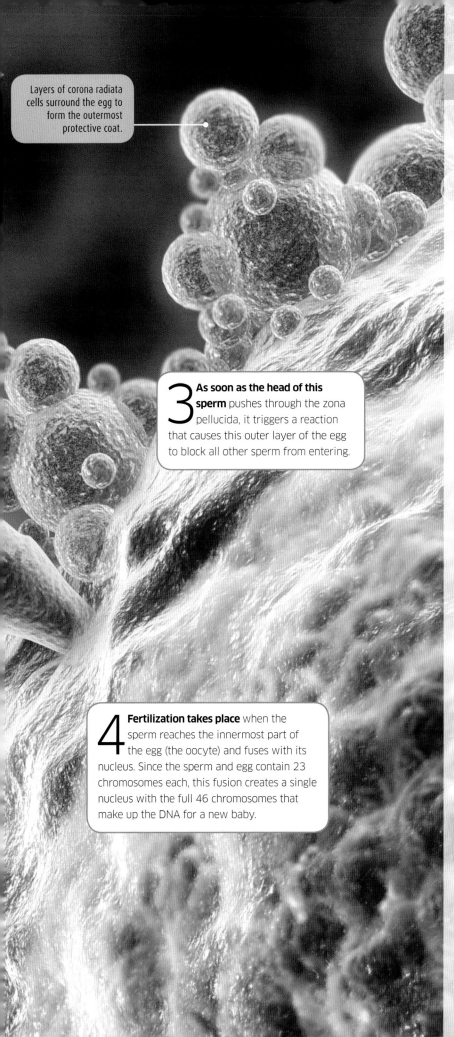

Layers of corona radiata cells surround the egg to form the outermost protective coat.

3 **As soon as the head of this sperm** pushes through the zona pellucida, it triggers a reaction that causes this outer layer of the egg to block all other sperm from entering.

4 **Fertilization takes place** when the sperm reaches the innermost part of the egg (the oocyte) and fuses with its nucleus. Since the sperm and egg contain 23 chromosomes each, this fusion creates a single nucleus with the full 46 chromosomes that make up the DNA for a new baby.

FASCINATING FACTS

About the size of a grain of sand, the egg is one of the largest cells in the human body. The sperm is one of the tiniest.

500 million

In one ejaculation there can be 200–500 million sperm, but only 200–300 will survive the journey to the egg.

7 million

This is the number of immature egg cells a female baby grows while in utero. She will have these by 20 weeks.

400,000

A girl's ovaries contain about 400,000 eggs by the time she reaches puberty. Each menstrual cycle, 1,000 eggs are lost.

100 days

The man's testicles generate a new complement of sperm cells every 100 days.

36 hours

The average life span of sperm is between one and two days.

Q When will my baby arrive? Can I find out before I see my doctor?

It is easy to calculate the estimated birth date of your baby as long as you know the first day of your last menstrual period.

Before your first ultrasound, your doctor will use the first day of your last menstrual period (known as LMP) as a marker for the start of your pregnancy. This means you can calculate the estimated date of delivery (EDD) yourself using a due-date calendar, such as the one below. It is wonderful to have an actual day to work toward, but try not to get too tied to it since the due date is only an estimate after all. Almost 50 percent of babies are born before the EDD and about the same again are born after the EDD. You will reach full term at 37 weeks and if you haven't given birth by 41 weeks you will be offered an induction to reduce the risk of having an overdue baby.

4%
of babies are born on their **due date.**

WHEN WILL YOUR BABY BE BORN?

To figure out your estimated date of delivery (EDD)—also known as the due date—find the date you started your last menstrual period (LMP) on the upper lines of the chart, then see the dates in bold below to discover when your baby is expected. For example, if your last LMP was August 16, then your baby will be due on May 23.

	1	2	3	4	5	6	7	8	9	10	11	12	13	14	15	16	17	18	19	20	21	22	23	24	25	26	27	28	29	30	31
JANUARY	1	2	3	4	5	6	7	8	9	10	11	12	13	14	15	16	17	18	19	20	21	22	23	24	25	26	27	28	29	30	31
OCT/NOV	8	9	10	11	12	13	14	15	16	17	18	19	20	21	22	23	24	25	26	27	28	29	30	31	1	2	3	4	5	6	7
FEBRUARY	1	2	3	4	5	6	7	8	9	10	11	12	13	14	15	16	17	18	19	20	21	22	23	24	25	26	27	28			
NOV/DEC	8	9	10	11	12	13	14	15	16	17	18	19	20	21	22	23	24	25	26	27	28	29	30	1	2	3	4	5			
MARCH	1	2	3	4	5	6	7	8	9	10	11	12	13	14	15	16	17	18	19	20	21	22	23	24	25	26	27	28	29	30	31
DEC/JAN	6	7	8	9	10	11	12	13	14	15	16	17	18	19	20	21	22	23	24	25	26	27	28	29	30	31	1	2	3	4	5
APRIL	1	2	3	4	5	6	7	8	9	10	11	12	13	14	15	16	17	18	19	20	21	22	23	24	25	26	27	28	29	30	
JAN/FEB	6	7	8	9	10	11	12	13	14	15	16	17	18	19	20	21	22	23	24	25	26	27	28	29	30	31	1	2	3	4	
MAY	1	2	3	4	5	6	7	8	9	10	11	12	13	14	15	16	17	18	19	20	21	22	23	24	25	26	27	28	29	30	31
FEB/MAR	5	6	7	8	9	10	11	12	13	14	15	16	17	18	19	20	21	22	23	24	25	26	27	28	1	2	3	4	5	6	7
JUNE	1	2	3	4	5	6	7	8	9	10	11	12	13	14	15	16	17	18	19	20	21	22	23	24	25	26	27	28	29	30	
MAR/APR	8	9	10	11	12	13	14	15	16	17	18	19	20	21	22	23	24	25	26	27	28	29	30	31	1	2	3	4	5	6	
JULY	1	2	3	4	5	6	7	8	9	10	11	12	13	14	15	16	17	18	19	20	21	22	23	24	25	26	27	28	29	30	31
APR/MAY	7	8	9	10	11	12	13	14	15	16	17	18	19	20	21	22	23	24	25	26	27	28	29	30	1	2	3	4	5	6	7
AUGUST	1	2	3	4	5	6	7	8	9	10	11	12	13	14	15	(16)	17	18	19	20	21	22	23	24	25	26	27	28	29	30	31
MAY/JUNE	8	9	10	11	12	13	14	15	16	17	18	19	20	21	22	(23)	24	25	26	27	28	29	30	31	1	2	3	4	5	6	7
SEPTEMBER	1	2	3	4	5	6	7	8	9	10	11	12	13	14	15	16	17	18	19	20	21	22	23	24	25	26	27	28	29	30	
JUNE/JULY	8	9	10	11	12	13	14	15	16	17	18	19	20	21	22	23	24	25	26	27	28	29	30	1	2	3	4	5	6	7	
OCTOBER	1	2	3	4	5	6	7	8	9	10	11	12	13	14	15	16	17	18	19	20	21	22	23	24	25	26	27	28	29	30	31
JULY/AUG	8	9	10	11	12	13	14	15	16	17	18	19	20	21	22	23	24	25	26	27	28	29	30	31	1	2	3	4	5	6	7
NOVEMBER	1	2	3	4	5	6	7	8	9	10	11	12	13	14	15	16	17	18	19	20	21	22	23	24	25	26	27	28	29	30	
AUG/SEPT	8	9	10	11	12	13	14	15	16	17	18	19	20	21	22	23	24	25	26	27	28	29	30	31	1	2	3	4	5	6	
DECEMBER	1	2	3	4	5	6	7	8	9	10	11	12	13	14	15	16	17	18	19	20	21	22	23	24	25	26	27	28	29	30	31
SEPT/OCT	7	8	9	10	11	12	13	14	15	16	17	18	19	20	21	22	23	24	25	26	27	28	29	30	1	2	3	4	5	6	7

Q How can I find out my stage of pregnancy?

You will have your first ultrasound, also known as a dating scan, at around 8–14 weeks. The due date is based on your last menstrual period, but does not tell you when you conceived. Ultrasounds are a more accurate indicator of your stage of pregnancy and due date. You may find you are further along than you thought.

Q Is it important to know which trimester I'm in?

It helps to understand the trimesters, so you know what to expect at each stage. The first trimester lasts from the first day of your last period to 12 weeks pregnant (you conceive at two weeks). During this trimester you may experience a lot of symptoms (see opposite). It can also be an anxious time because the risk of miscarriage is highest in the first trimester. In the second trimester—from 13 weeks to 25 weeks pregnant—you may have fewer symptoms, but will probably feel more pregnant because you will start to show. The final trimester, up to 42 weeks, can be very tiring, due to the weight of the baby, interrupted sleep, and symptoms such as backaches. While this can be a tough stage, it is exciting too since you begin all the preparation for your baby's arrival.

Did you know...

Twin pregnancies can bring additional nausea and vomiting. While it doesn't happen for every expectant mom of twins, there is an increased risk of nausea and vomiting due to the higher hCG levels (see p.39) in a twin, or other multiple, pregnancy. There are also higher levels of the hormone progesterone with twins, which can cause shortness of breath. In later pregnancy, carrying multiple babies can lead to more fatigue, constipation, heartburn, and back pain for mom-to-be.

Q I'm pregnant but I have no symptoms. Should I be worried?

It's normal for some women to experience few or no symptoms in early pregnancy, even though hormones are flooding the body and changes are underway. This is nothing to worry about—you are just as pregnant as a woman who has nausea and vomiting, for example, but just not as sensitive to the hormonal changes that are taking place.

Even though you may not feel the fatigue associated with early pregnancy, be sure to get rest and take good care of yourself.

Q Are there any pregnancy symptoms I should be concerned about?

Although concerning symptoms are not common in early pregnancy, seek medical advice if you have any of the following symptoms.

» Vaginal bleeding: light spotting is common but you must report it to your doctor. Heavy bleeding, especially if you also have abdominal cramps, can be a sign of a threatening miscarriage. Bleeding and lower abdominal pain can also signal an ectopic pregnancy (see p.308).

» Severe vomiting: seek advice if you are vomiting to the point of dehydration and can't keep any fluids down for more than 12 hours.

» A fever: you may have an infection.

» Vaginal discharge and itching: this may mean you have an infection such as yeast. It can be treated to offer relief from the symptoms.

Q I'm five weeks pregnant. I feel OK, but what symptoms might I get?

Most women experience some symptoms in early pregnancy due to the hormonal changes taking place. Thankfully many of these pass, especially nausea and sickness, by the end of the first trimester or early in the second trimester.

EARLY PREGNANCY SYMPTOMS

All women are different, but here are some of the symptoms you may experience in early pregnancy.

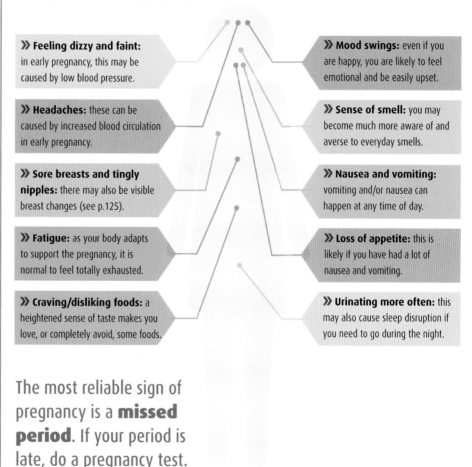

» Feeling dizzy and faint: in early pregnancy, this may be caused by low blood pressure.

» Headaches: these can be caused by increased blood circulation in early pregnancy.

» Sore breasts and tingly nipples: there may also be visible breast changes (see p.125).

» Fatigue: as your body adapts to support the pregnancy, it is normal to feel totally exhausted.

» Craving/disliking foods: a heightened sense of taste makes you love, or completely avoid, some foods.

» Mood swings: even if you are happy, you are likely to feel emotional and be easily upset.

» Sense of smell: you may become much more aware of and averse to everyday smells.

» Nausea and vomiting: vomiting and/or nausea can happen at any time of day.

» Loss of appetite: this is likely if you have had a lot of nausea and vomiting.

» Urinating more often: this may also cause sleep disruption if you need to go during the night.

The most reliable sign of pregnancy is a **missed period**. If your period is late, do a pregnancy test.

» A burning sensation when you urinate: this can be the sign of urinary-tract infection, which will need to be treated with antibiotics.

» Leg or calf pain, swelling on one side, and/or a severe headache: these are signs of a blood clot, which is more likely to occur in pregnancy, though it is rare.

» A flare-up of a current medical condition: let your doctor know of any symptoms that you have experienced since being pregnant.

7 in 10

women **experience nausea or vomiting** or both during pregnancy.

Q I've been taking the pill—but I'm pregnant. Will my baby be OK?

The risks to your baby are low. If you are on the pill or minipill, stop taking it if your pregnancy test is positive—you don't need to finish the cycle.

It's understandable that you may not have been aware you are pregnant for a while. Some of the side effects of this form of contraception, such as feeling nauseous and having tender breasts, can also be early pregnancy symptoms. The results of a pregnancy test won't be affected by the pill since the test only reacts to hCG readings.

Try not to worry, but take action immediately to stop whatever type of contraception you are using, as outlined in the chart, right. The hormones in the pill don't last long in your system and trials indicate that there isn't an increase in the risk of birth defects. There is, however, a slightly greater chance of an ectopic pregnancy (see p.308); the minipill can alter the motility of the fallopian tube–affecting the ability of an egg to move through it.

Make an appointment to see your doctor as soon as you can to let him or her know that you are pregnant and that you conceived while you were taking a contraceptive pill. Your doctor can do an ultrasound to rule out an ectopic pregnancy.

Did you know...

Some couples rely on the withdrawal method as a form of contraception. This is when the man pulls his penis out of the woman before he ejaculates. While this can be effective for some couples who are adept in the method, it shouldn't be relied upon to prevent pregnancy. Some experts claim that preejaculate can pick up sperm that's in the man's urethra from a previous ejaculation, which can lead to pregnancy.

CONTRACEPTION FAILURES AND EFFECTS

While some types of contraception are more effective than others, no single type is a foolproof barrier to pregnancy. This table explains what to do if your contraception has failed.

TYPE OF CONTRACEPTION	WHAT DOES IT DO?	HOW SHOULD I STOP?
Combined pill	Contains estrogen and progestogen. Estrogen inhibits ovulation and progestogen thickens cervical mucus to make it difficult for a sperm to reach an egg and an egg to implant in the uterus.	Stop taking the pills right away. There is no need to finish the cycle.
Minipill	Contains just progestogen, not estrogen. The progestogen thickens cervical mucus to make it difficult for a sperm to reach an egg and an egg to implant in the uterus.	Stop taking the pills right away. There is no need to finish the cycle.
Emergency contraceptive pill (also called the morning after pill)	Works by preventing or delaying ovulation.	Do not take any more emergency contraception.
Injections	Contains progestogen, which thickens cervical mucus to make it difficult for a sperm to reach an egg and an egg to implant in the uterus.	Simply stop renewing your injections.
Implants	Inserted under the skin of your upper arm, the flexible tube slowly releases progestogen to stop sperm from reaching an egg and the uterus from supporting a fertilized egg.	A specially trained doctor will need to remove the implant, and an ultrasound may be necessary to locate it.
IUD	Positioned in the uterus, it prevents a sperm and egg, or a fertilized egg, from implanting in the uterus or fallopian tubes.	There is a risk of miscarriage and ectopic pregnancy because of the presence of a foreign body in the uterus, possible inflammation, and an increased risk of infection. If the IUD is visible, it's best for a specialist to remove it; if not, it is best left where it is for the pregnancy.
Spermicide	Available in different forms (including gels and foams), spermicide contains chemicals that stop sperm from moving.	Do not use once you are pregnant.
Sterilization	The fallopian tubes are tied to prevent an egg from reaching the uterus.	N/A

WHAT ELSE SHOULD I KNOW?

There is no scientific evidence that the hormones estrogen and progestogen contained in this product affect a developing embryo and fetus.

There is no scientific evidence that the progestogen in this product affects a developing embryo and fetus.

This contains the same hormones as the combined and minipills, so there is no risk to the developing embryo and fetus. Neither does it cause an abortion.

There is no scientific evidence that the progestogen in this product affects a developing embryo and fetus.

There is no scientific evidence that the progestogen in this product affects a developing embryo and fetus. If the implant can't be located and removed, there is no need to worry.

You need to request an ultrasound to rule out an ectopic pregnancy. If the IUD stays in position while you are pregnant, it is usually delivered with the placenta after the birth.

There is no scientific evidence that this product affects a developing embryo and fetus.

You should make an appointment with your doctor promptly: your fallopian tubes are likely to have been damaged by the sterilization procedure and you may be at risk of an ectopic pregnancy (see p.308).

Q Is there anything I should do now that I know I am pregnant?

These practical steps are some of the first things to do on your pregnancy journey.
» Make an appointment with your doctor
» Start taking 400mcg folic acid a day (available from a pharmacy) if you're not already taking it
» Limit caffeine and avoid drinking alcohol, smoking, and taking drugs (see p.53)
» Eat healthily
» Exercise moderately
» Find ways to relax
» Become informed by reading about the stages of pregnancy, how your baby is developing, and understanding the tests and ultrasounds you will get in the coming months.

Q I didn't plan to get pregnant, but I am. What should I do?

You are probably deep in shock at the news, but It's worthwhile to remember that many women have mixed emotions when they find out they are pregnant, even when it is planned. First, take the pressure off yourself and your partner, if you have one, and take time to adjust to the situation. You will probably want to talk to trusted family members and friends for support, but if you feel anxious or fearful, tell your doctor. You may also want to seek professional advice about making changes to your housing arrangements or your finances when you feel ready. The magnitude of change may seem huge, but take a deep breath and start taking steps to make sure you have a healthy pregnancy.

Q I drank and smoked before realizing that I was pregnant. Will that have harmed my baby?

You probably didn't harm your baby if you had a couple of drinks and the occasional cigarette, but you must stop immediately to reduce risk of any damage to you and your baby.
Alcohol and drugs have their greatest effect during organ development, which doesn't begin until week five. As soon as you know you are pregnant, however, you should abstain from all alcohol and stop smoking during pregnancy. If

you drink or smoke heavily and you continue throughout your pregnancy, you are at risk of damaging both your health and that of your baby. Smoking can directly affect the placenta's growth, and in later pregnancy it can reduce the supply of oxygen and nutrients to the baby, resulting in a lower birthweight and more chance of a premature baby. Smoking doubles the risk of stillbirth. Regular or heavy drinking can lead to fetal alcohol syndrome (see p.325), which damages the baby's nervous system and inhibits his ability to thrive after birth.

Q I'm not as happy as I thought I'd be about being pregnant.

Whether planned or not, a pregnancy can raise deep emotional issues that you were not aware of before. You may be facing a whole range of emotions, including disbelief, feeling overwhelmed, and you may be at a loss about what to do next. Give yourself permission to go along with whatever you are feeling for the next few weeks until you have begun to adjust to this new role in life, and don't feel guilty. If you continue to feel negative about the pregnancy, seek support and reassurance from loved ones or speak to your doctor.

Q What if my partner isn't pleased about the pregnancy?

If you are in this situation, accept your partner's feelings and give him plenty of time to adjust to what is, after all, life-changing news. On hearing the news, he may feel upset and angry, and panic, especially if the pregnancy is unplanned. Try not to take his reaction personally. Hopefully it will become a constructive part of processing the news and coming to terms with the future. In the meantime, try to plan some short-term goals that you can enjoy together, or set aside time in your calendar for real time together to build your relationship as a couple.

Taken properly, the combined contraceptive pill is **more than 99 percent effective.**

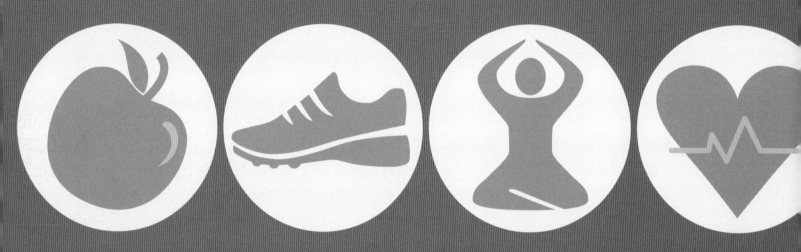

≫ In this chapter...

Nutrition, exercise, and well-being

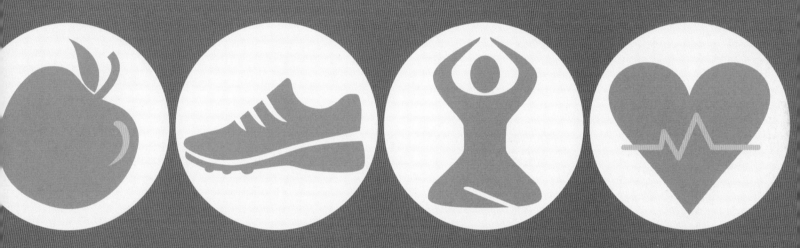

Knowing what to eat and how to exercise are both **beneficial to your health and that of your baby**. Pregnancy and childbirth will challenge your body more than anything you have experienced before. Being fully **prepared in mind** as well as in body is also important to maintain your well-being. This chapter gives specific **advice about a balanced diet**, which supplements to take, which food and drinks to avoid, and **how to exercise safely** during pregnancy and beyond.

From preconception to birth, what you eat and drink can **affect your pregnancy**: how quickly you **conceive**, **your health** during pregnancy, your experiences of **pregnancy** and **labor**, and the **health of your baby**—not only while he is growing inside you, but also long into his future.

Nutrition

Eating to stay healthy

There are few experiences in your life that will demand as much of your body as pregnancy and childbirth. Preparing yourself by eating as well as you can is hugely beneficial—a healthy body helps make your experience of conception, pregnancy, and labor a positive one.

Our diets have changed dramatically over the course of the last 50 years; it seems normal now to eat prepared, processed, and refined foods regularly rather than always making meals and snacks from scratch ourselves. However, eating enough of the right nutrients is one of the most positive things you can take control of. Good nutrition doesn't need to be any more complicated than the general principles of eating a healthy, balanced diet—just be aware that what you stock in your cupboards and fridge and put on your plate is even more important than usual, both for your fertility and energy levels and for the health of your developing baby. You don't have to follow a rigid diet or eat unpleasant foods: it's all about eating twice as well (and not twice as much) to ensure you receive the best nutrients from every mouthful.

Eating well at every stage

As soon as you conceive, you become the lifeline to your baby—everything you eat, drink, and breathe is broken down into molecules containing valuable nutrients and oxygen and transported through your bloodstream and placenta to the fetus. So it's important to have good habits in place from the start. This section gives advice on how you can prepare for and aid conception, including what supplements to take. Once you have conceived, you can read about eating for energy and health, what your baby needs, the best approach if you have an intolerance or you follow a special diet for personal or medical reasons, which foods to avoid, and advice on smoking and drugs. After the birth, you can learn about how to boost your recovery through good nutrition.

Q What is folic acid and why do I need to take it?

Folic acid is a B-group vitamin that is key to the formation of your baby's spine, brain, and nervous system. These organs are some of the very first to develop, which is why you are encouraged to take folic acid even before you conceive.

The neural tube is the part of the embryo that develops into your baby's brain and spinal chord. Making sure you have good levels of folic acid in your system throughout preconception, conception, and the first three months of pregnancy will help minimize the risk that your baby will develop neural tube defects by 72 percent. In dads-to-be, good folate levels can reduce the instance of sperm abnormalities.

Essential supplement

Folic acid is the synthesized version of vitamin B₉. When it occurs naturally in food, it is known as folate and is present in leafy green vegetables such as cabbage. Studies show that our bodies are better at using the synthesized version so look for supplements that contain 5-methyltetrahydrofolic acid, which is already "biologically active." When you are hoping to conceive, ideally both of you should start taking a daily supplement of 400mcg folic acid before you stop contraception. When pregnant, keep taking it until you are at least 12 weeks pregnant. If you are considered high risk (if either of you has a medical or family history of a neural tube defect; if a previous pregnancy was affected; if you are over 35; or if you are diabetic or epileptic), you may be advised to take a higher dosage of 5mg daily.

Somites run in pairs along the neural tube.

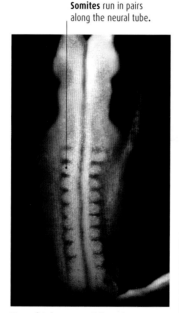

Neural tube By week five of pregnancy, there is a neural tube running down the middle of the embryo, complete with somites that will become vertebrae.

Whether you're already pregnant or trying to get pregnant, start taking **folic acid** as soon as you can.

NEURAL TUBE FORMATION

In the earliest stages, your baby forms from three primary layers of cells. These layers fold to create the basic structures of the body, including the important neural tube.

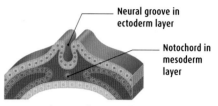

Neural groove in ectoderm layer

Notochord in mesoderm layer

1 **A neural groove begins to form** when the top layer (ectoderm) sinks toward a column of cells called the notochord in the middle layer (mesoderm).

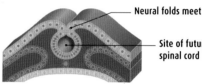

Neural folds meet

Site of future spinal cord

2 **As the groove deepens,** its edges come together to make a tube shape. This tube extends along the embryo's back, eventually forming the spine and brain.

Neural folds fuse and neural tube is complete

3 **Folic acid helps the folds of the tube to fuse.** If the tube doesn't close fully, it can result in birth defects such as spina bifida.

Q We are trying for a baby. Do we need to change what we eat or drink?

If you lead a healthy lifestyle and eat a good, balanced diet, you've already established the right pattern. If not, make positive changes to your nutrition now to help the health of your sperm and eggs (which each take three months to develop) and establish the necessary reserves of nutrients for a healthy pregnancy. Also eliminate, or reduce to within guideline levels, alcohol and caffeine, which have a detrimental effect on conception. Eat more phytoestrogens—found in linseed, whole wheat, and lentils—to balance hormones in both partners, and eat a colorful range of antioxidant-rich foods to boost the quality and motility of sperm.

Q Is it true that what you eat can affect how long it takes to conceive? We have fertility issues.

Anything—including diet—that can affect hormones and the health of the woman's eggs, the man's sperm, the fallopian tubes, and the uterus can have an impact on how long it takes to get pregnant. So yes, your diet can adversely affect your internal chemistry.

Your weight—whether you're overweight or underweight—is also an important factor if there are fertility issues, since it can determine whether or not you have too little or too much estrogen to ovulate. For a man, being underweight can affect the quality of his sperm. Eat the right balance of healthy, nutritious,

unrefined foods from the main food groups, avoid the "empty calories" of junk food, and have three regular meals a day to help you regulate your hormones and boost your chances of conception in the months ahead.

Some women may be advised to take a **prenatal multivitamin** in addition to folic acid, but in general you should be able to get all the **nutrients** you need from your diet.

Q What is a healthy, balanced diet and how can I eat enough nutrients?

A healthy diet is comprised of the right balance of nutritious foods from several main food groups: protein, fruit, vegetables, unrefined carbohydrates, and healthy fats. You should eat foods from these groups in their most natural, unprocessed state to receive the maximum number of nutrients.

Whether you are still at the stage of planning conception or are already pregnant, you need to make sure your diet includes the correct balance of the main food groups. A balanced diet allows your body to store enough of the right nutrients for a healthy pregnancy and feel in peak condition. Eating in a consistent and measured way also helps you to keep your weight within healthy limits, which is a factor for successful conception. Once you become pregnant, the benefit of eating a balanced diet is that you will be supplying your body with the best possible diet for fetal growth and development and providing yourself with enough energy to deal with the pregnancy.

HEALTHY EATING

Eat a variety of foods from each of these groups in the right proportions for optimum nutritional benefits at every meal. The breakdown of these healthy foods equates to approximately five to six portions of fresh vegetables, two portions of fresh fruit, and three portions each of protein and unrefined carbohydrates per day.

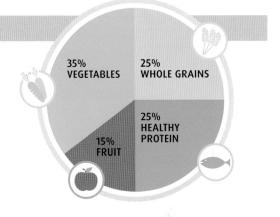

- 35% VEGETABLES
- 25% WHOLE GRAINS
- 25% HEALTHY PROTEIN
- 15% FRUIT

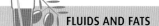

FLUIDS AND FATS

» **Stay hydrated:** often feelings of hunger are in fact symptoms of thirst. Water is best.

» **Enjoy healthy fats:** dairy (also a source of calcium) and oils (such as olive oil) are good for you in moderate amounts.

 VEGETABLES

The more vegetables—and the greater the variety—the better. Steaming is the best way to prepare vegetables if you don't eat them raw.

 FRUIT

Eat fresh fruit of all colors. Fruit contains fructose, a type of sugar, so a couple of portions a day will give you fiber and vitamins without overloading on sugar.

 HEALTHY PROTEINS

Choose fish, poultry, beans, and nuts; limit red meat and avoid bacon and processed meats. Steam, grill, or bake fish and meat.

 WHOLE GRAINS

Eat a variety of whole grains (such as whole-wheat bread, whole-grain pasta, and brown rice). Limit or avoid refined grains (such as white rice and white bread).

Fresh fruit and vegetables
When it comes to fruit and vegetables, the more colorful the better. Strong color is a sign that they are rich in vitamins and minerals, and high in protective antioxidants, which help to fight free radicals in the body. Eat a wide color range of vegetables and fruit for the maximum benefits.

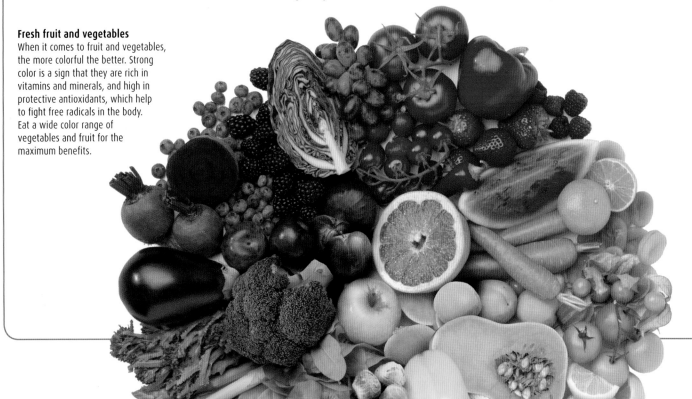

Q Should I take an iron supplement in case I become anemic?

It is usually better to get your iron needs from your diet. This is because iron supplements can have the side effect of causing constipation, which pregnant women are already susceptible to. Eating iron-rich, high-fiber foods is good for tackling both constipation and low iron levels. Include more lean red meat, green leafy vegetables, nuts such as peanuts, and dried fruit in your diet. It's usual during pregnancy to feel more tired than normal, particularly in the first and last trimesters. However, if you are extremely lethargic, pale, and suffering from heart palpitations and/or shortness of breath, you could be anemic. If you are, your doctor will discuss iron supplementation. In addition, consider cutting out caffeine entirely since this can hamper iron absorption.

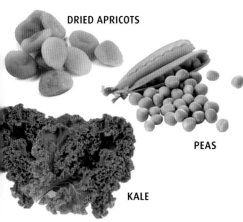

DRIED APRICOTS

PEAS

KALE

Iron-rich foods Dried apricots, peas, and leafy vegetables such as kale are great sources of iron. Vitamin C helps with iron absorption, so drink orange juice with your meal.

Q Do I need to take a multivitamin supplement now that I am pregnant?

The most important supplement you need to take is folic acid. Health-care professionals advise a vitamin D supplement (10 mcg daily) to help your body metabolize calcium for the benefit of maintaining your own bones and teeth as well as your baby's developing bones. The other elements in a multivitamin supplement aren't strictly essential if you are eating a balanced diet. If you do choose to take a supplement, make sure it is right for pregnancy. Never take a supplement containing vitamin A, since too much can harm your baby.

Q Could my weight affect my chances of having a healthy pregnancy?

Unfortunately, being either obese or underweight can have a negative impact on both your ability to conceive and your health in pregnancy. If you can, take action to make sure your weight is within healthy limits before getting pregnant.

It is best to achieve a healthy weight before you think about conception. For both partners, you need a certain level of body fat to produce the right levels of hormones for healthy sperm production and ovulation to occur. In obese people, excess estrogen can decrease sperm levels and hamper or even prevent ovulation, while underweight people can have too little fat in their bodies to conceive. If you are underweight, there is a greater risk of your baby having a low birthweight or being premature. Gain and maintain weight healthily by eating an extra 200–300 calories a day until your weight improves. During pregnancy, obesity can affect the health of your baby, and it is known to increase the risk of conditions such as gestational diabetes and preeclampsia (see pp.144–45)—factors that can cause complications during pregnancy and the birth.

BODY MASS INDEX (BMI) CHART

This chart is appropriate for women over the age of 18. Body mass index (BMI) gauges whether you are a healthy weight in relation to your height. A BMI of 30 or more is considered obese, while a BMI of less than 18.5 is deemed underweight.

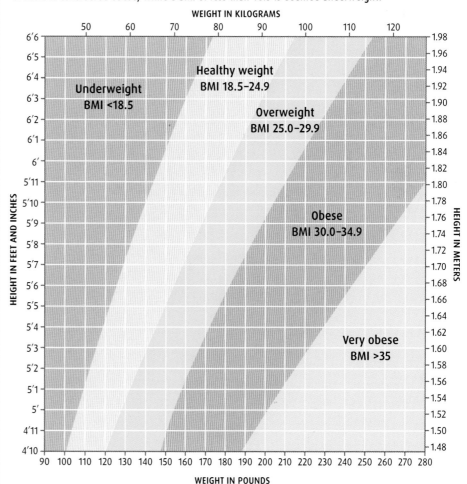

Knowing what foods and drinks to avoid helps your health and the safe development of your baby. Some foods contain, or may contain, bacteria or substances that may make you sick or be harmful to your baby. While this may seem very alarming, it's worth remembering that the risks are very low.

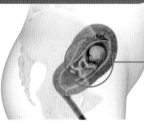

Health and hygiene

You are more vulnerable to infections while pregnant, so being aware of what you eat and drink and following good food hygiene principles are necessary precautions.

Food hygiene is straightforward if you are vigilant. Always check the sell-by dates on food product labels and reject any food that smells off or looks suspect. Wash your hands before and after handling food, and rinse fruit, salads, and vegetables to remove traces of soil and pesticides. Be extra careful with raw poultry and meat: use separate chopping boards and knives, and wash them afterward with detergent in very hot water. Defrost frozen foods carefully according to the instructions on the packaging, and if you reheat cooked food in the microwave, make sure that the whole dish is piping hot.

Avoid foods (listed below) that may carry harmful bacteria, parasites, or cause food poisoning; some herbal teas and sugar substitutes; smoking; recreational drugs; alcohol; and limit caffeine. If you drank alcohol or smoked before you discovered you were pregnant, don't be anxious but stop now. The fetus will start being supported by the placenta from 12 weeks, although it can't protect an unborn baby against all infections and bacteria.

FOODS TO LIMIT OR AVOID

Although there is usually only a small risk that foods such as these may prove harmful to your baby, they are best avoided or limited while you are pregnant.

Banned foods Cured meats and unpasteurized cheeses should be avoided.

FOOD	YOU SHOULD AVOID	RELATED PROBLEMS	YOU CAN EAT
Cheese	» Any unpasteurized cheese. » Soft mold-ripened cheeses (with a "white rind"), such as Camembert and Brie. » Uncooked soft blue cheeses, such as Roquefort and Gorgonzola.	In rare cases, cheese may carry the listeria bacteria. Listeriosis (listeria infection) may cause only mild, flu-like symptoms in you, but it can be harmful to your baby and in severe cases can lead to brain damage.	» Hard cheeses and hard blue cheeses (such as Parmesan, Gouda, Cheddar, and Stilton). » Soft cheeses made with pasteurized milk—for example cottage cheese, cream cheese, mozzarella, feta, and ricotta.
Meat	» Raw or undercooked red meat. » Cold cuts and luncheon meats. » Liver or other organ meats, and liver pâté—they contain high levels of vitamin A.	Undercooked meat may be infected with the toxoplasmosis parasite and cold cuts may contain listeria. Both may harm your baby. Too much vitamin A can cause birth defects and harm your baby's liver.	» Meat that has been cooked to a safe temperature is fine to eat. Cold cuts are fine, too, if they are served hot, or have been cooked.
Seafood	» Uncooked shellfish. » Avoid shark, marlin, and swordfish, which contain high levels of mercury.	Food poisoning from seafood is unpleasant for you, but it doesn't pose any health risks to your developing baby. High levels of mercury, found in certain fish, can be harmful to your baby's nervous system.	» Oily fish, but only once or twice a week, since it may contain toxins such as PCBs and dioxins (as well as lots of good nutrients). » Cooked shellfish.
Eggs	» Raw eggs and raw egg products such as mayonnaise and mousse. » Undercooked eggs—eat only if the yolk and white are solid.	There is a tiny risk that raw eggs may contain the salmonella bacteria. A salmonella infection is not thought to be harmful to an unborn baby, but can cause vomiting and diarrhea for you.	» Choose eggs stamped to show that they have been laid in conditions following the strictest hygiene.

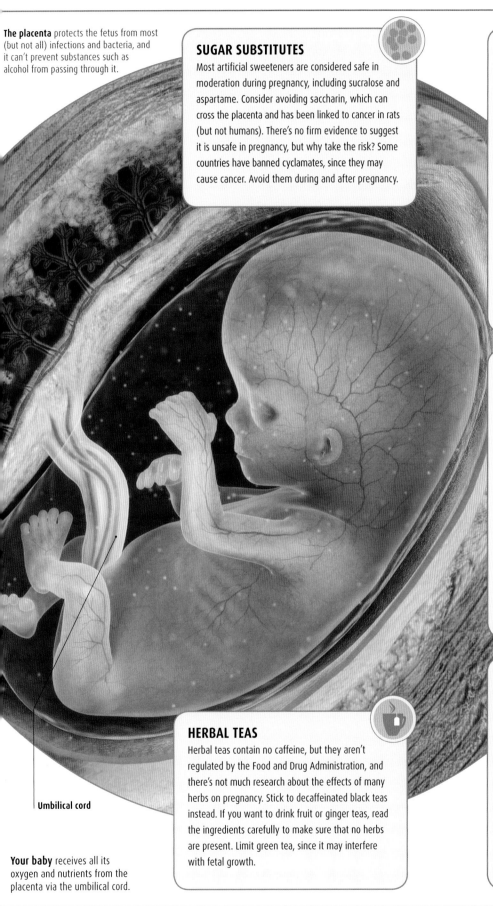

The placenta protects the fetus from most (but not all) infections and bacteria, and it can't prevent substances such as alcohol from passing through it.

Umbilical cord

Your baby receives all its oxygen and nutrients from the placenta via the umbilical cord.

SUGAR SUBSTITUTES

Most artificial sweeteners are considered safe in moderation during pregnancy, including sucralose and aspartame. Consider avoiding saccharin, which can cross the placenta and has been linked to cancer in rats (but not humans). There's no firm evidence to suggest it is unsafe in pregnancy, but why take the risk? Some countries have banned cyclamates, since they may cause cancer. Avoid them during and after pregnancy.

HERBAL TEAS

Herbal teas contain no caffeine, but they aren't regulated by the Food and Drug Administration, and there's not much research about the effects of many herbs on pregnancy. Stick to decaffeinated black teas instead. If you want to drink fruit or ginger teas, read the ingredients carefully to make sure that no herbs are present. Limit green tea, since it may interfere with fetal growth.

ALCOHOL

We know that alcohol crosses the placenta, meaning any alcohol you drink can make its way into your baby's system. Because the liver is one of the last organs to develop in the fetus, your baby can't detoxify the effects. This raises the concentration of alcohol in the baby's blood and starves the baby of oxygen.

⚠️ **Alcohol-related problems** in babies exposed during development include:
>> **low birthweight**
>> **premature birth**
>> **In extreme cases fetal alcohol syndrome**, which can cause malformed facial features, learning difficulties kidneys, and heart defects.

✔️ **Abstention from alcohol** is the only clear way to be sure you are minimizing the risks to your baby.

CAFFEINE

This is present in much more than just coffee and tea—chocolate, carbonated drinks, and energy drinks, to name a few. Guidelines are that, during pregnancy, women shouldn't drink more than two cups of instant coffee a day.

⚠️ **Caffeine-related problems** in babies exposed during development include:
>> **low birthweight**
>> **raised heart rate**
>> **raised blood pressure**
>> **miscarriage in rare cases**

✔️ **Switch to decaffeinated alternatives** for tea and coffee (at least 97 percent caffeine-free) and consider fruit teas—but proceed with caution, since they could contain herbs and not all herbal teas are safe (see left).

SMOKING, DRUGS, AND MEDICATIONS

⚠️ Cigarettes and recreational drugs (such as cocaine and marijuana) are known to pose significant health risks to an unborn child, resulting in:
>> **low birthweight**
>> **brain or lung damage**
>> **miscarriage**
>> **babies born with "addiction"**

✔️ **The advice is clear**—do not smoke or use drugs. Seek advice before using e-cigarettes, patches, or gum. Consult your doctor if you take prescription drugs, and don't take over-the-counter medicines without advice.

Q I am gluten intolerant. What does this mean for my baby?

A gluten-free diet can be low in calcium, iron, fiber, zinc, B-vitamins, vitamin D, and magnesium. If you're celiac, it's important that you continue with your gluten-free diet, since studies show that pregnant celiac women who reintroduce gluten to their diet can be at increased risk of miscarriage and low birth weight. There are no specific dietary guidelines to follow other than eating a healthy balanced diet, but the fact that you are gluten-free means you could be lacking nutrients–specifically iron, vitamin B_{12}, and calcium. You may require some supplementation in addition to what you eat in order to meet the recommended daily amounts of these missing nutrients. Talk to your doctor, who will be able to assess your diet and give you individual advice. In the meantime, increase quantities of potatoes, rice, corn, nuts, beans and lentils, red meat, chicken, fish, eggs, and dairy in your daily diet, all of which will help boost your intake of those nutrients that are otherwise present in gluten-containing foods.

Q Should I start shopping for organic foods now that I'm pregnant?

We are exposed to chemical pesticides and fertilizers in all kinds of ways–in the air, in cleaning products, and in the food we eat. Pesticides work by attacking the nervous systems of insects. Concern for unborn babies centers on the effects these chemicals may have on neural development, because studies have found tiny amounts of expressed sequence tags (ests) or DNA clones in amniotic fluid.

Although risks from food are smaller than those from airborne pollutants, anything you can do to minimize your exposure can only be a positive thing. If you aren't able to switch to an entirely organic diet, select wisely. For example, it's better to spend extra on organic meats as unorganic meats may have hormones and antibiotics within the flesh that are impossible to remove through cooking, than on organic fruits and vegetables, which you can wash and peel (in most hard fruits and vegetables, pesticides remain primarily on the outer skin and leaves). Do, though, choose organic soft fruits, which are less likely to have residues beneath the skin.

If you aren't able to switch to an entirely organic diet, select your organic purchases wisely and include meat and soft fruit.

Q I'm vegetarian. Can I continue eating as I usually do?

It is perfectly possible to remain vegetarian or vegan while pregnant and have a healthy baby, but be prepared to supplement any nutrients you may be lacking.

Make sure that you're aware of the nutrients your vegetarian or vegan diet does and doesn't give you, and discuss your diet with your doctor. If you need extra nutrients, he or she may advise you to take supplements for the duration of your pregnancy (especially important for iron). For your own peace of mind, check first that any supplements are not animal derived. You may also need to plan your meals a little more carefully, but you should remain in good health throughout your pregnancy.

PREGNANCY REQUIREMENTS

Combining fresh foods with supplements is a good idea if you are vegetarian or vegan.

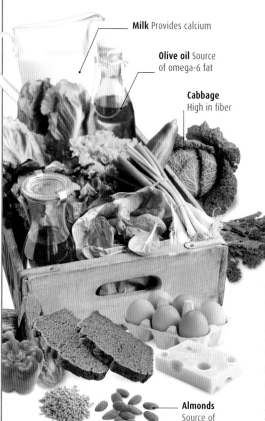

Milk Provides calcium

Olive oil Source of omega-6 fat

Cabbage High in fiber

Almonds Source of omega-3 fat

Balanced diet As a vegetarian or vegan, make sure you get all your major food groups: grains, protein, fruit and vegetables, dairy, and fats.

» **Iodine:** you may need to take supplements of iodine, which—among other things—is essential for maintaining pregnancy to term, a healthy birth, and improved brain function in your baby.

» **Vitamin B_{12}, essential fats, iron, and vitamin D:** these are all essential to take either through food or in a supplement form.

» **Essential amino acids:** daily quantities of beans, peas, or other legumes; corn or wheat products; grains; seeds; nuts; brewer's yeast and soy; cheese, milk, eggs or other dairy; and a broad color spectrum of vegetables should provide all the amino acids you need.

» **Iron:** if you don't need to supplement, good sources are leafy green vegetables (spinach and kale are good), fortified breakfast cereals, dried fruits, and whole-wheat bread. Drink orange juice at the same meal to help iron absorption from these foods.

» **Omega fats:** flaxseed, walnut oil, and soybeans are all good sources of omega-3 fats; nuts, grains, safflower, sesame, and sunflower oils are all good sources of omega-6.

» **Calcium:** if you're vegan, make sure you get enough calcium. Leafy green vegetables, sesame seeds (and derivatives such as tahini), and legumes are all sources. Look for calcium-fortified vegan products such as tofu, soy, rice, oats, and bread.

Q I am lactose-intolerant. What can I do about my calcium intake?

Your ability to digest lactose may actually improve while you are pregnant, or you may need to take a calcium supplement to make sure you get enough calcium.

Calcium is crucial: it helps to build your baby's bones and teeth and prevents your bones from weakening. Interestingly, studies show that lactose intolerance eases off in around 30 to 50 percent of pregnancies. So, to begin with, consult your doctor about how to reintroduce a tiny amount of cow's milk into your diet and measure its effects, and follow his or her guidance before you begin supplementation. If you remain intolerant, you may need to take a calcium supplement, as well as vitamin B12 and D supplements, which are also found in dairy products. In the meantime, increase your intake of other calcium-rich foods.

CALCIUM-RICH FOODS TO EAT IF YOU ARE LACTOSE-INTOLERANT

Include a few of these calcium-rich foods in your diet each day; the daily recommendation is 1,000 milligrams of calcium.

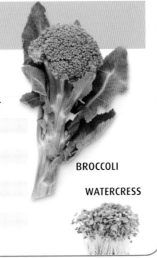

BROCCOLI

WATERCRESS

FOOD	SERVING AMOUNT	CALCIUM CONTENT
Canned sardines	2 oz (60 g)	240 mg
Water cress	4 oz (120 g) raw	188 mg
Wakame	3^1/$_2$ oz (100 g) raw	150 mg
Green beans	7 oz (200 g) cooked	132 mg
Tofu	4 oz (120 g) raw	126 mg
Broccoli	4 oz (120 g) raw	112 mg
Rhubarb	4 oz (120 g) raw	103 mg
Chickpeas	7 oz (200 g) cooked	99 mg

Q I'm Muslim and I plan to observe Ramadan. Will fasting harm my baby?

Any kind of fast is not recommended during pregnancy—your body and your baby need a constant supply of nutrition and water in order to remain healthy and develop properly. Studies show that fasting can lead to premature birth, low birth weight, and neurological problems in babies. However, many Muslim women choose to observe the Ramadan fast. First, consult your doctor to discuss your individual situation and your baby's health, and then fast only if you have a healthy weight, good energy levels, no known conditions, and you feel strong. Islamic law does permit pregnant women not to fast; you can make up the days after the birth or compensate by giving to charity. So, if at any time you feel dizzy, dehydrated, or otherwise unwell, or if you think your baby has stopped moving, stop the fast immediately and consult your doctor.

Q Is there anything special I need to worry about as a pescetarian?

This semivegetarian diet, which excludes meat and poultry and may include dairy products and eggs in addition to fish and shellfish, shouldn't exclude any natural nutrients from your diet. Fish is an ideal form of protein; it is rich in B-complex vitamins, calcium, potassium, iron, zinc, phosphorous, and selenium, and the omega-3 fats that oily fish such as halibut, salmon, tuna, mackerel, and sardines contain are crucial for heart and brain health. However, the current medical advice is that you should eat only two or three servings of fish per week (8–12 ounces), choosing fish varieties that are lower in mercury, like salmon, light canned tuna and tilapia. (Too much mercury can be harmful to your unborn baby's development. Avoid swordfish, tilefish, shark, and mackerel, which are high in mercury.) Limit white albacore tuna to 6 ounces per week. Avoid raw shellfish, too.

Q I've been following a low-carb diet. Is it safe to continue this diet?

Without good medical reason (such as an allergy, intolerance, or other food-related auto-immune condition), there is no justification for restricting or eliminating any major nutrient during pregnancy. Carbohydrates are an important source of energy, fiber, iron, and B-vitamins, which makes them essential for your health and that of your baby. If you're worried about weight gain, remember that, gram for gram, carbohydrates have fewer calories (1 g of carbohydrate gives 4 calories of energy) than fat-rich foods (9 calories per gram). Carbohydrates also keep you feeling fuller longer, so they will actually help prevent any tendency you may have to snack.

Q I'm overweight. Would it make sense to eat fewer calories now that I'm pregnant?

Usually, dieting to lose weight while pregnant is not advised because it can deprive your baby of essential nutrients, but if your BMI was over 30 to begin with (see p.51), it can be a good idea to manage your weight. If you were already obese, there are specific risks to pregnancy—such as gestational diabetes, preeclampsia, having a large baby, stillbirth, and increased likelihood of cesarean section. Work with your doctor to create a program to maintain your weight throughout your pregnancy. Too much calorie restriction is not ideal—especially if you were underweight before becoming pregnant—since this increases the risk of having a small, or low birth weight baby, which is linked to developmental issues.

Carbohydrates are essential: if your **body** doesn't get enough **fuel** from carbs, it begins to metabolize your fat reserves and release toxins called PCBs that may harm your **baby's development**.

Q I feel permanently exhausted. What can I eat to give me more energy?

If this is your first or third trimester, your body is working extra hard to either form a baby or enable it to grow enough to be ready for labor and the birth. Choose foods that are rich in protein or fiber to give your body the fuel it needs.

The primary energy-giving nutrients you need are iron, complex carbohydrates, and protein. Try mapping your energy needs over a day and eat appropriately to combat the times when you typically have an energy drain. Aim to load up with protein and complex carbs at breakfast and lunchtime to give you slow-burning energy for up to three to four hours at a time, and make dinner the lightest meal, but still nutritious—think healthy salads, for example. Include a healthy midmorning and midafternoon snack, and don't reach for caffeine and sugary foods. Aside from the fact that these aren't good for you, the energy hit they provide will be short-lived, and you'll soon feel more tired and depleted than you did before.

NUTRIENTS YOUR BODY NEEDS FOR SUSTAINED ENERGY

Include foods containing these energy-enhancing nutrients in your meals and snacks so that you can deal with your day. Eat little and often to stave off hunger pangs and maintain energy levels.

NUTRIENT	ENERGY EFFECTS	FOOD SOURCES
Iron	Improves the health of cells so that oxygen reaches all the body systems efficiently.	Leafy green vegetables (spinach, kale etc.); shellfish; lean meat; dried fruit; nuts and seeds; legumes; whole grains.
Complex carbohydrates	These foods release energy at a steady pace into your body in the short and medium term, preventing the energy spikes that refined carbs (simple carbohydrates) and sugary foods cause.	Whole grains (including brown pasta and rice); oats; fresh fruit and vegetables (particularly starchy vegetables, such as potatoes, corn, green peas, and parsnips); legumes (including beans, peas, and lentils).
Protein	The process of breaking down protein into energy is a long one—first your body separates the protein into its constituent amino acids, which it then converts into glucose (your body's fuel). This means that protein gives you a slow energy release over several hours.	Lean meat; fish; dried legumes (such as beans, peas, and lentils); nuts and seeds; eggs; milk; and yogurt.

Q I often feel thirsty. Is this normal? Can I drink what I want?

It's very normal to find yourself drinking more while pregnant, because your body requires extra fluids to deal with the demands of your growing baby. Your body needs water to flush out toxins and waste—both your own and those generated by your developing baby—from your body. You also need water to produce the extra healthy blood cells needed during pregnancy. These blood cells carry essential nutrients to your baby through the placenta. Staying

well-hydrated during pregnancy is also essential for helping to prevent water retention (edema), dry, itchy skin, fatigue, constipation, urinary-tract infections, and complications in pregnancy associated with dehydration.

Unless your body requires more, or it's a hot day or you live in a warm climate, around 2.3 quarts (2.2 liters) of fluid a day should be sufficient (this is the recommended amount for a healthy adult). If you feel thirsty—or even hungry—you're probably slightly dehydrated,

Stay hydrated Drink at least 8 glasses of fluid a day— water and milk both provide effective hydration.

An app is a great way to check if you are eating enough calories a day by **monitoring your calorie intake** if you want to stabilize your weight. There are lots of free food-journal apps available to help you log your food and beverage intake. Aim for **2,200 calories** a day in the first trimester and **2,300 calories** a day during the second and third trimesters.

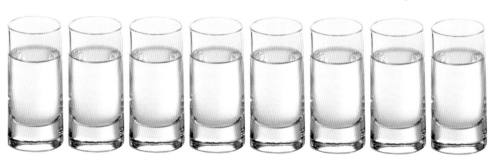

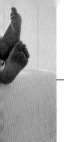

Dealing with exhaustion There may be times when you feel too exhausted to move, but try to eat for energy and stay hydrated.

TOP TIPS

Having a glass of freshly squeezed orange juice or eating other vitamin-C rich foods at the same time as eating iron-rich foods will help iron absorption.

Start your day with a bowl of oatmeal topped with a handful of berries, such as blueberries or raspberries; or with two slices of whole-wheat toast topped with a poached egg to keep you going through the morning.

Aim to have protein at breakfast and lunch, so that you feel the energy benefits during the day when you need them the most.

so take it as a sign to drink a glass of water immediately. Another sign of whether you are dehydrated or not is the color of your urine: the paler it is (ideally pale or straw-colored), the better hydrated you are. If your urine is dark, drink more water. Get into good habits to help stay hydrated: carry a water bottle with you and sip it little and often; put a glass of water beside you whenever you sit down; and drink a glass of water each time you go into the kitchen. Remember that milk, juices, and fruit teas (see p.53) count toward your daily intake, but caffeine and carbonated drinks don't.

Q I'm starving all the time—is it okay to eat more than I did before I became pregnant?

Healthy expectant mothers only need a small proportion of extra calories a day. To ensure optimal health for yourself and your baby, you should expect to increase your calorie intake by 200 calories per day in the first trimester, and by 300 calories per day after that. However, you are burning lots of energy while "building" your baby so it's not surprising that you feel hungry. Follow the advice given in the table (left) to try to stabilize your energy levels, and therefore any food cravings, so that you feel fuller longer. You should also be able to maintain more consistent energy levels if you remember to eat little and often—three meals, with two small (healthy) snacks in between. For quick snacks, try dried fruit with a few nuts, trail mix, rice cakes, oatcakes, or raw vegetable sticks (carrots or broccoli) with hummus, for example. If you feel hungry all the time, try switching to six small meals over the course of the day (see p.58), being careful not to overeat when you do so. Try to remember to check your weight gain at your next checkup (you might need to ask to be weighed, since this doesn't necessarily happen at every appointment) and increase your calorie intake appropriately if your weight is below healthy limits.

Q What can I do to change my eating habits? I want to lose my pregnancy weight after the birth.

Pregnancy, the start of a new life, is a great time to assess poor lifestyle choices and replace them with better ones—particularly when it comes to food. Imagine your plate of food as three separate sections to be filled. Allocate the biggest section of the plate—nearly half—to vegetables, which contain fiber (and so are filling) and are packed with nutrients, but are light on calories. Divide the remainder of your plate evenly between proteins (such as lean meat, fish, and legumes) and unrefined complex carbohydrates (such as potatoes, or brown pasta, or rice). It is a good idea to get your partner onboard with the new eating habits, too—now is a good time to reinforce the notion that you are in this together.

Clean out of your kitchen cupboards as well. Empty them of any refined foods that are high in fat or refined sugar, give the cupboards a thorough cleaning, and replace their contents with healthy alternatives, especially healthy snacks (see p.60). Do the same with your fridge and freezer, so that you are not tempted to indulge in the wrong kinds of food. If you find yourself reaching for a sugary snack, stop, and have a beverage instead: pour yourself a glass

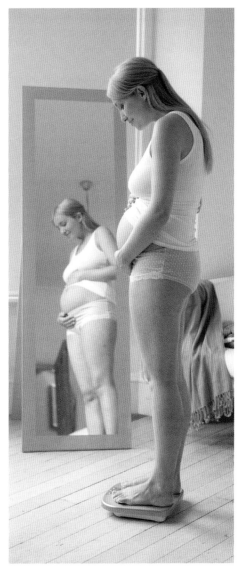

Weight gain You will put on most of your extra weight after 20 weeks of pregnancy. This is mainly due to your growing baby, but you will also be storing fat ready to produce breast milk.

of fruit juice, water, or fruit tea (as long as the tea is safe for pregnancy—see p.53). You could also try making juice ice pops, which last longer and can feel more satisfying than drinking juice.

🔍 Did you know...

Unless you are allergic to peanuts yourself, there is no evidence to suggest that eating peanuts while pregnant will contribute to your baby's chances of developing a peanut allergy (including having any impact on asthma or eczema risk). Although high in calories, peanuts are more filling than many other snacks; eat in moderation.

Q I feel so sick that I can only stomach dry crackers. Is my baby getting everything he needs?

If you are suffering from morning sickness and finding it hard to keep anything down, try changing what you eat and when. Your baby won't suffer.

Your hormones slow your digestive system during pregnancy so that your body can take the maximum nutrients from whatever food you eat. Furthermore, your body prioritizes your baby, drawing reserves of major nutrients such as calcium and protein from your own body if it needs to. As long as you eat a little, your baby should be fine. If you're worried or vomiting frequently, however, talk to your doctor.

EATING DURING THE DAY

If you are suffering from nausea and vomiting, try these suggestions to help you change the repertoire of what you eat or drink and when.

» **Eat little and often:** Try eating six small meals a day (right) rather than attempt three meals and two snacks.

» **Make your food starch rich:** In addition to being bland, which is all you might be able to face, potatoes, rice, pasta, and couscous contain good quantities of nutrients (B-vitamins, iron, protein, and fiber among them).

» **Eat raw foods:** Your queasy response to food often has to do with the smell of it rather than the taste. Raw (or cold) foods tend to have less of an aroma, which might make them more palatable for you.

» **Nibble on snacks:** Unroasted skinned almonds, which are nutrient-dense but plain to taste, are ideal.

» **Sip water:** Try adding a slice of lemon or two, or try hot water with a few mint leaves (which contain potassium, iron, and folate, among other nutrients). Drinking ginger tea can help to suppress nausea.

Sip water infused with a slice of lemon (which provides antioxidants and vitamin C).

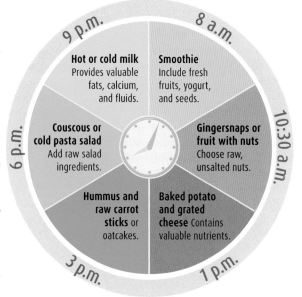

9 p.m.
Hot or cold milk Provides valuable fats, calcium, and fluids.

8 a.m.
Smoothie Include fresh fruits, yogurt, and seeds.

10:30 a.m.
Gingersnaps or fruit with nuts Choose raw, unsalted nuts.

1 p.m.
Baked potato and grated cheese Contains valuable nutrients.

3 p.m.
Hummus and raw carrot sticks or oatcakes.

6 p.m.
Couscous or cold pasta salad Add raw salad ingredients.

Six small meals Break your food intake down into more palatable, manageable minimeals such as these to help you consume enough nutrients each day.

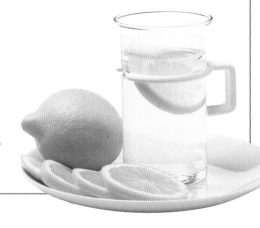

Q I love chocolate and I can't resist eating it. Does this mean my baby will have a sweet tooth?

If you like chocolate, your baby may have a preference for the smell and taste of chocolate. However, as long as your diet is healthy, with chocolate as a small and occasional indulgence (choose organic, dark varieties that are high in flavanols), your overall influence is a good one. A French study at the European Centre for Taste Science in 2012 concluded that what a mother eats, particularly during the final stages of her pregnancy, can significantly influence a newborn baby's preference for certain foods. It's thought that the flavors of foods pass through the amniotic fluid and into the baby's newly forming olfactory nerves so that when the baby is born, he will turn toward the smell of food that is familiar (and away from food that isn't). Perhaps the most important thing to remember is that any foods you consume that are high in saturated fat and sugar are low in nutritional value. Studies show that a pregnancy diet that is high in sugar and saturated fat can lead to higher birth weight babies and have a longlasting effect on your baby's own dietary choices.

Q Does the fact that I'm skinny and petite mean that I will have a low birth weight baby?

No, not necessarily. The evidence shows that as long as you eat healthily, you will have a full-term baby who is just perfect for his genes. Low birth weight is a medical term meaning that your baby weighs less than 5½lb (2.5kg) when he is born. In a healthy pregnancy without complications, there are two main influences on a baby's birth weight. The first is what you eat while your unborn baby is growing (and, in fact, what you ate before you got pregnant because your previous weight is a factor). A study conducted in Oxford, UK, in 2014 compared the birth weights of 60,000 babies from across the world and concluded that nutrition, even more than the mother's size or her ethnicity, impacted the size of her baby at birth. The second is due to genetics. If you're petite and were yourself a small baby, it's possible (and normal) that your baby will inherit your petite size. Of course,

Q What does "eating for two" mean exactly? If I'm having twins, do I need to eat for three?

The adage "eating for two" does not mean that you need to eat twice as much as you did before you got pregnant. You just need a small increase in calories, and slightly more still if you are carrying twins or triplets.

If you are pregnant with one child, your optimal calorie intake during pregnancy should increase by only 200 daily calories during the first trimester, and by 300 daily calories during the second and third trimesters. The list of suggested snacks (right) shows what 200 calories looks like in practice. If you are carrying multiples, you should increase your calorie intake per baby. So, for twins, you need to add 400 calories at the start of your pregnancy and 600 calories during the middle and the final stages of pregnancy. The other crucial thing to remember is that you need to optimize the nutritional value of the food you "share" with your growing baby, so try to ensure these extra calories are nutrient dense—don't forget quality in your quantity.

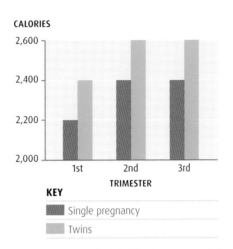

CALORIES

Optimum calorie intake The recommended guidelines on this chart ensure that you will give yourself and your baby enough nutrients and energy.

Make sure that the small increase in extra calories you need to eat during pregnancy are nutrient dense so that you have quality in your quantity.

CALORIE EQUIVALENT

How can I eat an extra 200-600 calories? Choose from these options or look for other healthy alternatives.

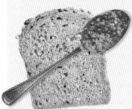

200 calories =
1 slice of bread and
1½ tablespoons of
peanut butter

APPROXIMATELY 200 CALORIES:

» **4 tablespoons of trail mix**

» **4 tablespoons hummus and 4 baby carrots**

» **Boiled egg and toast** without butter

APPROXIMATELY 400 CALORIES:

» **7 oz (200 g) low-fat yogurt and 1 apple**

» **7 oz (200 g) avocado on 1 slice of toast**

» **Grilled-cheese sandwich**

---

your baby's father's genes will come into play, too. If he is tall and broad, your baby may just as likely be long and heavy at birth—or somewhere in between the two of you. Tell your doctor if you or your partner were particularly small at birth and discuss whether anything in your family histories might be reason for concern in your own baby's weight.

Q Do I have excessive cravings? I seem to want foods and drinks I've never thought of having.

If you are suddenly desperate for foods you may previously have had little interest in, you are following a typical pattern in pregnancy. During early pregnancy in particular, your senses seem to be heightened due to your high hormone

levels: you may crave new foods and find that others—including tea, coffee, or fast foods—become repellent. This may be due to your sense of smell being more sensitive or a strange, perhaps metallic, taste in your mouth. Some experts suggest that your taste buds play a role in how you interpret you body's needs.

Nobody really knows what causes cravings in pregnancy since scientific studies cannot easily quantify or measure them. Some studies have suggested a potential link between certain cravings—salty foods such as olives, sour fruits like lemons, or vegetarians eating meat—and maternal diet deficiencies. However, researchers are unsure if a deficiency occurs because of abnormal eating habits in pregnancy, or the cravings occur because of a deficiency in your diet. Most cravings don't represent a threat to you or your baby unless you have the condition pica, when you crave nonfood items such as clay.

If you have persistent **morning sickness**, have food **cravings** such as drinking milk only, or have **lost your appetite** in late pregnancy, don't stress about whether your **baby is receiving enough** nutrients. **Stress** can prove to be more detrimental to you and your baby than **eating lightly** for a period of time.

Q What should I eat to optimize recovery after the birth?

The energy demands of new motherhood are immense, and yet at the same time you are still recovering from the birth and likely to feel sleep deprived and time poor. You may not have time to cook a complex meal, but you can eat well.

Making sure you get enough proper nutrition is immensely important. Your body is recovering from the tremendous physical exertion of the birth, and you are undoubtedly exhausted. You may even find you are anemic if you lost blood during the birth, or if you've had more than one baby. Although diet can't compensate for any sleep deprivation, eating enough nutrient-rich snacks and meals will help to quicken your physical recovery, help to combat any nutritional issues such as constipation, provide your body with fuel to give you the stamina to care for your baby, and help you feel better.

Healthy habits

If you established good shopping and eating habits in pregnancy, you should already be in the right mindset for continuing to eat a balanced diet. If not, this is a key time to avoid "empty calories" such as junk food and sugary snacks. They supply very little nutritional value and provide only a temporary boost of energy, leaving you feeling more tired than before. Include a wide variety of colorful fresh fruit and vegetables, whole grains, lean protein, and dairy products in your diet (see p.50). If you

are lacking iron, your doctor may recommend that you restore your iron levels through both diet and supplement, so choose iron-rich sources such as lean red meat, spinach, and chickpeas. If you have constipation, eat lots of fruit and vegetables, drink more water, and eat plenty of fiber: choose oats, whole-grain breads, brown rice, bran, and other high-fiber cereals. If you had a cesarean section or surgery after the birth, increase your intake of Vitamin C, which contributes to incision healing, and protein, helping your body to repair itself.

All this may sound good in theory, but in practice you might have little time to cook and rely on snacking instead. There's nothing wrong with snacking, as long as you eat healthily (see box, right). Your nutrient intake will be fine if you can eat a good breakfast— oatmeal with berries or poached eggs on whole-wheat toast—have nutritional snacks throughout the day, and sit down to one simple main meal—perhaps a bowl of pasta (with sautéed shrimp, garlic, oil, and lemon juice) with steamed vegetables. As you find your rhythm, the time and energy to cook will return.

Include a wide variety of **colorful fresh fruit** and **vegetables,** whole grains, lean protein, and dairy products in your diet.

Snacks and superfoods

Keep your snacks healthy and include plenty of "superfoods," such as blueberries, broccoli, tomatoes, oily fish, and oats. These give you much-needed vitamins, minerals, and antioxidants. Stock up on fresh fruit— especially bananas, which contain slow-release energy, and berries. Dried fruit, raw vegetables (carrots, broccoli, celery, etc.), cherry tomatoes, unsalted rice cakes, breadsticks, oatcakes, hummus, and guacamole are also great. Try making a tasty dip by blending cooked cannellini beans with olive oil and garlic in your food processor. Store it in the fridge, and eat with vegetable sticks or spread on oatcakes.

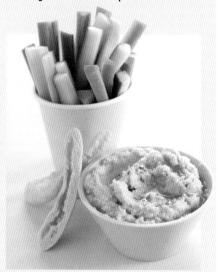

Finger food Easy to reach for and to eat with one hand, nutrient-rich snacks are ideal in the early days of taking care of your baby.

Sit down to **eat your meals;** eating on the run contributes to fatigue and can lead to overeating. If your **baby wants to be held**, put her in an infant sling so you are **hands-free** to eat.

Q I want to lose my baby weight. Is it okay to start dieting now?

Dieting too soon after the birth can delay your recovery and sap your energy levels, but if you eat sensibly and healthily, you will gradually lose your baby weight. You will find that you shed some weight fairly quickly after the birth as you lose "extras" such as the amniotic fluid and any water retention. Now that you are taking care of a baby, you should find yourself more active than in the last stages of pregnancy

and will be burning off more energy. However, it's recommended that you wait until you have had your six-week checkup before you start watching your calorie intake if you are not breast-feeding, and even then the advice is that you must not go on a crash diet. If you eat healthy, nutrient-rich foods in sensible amounts and exercise moderately every day so you lose fat and not muscle, you will gradually lose the weight and keep it off. Breast-feeding requires extra calories, so it's vital that you don't even think about restricting your calorie intake until after you have weaned your baby.

Q Do I need to change my diet now that I'm breast-feeding?

You don't need to eat any special foods while you are nursing, but everything you consume passes through to your baby, so there are some things to avoid.

The wonderful thing about breast-feeding is that you don't have to do or eat anything different or special to breast-feed successfully—once your baby has learned the art of latching on, your milk will naturally deliver the best possible nutrients to her. However, since you are the primary source of nourishment for your baby while you breast-feed her, it makes sense to eat a healthy diet and drink plenty of water.

Straight to baby

Everything you eat and drink passes through your breast milk to your baby in small amounts. Because of this, experts recommend that you take precautions with some foods, beverages, and other consumables. The advice for eating fish in pregnancy remains the same while you breast-feed: eat only two or three servings of fish a week to limit the amount of mercury you consume. It's best to avoid caffeine and alcohol along with nicotine and medications (unless prescribed by your doctor), although you might have a small drink during hours when you aren't breast-feeding.

Breast-feeding is demanding on your energy levels so you need plenty of fuel both to deal with taking care of your baby and to produce enough milk. You need to increase your calorie intake by 500 calories a day for as long as you breast-feed. You may want to incorporate an extra snack during the day to make sure you consume enough calories, or have a slightly bigger portion at mealtimes.

Spotting sensitivity

You may notice your baby develop a strong reaction to your breast milk. This could simply be a one-time dislike of the taste due to something you've consumed that day, or it could possibly be the sign of a food intolerance. Irritability after feedings, cold symptoms, and congestion are all possible symptoms of a food intolerance, although they are not all necessarily caused by diet. Other common symptoms are a rash, hives, itchy skin or eczema, digestive problems such as constipation or diarrhea, abdominal discomfort, swelling of the lips or eyes, and colic (see p.285), but again these are not always caused by food. If you think your baby is sensitive to or unsettled by certain foods you eat, talk to your pediatrician, especially if you have a family history of allergies.

It's useful to be aware of the most common food triggers so that you can watch your diet and keep a close eye on your baby for any signs that what you've been eating doesn't agree with him or her. Garlic, chili or spicy foods, cow's milk, orange juice, soy products, wheat, corn, eggs, peanuts, tomatoes, or shellfish are all common culprits. If you can identify a specific food that you think is causing discomfort, eliminate it from your diet for several days to see if that's the trigger, but be aware that some products, such as cow's milk, can stay in your body for up to two weeks. It's important that you continue to eat a balanced diet, so always consult your doctor before making significant changes to what you eat.

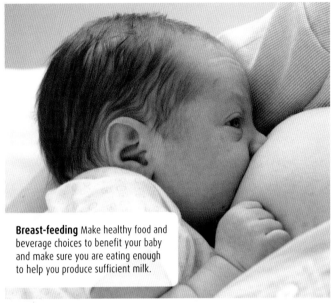

Breast-feeding Make healthy food and beverage choices to benefit your baby and make sure you are eating enough to help you produce sufficient milk.

WHAT TO AVOID

It's a good idea to avoid some substances so that your baby isn't affected in any way. Enjoy fruit teas, decaffeinated tea and coffee, mineral water, and an occasional glass of fruit juice instead.

AVOID	EXAMPLES
Alcohol	Alcohol is not advised in more than moderate, occasional quantities (1–2 units every now and then is unlikely to harm your baby). If you want to drink one night, express milk beforehand so your baby isn't affected.
Nicotine	Smoking is not advised near or around babies: breathing in secondhand smoke is known to be bad for your baby's long-term health and increases the risk of SIDS. If you smoke and breast-feed, you may slow your baby's weight gain, since nicotine reduces the amount of milk you produce.
Medicines	All medicines, including prescription drugs, over-the-counter drugs, oral contraceptive pills, and vitamin, dietary, and herbal supplements pass through your breast milk in small amounts, and while some may not have an effect on your baby, you should talk to your doctor before you take any kind of medicine, herbal or otherwise.
Caffeine	Caffeine is present in coffee, chocolate, tea, and some soft drinks and energy drinks, as well as some cold and flu remedies. Babies' bodies can't get rid of caffeine very well and may not be able to deal with you having too much caffeine in your diet.

Feeling **physically and mentally happy** goes a long way toward having a great pregnancy experience. Addressing any concerns you have about **life changes** and enjoying an **active pregnancy** safely is **beneficial** for both you and your unborn baby.

Exercise and well-being

A positive frame of mind

It's usual to feel apprehensive as well as excited about impending parenthood and such issues as the birth, money, and changing relationships. Accepting your worries as a first step can help you move forward and start to enjoy your pregnancy, and find solutions (see pp.69–73). Staying physically active contributes to your sense of well-being, helping to improve your moods, sleep patterns, and body image. Exercise also eases a range of pregnancy problems (nausea, aches and pains, and low energy) and lowers the risk of hemorrhoids, varicose veins, and even gestational diabetes.

Your pregnant body

During pregnancy, your musculo-skeletal system changes, affecting the way you exercise and the amount you do. To prepare for birth, the hormones relaxin and progesterone almost immediately begin to loosen the ligaments in your pelvic cradle (and elsewhere). This makes your joints more flexible so the baby can pass through, but you may feel unstable as you walk. As your belly grows, your "core"

abdominal muscles, which stabilize your back, stretch and become thinner to accommodate your baby, thus making them weaker. You may also feel off-balance as you adjust (and readjust) to a changing center of gravity as your baby grows and your weight shifts forward. In addition, a growing baby puts pressure on your bladder and pelvic-floor muscles, making certain types of exercise uncomfortable to do, and on your lungs, causing breathlessness even if you are normally very fit.

How much to exercise

You are the best judge of what level of exercise suits you, but as a rule of thumb don't exert yourself more than you were used to before pregnancy. If you haven't exercised before, you can start some gentle activites in your first or second trimester. It's also normal to feel very tired during early pregnancy, so get plenty of rest as well. Consult your healthcare professional before any exercise, especially if you have high or low blood pressure, are anemic, a heavy smoker, have a BMI greater than 40 or lower than 12, or are expecting more than one baby.

Q What are the best types of exercise during pregnancy?

Low- or no-impact exercise is ideal while you are pregnant, since it is easiest on your joints. Don't forget that any exercise that doesn't require you to try to maintain your balance over uneven or slippery ground is best.

The main goal of exercising through pregnancy is to strengthen your muscles, improve your circulation, ease any backache, and help you feel well. It's important to avoid any exercise or activities that require jumpy and jerky movements, take sharp changes of direction, or is so vigorous that it raises your core temperature or puts excessive strain on your cardiovascular system or joints. In addition, impact sports and sports that involve a risk of falling–such as cycling, horse riding, downhill skiing, and contact sports–are not advisable. Some good choices are listed below.

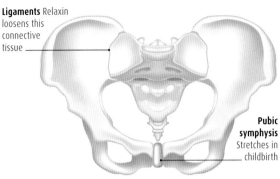

Ligaments Relaxin loosens this connective tissue

Pubic symphysis Stretches in childbirth

Softer joints The hormone relaxin acts on the soft tissues connecting the bones of your pelvic cradle. This is great preparation for labor, but can cause aching pain beforehand. Go easy on your joints when exercising.

GREAT WAYS TO EXERCISE

Keep supple and elevate your heart rate without causing stress to your body with these options. Warm up gently, and stretch after.

» Running, power walking, and walking: if you are already running regularly, continuing is perfectly safe. Don't try to train for an event though. Run just below your usual fitness levels, and listen to your body if it tells you you've had enough. If you haven't previously been a runner, walking and power walking are great alternatives.

» Cycling: a low-impact form of exercise, cycling is good for your breathing and circulation. Because there's a risk of falling off your bike, especially after your belly begins to grow and your center of gravity and sense of balance begin to shift, it's safer to use a stationary bike during pregnancy. It's just as good for you. A recumbent bike, on which you sit back, not upright, puts less pressure on your perineum, and may feel more comfortable as your baby grows and bears downward.

» Swimming: as long as the pool is a normal temperature (not higher than 90° F/32° C), swimming is fantastic, since the buoyancy of the water supports your body. Best of all, as long as you feel comfortable, you can keep swimming right up until the moment you go into labor. A water aerobics class will be especially suited to your pregnant body.

» Stretching and strengthening techniques: exercise such as Pilates and yoga, when specially adapted for pregnancy, can be gentle on your muscles and ligaments, increase strength and flexibility, and improve your breathing to help you through labor. They are also good for easing back and hip pain (normal side effects of loosened ligaments) and preparing your body for birth. Always find a qualified teacher, since there are certain yoga postures and forms of Pilates that aren't suitable during pregnancy.

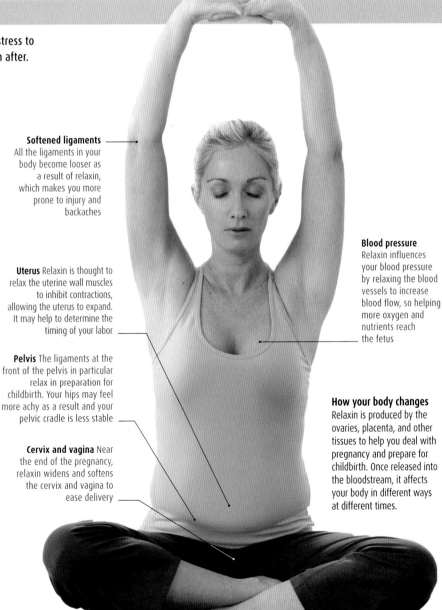

Softened ligaments All the ligaments in your body become looser as a result of relaxin, which makes you more prone to injury and backaches

Uterus Relaxin is thought to relax the uterine wall muscles to inhibit contractions, allowing the uterus to expand. It may help to determine the timing of your labor

Pelvis The ligaments at the front of the pelvis in particular relax in preparation for childbirth. Your hips may feel more achy as a result and your pelvic cradle is less stable

Cervix and vagina Near the end of the pregnancy, relaxin widens and softens the cervix and vagina to ease delivery

Blood pressure Relaxin influences your blood pressure by relaxing the blood vessels to increase blood flow, so helping more oxygen and nutrients reach the fetus

How your body changes Relaxin is produced by the ovaries, placenta, and other tissues to help you deal with pregnancy and prepare for childbirth. Once released into the bloodstream, it affects your body in different ways at different times.

Q How can exercise make my pregnancy easier?

If you are one of the 70 percent or so of women who experience backaches and other physical discomfort in pregnancy, you may think that resting will help. Instead, practice safe, low-impact exercises to decrease the muscle spasms.

It's not just the extra weight of your baby as she grows that puts a strain on areas such as your back. The aches you experience increase because the hormone relaxin loosens your ligaments, especially those in your pelvic cradle. This makes way for your growing baby and prepares for birth; in fact all your ligaments soften due to the high concentrations of relaxin required to loosen the pelvic joints. Your baby's increasing size also stretches the transversus abdominis (TVA) muscles, which act like a girdle to support and stabilize your lower back from the sides and front. As your center of gravity shifts forward with the baby's weight, it's likely that your posture will change to compensate, increasing the strain on muscles in your lower back. It may be tempting to lie down when you ache, but any exercise that helps you strengthen these deep transversus abdominis muscles will ease the pain or discomfort. Consider prenatal Pilates classes, which specifically target your "core stability"—strengthening these core muscles so that your back remains as steady and supported as possible—or try the exercises shown opposite. These gentle stretching and strengthening movements will decrease muscle spasms, release back tension, and improve your spinal flexibility.

Any exercise that helps **strengthen the transversus abdominis muscles** will ease pain and discomfort.

TRANSVERSUS ABDOMINIS MUSCLES

This "core" of deep abdominal muscles lies beneath the outer muscles (such as rectus abdominis, or the "six pack"). They wrap around the spine and help to stabilize your torso and lower back. The stronger the tranversus abdominis muscles are, the more support they give.

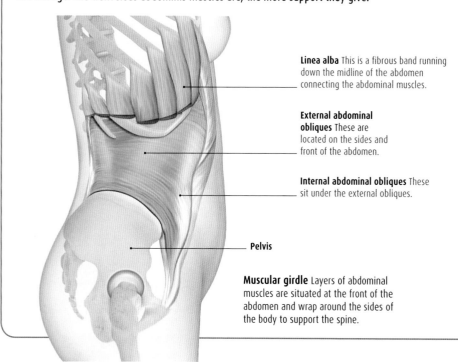

Linea alba This is a fibrous band running down the midline of the abdomen connecting the abdominal muscles.

External abdominal obliques These are located on the sides and front of the abdomen.

Internal abdominal obliques These sit under the external obliques.

Pelvis

Muscular girdle Layers of abdominal muscles are situated at the front of the abdomen and wrap around the sides of the body to support the spine.

Q How do I ease the symptoms of water retention?

There are a couple of options you can try if you are experiencing water retention, or edema, in your ankles, feet, and hands, or if your joints are feeling stiff. One of the best choices is to walk around for a while every so often during the day to get your circulation going (avoid sitting or standing still for long periods), or go for a daily walk outdoors, or swim. Swimming has the added benefit of cooling your body down in hot weather; becoming too hot can cause water retention. Elevating your feet can help, too. Use a foot stool if you work at a desk, or elevate your feet properly for a while: sit back in a chair, raise your feet right up, and rotate your ankles several times in each direction to get the blood flowing.

Complementary therapies

Massage can be very beneficial in helping to dissipate fluid and reduce tension. For a home massage, gently massage your feet, ankles, and lower legs with a lotion or cooling gel; use upward strokes working toward your knees. If you are heavily pregnant, you may find it easier to ask your partner to do this. When massaging your hands, press firmly from your nails to the base of your fingers. Reflexology and acupuncture can also help; your practitioner may be able to show you acupressure points to use in between visits.

Water retention often occurs during the last three months of pregnancy due in part to the extra blood—up to 50 percent more than usual—that you produce. It also occurs if you are dehydrated, as your body tries to retain as much fluid as possible, so drink plenty of water.

When you exercise, make sure that you wear clothing that gives you a **full range of movement** and choose suitable footwear that will **support** your ankles and feet. Keep drinking plenty of water and take regular rest breaks.

Q What simple exercises can I try at home?

Recommended by midwives, these exercises are easy to do at home. However, check with your doctor first that they are safe in your specific case. Stop if you feel any discomfort or dizziness.

HAND STRETCHES

Try these simple stretches if you feel pain, tingling, or numbness in your hands.

» **Shake your hands for one minute** as if air-drying them after just washing them.

» **For a deep stretch,** hold out one arm, keep your elbow straight, and drop your wrist so your fingers face the floor. Using your other hand, apply gentle pressure to the back of your hand to gently stretch your wrist and fingers for 20 seconds. Repeat with the other hand.

» **Put your hands together in a prayer position**. Spread your fingers, then pull your palms as far apart as possible while keeping your fingertips together. Repeat several times.

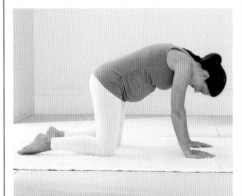

FOOT STRETCHES

Relieve foot cramps and ease any arch strain, or even plantar fasciitis, with this exercise.

» **Foot roll** Stand in bare feet on a nonslip surface. Roll a tennis ball or golf ball around under the base of one foot for two minutes to gently massage all the muscles. Repeat with the other foot.

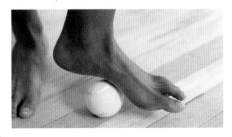

BACK STRETCHES

Keep your spine flexible by warming up and strengthening the muscles around it. Kneeling on all fours also helps to relieve tension in your spine.

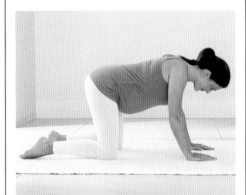

1 **Kneel on the floor,** then lean forward and support your weight on your straightened arms (don't lock your elbows), so that you're on all fours. Keep your hands, knees, and feet in line with each other. Keep your back horizontal. Relax your neck and inhale.

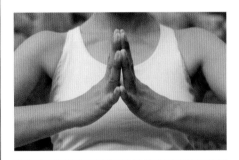

2 **Slowly draw up your abdominal muscles** as you exhale, tuck your pelvis under, and lengthen the base of your spine gently so your back is arched like that of a cat. Keep your elbows gently straight, but not locked. Inhale and release to straighten your back again; be careful not to hollow out your back.

3 **Repeat the arching movement ten times** altogether. When you've finished, sit back on your heels and breathe deeply a few times to relax. Get up slowly so you don't feel dizzy.

SPINE STRETCHES

As your baby grows heavier, it's beneficial to align and stretch your spine every day. Try these two simple exercises to relax and refresh you.

1 **Stand with your feet** hip-width apart just in front of a wall. Bend your knees slightly and rest the length of your spine against the wall. Breathe deeply.

2 **When you're ready,** breathe out and pull your belly button toward your spine. Your pelvis should tilt up and away from the wall slightly, so that your lower back presses into the wall. Hold briefly, then inhale and release. Repeat ten times.

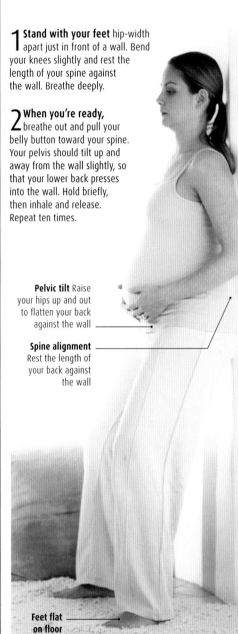

Pelvic tilt Raise your hips up and out to flatten your back against the wall

Spine alignment Rest the length of your back against the wall

Feet flat on floor

Ease discomfort and stabilize your back using these **stretching** and **strengthening** techniques.

Q I've heard I need to exercise my pelvic floor. Where is my pelvic floor and why is it important to my pregnancy?

Your pelvic floor is a group of strong, layered muscles that stretches like a double sling, or a hammock, from your pubic bone to your tailbone. This sling supports your abdomen and holds in your reproductive and pelvic organs. During pregnancy, the muscles support the growing weight of your uterus and baby; during labor, they help guide your baby out of your body.

Some muscles of your body, such as your heart, are involuntary, but most are voluntary, which means you can consciously tighten and release them. You do this with your pelvic-floor muscles when you "hold in" if you need to go to the bathroom (the double sling of muscle has holes in it that correspond to your urethra, rectum, and vagina).

How the pelvic-floor muscles work

During pregnancy, your pelvic-floor muscles are loosened by the hormone relaxin, and then stretched and weakened by the weight of your growing baby bearing down on them. Having strong pelvic-floor

muscles is crucial: an already weak pelvic floor can mean that during pregnancy and afterward you can leak urine when you cough, sneeze, laugh, jump, or run—a condition known as stress incontinence. Also, during labor your pelvic floor forces your baby to turn in the cavity of your pelvis. He is then able to fit into the birth canal so you can push him out during second-stage labor. A weak pelvic floor may make this process less efficient. A surge of relaxin loosens your pelvic floor further to enable the baby to move through the birth canal: the pelvic-floor muscles near the front of your body are forced downward and those near the back are forced upward, creating an opening for your baby.

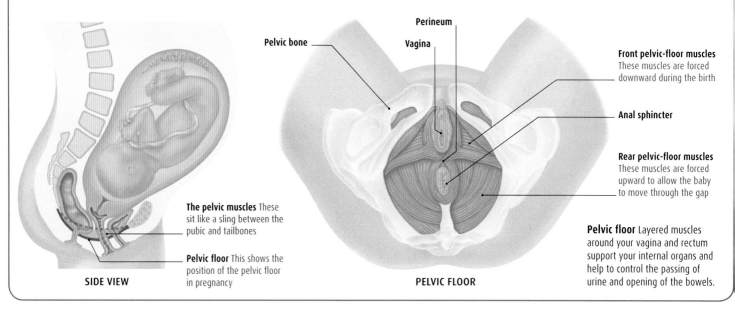

The pelvic muscles These sit like a sling between the pubic and tailbones

Pelvic floor This shows the position of the pelvic floor in pregnancy

SIDE VIEW

Perineum

Pelvic bone

Vagina

Front pelvic-floor muscles These muscles are forced downward during the birth

Anal sphincter

Rear pelvic-floor muscles These muscles are forced upward to allow the baby to move through the gap

Pelvic floor Layered muscles around your vagina and rectum support your internal organs and help to control the passing of urine and opening of the bowels.

PELVIC FLOOR

Q Are the pelvic-floor muscles permanently stretched after labor? What's a prolapse?

After labor, your pelvic-floor muscles should "ping" back into place relatively quickly, keeping your organs neatly tucked in as they were before. If the muscles are damaged during labor, however, you may suffer a "prolapse," when your abdominal organs bear down into your vagina. Often, it's not until later in life that any damage becomes apparent and a prolapse occurs. So it's important to practice Kegel (pelvic floor) exercises throughout pregnancy and afterward, trying to reverse the damage and give the muscles back as much strength as possible.

Q I have a toddler who still expects to be carried. Will I harm the baby— or myself—if I lift him?

As long as your doctor hasn't told you not to, careful lifting is fine—it poses no threat to the safety of your unborn baby. Your back and pelvic floor, though, can be a different matter. It's vital that you protect your back by lifting carefully, whether you are picking up your toddler or lifting and carrying grocery bags or heavy objects.

To lift safely, plant your feet shoulder-width apart and flat on the floor. Bend down from your knees (not your waist), tucking your buttocks under and keeping your back straight.

Wrap your arms around your toddler, asking him to lock on with his legs, or hold the grocery bags or heavy object firmly. Push up with your thighs (use one arm to hoist yourself up against something if you need to), rather than straining your back. Once you're standing, adjust your toddler's position so it's comfortable for you— his legs straddling your belly, for example, or on one or other of your hips (if you carry your toddler on the side, switch sides each time to balance out the strain). If you carry several shopping bags, make sure that you distribute the weight evenly between both hands. Lifting also strains your pelvic floor, so always engage your pelvic-floor muscles before lifting anything, and practice your Kegel exercises frequently (see opposite).

Q How do I do Kegel exercises? Is there a way to be sure I'm doing them correctly?

Pelvic-floor exercises or Kegels—named after US gynecologist Arnold Kegel—are the exercises that keep the pelvic-floor muscles toned so that they are strong enough to assist the second stage of labor (see opposite).

It's important to perform Kegel exercises daily while you are pregnant, since the pelvic-floor muscles work with your deep transverse abdominal and back muscles to stablize your spine, support your baby, and help prevent stress incontinence. However, don't overexercise your pelvic floor when you do this internal movement–more than 100 squeezes a day could make it difficult for the muscles to relax during the birth, which then makes it harder for the baby to make his way out.

First, find out what your pelvic-floor muscles feel like: imagine you are drawing up water into your vagina. Another way to find the muscles is to stop urinating toward the end of your flow (don't do this in the middle since it could lead to a urinary-tract infection). The muscles you tighten to do either of these actions are your pelvic-floor muscles. The movement is completely internal and not visible to other people.

Benefits of Kegel exercises

Do them anytime, anywhere, in any position. Practice them while you make coffee, wait in a line, or to the rhythm of a song. If you only do a few at a time, the cumulative effects will be worth every one, and may even help to improve your sex life. If you suffer from stress incontinence, you should notice a difference after about six weeks.

DO A SIMPLE KEGEL EXERCISE

Here is a simple routine you can follow. Try to do the whole sequence three times a day. You might find it helps to lift starting with the rear muscles and then moving forward to the front, before holding and then releasing.

1 SQUEEZE THE MUSCLES
Sit comfortably in a chair with your feet flat on the floor and your back straight. Keep your body and your face relaxed. Pull up and squeeze your pelvic-floor muscles as tightly as they will go and hold for ten seconds. Release the muscles.

2 SLOW SQUEEZE AND RELEASE
Repeat the squeeze 9–20 times, holding each for ten seconds. Do not use your abdomen or buttock muscles. Make sure you rest the muscles for ten seconds between contractions.

3 QUICK SQUEEZE AND RELEASE
Finally, do a set of quick squeezes. Following the natural rhythm of your breath, lift the muscles as you inhale. Exhale and release and briefly relax the muscles. Repeat ten times.

If you find it hard to know whether you are locating the right muscles, it can help to try doing the exercises in different positions. Below are some options that will help you focus all your attention on the correct area and relax the rest of your body.

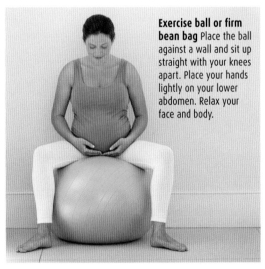

Exercise ball or firm bean bag Place the ball against a wall and sit up straight with your knees apart. Place your hands lightly on your lower abdomen. Relax your face and body.

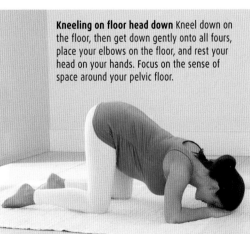

Kneeling on floor head down Kneel down on the floor, then get down gently onto all fours, place your elbows on the floor, and rest your head on your hands. Focus on the sense of space around your pelvic floor.

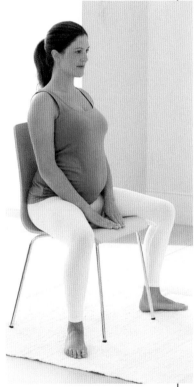

Astride a chair Sit upright on a chair with your knees wide apart and your feet at an angle that allows for maximum stability. Rest your hands on the front of the chair seat. Relax your face and body and focus on your pelvic area.

Q Will I have to give up running? I want to stay fit and feel my best throughout my pregnancy.

You can keep up some sports, such as running, for as long as feels comfortable and is medically safe; then switch to low- or no-impact sports later on so you can continue exercising.

Low-impact exercise This exerts minimal stress on your weight-bearing joints.

As long as you are a seasoned runner, continuing to run during your first trimester and into your second trimester is fine if you feel well and comfortable. You may find that the increasing weight of the baby and your changing center of gravity mean that you won't want to run as far or as fast as before, and you may tire more quickly. Avoid running on bumpy or icy ground so you don't fall. After 12 weeks of pregnancy, check with your doctor about how long it is safe for you to continue.

With any high-impact sport, you should follow a few rules while pregnant. Warm up and cool down gently and don't overstretch: unlike muscles, which regain their shape after the birth, ligaments will not recover if stretched excessively. Exercise moderately below your usual fitness levels; you should be able to talk easily while you exercise—so avoid pushing yourself too hard. If you overheat, the fetus may suffer, particularly in the first trimester when it can't regulate its own temperature. If you are out of breath for a period it may reduce the amount of oxygen the fetus receives. It's especially important to rehydrate properly afterward, since dehydration can lead to complications including premature contractions.

Do not attempt any high-impact, high-risk, or contact sports if you exercised intermittently before becoming pregnant, or are new to exercise.

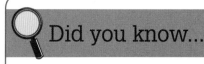

Did you know...

Exercise has the happy consequence of causing the brain's transmitters to release endorphins into the brain and nervous system. These hormones have a number of physiological functions, including triggering a positive feeling and reducing stress, helping to boost your mood.

WHICH SPORTS TO ENJOY AND FOR HOW LONG

Exercise is a wonderful way to maintain your energy levels and feel good, but you may need to exercise within a different set of parameters as you move through each trimester.

SPORT	PROS & CONS	FIRST & SECOND TRIMESTER
Swimming	Strengthens your heart and lungs and tones your muscles while supporting all your weight and keeping your body temperature stable.	Ideal for all levels of fitness. Sign up for water aerobics classes if available.
Badminton	A low-impact aerobic sport that promotes cardiovascular health.	As with most racket sports, unless you are a regular player, don't play while pregnant. Try other low-impact alternatives.
Cycling	Gives you a cardio workout while supporting your weight so there is less stress on your body.	Use a stationary bike and don't overexert yourself. Cool down afterward.
Golf	Low-impact golf works core muscles, helps to improve stability, and improves cardiovascular health if you walk the course.	Continue if you already play golf regularly, but stretch well first, adjust your game to "slow and easy," and be careful not to lose your balance.
Gym	Has a variety of equipment and exercise classes to give you a cardio workout and strength training (use light weights only).	Exercise at a moderate intensity on machinery. Sign up for pregnancy exercise classes.
Hiking & climbing	Hiking improves your strength and cardiovascular health. Climbing is not advised.	Consult your doctor first before going hiking, then choose even terrain and make sure you have supportive hiking boots and hiking poles.
Pilates	Focuses on core muscles—abdominal, pelvic floor, and back—to promote good posture, stability, and strength without straining other joints.	Ideal for all levels of fitness, but for safety, make sure your instructor knows that you are pregnant.
Walking & power walking	Strengthens your heart and lungs, tones your muscles, and is safe for your body.	Walk for 30 minutes three times a week if you are a beginner. If you are fit, focus on power walking—walking at a brisk pace—to raise your heart rate.
Yoga	Gives you techniques to help you breathe, move, stretch, and relax while pregnant. Also strengthens your muscles. Avoid hot yoga.	Ideal for all levels of fitness. For safety's sake, tell the yoga instructor that you are pregnant.
Dancing	Gives you a good cardio workout, but can stress the joints. Always keep one foot on the ground and avoid spinning, leaping, jumping, and so on.	Continue if you already dance regularly, but exercise below your usual fitness levels.
Running	Elevates your heart rate and works your muscles, but can cause stress to your joints.	Continue if you run regularly, but listen to your body during your second trimester in particular.
Tennis	Gives you a cardio workout, but rapid changes in direction can stress your joints and cause falls.	Unless you are a fit and very experienced player, don't play while pregnant. Try low-impact alternatives.

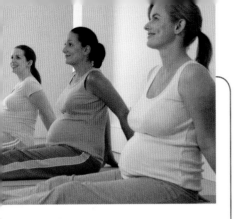

KEY

	No impact
	Low impact
	High impact

THIRD TRIMESTER	WHEN TO STOP
Listen to your body and slow down if need be.	You can continue swimming until the birth.
Change to a recumbent bike if you feel uncomfortable.	Stop if you feel too tired or get dizzy.
Try other alternatives unless your doctor says it's safe to continue.	Stop when you feel too tired and heavy.
Find out which equipment is safe to use. Continue pregnancy classes.	Stop if you feel too tired or get dizzy or light-headed.
Check with your doctor that it's safe to continue hiking.	Stop if you feel too tired or get dizzy or light-headed.
Focus on relaxation and breathing techniques.	Continue with gentle Pilates until the birth.
Listen to your body and slow down if you feel tired.	Continue walking until the birth.
Don't lie flat on your back after 16 weeks or you may feel faint.	Continue with gentle yoga until the birth.
Try low-impact options unless your doctor says it's safe to continue.	Stop if you feel too tired or get dizzy or light-headed.
Try low-impact options unless your doctor says to continue.	Stop if you feel too tired or get dizzy.

Q Will having sex affect the baby at all?

There is no medical evidence to suggest that having sex if your pregnancy is straightforward will harm your baby in any way—it's perfectly safe for you to enjoy sex in each trimester. Neither is there is any risk of miscarriage or premature birth when you have penetrative sex. Once you become pregnant, your baby is well protected: your cervix is sealed with a thick mucus plug, and as the fetus grows, the amniotic fluid around it helps to cushion it from any pressure. If you have complications, however, such as heavy vaginal bleeding or your water breaks, you are advised not to have sex and should seek medical attention straight away.

Increased libido
Making love during your first trimester shouldn't feel any different physically, but if you are nauseous or chronically tired, you may have a low libido. If you've had a previous miscarriage or assisted conception, you and/or your partner may feel nervous about having sex. Reassure each other and cuddle to maintain your intimacy until you want to make love.

During the second trimester, your body changes shape noticeably, which can make some women feel less sexually attractive. However, you should have more energy, feel more relaxed about the baby's safety, and find your libido has returned: the increase in blood volume in your body can heighten sensations, and help you reach orgasm more readily. If you feel your baby moving after sex, it may be due to the adrenaline release you receive at orgasm.

During your third trimester, you may have Braxton Hick's contractions if you reach orgasm and these can last from a few minutes to half an hour afterward, which is normal. However, if the contractions continue longer and you are concerned, contact your doctor.

Q I can't stop thinking about the birth. How will I handle labor, and motherhood?

It's hard not to leap ahead and think about the future, but as your body changes and the baby grows your emotional mindset will evolve. Your hormones are already responding to the new life inside you and gradually preparing and enabling your body to give birth, but it can be hard for your thought processes to fall in line with your natural instincts. Your well-being is of paramount importance so that you are in the best possible shape physically and mentally to give birth and take care of a baby. For now it's good to focus on the present and how best you can take care of yourself and the fetus. Keeping fit, eating healthily, and avoiding stress, anxiety, and fear are key. Try to relax and unwind as much as possible, talk to your doctor about any concerns you still have and, as much as you can, be aware of the miracle of pregnancy and how your baby is growing.

> Taking a **pregnancy exercise class** provides more than just physical rewards: it's a great way to meet other, like-minded **moms-to-be** to share your experiences and enjoy making some new friends.

Q I'm still in shock about being pregnant. Will I ever get excited and enjoy my pregnancy?

If you feel that you can't shake off your state of shock, be reassured. The first few weeks are an unusual time as you battle to cope with the onset of early pregnancy symptoms, wonder about the future, and yet see no real evidence of a baby. Sometimes negative feelings arise partly as a result of having to keep it all a secret for a while. As you open up about your news, and start to feel physically better, the shock should dissipate. Do positive things to make your experience of pregnancy as enjoyable as possible: pamper yourself with relaxing baths and massages, sleep in when you can, plan events to look forward to, and enjoy closer bonds with family members and friends and enjoy their excitement and good wishes, for example. If the feelings of shock or fear don't subside, talk to your doctor to ensure you don't have the condition tocophobia: a fear of pregnancy and childbirth.

If you want **extra support** throughout your pregnancy, try out a few of the online **social media forums** for expectant moms—you'll be joining a wonderfully empowering and reassuring **support network** that you may want to continue with after your baby is born.

Q I'm going to be a single parent. Will I be able to manage and how can I prepare properly?

All new moms worry about being able to cope, and those concerns are often heightened if you feel you have no one to share them with. But you aren't alone. First, discuss how you feel with trusted friends and family, and with your doctor, and ask them for reassurance.

Then, even before your baby is born, start building your support network. Identify a birthing partner and share your birth plan with him or her. Talk to the people you are closest to about who can be around to help you in the first few weeks after the birth—to do some practical essentials such as the shopping or cleaning, but also to provide some companionship and to take care of the baby occasionally, so you have time to yourself (your well-being is important for your baby, too). You may want to make a list of what chores you normally do so that your "support team" knows what to do and can divide up the tasks.

Ask your doctor if she can put you in touch with other single moms-to-be, or look online for single parent groups in your area. Never be afraid to ask for help, nor to accept offers of it.

Finally, well before your due date, be sure to get organized: prepare and wash clothes and bedding for your baby, and cook yourself some nutritious meals and freeze them—stews, casseroles, and soups that you can eat using just a fork or spoon are best. Leave yourself as little as possible to do after the birth so you can spend the time fully engaged with your new baby.

Q How expensive is having a baby going to be? I'm not sure I'll be able to afford it.

You may never feel financially ready to welcome a newborn into your life, but your baby doesn't have to be a money drain if you take a realistic approach.

Although every parent wants the best for their child, it is vital not to have sky-high expectations about what your baby needs, or insist on the best. You may have a clear vision of the life you want to give your child and be anxious that you won't be able to fulfill this desire, but all your new baby really wants is to be close to you and be warm, dry, and fed. There's no need to buy every piece of baby equipment brand new. Babies quickly grow out of clothes and equipment, so it's usually easy to find good-quality secondhand items via local sales or online forums. You might also be pleasantly surprised by how many gifts you receive—and by the money you save staying in.

It's true, however, that having a baby will impact your income if you intend to continue working and have to take child-care costs into consideration, and as your baby develops into a child and then a teenager, supporting him will become more expensive. If this is a concern, it's worthwhile to take advantage of the time you have now to make a clear financial plan. Discuss your household finances with your partner so you are both aware of the issues and responsiblities ahead and there are no misunderstandings.

You may want to discuss the idea of **setting up a joint "baby" account** and start saving for your child's future.

FINANCIAL CHECKLIST

Get your finances in order as soon as possible so that you have the right systems in place and feel in control of your money by the time your baby arrives.

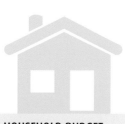 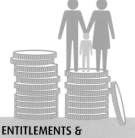 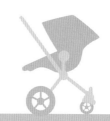

HOUSEHOLD BUDGET

Look at your monthly outgoings
Pinpoint where you can save money—perhaps gym memberships and subscriptions that you rarely use, for example, or unessential purchases. If you and your partner have separate bank accounts, figure out how to share the bills and seek out the most cost-effective way to pay them. You may want to discuss the idea of setting up a "baby" account.

ENTITLEMENTS & CREDITS

Your health insurance plan
This may or may not cover the cost of your prenatal appointments during your pregnancy, and you may qualify for other benefits at work. You may also qualify for the IRS's Child Tax Credit, depending on your income.

BABY EQUIPMENT

Make a list of baby equipment
Include essential items only, and think before you buy—a bulky, unwieldy carriage may prove impractical, or a diaper disposal pail may never get used. Ask friends and family if they have items you can borrow, or buy secondhand; you may just need to buy a few new items like a changing mat and a crib mattress. If you buy new, shop around first.

Q Will my relationship with my partner change forever with a baby around? How do we adapt?

There is no doubt that having a baby around will change the current dynamic of your relationship, but that in itself can have positive rewards.

It's normal to feel concerned about the impending changes ahead and worry that you may lose something of the precious intimacy you currently enjoy. Whether you have planned this baby or not—and even if you feel a sense of contentment about creating a family—your relationship with your partner will inevitably need to evolve as you become parents.

It's a good idea to define the feelings you have about a change in your relationship and becoming parents. If your relationship is strong, take heart from the fact that you already understand the process of getting to know each other, learning about each other's qualities and character so you can relate to one another and support and nurture each other in life.

Talk to each other

It's important that you find time to talk about issues on your minds. These may include worries about spending less time with each other after the birth, and maybe more time with your in-laws; the changes in your roles and how to manage household tasks; moving from two wages to one (even if it's only temporary) and the sense of dependence or pressure this may bring; and personal expectations about how you want to parent your baby.

If you worry about becoming parents, be reassured that it's not as difficult as you think. You will adapt to your roles, but give yourselves time. Researchers have estimated that it takes new parents at least four months to establish a routine and feel confident with their baby.

Keep **communicating** openly and **showing respect** to each other as you prepare for, and then **parent**, your child.

DISCUSSION POINTS

Talk through your expectations of life as a family so you understand each other's hopes and feelings and know how to keep your relationship a priority once you become parents.

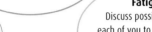

Parenting styles
You may have different ideas of what constitutes "normal" family life—talk through them now.

Work pressures
Brainstorm ideas about how you can both try to create a good work/life balance.

Fatigue
Discuss possibilities for each of you to take turns in having regular "time out" for yourself to relax or rest.

Time alone together
Sex and intimacy and effective communication are important discussion points.

Responsibilities
Delegate chores between yourselves so you have a clear understanding of who will do what and when.

Support
Talk about whether you can afford—and want—to have some extra support at home after the birth.

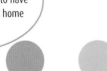

Q I feel stressed. Will the baby be affected?

It's perfectly natural to feel anxious about how you will cope with life—and a baby. There probably isn't a woman who hasn't felt worried, anxious, inadequate, or even fearful at some point during her first (or subsequent) pregnancy. Bringing a new life into the world is a magical time, but it's also one filled with unpredictability and change. And if you work or lead a busy life, the prospect of trying to process all you need to do before the birth can sometimes feel incredibly pressured.

If you feel stressed, your body produces higher levels of the hormone cortisol. Research is still being conducted as to whether prolonged bouts of cortisol affect your unborn baby: some studies have shown that the effects of chronic

stress on a fetus can be minimal; others that constant stress may put your baby at risk. We all experience stress at various times, but it's important that you don't let it overwhelm you. Try to live in the moment, learn to delegate and don't attempt to do everything yourself, rest when you can, and exercise moderately—it's a great way to release stress.

If your stress has turned into anxiety and you feel you can't cope, have no appetite, you're worried about going out, you cry much of the time, and feel lethargic and uninterested in life, you may have prenatal depression (PND). Although less well known than postpartum depression (see p.263), it probably affects more women than we realize simply because moms-to-be often feel ashamed of and are afraid to mention their negative feelings. If you're at all concerned, talk to your doctor, as well as your family and/or friends.

Q I am excited about our baby, but my partner isn't. How can I get my partner more enthused?

It seems obvious, but make an effort to involve your partner in as many ways as possible. Encourage your partner to feel your belly often, for example, and talk to your baby: around 24 weeks gestation the fetus begins to hear what's going on outside the uterus. Also consider whether what you see as lack of enthusiasm may in fact be anxiety about your partner's responsibilities, so ask your partner how they are feeling. Finally, while pregnancy is a living part of you, for your partner there's probably something a bit unreal about it. Hang in there; for many partners, full and enthusiastic engagement happens only when finally they hold their baby in their arms.

Approaches to childbirth have changed dramatically over recent decades: nowadays it is considered perfectly acceptable to try different techniques and positions in labor to help you manage pain and stay focused yet relaxed for a positive, calm birth. Practicing different techniques while you are still pregnant can help you feel in control when the time comes.

Physical preparation

Thanks to the pioneering efforts of some childbirth experts (see opposite), it is no longer standard procedure to be confined to a bed during labor. Moving around and staying in an upright position may help to shorten the length of your labor. So it's a good idea to practice safe squats, for example, while pregnant to strengthen your legs and thighs in preparation for birthing standing up. "Labor breathing" is another effective way of helping you to manage the pain of each contraction and keep a positive, relaxed attitude. Practice labor breathing regularly in pregnancy so you feel familiar with the technique once you are in labor.

Mental preparation

As your body goes into labor, your brain triggers the release of the hormone oxytocin, which increases the contractions of the uterus to ease labor along, and endorphins, which help you feel calmer and can alleviate pain. Staying as relaxed as possible during labor will let these body chemicals work effectively; if you feel scared or fearful, adrenaline, a stress hormone, will flood your body and limit their effects. For some women, techniques such as hypnobirthing, audio-analgesia, visualization (see pp.228–29), meditation, and relaxation will enable an easier labor and birth as well as offering a sense of spiritual well-being.

PATTERNED BREATHING

Consciously changing your breathing patterns as labor progresses helps to force oxygen into your bloodstream so you can stay calm and relaxed enough to handle the pain. Remember, breathing out properly is all-important.

1 Late first stage of labor During this early stage take deep, slow, even breaths at the start and end of a contraction, and light breaths during its peak.

IN — Deep, even breaths — Light breaths — Deep, even breaths — OUT

2 Transition stage As the contractions become intense, and to avoid pushing too early, take shorter breaths in groups of two to three, blowing out each time (see right). Breathe out gently when the contraction ends.

IN — Short breaths — Short breaths — Short breaths — OUT — Blow — Blow — Gently out

3 Second stage of labor Take and hold a deep breath while pushing down smoothly. After each push, take deep, even breaths.

IN — Deep, even breaths — Even breaths — OUT — Push — Push

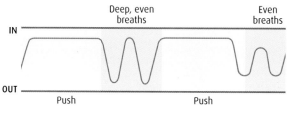

Breathing tips

>> Start practicing as early in pregnancy as you want, so that you are familiar with all three stages of breathing when you eventually go into labor.
>> Inhale calmly through your nose and concentrate on relaxing your muscles. Focus on your out breath: blow out slowly through your mouth and imagine you are exhaling the pain of a contraction. Everyone's pain threshold is different: don't be afraid to ask for medical pain relief if you feel you need it.

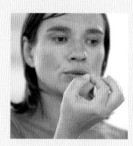

Breathing out properly Hold one hand about 12 in (30 cm) away from your mouth and join your thumb and index finger. You are exhaling properly if you can feel your out breath cooling your fingers. This may help especially with more intense contractions.

TYPES OF PREPARATION

If you are interested in practicing one or more of these approaches, look for dedicated childbirth classes in your area.

Mind

» Hypnobirthing is a form of self-hypnosis where you consciously take calm control of your birthing experience with breathing and relaxation techniques. You remain fully aware and focused throughout (you are not in some kind of hypnotic "sleep").

» Audio-analgesia uses a combination of music and white noise to help you control and dull the sensation of pain.

Spirit

» Relaxation, meditation, and mindfulness can clear your mind of thoughts and block out what is going on around you while you remain calm, aware, and centered (below). Find a warm, quiet space. Lie down. Gently stretch out your arms, legs, shoulders, wrists, shoulders, and neck. Get comfortable, close your eyes, breathe regularly, and focus on an object or the present moment.

Body

» Squatting opens out your pelvis to ease the baby's passage through the birth canal. Stand up straight with the back of a sturdy dining chair facing you. With your feet hip-width apart, toes pointing slightly outward, and hands on the chair back, bend your knees until you're in a sitting position. Push your weight into your heels. Push up from your thighs. Repeat five times.

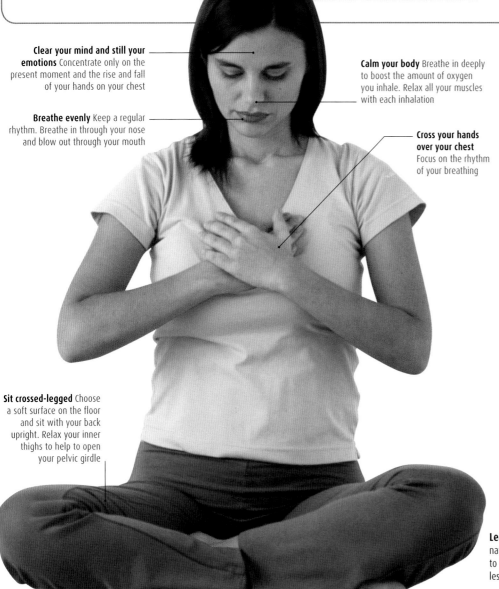

Clear your mind and still your emotions Concentrate only on the present moment and the rise and fall of your hands on your chest

Breathe evenly Keep a regular rhythm. Breathe in through your nose and blow out through your mouth

Calm your body Breathe in deeply to boost the amount of oxygen you inhale. Relax all your muscles with each inhalation

Cross your hands over your chest Focus on the rhythm of your breathing

Sit crossed-legged Choose a soft surface on the floor and sit with your back upright. Relax your inner thighs to help to open your pelvic girdle

CHILDBIRTH PIONEERS

You might find the writings of some of the different childbirth philosophers and practitioners inspirational when considering the type of birth you want.

» **Dr. Ferdinand Lamaze** investigated effective relaxation and breathing techniques, now known as "Lamaze breathing."

» **Frederick Leboyer** seeks to reduce the trauma of birth, saying that babies should be born into calm, softly lit surroundings and placed on the mother's skin before the cord is cut. He is also an advocate of water births.

» **Sheila Kitzinger** enabled women to reclaim some control over the way they want to give birth. She campaigned for the avoidance of unnecessary obstetric intervention where appropriate so that giving birth is a powerful, positive experience.

» **Michel Odent** endorses active childbirth techniques, thereby reducing the need for pain relief and the number of assisted deliveries and cesarean sections.

Learning to relax Try focusing your awareness on your natural breathing rhythm to link your emotions and thoughts to your physical sensations. The more relaxed you are, the less tension, and therefore pain, you will experience.

Q What exercises can I do immediately after having my baby?

You may be desperate to lose any excess pregnancy weight and tone up again after the birth of your baby, but you must take things gently until the six-week checkup, when your doctor should give you the all-clear.

Childbirth has a profound effect on your body and it takes a while to recover your pre-pregnancy strength and resilience. Although it's good to be active again as soon as possible after the birth, the general advice is that for the first six weeks you should not attempt to return to–or improve on–your pre-pregnancy fitness levels. Your transverse abdominal muscles (see opposite) may still be stretched apart, and levels of relaxin are still high in your body, so your joints will remain loose for a while yet; you may inflict serious long-term damage to your ligaments if you try any high-impact exercise. Your lochia (vaginal bleeding) may get heavier or turn bright red if you do exercise too hard too soon after giving birth–a warning sign that you need to dial down your activities again. If you want to swim, leave seven clear days without vaginal bleeding beforehand so you don't pick up an infection (and avoid it if you have had stitches or a cesarean section). Anything other than gentle exercise and Kegel exercises is off limits until at least after your six-week checkup. To get your circulation going, take a gentle walk every day, and gradually build your stamina. Remember to keep your back straight as you push the baby stroller.

Kegel and stretch exercises

Focusing on your Kegel exercises again after the birth is essential to retone the muscles as soon as possible, so practice them throughout the day, sitting, standing, kneeling, or lying down as often as you remember (see pp.66-67). If you can't feel the muscles, try practicing first on an exercise ball. Now that you don't have to limit the number of pull ups you do in order to be able to consciously relax the muscles during labor, do as many repetitions as you can manage–the more the better. You can also start gently exercising and stretching (see below) to begin toning major muscles, boost your recovery from the labor and birth, and help you get rid of any aches and stiffness.

GENTLE EXERCISES FOR THE FIRST SIX WEEKS

You can do these gentle exercises to tone your lower stomach muscles and stretch out your body after the birth, even if you have had a cesarean section. Start with just a few repetitions if you can manage them in the early days, and gradually build up your strength over six weeks with more repetitions.

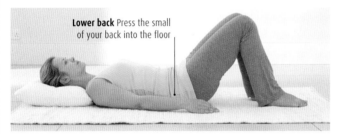

Lower back Press the small of your back into the floor

Pelvic tilt Lie on the floor and support your head and shoulders with a cushion. Relax your arms at your sides and press your back into the floor. Keep your knees bent and your feet flat on the floor. As you exhale, press the small of your back into the floor for 10 seconds. Then release and relax. Repeat this 3-4 times initially, building up to 12 and then 24 repeats.

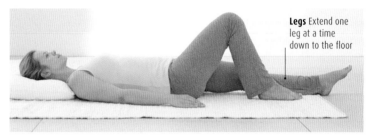

Legs Extend one leg at a time down to the floor

Leg slides Lie on your back with your head and shoulders supported, knees bent with feet flat, and arms at your sides. Exhale and slide one leg down until it is flat on the floor. Repeat with the other leg. Inhale and slowly bring one leg back up. Repeat with the other leg. Repeat the exercise 3-4 times. Increase gradually over the weeks until you can do 12 or more leg slides comfortably.

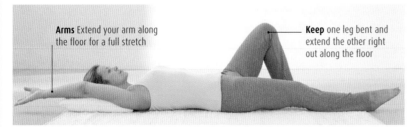

Arms Extend your arm along the floor for a full stretch

Keep one leg bent and extend the other right out along the floor

Spine alignment Lie on your back with your head and shoulders supported and knees bent with feet flat on the floor, and the small of your back pressed into the floor. Exhale and extend your right leg down so it is flat on the floor. Breathe in, then as you exhale stretch your right arm along the floor behind your head. On your next exhale, stretch from heel to fingertips. Repeat on the other side.

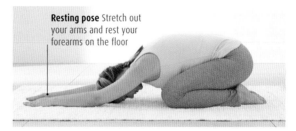

Resting pose Stretch out your arms and rest your forearms on the floor

Extended Child's Pose Get down onto all fours, then sit back on your heels, separate your knees, extend your arms out in front of you, and rest your forehead and your forearms on the floor. Your belly should rest between your thighs. Hold for 2 breaths or as long as it feels comfortable. This pose will enable you to elongate your back fully and release any tension in your hips.

Q I thought I'd get my stomach back quickly, but it's so wobbly! Will it ever recover?

Your stretched transverse abdominals and uterus mean that your belly won't recover its pre-pregnancy shape immediately. But fear not—the muscles will gradually recover and contract after the birth. The time it takes will be different for each person. Breast-feeding will help speed up the contraction of the uterus, as the hormone oxytocin, which is released when your baby latches on, contracts both the smooth muscles of the milk sacs in your breasts and the smooth muscle cells in your uterus walls.

You can start with some simple exercises to regain your waistline, but you must perform a simple check first on your abdominal muscles (see right). Once you feel a gap of just one finger-width between your transverse abdominals, begin with a simple head and shoulder lift. After your six-week checkup, move on to doing abdominal crunches and sit-ups.

Q How soon is it safe to start having sex after the birth?

Traditional advice recommends no sex until the six-week checkup, although there is no danger to your health if you have sex sooner. When you resume your sex life is a very individual issue, and something you should both take gently. If you feel ready to have sex again as soon as two to three weeks after the birth, that's fine. Penetrative sex may feel a little dry and painful though, so use a lubricant. However, don't feel pressured to resume your sex life until you feel ready. Exhaustion, soreness, and your physical recovery can all take its toll on your libido in the days, weeks, and even months following the birth. Take things slowly with your partner, discuss what you both want, and enjoy kissing and hugging until you are ready for sex. And don't worry if sex feels like it's out of the picture for the foreseeable future: a study conducted by the *British Journal of Obstetrics and Gynaecology* in 2013 found that only 41 percent of first-time mothers had had vaginal intercourse by the time their baby was six weeks old. The most important thing to be aware of is that you are potentially fertile again, even if you are breast-feeding, so take precautions and use contraception.

Q How do I get back into shape after the six-week checkup?

Your goal to regain your former level of fitness, or improve your fitness if you were previously quite sedentary, should be gradual, and you shouldn't start high-impact activity too soon. Let your body be your guide.

Once you have the all clear at six weeks, you can build your fitness levels again. However, before you hit the gym in a flurry, do a simple test. Lie on your back, place your hands behind your neck to support it, and slowly lift your head. As you hold that position, place a finger just above your belly button and press down gently to feel the gap between the muscles. If the gap is just one finger-width apart you can start exercising normally; workout moderately for 30 minutes or more a day for three to six months and then gradually work up to high-impact activity. If it is wider—two or more finger-widths apart—don't resume regular exercise yet.

TRANSVERSE ABDOMINAL MUSCLE CHANGES

The natural changes that occur to your muscles in pregnancy need time to revert to normal before you can begin exercising again.

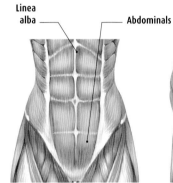

Linea alba — Abdominals

Pre-pregnancy The muscles are aligned at the front on either side of the linea alba.

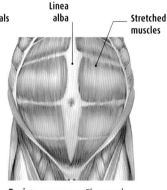

Linea alba — Stretched muscles

During pregnancy The muscles stretch and usually split apart to allow the fetus to grow.

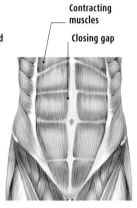

Contracting muscles — Closing gap

Postpartum The stretched muscles take time to close up again. You must wait until the gap has almost closed before resuming normal exercise.

Q I still have a backache. Why hasn't it gone away yet?

You need to continue to protect your back to prevent backaches from bad posture and injury from lifting and carrying. Your loose ligaments, which still haven't tightened up yet, account for some of the pain. But constantly bending down to lift a baby can strain your back muscles. When you pick him or anything else up, bend from your knees, keep your back flat, hold him close to you, and lift up by straightening your legs. Check your posture, too, and keep your back straight and your shoulders back. Ideally your baby should be the heaviest thing you lift for at least the first six weeks after the birth.

In the early weeks after the birth, **resting** when you can and slowing down are two of the most **positive things** you can do, so **don't feel guilty.** Concentrate on your recovery and your baby, exercise gently, eat healthily, and your **energy levels will gradually return.**

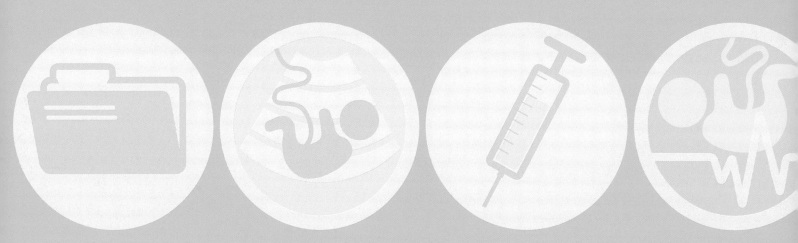

Prenatal care

Prenatal care appointments steer you through your pregnancy journey. This chapter explains where your care will take place, who your **doctors** will be, and what is likely to happen at your **prenatal appointments**, from your first appointment through to your final visit just before you give birth. Find out about all the **tests and scans** available and start thinking about your **birth choices** and who you would like to be your birth partner.

The care that you receive during your pregnancy will be a mixture of **routine checkups** and **personalized care** that works to take care of the **health** of you and your baby. Your appointments are also an opportunity to **ask questions** that will inform your choices when you **plan and prepare** for the day your baby will arrive.

Your care explained

What your prenatal care involves

Once you've absorbed the news of finding out that you are pregnant, you'll probably start to focus on the practicalities of what happens now. Should you go to see your doctor? How do you get yourself into the system of prenatal care? Who will take care of your health and the health of your unborn baby?

For most women, there will be a standard number of regular appointments to check their progress; for others there can be extra appointments if their doctor needs to keep a closer eye on them and their baby as they progress through pregnancy. You'll be given routine blood and urine tests and your blood pressure will be checked. Advice on lifestyle and well-being will also be given by your doctor. You can opt to be screened for infections and complications that could affect you or your baby, and there are ultrasounds and tests to assess your baby's health (see pp.92–103).

Prenatal appointments are a great opportunity to seek advice about the many changes you are experiencing, as well as to connect with your pregnancy, and with your baby (you'll find out how much she's growing and you might get to hear her heart beating). You can even go to childbirth preparation classes if you want to learn more about what happens during labor and birth, and how to take care of your new baby afterward.

Your birth, your choices

Your doctor will lead your care so that you have a pregnancy that is as healthy and safe as possible, but he or she should take into account your needs and preferences. There will be some decisions about which tests you do and don't want, how and where you'd like to give birth, and whom you'd like with you when you do.

When planning your birth you might consider: Are you more comfortable with the idea of a giving birth at a hospital or birth center? How would you describe your pain threshold? Does the idea of giving birth in water appeal or fill you with dread? What about giving birth standing up, sitting in a birthing chair, or lying down? Your answers to these questions might change over the course of your pregnancy—and that's fine, too. Mapping out your wish list is a good way of honing in on specific aspects of your pregnancy, but don't let yourself get too frustrated if things don't always go according to plan. Nature sometimes has different ideas, which is all part of the adventure.

Q What should I do when I first find out that I am pregnant?

Call your OB/GYN's office and make an appointment. They will schedule your first appointment when you are six to eight weeks pregnant. If you have any abnormal bleeding or other concerns, they may want to see you sooner than that.

You may be asked when the first day of your last menstrual period (LMP) was, in order to calculate an estimated date of delivery (EDD), or due date. Give your doctor a rough idea if you don't know this date for sure; you'll be offered an ultrasound at around 12 weeks pregnant to assess the due date more accurately (see p.95).

You will need to tell your doctor about the history of any previous pregnancies (including terminations), any health issues you have, and any relevant family medical history for both you and the baby's father. If you're taking medications, have them with you, so he or she can tell you if it's safe to continue taking them. Be prepared to say how long it has taken you to get pregnant (if you've been trying), and if you had fertility treatment. In the latter case, you will have an early ultrasound to confirm the pregnancy and make sure all is well (see p.94).

You can be asked about your diet, alcohol consumption, and any smoking or drug use. It's important to be honest in your answers since this appointment is an opportunity to ensure that you get the best available care for yourself and your baby. Everything you tell your doctor is confidential—and it will benefit the health of your baby.

Finally, you will be given information on nutrient supplements to take (including folic acid and vitamin D), food safety, nutrition, and the various screening tests available to you in pregnancy.

> Your doctor can answer **any concerns** you have about your pregnancy at any time **throughout your nine months,** whether about your own health or that of your baby.

Q Who will take care of my health, and that of my baby, during pregnancy?

If you have a straightforward pregnancy, your regular checkups will be done at your doctor's office by an OB/GYN rather than at a hospital. In some cases you will have one primary contact. Other women see several doctors.

Your OB/GYN (the doctor you see at your initial pregnancy appointment) may be your primary caregiver throughout. He or she will take your blood and urine samples, measure your blood pressure, and check the growth and well-being of your baby. He or she will also book your ultrasounds and be a regular point of contact for support and advice.

If your pregnancy is not straightforward, (if you have a multiple pregnancy, preexisting conditions, or risk factors, or if any factors develop during your pregnancy), you may be referred to a specialist for additional care.

If your doctor is part of a practice with two or more OB/GYNs, he or she will want you to have at least one prenatal appointment with each doctor in the practice, so that you'll get to know each one. You don't know who will be on call at the hospital when you go into labor.

Health-care professionals you may meet during your pregnancy include:

≫ Your OB/GYN is the first person to see when you become pregnant. You should continue to consult your OB/GYN during pregnancy about other health problems and medication.

≫ The other doctors in your OB/GYN's practice (if you're not seeing a solo practitioner) will conduct some of your prenatal appointments. The doctors should take turns monitoring you throughout your pregnancy so that you meet everyone.

≫ A sonographer is someone who is specially trained to use and take readings from an ultrasound scanner in order to monitor the intrauterine health of your baby.

≫ A maternal-fetal medicine specialist is an OB/GYN who treats women with high-risk pregnancies. If you have a preexisting chronic health condition or you're carrying multiples, your doctor may refer you to this specialist for some or all of your appointments.

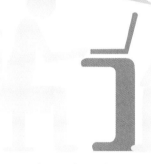

Q Can I make sure I've understood?

Q Can you explain it again?

Q Is there a pamphlet I can take home?

You can always ask questions Quiz any health-care professional you meet. There is often a lot of new information to absorb; asking the three questions suggested above can help make things clearer.

≫ A midwife may be an alternate caregiver to an OB/GYN. A certified professional midwife may be your primary caregiver during your pregnancy if you are healthy, expect to have a normal, uneventful pregnancy and know that you'd like to have your baby at a birth center. A certified nurse midwife may do hospital deliveries.

≫ An anesthesiologist is a doctor who specializes in pain relief and anesthesia. You'll see an anesthesiologist if you ask for an epidural in labor, or if you have a C-section.

≫ A nurse practitioner may work in your OB/GYN's office and see you for routine prenatal appointments. She can take your measurements and give you routine tests but won't be available when you go into labor.

Q What will happen at my first appointment with the doctor?

The first appointment is a chance to identify your needs (such as additional care for preexisting conditions, extra monitoring for risk factors, or support for personal circumstances), discuss your options for screening tests, and do a health checkup. You and your doctor have a lot to discuss, so allow a couple of hours for the first appointment. He or she will:

» **Discuss your general medical history.** Give your doctor details of any illnesses or surgeries you've had, and about any medications you're taking.

» **Ask you questions to get to know you,** your circumstances, and your family history.

» **Take a history of your gynecological health**, including your menstrual cycle, use of birth control, and details of any previous pregnancies (including your labors and your babies' health and weight at birth.)

» **Ask about your pregnancy symptoms** (fatigue, nausea, and so on) and whether you've had any bleeding.

» **Ask about how you're feeling emotionally.** It's normal to feel anxious—even terrified and confused!—so don't be worried about saying so.

» **Do a basic health checkup** to check for general well-being, including taking your BMI (see p.51) and blood pressure, and a urine test to check for infections. Your doctor may take blood samples if you opt for screening tests.

» **Advise you about optional screening tests for your baby,** such as screening for spina bifida and Down syndrome (see pp.95-9).

» **Give you information** about nutrition and diet, exercises (including Kegel exercises), your baby's development, childbirth classes, planning your labor and place of birth, and breast-feeding.

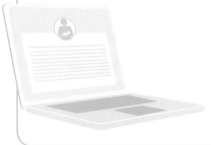

You can ask your doctor any **pregnancy-relation question,** at this appointment, from diet concerns to questions about having sex.

Q How often will I have follow-up appointments?

In a straightforward pregnancy, you will have your regular prenatal appointments at 8, 12, 16, 20, 24, 28, 30, 32, 34, 36, 37, 38, 39, and 40 weeks. If you opt for them, there will also be two ultrasounds—one at 11 to 14 weeks, and another at 18 to 22 weeks. (Your doctor may also offer you an ultrasound at your initial appointment at 8 weeks.) Whether this is your first, second, or third pregnancy, your doctor will see you the same number of times and offer ultrasounds on the same schedule.

Every prenatal appointment will involve a urine test and a blood pressure check. Your doctor will measure your belly (from 24 weeks) to check your baby's growth, and also feel your tummy to establish the position of your baby (from 36 weeks).

You'll be able to talk through any ultrasound or screening test results and implications with your doctor where necessary. Over the course of your appointments, your doctor will discuss with you such topics as labor expectations, the importance of flu shots while you're pregnant, postpartum depression, and breast-feeding.

Q I told my doctor that I was pregnant, and he did tests to confirm this.

Even if you've had a positive home pregnancy test, your doctor may want to confirm your test results with a urine or blood test in the office when you come in for the first appointment. This may simply be standard procedure in your doctor's office, or they may need to measure levels of hormones in your urine or blood when you come in for the appointment. Finding out you have conceived, whether it's planned, unexpected, long-awaited, or quick, can feel instantly life-changing for you, and the extra confirmation you get at your doctor's office may be thrilling.

Q I have a nine-month-old baby and I'm pregnant again. Are there risks?

It's important that you see your doctor as soon as you know you are pregnant because your body can take at least a year to recover before safely undertaking pregnancy again. Problems are, of course, relatively rare, but it's important that you are carefully monitored from the start and advised about how best to manage with both the demands on your body and taking care of a small baby during the tiring early stages of pregnancy. Pregnancies that occur in quick succession raise the risk of placental abruption (see p.147), low birthweight for your baby, and your own nutritional deficiency.

Q My doctor has said that our relationship is confidential. Can I really trust her?

It's important that you and your doctor develop a mutually trusting relationship that enables you to get the appropriate advice and care. You can feel confident that almost anything you could tell your doctor will not be shared with anyone else. Doctor-patient confidentiality requires that your doctor keeps your health information private, unless there's a concern for someone else's safety, including your own. If you have a sexually transmitted disease, a dependency on drugs or alcohol, or you feel especially anxious or depressed, it should remain confidential.

Q Will my health insurance cover a midwife instead of a doctor?

It depends on your health insurance company and the state where you live—there are no national guidelines. If you're eager to see a midwife, call your insurer and check before you go to your first appointment. Only a small number cover costs for appointments with midwives and births at birthing centers, rather than hospitals. If you want to pay out of pocket to see a midwife, it should be considerably less than if you paid out of pocket for a doctor, partly because midwives tend to order fewer tests than doctors.

Q What blood tests are taken at my prenatal appointments?

A range of tests can check for blood type, infections, genetic diseases, and anemia. Your doctor may take samples for the following:

» Your blood type and rhesus status Tested once in early pregnancy. Your blood type (A, B, AB, or O) will be recorded in your records in case for any reason you need a transfusion during delivery. If you are rhesus negative (see p.82) you will need one or two additional injections.

» Hepatitis B Tested once, in early pregnancy. This viral infection can cause liver damage in the baby, and the baby needs treatment at birth.

» Anemia Tested at the first appointment and at 28 weeks. A full blood count can suggest anemia if your hemoglobin levels are low. It also tests levels of blood folate and vitamin B_{12}, blood platelets, and white cell count (to check that you aren't fighting an infection).

» Rubella immunity Tested once in early pregnancy. The rubella virus can cause serious congenital abnormalities in babies (see p.139). If you're not immune, you can't be vaccinated in pregnancy so your doctor will advise on how to minimize your risk of exposure in pregnancy.

» HIV and syphilis Tested once in early pregnancy. These diseases pose a significant risk to your baby if you don't know about them—but your baby can be protected if you do. You have the right to refuse an HIV/AIDS test.

» Sickle-cell disease and thalassemia Tested once in early pregnancy. This is a test for genetic blood disorders that can be passed to the baby. Usually offered to those at risk of being carriers.

» Other tests If you're at high risk, you may have blood tests for hepatitis C, vitamin D deficiency, toxoplasmosis, and for chicken pox immunity if you're not sure of your history.

Q Will I be screened for Group B streptococcus (or GBS)?

Yes. Women are tested for GBS late in pregnancy, typically between 35 and 37 weeks. You'll have two swabs, one vaginal and one rectal, and if you carry the infection, you may be offered intravenous antibiotics during your labor, or the baby will be given antibiotics as soon as she is born. If you were GBS-positive during a previous pregnancy, your doctors will treat you with antibiotics again this time.

Q Why do I need to provide a urine sample at each appointment?

Your doctor tests urine for protein (high levels indicate high blood pressure, preeclampsia, urinary tract infection, or kidney disease). If you have gestational diabetes, your doctor may also test your urine to ensure that your condition is under control. Plan to give a sample at each visit.

Q Will I need a whooping cough vaccine? Why?

You will be offered a whooping cough vaccine between 27 and 36 weeks. Cases of whooping cough have gone up in recent years. Babies are routinely vaccinated against the virus at two months, but before this time they're vulnerable to infection. If you are vaccinated in pregnancy the immunity crosses the placenta and protects your baby in the weeks after birth.

Q Why is my blood pressure measured at every checkup? What are they looking for?

Pregnancy-induced hypertension (high blood pressure) (see p.144) can restrict the flow of blood to your baby, interfering with his growth. Your doctor will take your blood pressure throughout your pregnancy in order to be vigilant.

If your blood pressure rises too much, it also carries risks for you (the same risks as high blood pressure in nonpregnant people). It can also be a symptom of preeclampsia (see p.144), along with protein in your urine. Average pregnancy blood pressure is actually a little lower than normal nonpregnancy blood pressure for most of pregnancy, because hormones dilate your arteries to deal with the extra blood volume your pregnant body creates to grow your baby. By the end of pregnancy, you have about an extra 1¾ pints (1 liter) of blood pumping around your body.

Blood pressure readings These have an upper number (systolic) that denotes the pressure in your arteries when your heart pumps, and a lower number (diastolic) for the pressure between pumps when your heart rests.

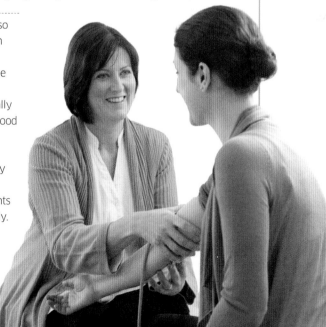

Q Why am I being tested for rhesus status? What is it?

In addition to having a blood type (A, B, AB, and O), all blood is either rhesus positive or rhesus negative.

A blood test early in pregnancy checks rhesus status. About 15 percent of people have rhesus negative blood. If your blood is rhesus negative and your baby's blood is rhesus positive, you may develop antibodies (defensive cells) if the baby's blood leaks into your blood. This contact can happen during a miscarriage or termination, at birth, or if you fall on your abdomen. It doesn't usually affect first babies, but once you develop antibodies, they can attack a subsequent rhesus-positive baby, causing anemia. In a first pregnancy, you'll have an Rh immunoglobulin (RhIg) injection to prevent antibodies from developing if you're rhesus negative. If your blood already has antibodies, extra ultrasounds will monitor the baby, and treatment may be needed.

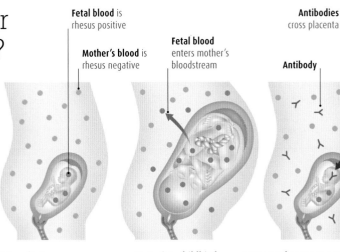

Fetal blood is rhesus positive

Mother's blood is rhesus negative

Fetal blood enters mother's bloodstream

Antibodies cross placenta

Antibody

1 In a first pregnancy, a rhesus-positive baby's blood will not cause issues unless it leaks into the rhesus-negative mother's body.

2 During childbirth the mother's rhesus negative blood creates antibodies in reaction to the "foreign" blood.

3 In a subsequent pregnancy, the antibodies can destroy a rhesus positive baby's blood cells, causing anemia in utero and jaundice after birth.

Q How will my doctor know if my baby is growing properly?

Your baby's growth is usually monitored by the growth of your uterus from its highest point (fundus) to the top of the pubic bone (symphsis pubis). This is called the "symphysis fundal height" (SFH) and, interestingly, the measurement in centimeters often corresponds to your baby's gestational age in weeks. Your doctor will check your fundal height at every prenatal appointment from 24 weeks until birth, using a tape measure placed over your belly as you lie on your back. The fundal height is recorded on a percentile chart that plots this measurement against your baby's gestational age. At your next appointment a new fundal height measurement will indicate whether or not your baby is growing as expected. Before you are 24 weeks pregnant, your first ultrasound (see p.95) indicates how your baby is growing, and your doctor might listen to your baby's heartbeat at your checkups. Toward the end of pregnancy, your doctor will palpate your abdomen (see opposite) to check your baby's position as well as growth.

Q Do I need to go to childbirth classes? How do I choose them if I do?

Whether or not you go to classes is entirely up to you. However, there are great benefits if you do—including learning about your pregnancy, labor, and birth, and how to take care of your newborn baby. You will also meet other moms- and dads-to-be in your area due at the same time, which can be a great support when you are a new parent.

Your doctor will give you details of local childbirth classes—which may be run by labor and delivery nurses or midwives who work in your area. You can take more than one class, if you'd like to. Most childbirth classes begin at around eight to 10 weeks before the baby is due (at 30 to 32 weeks pregnant). If you are expecting twins or more, you should book your classes to begin when you are around 24 weeks pregnant, because your babies are more likely to be born early. Classes usually run for between three and six weeks, with one class every week, and each class lasting up to two hours.

You might find a six- or eight-hour class on a weekend for busy couples who don't have time to attend shorter evening classes over the course of several weeks.

Childbirth classes You are encouraged to bring along your birth partner, so that he or she can learn some specific techniques to relax you during labor.

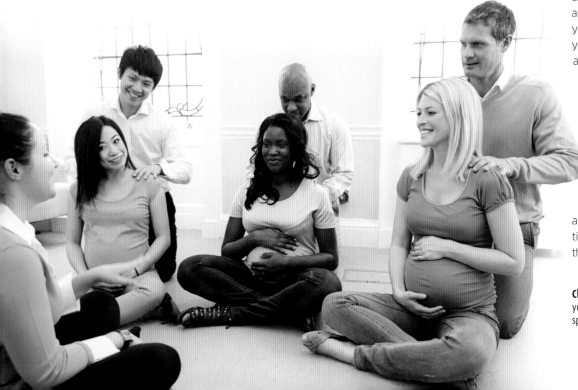

Q Is it safe to use complementary therapies in pregnancy?

There are certain complementary therapies, or aspects of them, that are not safe for you or your baby during pregnancy. Your doctor is trained to support you in your decisions about your care and will guide you on what is appropriate and what's not, based on medical evidence. Avoid buying over-the-counter remedies, and consult a practitioner qualified in prenatal care before using any oil or herb.

» Chiropractic: useful for back and joint pain. Always look for a practitioner with a qualification in prenatal care.

» Acupressure, acupuncture, and shiatsu: can help with nausea and morning sickness in early pregnancy. Always go to a practitioner qualified in pregnancy care.

» Bach flower remedies: may help with stress or anxiety, if your doctor allows them. Clinical studies consider them to have a psychophysiological effect only–that is, feeling that you're taking control of an issue is the effective part of the treatment, rather than any active ingredient in the treatment itself.

» Osteopathy: useful for back and joint pain. Always choose an osteopath trained to treat pregnant women.

» Homeopathy: may help with nausea and vomiting, and fatigue. It is a matter of continuing medical debate as to how and why homeopathy works, so be sure that your doctor supports your decision before you move forward.

» Hypnotherapy: can help you manage labor pain. See a practitioner who can teach you self-help techniques to keep you relaxed and focused during your labor and birth.

» Moxibustion: reported to help turn a breech baby. Moxibustion is a form of traditional Chinese Medicine–use only if you receive your doctor's go-ahead.

» Massage: useful for stress, anxiety, back and joint pain. Find a masseuse trained in pregnancy care. You shouldn't lie on your back in the third trimester–instead lie on your side or try a foot, facial, or hand massage. Avoid essential oils.

Q What's my doctor feeling for when she presses on my belly?

Your doctor's pressing, stroking, and pushing movements across, above, and below your belly are known as "palpation." He or she will do this primarily to determine the position of your baby from around 36 weeks onward.

By palpating your belly, your doctor will be able to tell when your baby has moved into the head-down position ready for birth, when your baby's head has "engaged" (moved downward into your pelvic area), whether your baby is curled over, head to chest (the ideal position for birth), or is more extended, and the position of the baby's spine compared with your spine. As you lie on your back, your doctor will use both hands to smoothly and firmly feel all over your belly with the pads of his or her fingers. Try to stay relaxed throughout the procedure, since this makes the palpation more accurate. Let your doctor know if anything causes you any discomfort.

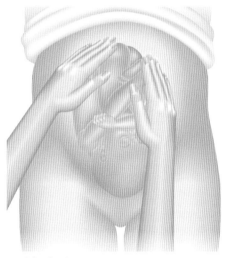

Fundal palpation This maneuver checks what part of your baby's body is at the top of your uterus. At 36 weeks, it's hoped to be your baby's bottom.

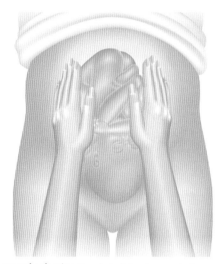

Lateral palpation Your doctor's hands move to the side of your abdomen so that he or she can check the position of your baby's spine.

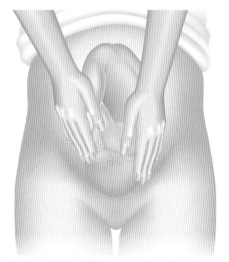

Pelvic palpation This helps your doctor determine what part of your baby is in your pelvis. It's the most important maneuver in the palpation sequence.

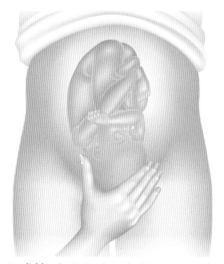

Pawlick's grip This is a form of pelvic palpation and it tells your doctor whether your baby's head faces downward and is engaged in your pelvis.

Q My mother is a twin. Should I tell my doctor about that?

Yes, if your mother has a family history of nonidentical twins say so. In some cases, you may go for an ultrasound as early as five weeks to see if you are carrying more than one baby. However, about 20 to 30 percent of twin embryos seen early on become single pregnancies before the next ultrasound–known as "vanishing twin syndrome." The causes are not known but there are no ill effects on the remaining embryo.

Q Will my symptoms be twice as bad if I'm carrying twins?

Some pregnancy symptoms may be more severe (but not twice as bad) than if you were carrying a singleton, but thankfully this is not the case for everyone. Nausea can be worse because you'll have higher hCG levels than in a single pregnancy. You may also put on more weight, and more quickly; in later pregnancy this can put added strain on your back. You might be more breathless as your babies grow and push against your diaphragm. You are also more likely to experience swelling, heartburn, constipation, and indigestion.

When it comes to labor and birth, having twins (or more) should not take much longer than if, under the same circumstances, you were to give birth to only one baby. Very rarely, "deferred labor" of the second baby can occur: the first baby is born, then labor stops and there is a significant gap (a day or more) before the second baby arrives. Your hospital would offer you support and careful monitoring until the second baby was born.

Q Are my twins identical or nonidentical?

You're not the only one who is curious to know the answer—your doctor will want to find out whether your twins are identical, and more importantly whether they share a placenta or even an amniotic sac.

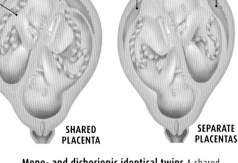

SHARED PLACENTA   SEPARATE PLACENTAS

Mono- and dichorionic identical twins A shared placenta may cause unequal blood circulation, thereby restricting the growth of one twin. Babies with separate placentas, and separate blood circulation, are more likely to grow to equal size.

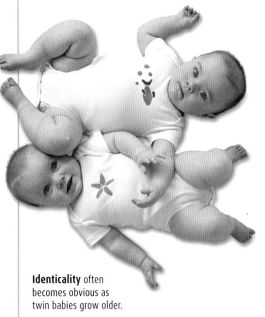

Identicality often becomes obvious as twin babies grow older.

You will usually find out if you are carrying multiple babies at your first ultrasound, when you are between 8 and 14 weeks pregnant. At this ultrasound, the sonographer will assess what type of placenta the babies have (chorionicity) and what type of amniotic sac (amnionicity), since this is critical for their care.

Chorionicity and amnionicity

All nonidentical twins have separate placentas (dichorionic) and amniotic sacs because they come from two different eggs that each attach separately to the uterus (see p.33). Sometimes the two placentas can fuse, but they are still considered dichorionic. Identical twins may or may not have separate placentas and amniotic sacs, depending on how early the initial fertilized egg (zygote) divided. A split within three to four days of fertilization creates a placenta and amniotic sac for each twin (one-third of cases); a split during days four to eight forms one shared placenta (monochorionic–the majority of identical twins) and two amniotic sacs (diamniotic); after eight days, the babies will share both a placenta and an amniotic sac (monochorionic and monoamniotic).

Twin-to-twin transfusion syndrome

A shared placenta can result in "twin-to-twin transfusion syndrome" (TTTS), when one baby "donates" blood to the other, but fails to thrive properly itself. Furthermore, the extra blood can put a strain on the receiving twin's heart. This condition occurs in about 15 percent of identical twin pregnancies. If you have monochorionic twins, you may have ultrasounds every two to three weeks from 16 weeks to keep an eye on how the babies are growing. Recent obstetric advances have improved the survival rates of twins with TTTS, with laser surgery helping to ensure a better flow of blood between the babies.

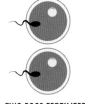

ONE EGG FERTILIZED

egg divides

TWO BABIES

Identical twins (monozygotic) When a single egg that is fertilized by a single sperm splits in two, it forms twins that share the same DNA: identical. They are always the same sex.

TWO EGGS FERTILIZED   **TWO BABIES**

Nonidentical twins (dizygotic) If two eggs are fertilized by two different sperm, your twins will have different DNA: nonidentical. They may be the same sex or different sexes.

Q I'm carrying twins. Will my prenatal care be different from someone carrying a single baby?

You'll be more closely monitored than a woman carrying just one baby. You won't necessarily have complications, but since there is higher risk with multiple pregnancies you will have more prenatal appointments and ultrasounds than for a single pregnancy. Your checkups may be with a maternal-fetal medicine specialist in a separate office, rather than solely at your OB/GYN's office. The specialist can give you support and advice about multiple births.

Q I wanted to have a home birth. Can I still do that if I'm carrying twins?

Multiple births generally happen at the hospital because there is a greater risk of complications during labor, and thus they need larger medical teams. It's more likely that your babies will be in a difficult position for birth or have a cord prolapse (when the umbilical cord starts to protrude from your uterus ahead of the baby). It's also more likely that one or both of your babies will have a low birth weight, which requires special care in a hospital immediately after birth.

Q I feel a bit daunted about having twins. Is there someone I can talk to?

Your doctor can put you in touch with local twin (and multiple) support groups and other recent mothers of multiples. Try to gather as much information and reassurance as you can—and also any practical tips about how to best take care of yourself and your babies in pregnancy and after the birth. Organizations such as the National Organization of Mothers of Twins Clubs (see pp.338–39) are a good source of information and advice for parents of twins. You should also be able to start childbirth classes earlier than women carrying singletons, usually around 24 weeks, rather than the usual 30 or 32 weeks. Encourage your partner to come to these classes, too—although the role of a partner can never be underestimated for any mother and baby, when it comes to multiple births, the practical and emotional support of your partner will be more significant than ever.

Q Is it possible to have a vaginal birth if I'm carrying multiples?

If you are having three or more babies, a cesarean section will be recommended as the safest option. With twins, a vaginal birth is possible if your pregnancy is uncomplicated and the babies are in good positions at labor.

Toward the end of pregnancy, multiple babies have less space in the uterus and the placenta(s) can become less efficient. For these reasons, unless the babies arrive prematurely, you'll have a scheduled early C-section for triplets or more; twin pregnancies are offered induction at 37 weeks plus for monochorionic twins, and 38 weeks plus for dichorionic twins (see opposite and pp.224–25). You could be offered an elective C-section for a twin pregnancy if there are known complications such as a shared placenta or amniotic sac, one or both of your babies are especially small, the placenta is low-lying, you have had a previous C-section, or if you've had complications such as preeclampsia. If your pregnancy has been a healthy one, you may be able to have a natural birth. Your options will depend on how the twin who is closest to the birth canal (the "presenting" twin) is positioned in your uterus.

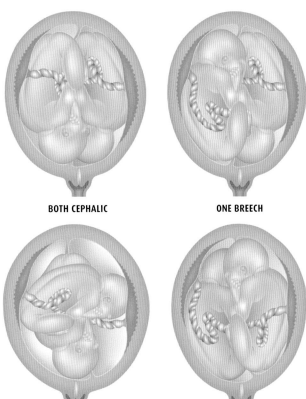

BOTH CEPHALIC   **ONE BREECH**

ONE TRANSVERSE   **BOTH BREECH**

Both cephalic (head down)
When both babies are head down, there is a good chance of successful vaginal birth for both. Around 45 percent of twins present in this position.

One breech (bottom first)
About 25 percent of twins present with the first baby head down, and the second breech. In this case, vaginal birth of the first twin is possible. If the presenting twin is breech, a cesarean section is advised.

One transverse (horizontal)
Babies who lie transverse can turn, so if the presenting twin is head down, vaginal birth may be possible. If the presenting baby is breech, a cesarean section is more likely.

Both breech When both babies are bottom first, in most cases you will be offered a cesarean section because the babies are less likely to turn.

Women pregnant with multiples are at a slightly increased risk of preeclampsia, **anemia**, low-lying placenta, and **midterm bleeding.** For all these reasons, your **doctor** will be **extra vigilant** throughout your pregnancy.

{Q Is it possible to choose where I have my baby?

Once you've chosen your health-care provider, there often isn't much choice in the matter, but there may be. The majority of babies born to women in the US are delivered in hospitals by doctors. If you have a doctor, it's very likely that your OB/GYN is affiliated with one or more hospitals in your area. If you've chosen a midwife, you'll likely give birth in a local birth center.

Visit each venue

In order to make an informed decision, it's advisable to take a tour of all the places you can give birth at. When visiting a venue bring a notepad with you to jot down answers to your questions. Don't be afraid to trust your instincts. If you're considering a home birth, meet with your doctor as well to discuss this option. Your midwife will give you a list of what you will need to have for a home birth.

What to ask at every venue

- Who will manage my birth plan?
- How easy is it to park and how far away is the parking?
- If I felt unable to travel once I went into labor, how would you recommend that I get to your location? Is getting a ride from an ambulance a reasonable option?
- Do you have exercise balls, mats, and chairs available in every birthing suite?
- Can I give birth in water?
- How many birth partners can I have?
- Can I bring my other children?
- Can my partner stay with me overnight after the baby has been born?
- How soon will I be able to go home?
- What pain relief will be available to me when I'm in labor?
- Other than my birth partner, who will be in the room with me?
- Will the baby stay with me all the time?
- What help will I have with starting to breast-feed?

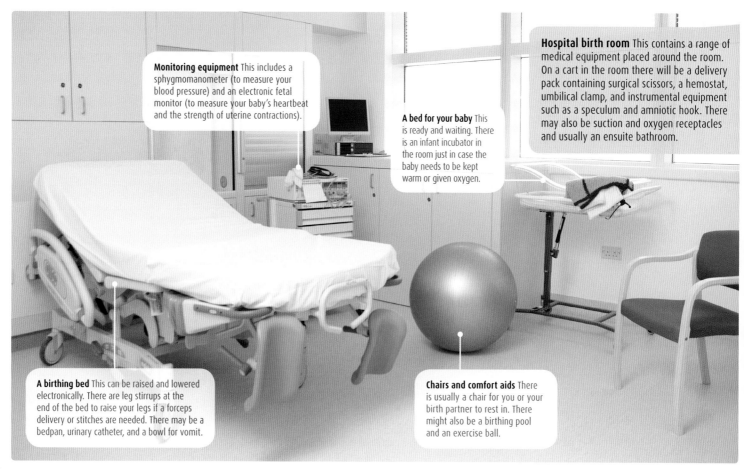

Monitoring equipment This includes a sphygmomanometer (to measure your blood pressure) and an electronic fetal monitor (to measure your baby's heartbeat and the strength of uterine contractions).

A bed for your baby This is ready and waiting. There is an infant incubator in the room just in case the baby needs to be kept warm or given oxygen.

Hospital birth room This contains a range of medical equipment placed around the room. On a cart in the room there will be a delivery pack containing surgical scissors, a hemostat, umbilical clamp, and instrumental equipment such as a speculum and amniotic hook. There may also be suction and oxygen receptacles and usually an ensuite bathroom.

A birthing bed This can be raised and lowered electronically. There are leg stirrups at the end of the bed to raise your legs if a forceps delivery or stitches are needed. There may be a bedpan, urinary catheter, and a bowl for vomit.

Chairs and comfort aids There is usually a chair for you or your birth partner to rest in. There might also be a birthing pool and an exercise ball.

THE PROS AND CONS OF WHERE TO HAVE YOUR BABY

Remember that it's never too late to change your mind and if your circumstances change you may have to rethink your decision. This table sets out some of the points to consider when you are deciding where to have your baby.

  Hospital

 Instant specialized medical attention if necessary.
» All forms of pain relief available.
» All technical gadgets and gizmos to react quickly in a changing labor situation.
» Baby unit (NICU) usually available if your baby needs medical attention immediately after birth.

Lack of continuous care
» The doctor on call who supports you in labor may not be your main OB/GYN.
» There may be changes of shifts during your labor, so you may see several hospital nurses before you have your baby.
» Count on spending a night or two after your baby is born.

  Birthing center

Midwife-led care in a low-tech envrironment.
» Although the unit is independently run, full medical care is close by.
» More relaxed birthing environment.
» More opportunity to let your labor run its course without intervention.
» Lower rates of assisted birth (use of forceps or vacuum extractor).
» May lead to a shorter labor.
» Fewer cesarean sections.
» Greater chance that your birth partner can stay overnight.

 40 percent of women giving birth to their first baby have to go into the hospital anyway (and about 10 percent for second or subsequent babies), although there is more immediate access to full medical care.

  Home

Continuous care.
» Your chosen midwife is likely to be the person who supports you in labor.
» You won't have to endure traveling during labor.
» Statistically reduced risk of assisted birth.
» You're at home with your baby right from the start.

 40 percent of women giving birth to their first baby have to go to hospital anyway (and about 10 percent for second or subsequent babies).
» No access to pain relief.
» Your birth partner may not be allowed to come in the ambulance with you if you have to go to the hospital.
» Home births are opposed by the American Medical Association and the American College of Gynecologists and Obstetricians because of the potential for complications, even in low-risk pregnancies.

■ Will someone show me how to change a diaper, sponge bathe, and bathe the baby?
■ What happens if I decide to bottle-feed—do I have to bring the bottles and formula with me?
■ Can we buy snacks and drinks here during labor, or should we bring them with us?
■ What facilities do you have for playing music in the birthing room?

What to ask at the hospital
■ Will I be moved to a ward after I've had the baby?
■ Is an anesthesiologist always available if I want an epidural?

■ What are the visiting hours and do they apply to my partner? What are the visiting hours for siblings?
■ Are there any single rooms and, if so, how are they allocated? Do we have to pay for them?

What to ask at a birthing center
■ How quickly could I get to a hospital if I needed to, and would I need to go in an ambulance?
■ For what reasons would I need to go to a hospital and which hospital would I go to?
■ Is a medical doctor able to come to the center in an emergency?

 Did you know...

In 1900, almost all babies in the US were born at home. Gradually, births moved to hospitals and the percentage of home births fell: 44% by 1940 and 1% by 1969. Although that number has been rising since 2004, it's still below 1% per year. A home birth isn't recommended by the American Medical Association because there could be complications, even in healthy women who could need to be transferred to a hospital.

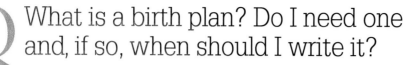

Q What is a birth plan? Do I need one and, if so, when should I write it?

A birth plan is your opportunity to put down on paper your preferences for labor and birth. You don't have to have one, but it's a good idea to at least think through what you would like. You can create it at any time.

A birth plan is a means of thinking through what's important to you about the process of having your baby and to highlight any queries you might have for your doctor. It can include anything and everything, from what music you'd like to have playing to the type of pain relief you'd prefer. You can start writing a birth plan as soon as you like, and amend it and add to it as your pregnancy progresses, gathering wisdom and ideas from doctors, medical staff, family, friends, and other moms-to-be. It is a good idea to remember, though, that labor does not always go as planned; you need to be flexible in the

event that you or your baby need medical assistance at any time that means you may need to deviate from your birth plan.

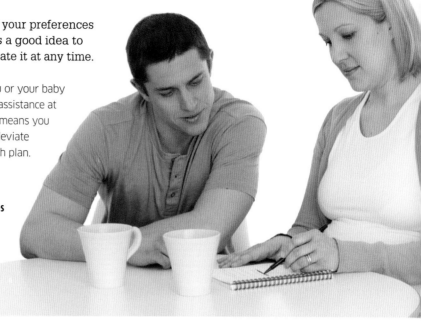

Your preferences
Go through your wishes with your partner.

STRUCTURING YOUR BIRTH PLAN

Use the following headings and ideas as a guide to writing your birth plan.
Remember that it can be more or less detailed than this.

 » My birth environment: Where you want to labor and give birth; what music (if any) you want playing; any other ways in which you want to set the right mood.

 » Emotional support and your personal care: Who you want with you and how you want them to support you; whether you want your birth partner near your head, or at the birth end; whether you want photos of you in labor.

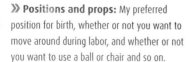 **» Positions and props:** My preferred position for birth, whether or not you want to move around during labor, and whether or not you want to use a ball or chair and so on.

 » Pain relief and physical care: Whether you'd like to have pain relief and if so, what kind; if there are any forms of pain relief you want to avoid; whether or not it is OK to have an episiotomy if your doctor thinks it would ease your labor.

 » Taking care of my baby during birth: Whether you want to stay upright and mobile while your doctor is checking your baby's heart rate; if you have any objections to your baby's heart rate being monitored continuously.

 » Assisted birth: If you are given a choice, whether or not you have a preference for forceps or vacuum extraction; whether you are OK to be given medicine to increase the strength of your contractions.

 » The moment of birth: Whether or not you'd like your baby placed on your tummy; who holds your baby first; whether you or your partner would like to announce the sex; who will cut the umbilical cord, and if you'd like to delay cord-cutting.

 » My placenta: Whether you want to deliver the placenta naturally; whether you'd like to see your placenta, or even keep it.

 » Caring for my newborn: Your wishes for feeding and skin-to-skin contact; who holds the baby while you deliver the placenta or have any stitches.

 » Telling the world: Who you'd like told first about the birth and even in what order; whether there are certain people you'd like to tell yourself, or whether you're happy to let your birth partner spread the news to everyone.

 » Emergencies: If you're having a home birth, which hospital you want to go to (if you have a choice) in an emergency; if you're having your baby at an independent birthing center, where you'd like to be transferred if you have an emergency.

 » Special requirements: Whether English is your first language; if you need a sign language interpreter; if you have special dietary requirements; if you or your partner has special needs; if you would like certain religious customs to be observed.

Write your **birth plan** using broad headings—see the box below for **some ideas**. Make the plan as **detailed** or as **vague** as you want. Read about the birth and all the options available to help you think ahead to what you might want. It's important to make sure you feel **confident** and **fully informed** about all of your choices beforehand.

» Cesarean sections: Who you want with you in the operating room; what music (if any) you want playing there; whether you would like the screen lowered at the moment your baby is born so that you can see the obstetrician lift the baby out; if you would like silence among the medical staff as your baby is lifted out so that yours can be the first voice your baby hears; who you would like to hold your baby if you have to have general anesthesia, and whether you are OK for your birth partner to tell anyone else about the birth and baby before you've woken up from the anesthesia. Also, if you've had general anesthesia, whether you'd like your baby to be bottle-fed from the breast milk bank, or to have formula if he needs to be fed before you wake up. Whether you would like a video or photographs taken of your baby as he's lifted out of your uterus; whether you'd like to have skin-to-skin contact and to try to breast-feed while your uterus and abdomen are being sewn up, or you're fine with your partner holding your baby until you're settled in the post-op room.

Q My partner has some ideas for the birth plan, but I don't agree with them all. Should I try to fit them in?

Your birth plan is about your care during your labor, so ultimately it should reflect your wishes. However, parenting is something that you are going to do together, so if there are things he feels strongly about that matter less to you, then in the spirit of this new and exciting joint venture, make sure you give his views consideration. When it comes to anything that might happen to your body your wishes and the advice of your doctor always come first.

Q Will I need to have my birth plan with me while I'm in labor? What if I'm too distracted to remember what's in it?

Your doctor will put a copy of your birth plan in your records so that it is available to whoever is caring for you at the time of your labor. It's also a good idea to give a copy to your birth partner, who can represent your wishes if you aren't able to articulate them yourself. Make sure to brief your birth partner, though, that although you might have said you want to avoid an assisted birth, for example, if the situation dictates that this is the safest way for your baby to be born and you understand why, your doctor's advice is paramount and so the birth plan would change.

Q What does VBAC stand for and is it something I should consider?

VBAC stands for "vaginal birth after cesarean section" and it means exactly what it says: if you had a C-section for your last birth, you might be able to have a vaginal birth instead this time. Assuming that you are able to have a VBAC, whether or not you want one is entirely a matter of personal choice and practicality. For example, you will recover more quickly from a vaginal birth than from a C-section, which can make it easier to take care of your other children with a newborn in tow, too. A VBAC can have fewer complications than a second C-section, but this is not always the case.

Q Are there any reasons that I wouldn't be able to have a VBAC?

You will be able to have a VBAC as long as your previous cesarean section was straightforward, and for pregnancy rather than anatomical reasons. So, if you had a complication during labor that made C-section a safer way to deliver your baby, there's no reason why you wouldn't be able to have a VBAC this time. However, if you weren't able to give birth vaginally because, for example, you have a small pelvis that makes it hard for your baby to get through, you will probably have to have a second C-section. If the cut in your uterus was a standard horizontal incision, you should be fine for a VBAC, but cuts elsewhere into your uterus will need to be considered on a case-by-case basis.

Q What's the likelihood that I'll end up having another C-section, even if I start out with the hope of a VBAC?

Assuming you had a straightforward, nonanatomical-related previous cesarean section (see above), there is a 70 to 85 percent success rate for VBAC. Specifically relating to your previous C-section, the main obstacle to success is that there's around a 0.5 percent chance that you develop a tear along your scar line during your contractions. The risk of a tear occurring during VBAC rises to 1 percent if you have had two previous C-sections; there is little data on the risks after three or more C-sections. It's often a case of waiting to see what happens.

70–85% Most hospitals record VBAC success rates of 70 percent to 85 percent.

Q What should I look for in a birth partner?

Ideally the person you have by your side during labor and birth will be incredibly patient, cool under pressure, and extremely caring. Here's a list of the qualities your perfect birth partner would possess:

» **A sense of calm:** a natural ability to stop you from getting worried or stressed.

» **Confidence:** to support your wishes and to support your medical team if they offer advice that will speed your birth and is in the interests of the best health for you and your baby, even if that's at odds with your birth plan.

» **Being able to respond:** and take comments or wishes from you without judging them—or taking offence.

» **Reasonable lack of squeamishness:** at the sight of blood or vomit.

» **Empathy:** someone who can respond to your mood without even being asked to, and in the right way.

» **A firm respect for medical care:** knowing when to step aside to let the medical team work with you unimpeded and unchallenged.

» **Someone without any time restrictions:** a person who can give you all of his or her attention, unselfishly and unequivocally throughout your labor, however long it may take.

» **Someone who will talk through any decisions:** while you're in labor, he or she can give you sensible, sound advice with the interests of you and your baby in mind.

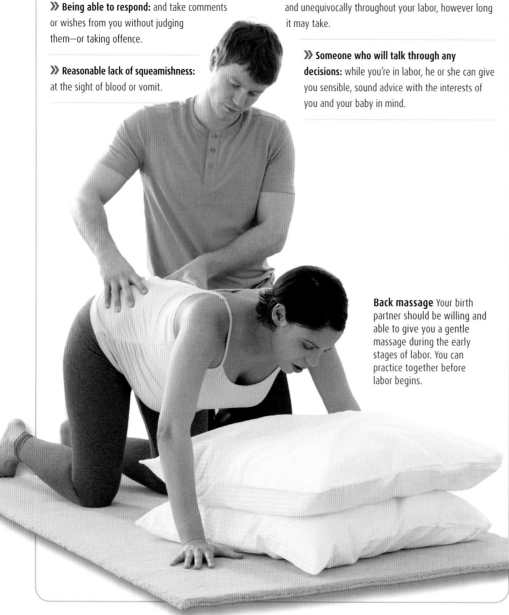

Back massage Your birth partner should be willing and able to give you a gentle massage during the early stages of labor. You can practice together before labor begins.

Q What is a doula and how can they help with my labor and birth?

From the Greek word for "caregiver," a doula is a birthing companion whom you choose to help prepare you for labor and birth, stay with you throughout birth, and, sometimes, help after the birth. This can be in practical ways (with household chores, for example) and by giving advice on baby care and breast-feeding. Some doulas offer only prenatal care and birth support, and others specialize in postpartum care. Some will do both. Research in the UK suggests that C-section rates fall by as much as 50 percent for women who have a doula as a birth partner, and that labor may be up to two hours shorter. If you employ a doula as a birth partner, she can also support your partner if you wish—talking him through what's happening, reassuring him, and guiding him on how best to help you.

Q Will I still need a doctor if I have a doula?

Yes, since doulas work alongside doctors and do not replace a doctor's role, but rather provide extra support and continuity of care. A doula isn't necessarily medically trained, though she will have completed a doula course that means she can support pregnancy in safe, medically recognized ways. If you want to use a doula, you will need to hire one privately. Look for a doula who has a qualification that is accredited by the governing body in your country (such as DONA International).

Today more **fathers** than ever attend the births of **their babies**. However, a close family member or friend, a **private midwife**, or **a doula** are also all good choices to **support** you, or both you and your partner through **labor and birth**.

Q I have more than one person in mind as a birth partner. Am I allowed to have two?

Some hospitals will allow two birth partners to be present in the delivery room with you (you may be able to have more, as long as none of them interferes with the medical staff). Talk to both of your potential birth partners and make sure they each understand that the other will be there. Check, in particular, that your partner is happy about the arrangement—this is an intimate occasion and he or she may feel strongly that it's something that needs to happen only between the two of you. It can be good to assign roles to each person attending—perhaps you can ask one birth partner to be there to support you emotionally, while the other one takes a more practical role, ensuring you have well-plumped pillows and creating the right ambience in the room for you. Be clear about whom, if anyone, you want to be at the birthing end of the event. The last thing you want is for each of them to start jostling to get the best view.

Q Can I have my older children present at my home birth?

Talk to your midwife in advance of your labor and establish what the rules are for accommodating other children. If your older children are with you, it's a good idea to assign someone else to take care of them for snacks and general entertainment (remember, labor can be a long process). That person may be your partner or another adult who has come to help. Your children shouldn't be a distraction for you or source of worry. They shouldn't get in the way or interfere with the procedure. Also, consider your children's ages and personalities and whether or not you think they will be able to cope with seeing their mom go through labor and birth. Even an easy birth can be traumatic for young children to witness. Talk through with them what's going to happen, and tell them that giving birth hurts the mommy, but it's safe pain and goes away as soon as the baby is born. Use words suitable for your children's level of understanding and encourage lots of questions. If you decide, on reflection, that it might be too much for them, ask a close friend or a grandparent to occupy them nearby (in the yard

if it's nice weather or in another room in your home) and invite them in only once (even as soon as) the baby has been born. It will be an unforgettable experience for everyone involved.

Q My partner doesn't think he'll be able to deal with seeing me in pain during labor. What can be done to help?

Many men confess that the hardest part of being with their partners as they give birth is seeing them go through pain and feeling helpless to do anything about it. The person you have with you during labor and birth needs to be calm, composed, and authoritative (with you and perhaps with the hospital staff); sometimes making decisions for you based on your birth plan. If your partner thinks he's likely to panic or faint, perhaps he may indeed be better waiting outside the delivery room until after your baby is born. You have several options:

Q Is the baby's dad less likely to bond with the baby in the long term if he isn't at the birth?

Studies show that his presence at the birth doesn't make a difference to a dad's ability to bond with his baby.

As long as he is fully engaged in the newborn's care once he or she has arrived in the world, a dad will definitely bond with his baby in the long term. Bonding is an intense attachment between parents and their baby. Bonding with a baby takes time and is a process that takes place as a mom or dad gets to know and takes care of their newborn baby. It gives parents the desire to nurture and take care of a baby. The only measurable difference is that fathers who are present at the birth tend to be more confident handling the baby; fathers who feel really positive about watching the birth tend to be more willing to take care of the baby independently of the mother (which gives you the opportunity to have a break every now and then).

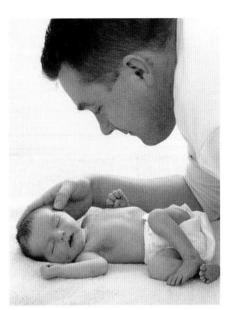

Doting dad Make sure dad is just as involved as you with diaper changing and outfit changes from the start. Also, encourage him to have skin-to-skin contact and make sure he gets to hold your new bundle of joy.

>> **Separate birth partner** Choose someone whom you trust entirely as a birth partner and who can support you fully to stay in the delivery room from start to finish, calling your partner in only when the baby is born.

>> **The early part** Have your partner in the room with you, but have someone else available to come in as soon as your partner finds it's getting too much for him to be present.

>> **Time limit** Ask your partner to stay with you for as long as he can stand it, and then to step out and let the hospital's labor nurses support you until the baby is born.

>> **Stay throughout** Ask your partner to stay the whole time, but tell him that it's fine if he stays at your head end (in which case it's unlikely that he'll see anything too gory) and turns away if he wants to during any stressful moments. Practice breathing techniques together so that you can both use them to relax during labor—for you to cope with the pain, and for him to cope with you being in pain.

During your pregnancy, you will be offered a series of **ultrasounds and tests** to monitor the **growth** and **development** of your baby, and to ensure that your own body is dealing well with your pregnancy. **Ultrasounds** provide a wonderful opportunity to **"meet" your baby,** and various **tests** check for abnormalities.

Ultrasounds and tests

What you might expect to happen

The blood, urine, and blood pressure tests that are routinely offered throughout your pregnancy are there to keep a close eye on you and your baby. The goal of these tests is to identify warning signs before they turn into problems. For example, if a blood test shows low levels of hemoglobin, this can indicate low iron levels, a sign of anemia; high blood pressure and/or protein in the urine are symptoms of preeclampsia.

You will also be given ultrasounds, which use sound waves to visualize your baby in the uterus. They are painless and carry no known risks to you or your baby. Aside from enabling you to see your baby, they also give a good assessment of how he is growing and developing, even down to checking the structure of his heart. They also indicate any issues that you might have, such as fibroids or a weak cervix. You will usually be offered a minimum of two ultrasounds, one between 8 and 14 weeks, the first ultrasound, and a second at around 18 to 20 weeks called the anatomy scan (ultrasound).

During your pregnancy you will also be given the option of having prenatal tests that check for various genetic or chromosomal abnormalities such as Down syndrome. Some of these assess your risk of carrying a baby with an abnormality and involve a blood test combined with measuring fluid at the back of the neck known as the nuchal translucency test via ultrasound. If there is any concern that your baby might have a congenital abnormality of any kind, you'll be offered further tests that are more invasive, such as chorionic villus sampling or an amniocentesis. These ultrasounds and tests enable the doctor taking care of you to gain as clear a picture as possible of your baby before he is born.

You will always have a choice as to whether you consent to the ultrasound or test in question; none of them is compulsory. However, all the tests are there to ensure that the appropriate care is given to you and your baby. Feel free to discuss any concerns you have with your doctor before a test takes place. He or she will be able to talk you through the details and risks of all the procedures so that you can make an informed decision.

Your time line of care

On the opposite page is a time line of tests and ultrasounds that you can expect during the course of your pregnancy. Unless there is a specific reason (such as a family history of twins) for having an early ultrasound, the tests and ultrasounds usually begin with the first appointment (see p.80). Some of these are ultrasounds and tests that every pregnant woman will be offered; others are exceptional, depending upon your circumstances. All of the tests are to monitor the health and well-being of you and your baby.

Q When might I be offered the different ultrasounds and tests?

The table below sets out the expected pattern of ultrasounds and tests during the course of your pregnancy. Some of these are offered to all pregnant women, others are for those in certain situations.

TIME LINE OF TESTS AND ULTRASOUNDS

WEEKS PREGNANT	TEST/ULTRASOUND	WHAT IS IT FOR?
4–5	Ultrasound if family history of twins	Check growth and heartbeats
8–14 *	The first ultrasound	Measure growth and estimates delivery date
11–14 *	Nuchal translucency test	Assesses risk of abnormalities
10–20	Blood tests	Assess risk of abnormalities
10–15	Chorionic villus sampling (CVS)	Diagnostic test for abnormalities
18–20	Fetal anatomy scan (ultrasound)	Diagnostic test for abnormalities
from 14	Amniocentesis	Diagnostic test for abnormalities
22–23	Repeat of anatomy scan	Take detailed fetal measurements
from 18–24	Cordocentesis	Diagnostic test for abnormalities
28–40	ultrasound or ultrasounds	Check growth and development

* The nuchal translucency test may be combined with the first ultrasound if the latter is done around 11 to 14 weeks.

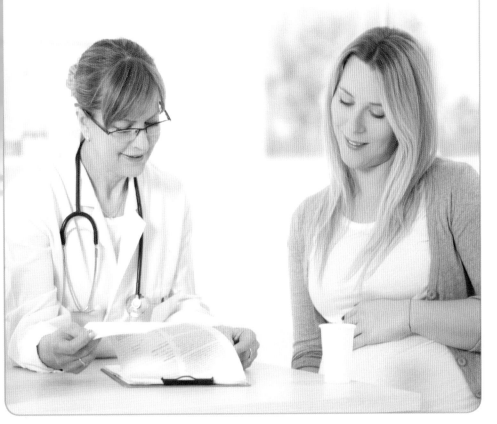

Q I've never had an ultrasound before. What does it involve?

During an abdominal ultrasound appointment, you will be asked to lie down on a raised bed. The room will be dark so that the images show up clearly on the screen—sort of like dimming the lights at the movies. The sonographer will apply gel to your stomach and then move a handheld scanner over your abdomen. Don't worry if he or she has to press hard from time to time to get the right position. A sonographer is a medical professional who may also be a radiographer (a person who takes X-rays), with training in skeletal anatomy, who likely specializes in prenatal ultrasound. He or she will make assessments of your baby's health according to certain statistics (the length of the baby's spine and femur, head circumference, abdominal circumference etc.) and what observations he or she can make from the images on the screen. When you go to the appointment for your 20-week ultrasound, a sonographer will be the person who's examining your baby's anatomy to make sure that all of the body parts look normal and healthy. This is the appointment when it may be possible for you and your partner to finally learn the sex of your baby on the way, if that's of interest to you. If you don't want to know the gender before your baby is born, be sure to tell the sonographer at the start of your ultrasound appointment, well before he or she starts describing what's in view onscreen!

Q Is an ultrasound safe for my baby? Are there any risks?

As far as it's possible to tell, it is perfectly safe for you and your baby. The ultrasound is performed using a handheld device that uses sound waves to build a picture of your baby. Unlike X-rays (which use radio waves), sound waves have no link to increased risk of childhood cancer or congenital abnormality in babies. The "beams" of sound penetrate your amniotic fluid and bounce off your baby's tiny body to create a moving image. Some people worry that sound waves will raise your core temperature, but actually the temperature rise from using an ultrasound is usually no more than 1.8°F (1°C), which is well below any level for concern.

Q I've got an early ultrasound appointment because I've been bleeding. Should I rest until then?

It's estimated that 10 percent of women experience some spotting or bleeding in the very earliest stages of pregnancy and most of them go on to have full-term, healthy babies.

While you're waiting for your ultrasound appointment, avoid heavy lifting and sexual intercourse and try to rest as much as possible, but don't fret about doing so—as long as your normal day is unstrenuous, there's no reason to imagine that it will make your bleeding worse, and you can continue as usual. Keep well hydrated and try to eat normally (even if you don't feel like eating). If your bleeding worsens, call your doctor and ask for advice. He or she may ask you to go to your local emergency room so that you are seen immediately. If your ultrasound shows

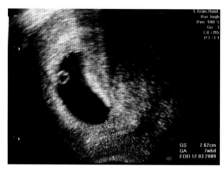

Six-week ultrasound The embryo will only be between ¼-⅜ in (5-9 mm) long at this stage of pregnancy.

that things are normal, you'll be sent home. Usually the bleeding will stop within 10 days, but if it doesn't, call the hospital. If the ultrasound shows that something is wrong, your sonographer will advise you about what to do next.

Q Can I take someone with me to my ultrasounds, and can I have a picture?

Most doctors recommend that you have someone with you to enjoy the experience of seeing your baby, but also so that you have support if something is not as you'd hoped or expected. It can be useful to have someone there to ask questions. Your partner, or a close family member or friend are the obvious choices. Sonographers are usually very happy to give you a photograph taken from the ultrasound. There may be a small charge for this—check at the reception desk beforehand.

> **Early ultrasounds** at **six to seven weeks** are usually **transvaginal.** Vaginal ultrasounds give a clearer picture at this stage than transabdominal ones and also use **sound waves.**

Q What's an EPU? My doctor mentioned it if I need an early ultrasound.

An EPU is an Early Pregnancy Unit (sometimes known as an Early Pregnancy Assessment Unit or Early Pregnancy Assessment Center; EPAU and EPAC respectively). It is a specialized unit in a hospital dedicated to detecting and treating concerns in early pregnancy. If you need to have an early ultrasound and your local hospital has one of these units, this is probably where you'll go. Not all hospitals have an EPU, in which case early ultrasounds are performed in the regular prenatal hospital clinic. There are often strict criteria for referral (from your doctor) to the EPU, including how far along your pregnancy is ("early" usually means within the first trimester, but not usually earlier than seven weeks along), whether or not you've had a positive pregnancy test recently, and the nature of your concern. EPUs can be reluctant to give women an ultrasound to assess the viability of their pregnancy if there's no immediate cause to suspect that the pregnancy is anything but viable. Straightforward referrals include a family history of twins, having period like bleeding, or spotting that has lasted over a week.

Q I've been having fertility treatment. When will I have my first ultrasound?

Systems differ depending on the doctor. You may have an ultrasound as early as three weeks pregnant to locate the embryo sac in your uterus. Other doctors wait until you have a positive pregnancy test result and give you an ultrasound at around six weeks pregnant (about four weeks after collecting your eggs), because it's around this time that the ultrasound can detect your baby's heartbeat. If it appears that your treatment has been successful, you'll have an ultrasound two weeks or so later (around eight weeks pregnant) to check that the embryo is growing as expected. You will probably then stop going to your fertility specialist and be asked to make an appointment with your OB/GYN so that you can start prenatal care.

Q I don't want to wait for my 12-week ultrasound to see my baby. Can I pay to have a private ultrasound?

Absolutely. You can pay for an ultrasound from as early as seven weeks gestation (before this, there is very little an ultrasound can show). Most sonographers will begin by giving you an abdominal ultrasound (using the handheld scanner over your growing baby), but at such an early stage in pregnancy, it's possible that he or she may switch to using a vaginal ultrasound to get a better picture of your baby. In this case, a long, thin sonograph device is inserted into your vagina to get closer to your uterus.

Q Why would I need an early ultrasound?

If you struggled to get pregnant, have a history of recurrent miscarriages or a multiple pregnancy, are at risk of an ectopic pregnancy, have an incompetent cervix, or have had some vaginal bleeding or uterine pain unrelated to your last menstrual period, your doctor may refer you for an ultrasound at around seven weeks pregnant. Similarly if you already know that you suffer from fibroids or you're suspected to be carrying twins or multiples, your doctor will want to check that everything is as it should be.

Q What happens at the first ultrasound?

The ultrasound at 8 to 14 weeks confirms your estimated delivery date, ensuring you get the right prenatal screening tests at the right time.

You may be asked to drink water before the ultrasound since a full bladder makes the ultrasound images clearer. During the ultrasound, the sonographer will determine the exact gestational age of your baby and estimate your delivery date. At this stage all babies develop at the same rate, regardless of their future size. The measurements taken at this ultrasound are used to ensure that your baby is growing normally. Two key measurements are taken: the crown–rump length (the length from the top of the baby's head to the base of the spine), and the diameter from one bone across to the other on each side of your baby's head. The heart rate will also be measured and the position of the placenta will be checked.

This may be your first glimpse of your baby and it is a particularly exciting moment if she is moving around. You can ask to take a photograph from your ultrasound to share with others; you may have to pay for it.

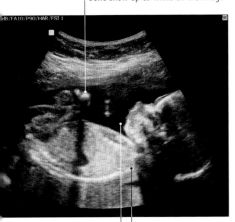

White areas Hard tissues such as bone show up as white on the image.

Black areas These identify the fluids such as the amniotic fluid that the baby lies in.

Gray areas Soft tissues appear gray and speckled on the image.

First ultrasound This is the first of your routine ultrasounds. This will indicate how your baby is growing and developing.

Having the ultrasound The sonographer will move a small handheld transducer or probe across your skin to get a view of your baby (below).

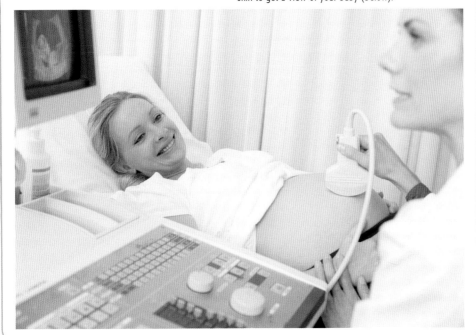

Q What tests are available to check for abnormalities?

There are various tests that can be performed at different stages of your pregnancy to check for abnormalities. Some provide information on the risk of your baby being affected by an abnormality. These involve an ultrasound and blood tests. If these tests indicate that your risk is high, you will be offered further diagnostic tests, which allow specific conditions to be confirmed. Knowing for certain can help parents decide how to proceed, but these tests are invasive and do carry a 1 percent chance of miscarriage.

Q What is the combined test and when is it done?

To give you the most accurate risk calculation of various abnormalities, including Down syndrome, you should be offered the combined test, which involves a blood test and the nuchal translucency test. The blood samples are measured for levels of beta-human chorionic gonadotropin hormone (beta-hCG), which are usually higher in the blood of a mother carrying a baby with Down syndrome, and pregnancy-associated plasma protein (PAPP-A), levels of which are usually lower. The blood samples are usually sent for analysis, so it can take up to two weeks to receive the results. The blood samples must be taken between 10 and 14 weeks of pregnancy.

Q What are the quadruple and triple tests and when are they done?

You may be offered a quadruple test if you are between 14 and 20 weeks pregnant, when the combined test would no longer produce a reliable result. The quadruple test measures blood levels of beta-hCG, alpha fetoprotein (AFP; a protein produced by the fetus), unconjugated estriol (uE3: a form of estrogen that shows a lower level in babies with Down syndrome) and the hormone inhibin-A. The blood levels are analyzed in light of your age and how old the fetus is to produce a calculated risk. The triple– or Bart's–is the same as the quadruple test but does not look at levels of inhibin-A.

Q What's the nuchal translucency (NT) test?

This is an ultrasound used to estimate the risk of Down syndrome. Although it cannot tell you for certain whether your baby will have Down syndrome, it will inform you if he is at high risk. All women are offered the NT test.

Your baby's nuchal translucency is the pool of fatty fluid beneath the skin at the back of the baby's neck. A sonographer can measure the thickness of the nuchal translucency during an ultrasound at around 11–14 weeks' gestation. After your ultrasound, this measurement is considered in relation to your own age, the baby's length from crown to rump, and the results from the combined blood test (see p.95). Analyzed together, these results can tell you what risk your baby has of being born with Down syndrome.

Comparing the nuchal measurement, your age, and your blood test results has an accuracy of more than 90 percent. Don't worry if your doctor doesn't offer a combined test–a nuchal translucency test combined with your baby's measurements and your age is still a good indicator of risk. If your risk is high, remember that the test is not a diagnosis. You'll be offered diagnostic tests (choronic villus sampling or amniocentesis, see opposite) that will give you a definitive result.

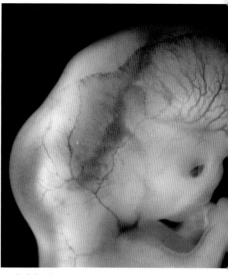

Nuchal fluid While all babies have some fluid at the back of their necks, babies with Down syndrome or other genetic disorders have more. The test is usually scheduled at your 12-week ultrasound.

UNDERSTANDING THE NUCHAL TRANSLUCENCY RESULT

The thicker your baby's nuchal translucency, the greater the risk of your baby having Down syndrome. It is important to note that the measurement is only one part of the test and should be assessed alongside blood test results and your age.

The result is expressed as a ratio. For example, you might be given the result 1:1,500, which means your baby has a one in 1,500 chance of being born with Down syndrome (or, expressed as a percentage, this means a risk of 0.07 percent). A ratio of 1:150 or greater is considered high risk, although even then it's still more likely that you won't have a baby with Down syndrome, (expressed as a percentage 1 in 150 is only a 0.67 percent chance). It's also worth remembering that even if you fall into the low-risk category, there is still a chance (albeit a very slim one) of your baby being born with Down syndrome. If you have a low risk of having a baby with Down syndrome you'll be given the results of the ultrasound within two weeks. If your risk is high, you'll normally get your results within a week, and often within two or three days, so you have as much time as possible to consider whether you would like further diagnostic tests such as an amniocentesis. Whether or not you take these tests is entirely your choice.

When making your decision, keep in mind that some physical indicators of Down syndrome can become apparent at later ultrasounds in your pregnancy, and in these cases your sonographer will tell you what he or she has discovered and what it means in terms of your baby's health.

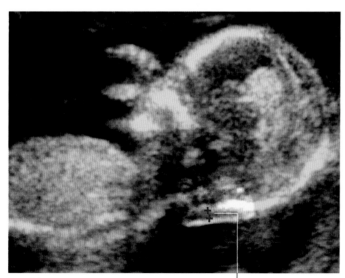

Low risk If the measurement is under 1/16 in (2 mm) at 11 weeks, or under 1/8 in (3 mm) at 14 weeks, your baby is unlikely to have Down syndrome.

| **Normal nuchal fold**

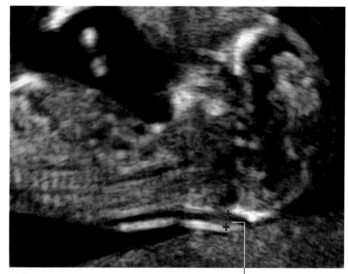

High risk If the nuchal fold measures more than 1/8 in (3 mm), there is an increased risk of your baby being affected by Down syndrome.

| **Larger nuchal fold**

Q I've been offered a chorionic villus sampling (CVS) test. What's a chorionic villus?

The term chorionic refers to your placenta, which is covered in tiny fingerlike fronds known as villi (singular, villus). These fronds increase the surface area of your placenta, maximizing the transfer of nutrients to your baby's body and waste out of it. The villi contain genetic material that is identical to your baby's, so the CVS test harvests some villi to analyze your baby's genetic makeup.

Q What are the risks associated with invasive tests?

Any invasive procedure carries with it a risk of infection, so be aware of any swelling, heat, or redness at the puncture site on your abdomen, if relevant, and if you develop a raised temperature. Both CVS and amniocentesis have a small increased risk of miscarriage above the normal risk of miscarriage at this gestation—around 1 percent each—with a slight increased risk for a CVS if performed earlier than 10 weeks and amniocentesis performed earlier

than 15 weeks. Some figures show that in general the miscarriage risk with CVS is slightly higher than it is with amniocentesis, particularly if your baby is small for his gestational age. Most miscarriages relating to these procedures occur within 72 hours of the test, but may occur up to two weeks later. Some people worry that those babies whose mothers have undergone CVS are at risk of being born without some of their fingers or toes. This risk is believed to exist only when CVS is performed at less than nine weeks pregnant. Your doctor should make you aware of all the risks before you consent to tests, and it is up to you as to whether or not to proceed.

Q What diagnostic tests are available? Can they detect all fetal abnormalities?

CVS, amniocentesis, and cordocentesis, are diagnostic tests that will confirm whether or not your baby has specific abnormalities. As these tests are invasive, it is vital to know which one is right for you and what they involve.

Performed between 11 and 15 weeks, CVS can detect some chromosomal abnormalities, genetic abnormalities (such as in cystic fibrosis), musculo-skeletal disorders (such as muscular dystrophy), blood disorders (such as sickle cell anaemia, hemophilia or

thalassemia) and nervous system disorders (such as Tay Sachs disease). It can't tell you if your baby has a neural tube defect such as spina bifida. This is usually diagnosed through your anatomy scan (ultrasound) (see p.100), and it can be detected through amniocentesis.

CVS, AMNIOCENTESIS, CORDOCENTESIS, OR NIPT

The table below lists the diagnostic procedures, the window of time in which they are performed during your pregnancy, and the general conditions that they are testing for. Before undergoing any of these procedures talk to your doctor about the pros and cons.

PROCEDURE	WHEN	TESTING FOR
CVS (Invasive)	11–15 weeks	Chromosomal and genetic conditions, blood disorders, nervous system and musculoskeletal disorders.
Amniocentesis (Invasive)	from 14 weeks	Chromosomal and genetic conditions, blood disorders, neural tube defects, and musculoskeletal disorders.
Cordocentesis (Invasive)	18–24 weeks	Chromosomal and genetic conditions, blood disorders, neural tube defects, and musculoskeletal disorders.
NIPT (Noninvasive)	from 10 weeks	Chromosomal and genetic conditions. CVS and amniocentesis may be offered after this test.

Allow yourself time to **think about** which test you will have, if any, since this is an **important decision** and you need to be **prepared** as much as possible for the result.

Q Is there a safer noninvasive alternative to CVS or amniocentesis?

Noninvasive prenatal testing. (NIPT) is a blood test that analyzes tiny amounts of fetal DNA in the mother's blood. It is a simple test and the sample is sent for analysis. Early indications are that NIPT is around 99 percent accurate in the identification of babies who have chomosomal abnormalities. In the US this test is mainly offered to women who are at high risk for having a baby with Down syndrome or other abnormalities. It's typically offered from 10 weeks. The results take up to two weeks to come back. However, it's worth knowing that present statistics reveal that up to 5 percent of blood samples won't contain enough of the baby's DNA for proper analysis.

Q Did you know...

Doctors use the following generalized statistics as a measure of how age might affect your risk of having a baby with Down syndrome. The risks are:

Age 20 the risk is **1 : 1,500**
Age 30 the risk is **1 : 800**
Age 35 the risk is **1 : 270**
Age 40 the risk is **1 : 100**
Age **45** the risk is greater than **1 : 50**

Q What's the procedure for CVS and how long will it take?

Chorionic villus sampling (CVS) is performed at 11 to 15 weeks to check your baby for certain disorders and abnormalities. The test is offered in pregnancies where a screening test shows there is a high risk of the baby having a condition.

Your doctor will remove the villi sample either by inserting a syringe needle through your abdomen into your placenta, or by inserting a tube via your vagina and entering your uterus through your cervix. In the latter case, a small amount of suction is passed through the tube to remove some villi from the placenta. The procedure your doctor uses will depend upon the position of your baby and the placenta.

You will be asked to go to your appointment with a full bladder, since you will need to have an ultrasound first to establish the position of the placenta in your uterus, and then to guide the doctor as he or she

takes the villi sample, (although in some circumstances your placenta may be positioned in such a way that you need to empty your bladder before the test continues). Including preparation, the whole procedure should take no more than 30 minutes, of which removing the villi will take only five to 10 minutes. The villi are then sent for testing. Your doctor will check your baby's movement and heartbeat after the procedure to make as sure as possible that all remains well.

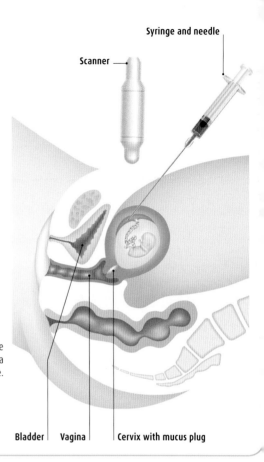

Syringe and needle

Scanner

Having the test A minute sample is taken from the placenta using a syringe with a long needle.

Bladder | Vagina | Cervix with mucus plug

Before you decide to have the test, the possible **risks** will be **discussed** with you and your partner.

Q What's the procedure for amniocentesis and how long will it take?

Syringe and needle

Scanner

Amniotic sac

Offered to pregnant women from 14 weeks, this is another invasive diagnostic test. As with any diagnostic test, careful consideration needs to be given as to whether you need it and the result you might be given.

At the beginning of the procedure, your doctor will use an ultrasound to determine the position of your baby, your placenta, and the umbilical cord. He or she will then insert a needle with a syringe attached into your abdomen, through the wall of your uterus, and into your amniotic sac. The goal will be to draw out around ¾ fl oz (20 ml) of fluid with the syringe. Amniotic fluid contains cells from your baby's skin, and these cells

contain DNA, which reveals details about your baby's genetic makeup. The fluid is then sent away for testing.

As with CVS, you'll need a full bladder so that your doctor can get a good ultrasound picture. (If you're more than 20 weeks pregnant, you may be asked to have an empty bladder.) Once the procedure is over, the doctor will also check your baby's movements.

The whole procedure should take 20 to 30 minutes. If your doctor doesn't draw enough in the first instance (this happens in around 8 percent of cases), he or she will reinsert the needle and take some more fluid.

Bladder | Vagina | Cervix with mucus plug

Having the test Guided by the ultrasound probe, a needle is inserted to remove a small amount of amniotic fluid.

Q I have heard of the cordocentesis test. Should I be having it?

Like CVS and amniocentesis, this test detects chromosomal abnormalities. It can be performed after 18 weeks of pregnancy and is most commonly done if the other tests have not provided a reliable diagnosis. It is conducted in the same way as an amniocentesis, but with this test a tiny sample of the umbilical cord is taken. The results are usually available within three days. Careful consideration needs to be given before any of the diagnostic tests.

Q Will I be able to drive after I've had an invasive procedure? Can I go right back to work?

Whether you've had CVS or an amniocentesis, it's a good idea to have someone drive you home afterward. Although there are no risks involved with driving, you may feel shaky and experience some stomach cramping for a few hours, which can make driving uncomfortable. You'll be asked to rest for 24 hours, which means you should certainly take the following day off from work, and then take it easy for the next few days. Whether or not you take more time off depends upon your job; you should avoid doing any strenuous activity and any heavy lifting.

Q How quickly will I get the test results? How will they be given to me?

Processes differ from doctor to doctor, but in many cases you will be offered the option of having the results of the three main chromosomal abnormality tests (Down, Edwards', and Patau's syndromes, see box right) within two to three working days—this is called the Rapid Test, and you may have to pay for it. The results of a full chromosomal analysis (known as full karotyping) and genetic and blood analysis will usually take two to three weeks. You'll be given the option of finding out the results on the telephone or face to face (in both cases your doctor will write to you afterward confirming what he or she has told you). Remember that you have had these tests because you are considered at "high risk" of

your baby being born with genetic abnormalities, which means you may be faced with difficult news about your baby's health. However you choose to receive the results, make sure someone is with you to support you if necessary.

Q What happens if my test confirms that my baby has a genetic or chromosomal abnormality?

Once you have absorbed the initial diagnosis, your doctor will arrange another appointment for you to talk through the options in more detail if you need to. Make sure you understand the results in layman's terms—keep asking for clarification until you do. Some of the main things to consider are: whether the condition can be treated while your baby is still in the uterus, or when she is born; what type of special needs your baby might have and to what extent; and will the condition be life limiting, and, if so, what is the baby's life-expectancy. There is no doubt that these are questions no prospective parent wants to ask. Make a list and take someone with you to the appointment who can support you and be a second set of ears to hear what you're being told. Depending upon the diagnosis, you may be offered a termination, although ending a pregnancy is a huge and emotional decision. Take your time. You won't have to make a decision there and then. Your doctor will offer you counseling to help you to come to terms with the situation before you do. Accept the offer if you think talking to an independent person will help you. In the end, though, no one but you can make the decision about what is right for your family. Surround yourself with people who will love and support you through your decision.

Q I know that Trisomy 21 is another term for Down syndrome, but what are Trisomy 13 and Trisomy 18?

Chromosomal abnormalities occur when there are either too few or too many of a specific chromosome. There are hundreds that are incompatible with life, meaning the pregnancy might end or the baby might survive for only a short time after birth.

All three of these conditions relate to chromosomal abnormalities. Healthy humans have 23 pairs of chromosomes, each numbered 1 to 23. Occasionally, a baby develops with an extra chromosome on one of the pairs, making a group of three (trisomy). Trisomy 21 (Down syndrome) means that there is an extra chromosome 21. Trisomy 18 indicates an extra chromosome 18, resulting in Edwards' syndrome; Trisomy 13 results in Patau's syndrome. Edwards' and Patau's syndrome are both extremely rare and life-limiting conditions, in which the baby is born with severe neurological and physical abnormalities. In either case babies aren't expected to live for more than a few days after birth. Both CVS and amniocentesis can detect whether or not your baby has any of these extra chromosomes.

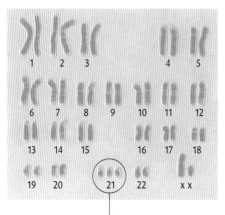

Chromosome 21 In this intance there are three copies of this chromosome.

Chromosomal abnormalities When an abnormality is found, it can be an error in the number or structure of the chromosomes or a problem with a gene. This can be caused by various factors.

{Q What is the anatomy scan?

Between 18 and 22 weeks pregnant you'll be offered a midterm (or midpregnancy) ultrasound. It is known as the anatomy scan. This is the first point in your pregnancy when a sonographer can make a detailed assessment of your unborn baby's health. A series of measurements are taken and physical features are checked to ensure there are no defects.

Seeing your baby

This is an exciting, but also potentially anxious time for prospective parents—the image you see of your baby on the ultrasound screen will, possibly for the first time, really look like a baby now. Even without specialized training, you'll be able to make out his eyes, ears, nose, fingers, vertebrae, and even perhaps some fingers and toes. At the same time, you will hear whether your baby is developing healthily. If you're worried, remember that most anatomy scans turn out to be happy, reassuring occasions. Only very rarely are parents faced with news that dramatically affects the care a baby might need after birth, or a difficult decision about whether or not to continue with the pregnancy at all.

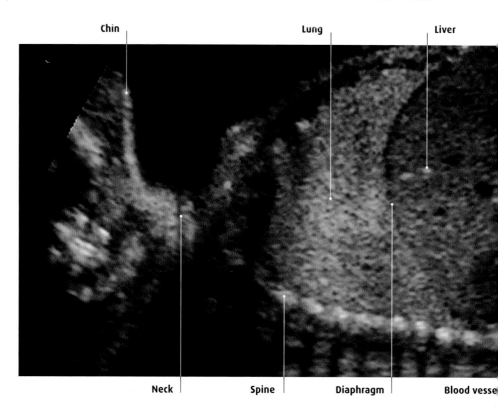

Chin   Lung   Liver

Neck   Spine   Diaphragm   Blood vessel

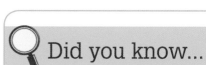 Did you know...

The heartbeat of a healthy adult at rest is around around 60-90 beats per minute (bpm). The following are the beats per minute (plus or minus 20 beats) that a sonographer or your doctor would expect for your baby's heart at various stages in your pregnancy:

» 155 bpm at 20 weeks pregnant

» 144 bpm at 30 weeks pregnant

» 140 bpm at full term (around 40 weeks) pregnant

Heart ventricles and atriums

Leg

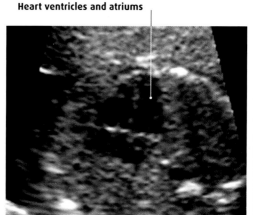

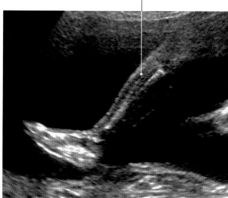

Your baby's heart The four chambers of the heart are checked to see if they are roughly the same size as each other, making sure the valves between them are working. If any problem is detected, you will be referred to a heart specialist for more detailed checks on your baby.

Your baby's leg A measurement is taken of your baby's femur (thigh bone), which gives a good indication as to how he is growing. Your baby's feet, toes, hands, and fingers will also be examined, checking that the digits are present—although they won't be counted now.

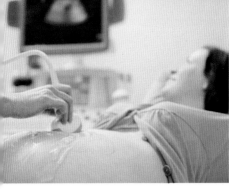

Taking a look The sonographer will need to change the position of the handheld sonograph as the ultrasound takes place—getting a good look at your baby from all angles.

Bowel

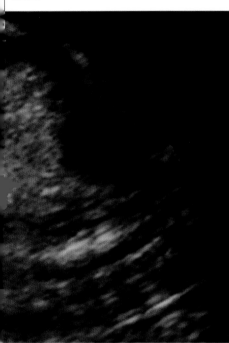

Looking at your baby's ultrasound At the 20-week ultrasound the sonographer will look closely at the structure of your baby's organs, and will also study external features, such as your baby's facial features.

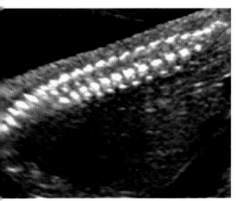

Your baby's vertebrae and spinal cord All the bones along the length of your baby's spine will be checked to see that they are properly aligned and that the spinal cord is fully enclosed in skin to eliminate the possibility of a neural tube defect such as spina bifida.

POSSIBLE ANOMALIES

The table below details specific checks your baby will be given. It's important to remember that the anomalies are all very rare. The chance that problems are detected—the pick-up rate—is affected by factors such as obesity, scar tissue from a previous C-section or surgery, and the baby's position.

CONDITION	DESCRIPTION	PROGNOSIS	PICK-UP RATE
Neural tube defects (occur in six out of 10,000 births)	Anencephaly and spina bifida are neural tube conditions in which the skull, spine, and/or brain don't develop fully.	There is no treatment for anencephaly and the baby will die before or shortly after birth. Spina bifida can be a limiting condition, but with considerable support, children can go on to lead active lives.	98 percent for anencephaly; 90 percent for spina bifida
Hole in the abdominal wall (occurs in 4–5 out of 10,000 births)	This can result in gastroschisis or exomphalos where part of the intestine and possibly the liver develops outside the baby's body.	Both conditions are potentially treatable with surgery as soon as the baby is born. Some babies with exomphalos also have heart defects.	98 percent for gastroschisis; 80 percent for exomphalos
Diaphragmatic hernia (occurs in 4 out of 10,000 births)	A hole in the baby's diaphragm means that his lungs aren't able to develop properly.	Around 50 percent of babies with this will die as soon as they are born, because their lungs are simply too underdeveloped even for emergency surgery at birth.	60 percent
Cleft lip and cleft palate (occurs in 1 out of 1,000 births)	Your baby's lips grow in two parts, sometimes including the palate inside the mouth. If the parts don't join together properly, or at all, the baby will develop a cleft lip and palate.	Neither cleft lip nor palate are life-threatening. Your baby will have surgery usually within six months after birth, to knit the two parts together, often with little scarring.	75 percent
Major heart defects (occur in 3–4 out of 1,000 births)	Enlarged heart chambers, valves that allow a two-way flow of blood and holes in the heart are some of the congenital heart problems that are classified as major defects.	Only when a specialist has diagnosed the nature of the baby's heart problem can any real indication be given of his likely prognosis.	50 percent
Lack of kidneys (occurs in 1 in 10,000 births)	Medically known as bilateral renal agenesis, this means that the baby has developed without any kidneys, and possibly a bladder.	Sadly, we need our kidneys to survive so babies with this condition die as soon as or before they are born.	84 percent
Lethal skeletal dysplasia (occurs in 1 in 10,000 births)	With this, the baby's bones don't develop fully, making the torso of the body very short, as well as giving the baby short limbs.	The short torso means that the baby's lungs don't develop fully, making it very hard for a baby to survive after birth.	90 percent

Q I'm 26 weeks pregnant and my doctor is worried about the size of my baby. What will happen?

When a baby's growth slows or ceases in the uterus, this is known as intrauterine growth restriction (IUGR), which can be the result of a variety of factors. If your doctor is concerned about your baby's growth, he or she will arrange extra ultrasounds to see what the problem is and how it can be treated.

The size of a developing baby is measured according to percentile graphs (you'll have these to keep track of your baby's length and weight once she is born, too). From 24 weeks onward, these graphs can plot the average growth rate of a baby according to the height of the mother's fundus. This is the measurement your doctor makes during your prenatal appointments using a tape measure and is taken from the highest point of your belly under your sternum, over the top of the belly to your pubic bone.

If this measurement falls beneath the tenth percentile when you are between 26 and 28 weeks pregnant, your doctor will probably send you for additional ultrasounds so that your baby's skull diameter and abdominal circumference can be checked directly over a given amount of time (and these measurements plotted on relevant percentile graphs). The height of your fundus is influenced not only by your baby's

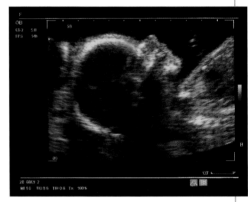

An ultrasound If your baby's growth appears to be slowing down, you may be offered more than one to assess progress more accurately.

size, but also by the amount of amniotic fluid you have—too little or too much fluid can also, rarely, be cause for concern. Having these growth ultrasounds is a precaution intended to reassure you and your doctor that all is well.

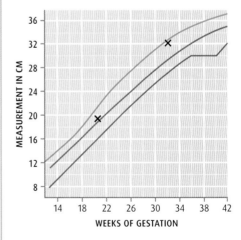

HEAD CIRCUMFERENCE

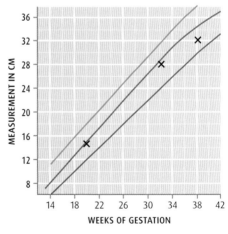

ABDOMINAL CIRCUMFERENCE

Growth graphs The graph on the left shows that a baby's head is growing steadily. The graph on the right indicates that the growth of the abdomen is showing decline possibly due to blood and nutrients being pumped to the heart and brain.

KEY
— 90th percentile ✕ Test results
— 50th percentile — 10th percentile

Q What kind of situations mean that I will need to have additional ultrasounds and checks?

Some pregnancies require extra monitoring to ensure that the baby is growing well. Sometimes this is because of issues identified at the beginning of pregnancy, and extra ultrasounds and checkups can be planned. Other problems arise during the course of pregnancy. The following conditions mean that extra checkups may be planned at your first appointment:
» Complications in a previous pregnancy, such as a small baby or a stillbirth.
» A preexisting medical condition, such as diabetes or a heart condition.

Situations that develop during pregnancy that may require additional monitoring include:
» Being pregnant with multiples, which you are most likely to find out about at your first ultrasound.
» Developing gestational diabetes.
» If you are rhesus negative and you have developed anti-D antibodies.

The following situations mean that you may need extra ultrasound(s) toward the end of pregnancy to check your baby's well-being:
» If your water breaks before your due date.
» Having too much or too little amniotic fluid.
» Being two weeks past your due date.
» If your baby stops her normal movements.

Q My doctor mentioned a Doppler ultrasound. Why would I need this?

If you have complications in your pregnancy, or an ultrasound confirms that there is a problem with your baby's growth, you may be given a Doppler ultrasound. This scan measures blood flow in the umbilical artery and uterus and determines the placental health. You may have more than one Doppler ultrasound during your pregnancy to monitor your baby's growth over a period of time. If there are concerns about your baby's movements, a type of Doppler ultrasound known as a cardiotocograph may be done that traces your baby's heartbeat, and depending on the results, an early induction of labor may be advised. Cardiotocographs are typically done in the third trimester, but can be done earlier.

Q At what stage can I have a 3D ultrasound of my baby?

3D ultrasounds can be done at any stage of your pregnancy. They show still pictures of your baby in three dimensions. 4D ultrasounds show moving 3D images of your baby, with time being the fourth dimension. With these, you will see your baby's skin rather than her insides.

In the US, standard prenatal care usually offers only a 2D image of your baby. However, there are many private clinics that will offer 3D (and even 4D—with sound) ultrasounds, if you're happy to pay for them. Ask your doctor for recommendations of reputable private prenatal clinics near you. Some women worry that creating the 3D image must mean using rays that could be harmful to the baby, but a 3D (or 4D) ultrasound is no more dangerous than one that is 2D—the sound waves are just put together from more angles to create the 3D image. If you are carrying more than one baby this type of ultrasound is really useful since it can show whether fetuses share a placenta or amniotic sac and can provide valuable information about the state of a pregnancy.

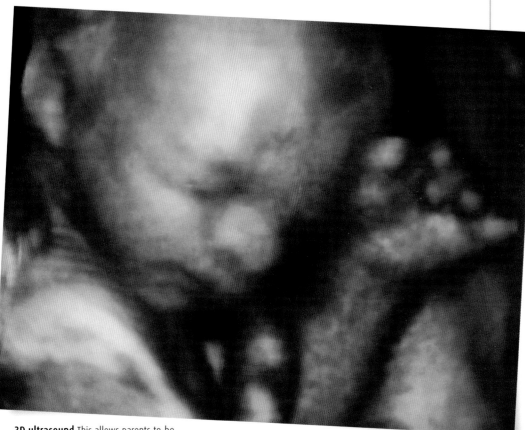

3D ultrasound This allows parents-to-be to see what their unborn baby looks like.

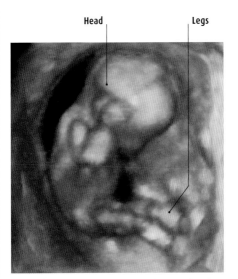

Head · Legs

14 weeks By 12 weeks a fetus is fully formed, and may be possible to tell the gender of a baby at 14 weeks. If you want to see your whole baby on a 3D ultrasound photo, then make sure you have one earlier on in your pregnancy. Space gets tighter as the weeks go by.

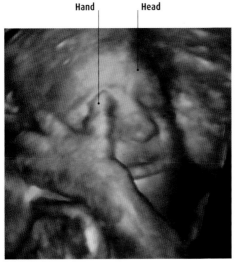

Hand · Head

Close-up 3D ultrasounds reveal a vast range of expressions on the face of a fetus, for example, frowning and smiling. Sometimes a fetus can be seen opening its mouth. This 38-week-old fetus is rubbing her eyes.

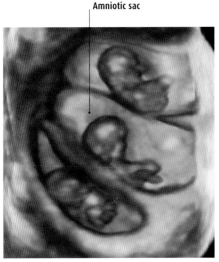

Amniotic sac

Triplets In this amazing 3D image of triplets, each fetus has its own sac. In between the sacs a small amount of placenta is seen as a V-shape. This indicates that each fetus not only has its own sac, but also its own placenta.

All about you

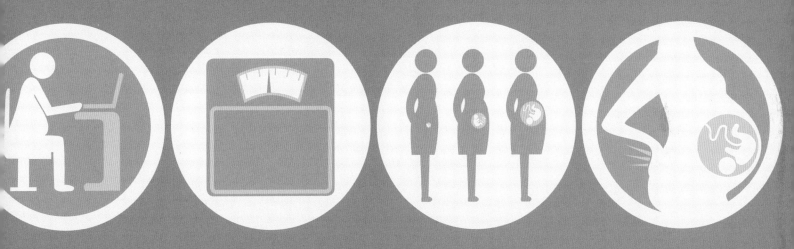

Your body will undergo **incredible changes** over the next nine months. Some of these will affect the way you live your life, and this can feel both bewildering and exciting as you watch your belly grow. Learn about the **lifestyle adjustments** you will need to make and read about the physical and **emotional changes** you are likely to experience. Find out how to deal with **common complaints** and any complications that might arise.

People often tell you that when you're pregnant **your life** will take on new meaning—but you may also be **wondering** how life will change on a more **day-to-day** basis now that you're expecting. There's a lot you can do to give you and your baby the **best possible chance** of enjoying a healthy, safe, and manageable pregnancy.

Lifestyle changes

The world around you

Now that you are pregnant you may be more conscious than ever before of how the environment we live and work in has a direct impact on our health and well-being, and you may wonder how it affects your developing baby's health and well-being, too. In this chapter we'll look at some of the questions you might have about the environment you live in and the chemicals you come into contact with and how you can minimize their effects (if there are any) on your own and your unborn baby's health. We consider the effects of air pollution if you live in a city and exposure to toxic heavy metals, and what to do if you have lead water pipes in your house.

The world of work

How pregnancy affects your working life will depend on the type of work that you do. In this section, we look at any aspects of your job that might be hazardous to your unborn baby or particularly debilitating for you while you're pregnant, so that you can take steps to protect yourself and your growing baby during this important time. We'll also investigate what maternity benefits you,

and also your partner, may be eligible to receive through your employer since more companies today are offering paternity leave to their male employees. We'll also discuss other benefits that you may be eligible for if your company doesn't offer employees paid maternity leave.

Lifestyle matters

We'll look at issues such as pets, the cosmetics you use, and leisure activities such as gardening. We'll answer some of the most commonly asked questions to guide you on where to make changes in your lifestyle. We'll put your mind at ease where you might have concerns. We all need our rest and probably no one needs it more than an expectant mother. Perhaps you want to take a vacation before your baby is born—how late can you fly? What happens if you need vaccinations? How can you make car travel comfortable? What vacation insurance coverage should you get? Finally, we'll take a look at sleep—more precious now than it might ever have been. How can you make sure that you get all the rest you need when being pregnant? We suggest the best time to sleep and how to limit naps to your body's natural sleep cycle.

Q Is it safe to have sex now that I'm pregnant, or could it harm the baby or even break my water?

It is safe to have sex in a straight forward pregnancy. It won't harm your baby as he is well cushioned in his amniotic sac and research has shown that it's highly unlikely that penetration can rupture your membranes and cause your water to break.

The biggest challenge to having intercourse when you're pregnant is accommodating your growing abdomen, but there's no health reason why you should stop having sex. In fact, later in pregnancy, the uterine contractions of an orgasm can help prepare you for birth. Many couples enjoy the freedom of having sex without using any contraception or without having to give thought to the consequences. However, remember that you can still contract sexually transmitted diseases, so if this is a concern use a condom.

Although sex is safe for your baby, it might not be all that comfortable for you, due to breast tenderness, cramping, nausea or increased fatigue. You might find gentle lovemaking more comfortable and you may need to adapt or experiment with different positions at various stages of your pregnancy. Many couples report that a side position works best of all, either facing or in spooning position with your partner behind you.

Many women experience swings in their sex drive during pregnancy. You may feel more sensitive due to the increased blood flow to the breasts and vagina, and the rise in progesterone and estrogen in your body, which can increase your libido. Your changing body might be incredibly exciting to your partner, or he might be too fearful of hurting the baby to relax. If you don't want to have sex, find other ways of being intimate with your partner. Communication and touching are essential for keeping you close and connected as a couple. For many couples the knowledge that they have created a life together helps to enhance their lovemaking.

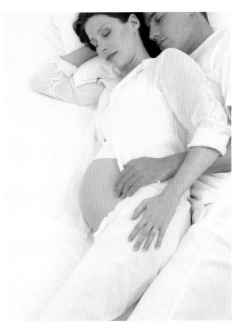

Take time to rest together By cuddling you can feel connected with your partner. Take a nap together or just have a lazy afternoon relaxing.

WHEN TO AVOID SEX

There are a few cases where it is best to avoid penetrative sex and your doctor may advise it for some medical situations. If you have any signs of infection, such as an unusual discharge, itchiness, or pain when you have sex, consult your doctor.

» **Bleeding:** If you've had any heavy bleeding during pregnancy, there may be an increase in the risk of more bleeding.

» **Previous miscarriages** or premature births.

» **Water has broken:** Once this happens, sex could introduce infection.

» **Cervical insufficiency** (see p.147)

» **Placenta previa** (see p.147)

Q Did you know...

Later in pregnancy, an orgasm can set off Braxton Hicks contractions (see p.201). Don't worry—this is a fairly common occurrence but if you're uncomfortable, try slow, deep breathing or relaxation techniques until they pass.

Q I'm worried about radiation harming my baby. Can I still use my cell phone or microwave?

There is no evidence to suggest you should stop using your cell phone—or microwave—during pregnancy. Studies into the long-term effects of cell phones on our health (whether we're pregnant or not) are still in their infancy, so for the time being, it's impossible to be definitive about possible hazards. Cell phones send out radio waves, just like (and no more dangerous than) the waves that come from your computer or your television. People worry more about phones because we hold them against our heads while we're using them. If you keep yours in a pocket close to your abdomen when you're not using it, from current evidence there's no danger to your baby. But if you're worried, carry your cell phone in your handbag or breast pocket and when you talk, use speakerphone and hold the phone away from your body.

Modern microwave ovens are built to strict guidelines that ensure any radiation "leakage" falls well below levels known to harm humans. If you're pregnant and you use a microwave, make sure it's up to modern safety standards. Stand back while the microwave is in operation.

Q Can I have a dental X-ray while I'm pregnant?

Most dental X-rays are too short, far enough away from your abdomen, and of low enough strength to be perfectly safe during pregnancy. However, make sure you tell your dentist you're pregnant so that he or she can advise you. Similarly, most chest and limb X-rays are safe during pregnancy. In almost all cases, if your doctor thinks you need to have an X-ray despite your pregnancy, it's because the benefits of doing so far outweigh the risks to you and your baby.

Q I live in a city. Will the air pollution harm my baby?

If you minimize your outdoor activities during peak pollution times then you will also lower the chances of pollution affecting your baby. You would have to be exposed to excessive amounts to cause serious harm to you or your baby.

In 2014, a study at the University of Florida concluded that women living in heavily polluted urban areas were more likely to suffer high blood pressure and resulting preeclampsia during pregnancy. Another study in Poland, which followed children from birth until the age of five, concluded that high pollution levels during fetal development and in the first years of life led to a small drop in the child's IQ. The Harvard School of Public Heath has also recorded links between fine particulate pollution (emitted by fires, vehicles, and industrial smokestacks) and autism during the third trimester.

Although these findings seem alarming, we already know that air pollution is bad for our health, so, while we need much more research to be certain of the effects on a pregnant woman and her unborn baby, it makes sense to exercise caution whenever you can. Walk down the street at times of low traffic, avoiding rush hour, for example, and keep the windows at home closed at these times, too. If you can, invest in a home air purifier. Walk along quiet streets with traffic that keeps moving, or, ideally, through parks, rather than walking beside stationary traffic. And drink plenty of fluids to keep flushing out your system.

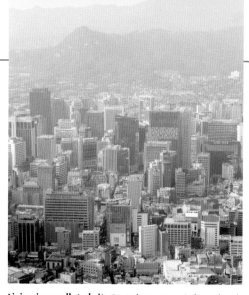

Living in a polluted city Try to keep your windows closed during peak pollution times and follow any instructions from health officials for residents.

AIR QUALITY CHART

An air quality index is used by many government agencies around the world to notify the public of pollution forecasts on a daily basis. Although each one varies slightly, they usually cover measurements of ground-level ozone, particulate matter, carbon monoxide, sulfur dioxide, and nitrogen dioxide. Check local news media for air quality forecasts and plan outdoor activities for days when particle and ozone levels are low. Pregnant women should always follow the advice for at-risk individuals.

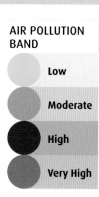

AIR POLLUTION BAND	HEALTH ADVICE FOR AT-RISK INDIVIDUALS
Low	Enjoy your usual outdoor activities
Moderate	Consider reducing prolonged or heavy outdoor activity
High	Reduce or reschedule outdoor activities
Very High	Avoid all outdoor exertion

Q I've got cats. Is it safe for me to clean out their litter box?

Ideally not. Cat feces can carry the *toxoplasma gondii* parasite, which causes toxoplasmosis in humans. If you're pregnant and you become infected, it can cause miscarriage or stillbirth, brain damage, sight or hearing loss, or an enlarged spleen or liver in your baby. The earlier in your pregnancy you're infected, the less likely it is that you'll pass the parasite on to your baby, but if you do, the risks are greater. Later in your pregnancy you're more likely to pass on the infection, but the risks for complications are much lower.

Signs of toxoplasmosis infection in a baby only become clear over time, although babies may have a low birthweight, or show signs of jaundice or anemia. Most women who own cats have had the infection, and as long as they were infected more than three months before conception, there's no risk to the baby. It's best to err on the side of caution, so ask someone else to clean the litter box. If that's not possible, wear rubber gloves and wash your hands immediately afterward. The parasite is also found in soil and raw meat so it is vital to wash your hands after gardening or handling raw meat and wash fruit and vegetables before you eat them. If you think you are at risk of toxoplasmosis, ask your doctor to test you.

Q I live in an old house that still has lead water pipes. Will drinking the tap water harm my baby?

For health reasons, even when you aren't pregnant, you should avoid contact with toxic "heavy" metals as much as possible. Lead in water can leach from your blood and bones and enter your unborn baby's system, and has been known to slow brain development in some children, both before and after birth. Some countries have local government programs that subsidize (or even provide free) replacement of domestic lead water pipes. Talk to your local government about programs in your area and have the piping replaced if you can. Meanwhile, drink filtered water (a simple filter pitcher does a great job of removing impurities—including mercury and aluminum, as well as lead—from tap water) and use filtered water in cooking. If you prefer, use bottled mineral water, but make sure that it has the lowest available sodium levels.

Limit your exposure to toxic heavy metals by using **glass, stainless steel,** or **ceramic cookware** rather than pans and dishes made from aluminum or lead.

Q **I usually dye my hair. Are there certain dyes that I shouldn't use?**

If you want to be extra safe, you can switch to plant-based hair dyes, including henna. However, there are only very low levels of harmful chemicals in hair dyes, and dying your hair once every three months or so during pregnancy is generally considered safe for your baby. What is more likely to happen is that your skin, which is especially sensitive at this time, will have an adverse reaction to the dye, or that your hair will behave erratically—perhaps the color won't take properly or your hair becomes frizzy or brittle. If you're using a chemical dye, even if you've used it before, do a test patch on one small section of your hair first. You might also consider highlights rather than a full dye—highlights will limit the amount of contact your skin will have with the chemicals, minimizing the risk of an adverse skin reaction and reducing the quantity of chemicals that enter your bloodstream.

Q **Can I still have a spray tan now that I'm pregnant?**

Although there's no concrete evidence either way, in general it's better to avoid inhaling any chemicals, including those in a spray tan, while you're pregnant. Instead, use a tanning cream or foam that contains the same tanning agents, but is applied directly to your body, removing the likelihood of you breathing in any chemicals. Also, cream and foam tans only penetrate the upper layers of your skin, so there is limited risk to your baby.

60 million

people in the United States carry the **toxoplasma parasite**, but few show symptoms since the immune system stops the parasite from causing any illness.

Q **I love gardening, but are there any hazards that might affect my growing baby?**

There are several hazards in the garden, such as working with chemicals, exposure to toxoplasmosis in the soil and on unwashed fruit and vegetables, heavy lifting, and getting up from a kneeling position.

A little light gardening is an excellent way to get outdoors and enjoy nature when you are pregnant, but there are some potential dangers lurking out there in the yard. You need to protect yourself from exposure to toxins such as fertilizers and pesticides, and follow good work practices to avoid injury. Follow the advice here to be sure you and your baby stay safe.

 » Remember to kneel and stand up safely; lower yourself and push up using your knees and thighs rather than your back or abdomen.

 » Always wear gardening gloves and try not to get soil on your hands; cats and other animals may have done their business in your yard.

 » Lift garden debris and heavy pots carefully, lowering yourself using your knees, instead of bending from your waist. Ask for help if something is too heavy for you to lift.

 » Wear a hat if it is warm and make sure to drink lots of water—gardening can be thirsty work. Try to do your gardening during the cooler part of the day.

 » Don't spray your plants with insecticide—leave that to someone else. If there's only you to do it, wear a mask that covers your mouth and nose.

 » Leave the really heavy work (such as mowing a large lawn or cutting back trees) for someone else and, whatever you're doing, if you feel dizzy or tired, stop.

 » Always wash your hands with antibacterial soap as soon as you've finished in the yard—even if you've been wearing gloves the whole time.

 » Wash vegetables and fruit thoroughly before eating them (even if you are picking them from your own garden) as the soil may contain animal feces.

Q **Where can I find out about maternity (or paternity), benefits at work?**

In the US, there are no laws in place ensuring that women receive paid maternity leave. The same goes for paternity leave. Policies vary at different companies, so it depends on your individual workplace as to whether or not you'll be eligible. Even if you are, the percentage of your salary that you'll receive, and the number of weeks you'll receive it, will vary by the company. Sometimes it depends on your length of tenure with your company. Your company may also allow you to use sick days or vacation days that you've accumulated to stay home with your baby. During your pregnancy, speak with your boss and/or your human resources manager to determine your eligibility for paid maternity leave and/or using sick or vacation days. A handful of states, including California, offer paid maternity leave for new parents. This may be partial pay for a few weeks' time.

Q **When should I tell my employer that I'm pregnant?**

Many women wait until they're 12 weeks pregnant before they share the news with anyone but immediate family. However, you may work in an environment that could be hazardous to your pregnancy. For example, if you're a dentist or doctor working with X-rays, or a hairdresser coming into contact with lots of chemicals, or if you're suffering from severe morning sickness and it's stopping you from doing your job properly, it's a good idea to tell

Did you know...

As soon as you let your employer know you're pregnant, ask for a copy of your company's maternity policy. If your company doesn't offer paid maternity leave, go online to read about the Family and Medical Leave Act (FMLA), which you can use to spend time with your baby without fear of losing your job.

Q **What is the Family and Medical Leave Act (FMLA)?**

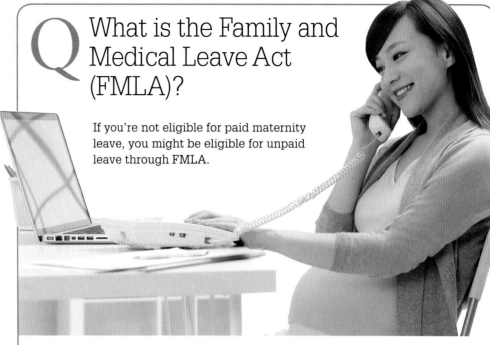

If you're not eligible for paid maternity leave, you might be eligible for unpaid leave through FMLA.

You'll be able to take time off from work–up to 12 weeks in a 12-month period. Your employer is required to hold your job (or a similar one) for you during that time frame and continue your health insurance coverage at the same rate. To qualify, you'll need to have worked for your company for at least 12 months and at least 1,250 hours during the past 12 months. You'll also have to work within 75 miles of offices where 50 or more of your company's employees work. (FMLA does not apply to very small companies.) If you meet the FMLA criteria, you're eligible for these benefits–whether you're male or female and whether you work for a private company or state or local government. (Some federal employees are also eligible.)

your employer sooner. Many women don't feel comfortable sharing the news about their pregnancy until their belly shows, around 20 weeks. Share your news with your boss before your friends. You need to remain on excellent terms with your boss, whom you'll work with when it's time to delegate your responsibilities to others when you need time off when your baby arrives. Don't let your boss learn about your pregnancy through the grapevine, if the office gossips hear about it first.

Q **What can my partner expect in terms of paternity leave?**

Although more companies offer paternity leave to their male employees than a decade ago, paternal leave still isn't a widespread practice at businesses nationwide. Of course policies vary by the company. Some may offer paid time off, while others may offer unpaid or reduced pay during paternity leave.

Most fathers-to-be who want to take time off from work to spend time with their newborns when they arrive have to use their accumulated vacation days or sick time. Have your partner check with his boss or human resources department representative to see if he can use vacation or sick leave in this way. Even if your partner is able to do this, his company may not want him to take more than a week or two off from work at a time for this purpose

Q **My job is really high pressure. Is stress bad for my baby?**

It is always a good idea to take steps to manage stress and anxiety. It is thought that the stress hormones cortisol and adrenaline can pass from you to your baby (studies have found both of these hormones in the amniotic fluid of stressed mothers). Some studies show that stress can increase the risk of premature birth, or of

12 weeks

is how much **unpaid time** off of work **new parents** can take if eligible for the Family and Medical Leave Act.

having a baby with birth defects or with a low birth weight. One study has also made a link between mothers who were stressed during pregnancy and introversion or hyperactivity in their children as they grow up. To help reduce stress levels, be sure to take your lunch break (rather than working through it), walk around the block to clear your head, and leave on time—at least for some of the week. You could also ask for extra help and delegate tasks where you can, in order to manage and streamline your workload effectively.

Q I want to go back to work after the baby is born—can I do that right away?

There are no US guidelines about when you can return to work, because there are no nationwide rules on maternity leave. In the UK, mothers can't return to work during the aptly named "recovery period," two weeks after the baby is born. (This gives women time to recover from childbirth.) If you can afford a few weeks off, take it.

Q I told my employer that I wanted 6 weeks off after birth, but now I'd like 12 weeks. Is this a problem?

Decisions about your maternity leave are very individualized, since they're made between you and your boss or human resources representative. You'll need to speak with your boss or HR representative as soon as you change your mind about the time frame for returning to work to see if they'll agree to your plan. If your company offers paid maternity leave for six weeks, you may be able to use sick or vacation leave for the additional time, or you might use unpaid FMLA leave for the remainder.

Q How can I keep healthy during a long, exhausting day at the office?

It is likely that a typical eight-hour work day will affect you differently when you are pregnant, particularly during the most tiring first and last trimesters. Fortunately, a few minor adjustments in the way you work can help.

 » Use your lunch break to eat and rest, not run errands. Take time to sit in a park or café in order to switch off from any stress at work.

 » Set up your workstation correctly and adopt good posture. You may need to readjust the position of your chair and computer as your pregnancy progresses.

 » Take frequent, short breaks away from your desk. A short stroll every 45 minutes can help you avoid acidity and heartburn. Stretching can prevent aches.

 » Drink water and eat small healthy snacks, such as fruit and nuts, throughout the day. This will keep energy reserves high and combat any nausea.

 » Choose comfortable clothing and footwear. Wearing layers of natural, breathable fabrics will help you adjust to any fluctuations of body temperature.

 » Stagger your commute by asking your employer if you can work slightly different hours to beat the rush hour— which can be challenging whether you are driving or using public transportation.

 » Keep housework and cooking to a minimum in the evenings—this time is essential for relaxation so ask your partner or family members to help you out.

 » Go to bed early whenever you are able.

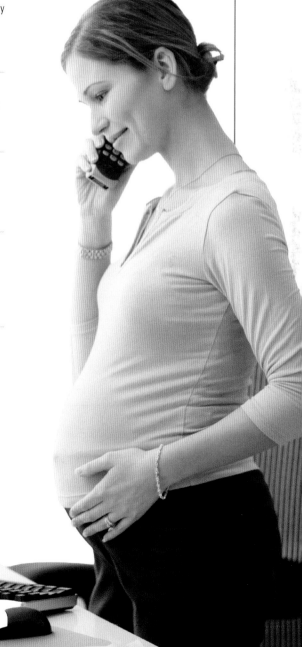

Q I want to take a vacation. What's the best time for me to go?

For most women, the best time is during their second trimester. This is when you're most likely to be enjoying your pregnancy, have increased energy, and feel sick less often. You're more likely to feel comfortable with the idea of traveling and leaving your creature comforts behind. During your first trimester you might feel nauseous and tired, and there is generally a greater risk of miscarrying your baby. During your third trimester you're likely to feel more uncomfortable during travel and most tired. On top of that, if anyone thinks there's a risk you might go into labor, you may have trouble arranging travel to and from your destination since airlines might be reluctant to have you on board a flight.

Q What's the latest point in my pregnancy that I can fly?

There's generally nothing dangerous about flying during pregnancy, as long as you're in a pressurized air cabin (all large planes are pressurized, but small island hoppers might not be). If you have high blood pressure, are very anemic, or you've had a previous miscarriage, you may be advised to avoid flying. It's best to ask your doctor for advice that's right for you.

There are also the airline's rules, which vary depending on the company. In general, they won't take you after around 36 weeks pregnant—although this isn't a hard-and-fast rule—or a few weeks earlier if you're pregnant with twins or multiples (remember, these are the dates for your return). Some airlines will make an exception. If you're traveling during

your third trimester, almost all will ask for a letter from your doctor to say that you can travel. Make sure you carry this letter with you if this applies to you: the airline has the right to refuse to let you board the plane if your due date or health are in doubt. They want to avoid having a pregnant woman in labor midflight.

Q Are there any types of vacation I should avoid while I'm pregnant?

Avoid any vacation that might put a lot of physical strain on your body, for example those involving activities that place you in danger of high impact, that restrict your oxygen intake, or that raise your core body temperature. This means that scuba diving vacations are temporarily off the agenda, as are skiing

Q Is there an increased risk of thrombosis for me during a "long-haul" flight?

Any flight longer than five hours is considered "long haul" for people at risk of thrombosis (blood clots)—which includes pregnant women.

During a long flight, blood can pool in your veins (usually in your legs) and cause clots. Before you book, check with your doctor that you're not at an especially high risk of developing thrombosis when you fly, for example if you suffer from diabetes, high blood pressure, or high cholesterol. During any flight, whether or not it's long haul, call a member of the cabin crew immediately

if you feel dizzy—the oxygen circulating in the cabin can be a bit thin and you may need a boost from an oxygen mask. To minimize the risk of thrombosis when you're in the air, follow these tips (see right).

Formation of blood clots This begins when fatty deposits called atheromas form. The growing atheroma reduces blood flow and oxygen to the tissues and then ruptures, causing a clot to form.

» Wear support hose or compression flight socks to help keep your circulation flowing while you're airborne. Most pharmacies sell these.

» Walk up and down the aisle every 30 minutes if the seat-belt sign is off. Do gentle stretches if there is space to do so at the end of the aisle.

» Drink plenty of water during the flight. It will keep you hydrated and force you to take regular trips to the bathroom (making you get up and move around).

» Ask for an aisle seat so you can stretch your legs (or, even better, pay for extra leg room if your airline offers it as an option).

» Point and flex your ankles from time to time while you're sitting. Move each foot round in a circular motion to help keep your circulation flowing.

» Wear loose clothes and shoes or sandals that will accommodate swollen feet. Take your shoes off while you're seated to make your feet less constricted.

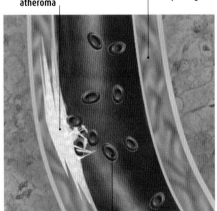

Damage from atheroma

Artery lining

Platelets (clotting agents)

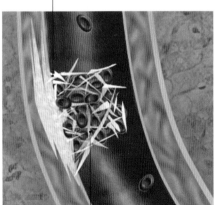

Ruptured atheroma attracts platelets

Blood clot blocking artery

Q I'm planning to drive rather than fly to my vacation destination. Can you give me advice on long car trips?

First, always wear your seat belt: put the lap strap under your abdomen, across your thighs, and over the top of your abdomen. Adjust your seat a little or invest in a cushioning pad if the strap cuts into your neck.

If you're driving and find the driving seat a squeeze, tilt the steering wheel back if you can, or recline your seat slightly to give you more space. Never move your seat backward so much that you can't reach the pedals properly and always make sure you can still see over the top of the steering wheel. If you adjust your seat, don't forget to adjust your mirrors, too. Take frequent rest and bathroom breaks. Sitting in the same position for long periods of time can be uncomfortable during pregnancy. When you get out of the car, swing your legs out first, and try not to twist awkwardly. Push up from a seated position using your thighs rather than your back.

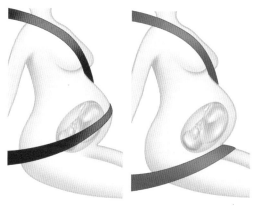

Comfort in the car Three-point seat belts with the straps placed above and below your belly will allow you to feel comfortable, while still being safe.

INCORRECT POSITION   CORRECT POSITION

vacations—not only because of the altitude you should not go more than 6,500 ft/2,000 m above sea level), but because of the risk for impact, too. Walking vacations on low, gently undulating foothills, or forest or seaside walks ould be good for you, especially during your second trimester, but don't make each day's activity any more strenuous than your pregnant body can deal with. Take frequent rest stops. If you are going to a sunny climate or intending to be outside frequently, always practice good sun safety by wearing a high-SPF, broad-spectrum sunscreen that doesn't contain oxybenzone (a chemical linked to low birth weights).

you and your baby. If you can't avoid traveling to a high-risk country, talk to your doctor well in advance about the immunizations you'll need and, if relevant, about malaria pills. On balance it's usually better to vaccinate than risk contracting disease, but you should always seek individualized medical advice.

Q Is it safe to have vacation vaccinations while I'm pregnant?

Most vaccinations are made using small amounts of the disease you're vaccinating against, so in general it's better to avoid going to countries that require you to have immunizations. In addition, avoid malaria-risk countries. Although there are malaria medications that are safe to take during pregnancy, malaria itself poses a high risk of death for

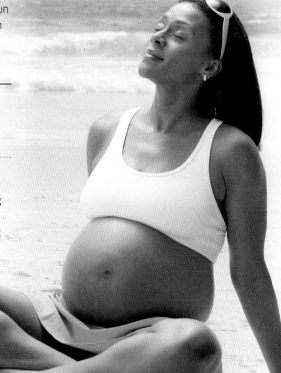

Q Should I get special travel insurance that covers treatment for my pregnancy?

You won't necessarily need pregnancy-specific travel insurance, but check your policy to see what pregnancy issues are covered. Look for what will happen if you go into labor, have to cancel your vacation because of a pregnancy-related issue, or you need repatriating. Make sure your insurer knows that you're pregnant before you travel and that you are complying with any stipulations that keep your cover safe, such as carrying a letter or certificate from your doctor to say you're fit to travel. Some insurers won't cover you if you travel beyond a certain week of pregnancy, which may be different from the week the airline stipulates, and often insurers don't cover the neonatal period, for example if your baby is born early and needs medical care.

Bring your **medical records** when you go on vacation so that any doctor **treating** you knows your pregnancy **history** and can take care of you safely.

Fatigue is inevitable in pregnancy. During the first trimester, it is caused largely by your body's effort to nourish your developing embryo, and a massive surge in progesterone. During the last trimester, it's the result of the general discomfort of carrying an ever-growing baby. However, there are techniques you can use to minimize fatigue.

Scale back

A busy social life is fantastic when you aren't pregnant, but during pregnancy you may need to be more selective about what you do. Try to cut back on events that are going to require very late bedtimes or long periods of time on your feet. Don't be afraid to cancel plans if you feel too tired to attend—your friends will understand. Figure out what your social limits are and work within them. Scale back on your chores, too—consider getting groceries delivered, for example.

Don't toss and turn

If you wake up in the night and can't get back to sleep, do something quiet but positive, rather than lying there ruminating. Keep a pen and paper beside your bed and write down a to-do list for the following day; read a few pages of a book; take a short walk to the bathroom and back. You could even listen to some soothing night music through headphones (quietly) to give your mind something else to focus on.

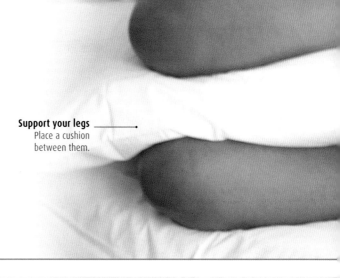

Support your legs
Place a cushion between them.

WAYS TO HELP YOU SLEEP

 Nap

Give your body (and brain) a chance to recuperate. If you're working, be unabashed about taking a nap at lunchtime (this is easiest if you have your own office, but a lounge may work). On the weekends, set an alarm for a 50-minute nap. This will give you five minutes to fall asleep, but should wake you during your lightest sleep stage (see top right for explanation on sleep cycles), so that you don't feel groggy.

 Rest

Even if you can't have a full nap during the day, make sure you make time to rest. That means, sitting comfortably in a chair with your eyes closed. According to research, being fully at rest and with your eyes closed is almost as restful as sleep itself. If you're at work, put some earphones in and listen to some music that you find deeply relaxing, or even simply take earplugs to block out the white noise around you.

 Rehydration

Dehydration compounds the effects of feeling tired, making you feel even more drained and lethargic. It's really important that you keep up your fluid intake every day. You don't need to drink more than nonpregnant people, but you do need to make sure you drink enough, which is around 74 fluid ounces (2.2 liters) of fluid a day.

 Food

Your body is best at sleeping when it is relaxed. If you have a light dinner, not later than 8 pm, by the time you go to bed a couple of hours later the hard work of digestion will be over and your body can concentrate on sleeping rather than digesting. See p.57 for advice on how to distribute your meals and snacks throughout the day.

Awake
REM
Stage 1
Stage 2
Stage 3
Stage 4

0 1 2 3 4 5 6 7 8 9
8-HOUR SLEEP CYCLE

SLEEP CYCLES

When you sleep, your body goes through "sleep cycles," each taking you through five stages, from light to dreaming to deep and back to light again. Each full cycle lasts around 90 minutes, although the time you spend within each stage varies depending on your overall level of fatigue. For a nap to be effective, you should aim for 50 minutes. If you're tired, you'll spend longer in deep, restorative sleep than any of the other stages, but by allowing yourself to come full circle into the light sleep that characterizes the end of a sleep cycle, you'll wake up feeling refreshed.

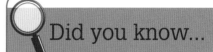

Did you know...

During each sleep cycle, we experience a period of REM or "dreaming sleep." Periods of REM sleep increase for pregnant women from about 25 weeks pregnant onward, spiking at around 33 to 36 weeks. Your dreams aren't necessarily more vivid, but you are more aware of them.

Sleeping comfortably This will become more difficult as your baby grows. Use pillows and cushions to support your body while you get some rest.

Best practice

Sleep experts call the rituals and practicalities of sleeping our sleep hygiene. Good sleep hygiene is essential to good sleep. So, keep your bedroom dark and cool. Create a bedtime ritual so that your brain learns what the forerunners to sleep are and gets itself ready to switch off. Keep noise and activity levels low in the hour before bedtime—turn off the television, laptops, cell phones, and tablets.

IMPROVE YOUR SLEEP POSITION

Sleeping with sore hip joints, nagging back pain, nasal congestion, heartburn, and a growing baby (not to mention other pregnancy issues) is a challenge in itself. Try these sleeping positions to maximize your chances of a restful night:

» If you have heartburn or congestion, sleep on your left side. Raise the end of your mattress so that your chest and head are raised slightly.

» Avoid rolling onto your back, which in the second trimester onward can restrict blood flow to your baby—put a pillow behind your back to stop you from rolling over, if necessary.

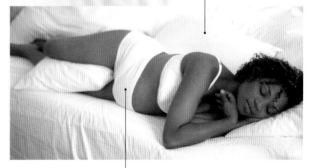

Pillow at your back This stops you from rolling onto your back.

Sleep on your left side This helps to avoid heartburn or congestion.

FASCINATING FACTS

As your belly grows, your body takes on many interesting changes, some of which are absolutely incredible.

23%

This is the amount of extra blood pumped into your uterus while you're pregnant.

30–50%

By 28 weeks your cardio output has increased by 30–50 percent.

20 in (50 cm)

This is the average length that the umbilical cord will grow to during a woman's pregnancy.

45%

By week 16, your body will contain 45 percent more blood than it did before you were pregnant.

99.5°F (37.5°C)

The temperature of the amniotic fluid that surrounds your baby.

50%

You breathe 50 percent more deeply in pregnancy.

A CLOSER LOOK
Your growing belly

Being pregnant is amazing. Not only does your body change to meet the demands of growing a baby inside you, but also it all takes place in just 40 weeks. When you're pregnant your body creates a whole new organ, the placenta. Your heart and liver might grow in size to help meet the demands of your pregnancy and your uterus expands to accommodate your baby as she increases in size.

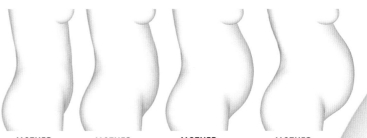

MOTHER AT 12 WEEKS   MOTHER AT 20 WEEKS   MOTHER AT 28 WEEKS   MOTHER AT 40 WEEKS

Growing belly As your uterus expands, so does your belly. The distance from the pubis to the top of the uterus is measured regularly from the second trimester of pregnancy. It's called the fundal height and is monitored as a marker of fetal growth. The measurement in centimeters usually matches the week of pregnancy that you're in.

1–4 weeks During the early weeks your baby is no bigger than the size of a grain of rice, so your uterus has only started on its growth spurt alongside your baby's. At four weeks, your uterus is pretty much the same size as before you were pregnant (about the size of a plum) and it measures between 2½–4 in (6–10 cm) in length (not height, since it's horizontal). **GRAIN OF RICE**

9–12 weeks At this stage your baby is about the size of a lime. You may notice that you've had more trips to the bathroom as your growing uterus puts pressure on your bladder. Frequent urination can also be a sign of a urinary infection, so speak to your doctor if you feel any pain. Your hands and feet may feel warmer because of the increased blood flow to your skin.

LIME

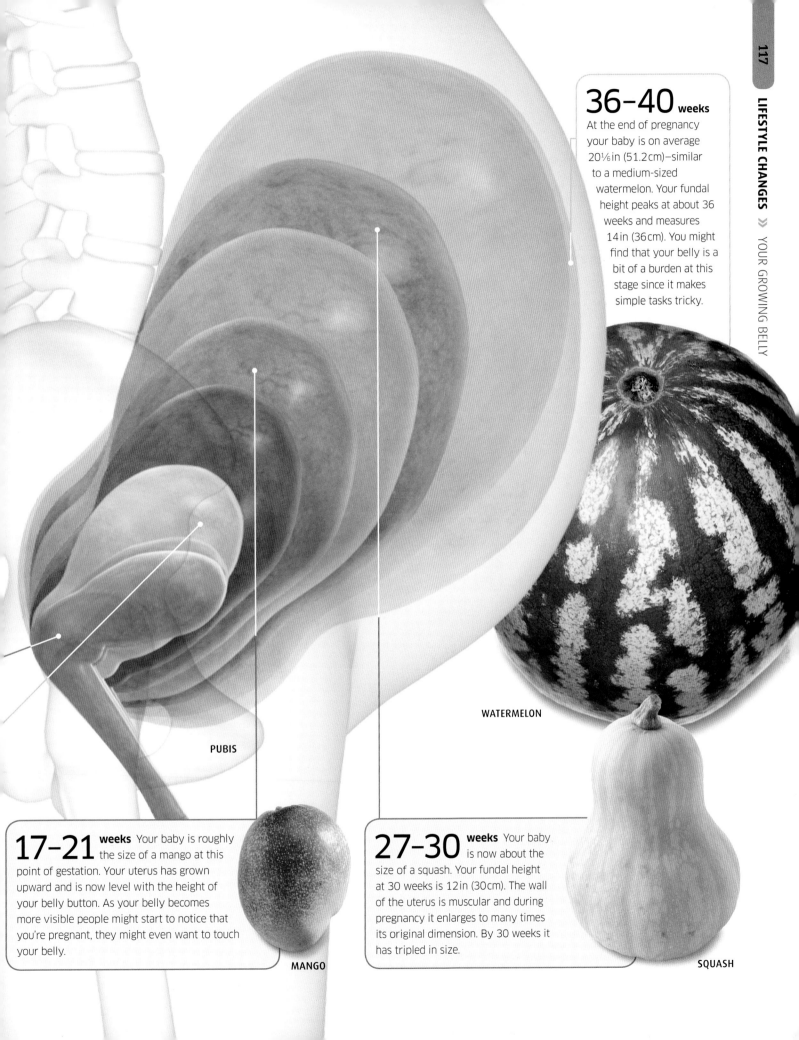

36–40 weeks

At the end of pregnancy your baby is on average 20⅛in (51.2cm)—similar to a medium-sized watermelon. Your fundal height peaks at about 36 weeks and measures 14in (36cm). You might find that your belly is a bit of a burden at this stage since it makes simple tasks tricky.

WATERMELON

PUBIS

17–21 weeks

Your baby is roughly the size of a mango at this point of gestation. Your uterus has grown upward and is now level with the height of your belly button. As your belly becomes more visible people might start to notice that you're pregnant, they might even want to touch your belly.

MANGO

27–30 weeks

Your baby is now about the size of a squash. Your fundal height at 30 weeks is 12in (30cm). The wall of the uterus is muscular and during pregnancy it enlarges to many times its original dimension. By 30 weeks it has tripled in size.

SQUASH

During pregnancy, your body goes through myriad **changes** that influence your emotional and physical **well-being.** There's more than just the **stretching** of your belly as the uterus grows; **you might notice** changes to skin, hair, feet, nails, and teeth, not to mention parts of the body you can't see.

Physical and emotional changes

How you change physically

Some of the physical changes that occur to your body during pregnancy might be ones that you are happy with; for example, you might enjoy having a fuller bust, more rounded hips, thick, glossy hair, and a translucent sheen to the skin. Other changes, though, such as stretch marks, may be less welcome and can feel like unpleasant side effects. You may also find that the arch of your foot drops and that you go up a shoe size, which may be a permanent change. Not all women experience all of these changes, but however you're affected, try to keep in mind that they're positive signs that your pregnancy is progressing. Almost without exception, changes to your skin, hair, and nails will reverse once your baby is born.

Understanding your hormones

All the changes that take place in your body during pregnancy are the result of messages that your hormones send to your brain. Pregnancy hormones affect you both physically—changing your body and helping your baby to develop—and emotionally, too. Pregnancy is known for triggering mood swings, and your hormones, combined with a heavy dash of fatigue and probably some anxiety, are to blame. If you have a partner, these moods may take a toll on him or her; make sure the two of you stay connected and find ways to both enjoy pregnancy. It is worthwhile to learn about pregnancy hormones and how they affect your emotions. Then having a few strategies that help avoid arguments and allow you to express your feelings constructively will help to steer you through the emotional minefield of this amazing time.

The hidden changes

If the outward signs of pregnancy and the hormonal changes weren't enough to come to grips with, there are lots of internal changes taking place that you may not even notice, but which are essential for nourishing your baby and maintaining your pregnancy. As you'll see, being pregnant affects the functioning of all your internal organs—your heart and liver have to work harder, and your lungs have to adapt to increase their efficiency in a much-reduced space. Within your breasts, long before your baby is born, changes take place that turn them into perhaps the most efficient food source we know of.

Q I've heard about pregnancy hormones, but what are they and what do they do?

At the beginning of your pregnancy, there is a surge of two hormones, estrogen and progesterone, which have an essential role in maintaining pregnancy. The rise of these hormones is the result of human chorionic gonadotrophin (hCG) signaling to the corpus luteum (the ruptured egg follicle) that pregnancy is underway.

At around six to nine weeks of pregnancy, the placenta takes over the production of estrogen and progesterone for the rest of your pregnancy. Other key hormones during your pregnancy include relaxin, oxytocin, prolactin, and endorphins. These, along with androgens (the male sex hormones), are collectively known as sex steroid hormones. The right balance of hormones is essential for a successful pregnancy.

The body system that regulates all of your hormones is called the endocrine system. This includes various glands and organs throughout your body, including the thyroid, adrenal, and pituitary glands, and the hypothalamus, the pancreas, and the ovaries. All your body systems are affected by the action of your endocrine system.

hCG levels almost double every **48 hours** at the beginning of your pregnancy.

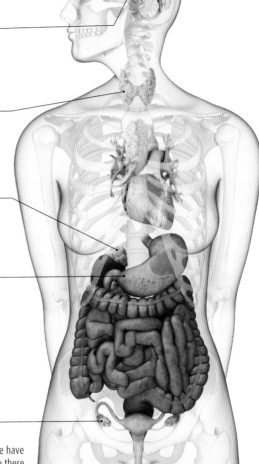

Pituitary gland
Known as the "master gland," it controls the acitivity of other hormonal glands.

Hypothalamus
Part of the brain, it is responsible for keeping the body in a constant and stable condition.

Thyroid
This gland secretes hormones that regulate the body's metabolic rate.

Adrenal glands
Hormones secreted by these glands act on body tissues to enable them to function.

Pancreas
The pancreas makes digestive juices and hormones such as insulin that control blood-sugar levels.

Ovaries
These produce eggs and the reproductive hormones progesterone and estrogen.

Hormones during pregnancy These have powerful and varied functions and are there to regulate the many changes taking place to enable your baby to develop and be born safely.

ESTROGEN

Initially secreted by the ovaries, estrogen prepares the lining of the uterus for a potential pregnancy. It also has the following key roles during your pregnancy:

» **Ensures the developing embryo** remains embedded in your uterus.

» **Dilates your blood vessels** so that blood can flow more easily and in greater quantity.

» **Stimulates the milk glands** in preparation for breast-feeding.

» **Improves bone health** while your body is under more pressure.

PROGESTERONE

This hormone plays a vital role in the early stages of pregnancy by preparing the body for fertilization and then establishing the placenta. It does the following:

» **Prepares the lining of the uterus** for implantation and encourages it to thicken.

» **Helps to regulate** the changes in your metabolism.

» **Thickens the "plug"** that forms in the cervix to keep bacteria from entering the uterus and causing infection.

» **Strengthens muscles** in the pelvic wall in preparation for labor.

OTHER HORMONES

Your pregnancy is also specifically influenced by the action of:

» **Oxytocin,** the "love" hormone that triggers labor and helps you to bond with your baby.

» **Endorphins,** the "feel-good" hormones that help to mitigate your experience of pain during labor.

» **Prolactin,** the hormone that stimulates your body to produce milk for your baby.

» **Relaxin,** the hormone that helps to loosen your muscles and ligaments to make space for your baby.

Q My mother had terrible varicose veins when she was pregnant. Will this happen to me?

Varicose veins are one of the most common side effects of pregnancy and they usually occur in the third trimester. If you do get them, your doctor can tell you how they can be treated after your baby is born.

A little under half of all pregnant women get varicose veins or hemorrhoids which are varicose veins in the anus (see p.132). You're more likely to suffer from them if a close member of your family has had them. They develop when progesterone levels in your body during pregnancy relax the walls of your blood vessels so they lose muscle tone. At the same time, your circulation is under greater strain from the increase in blood pumping around your body. Your veins are less taut and they also have more work to do. Aching in your legs is often the first sign that you might have varicose veins, as well as some itching around the affected veins.

If you think you might be at risk of varicose veins, your doctor can give you compression hose, which help to keep your veins "tightened." It is a good idea to exercise regularly and to avoid excessive weight gain, since this can exacerbate them.

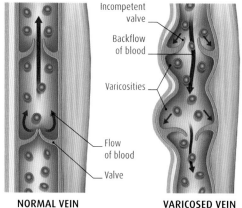

NORMAL VEIN   **VARICOSED VEIN**

Incompetent valve

Backflow of blood

Varicosities

Flow of blood

Valve

How varicose veins form
Valves in the vein walls stop your blood from flowing back down your veins between pumps. During pregnancy, the valves, with only weakened vein walls to support them, can fail to work. Blood starts to pool, which makes the veins distended and swollen.

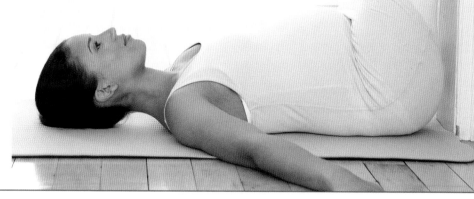

Relieving the symptoms Lie down and raise your legs so that they are higher than your hips. Avoid standing for long periods.

Q I had terrible acne as a teenager and now it's back. Why is pregnancy doing this?

When you were a teenager the surge of hormones during puberty caused your body to create excess sebum—the skin's natural lubricating oil. Now that you're pregnant, the same thing is happening again. Follow a strict cleansing routine for the skin on your face, morning and night, using a gentle, hypoallergenic cleanser. Avoid using a highly scented soap, which can dry out and irritate your skin. You can use an astringent if this has helped you in the past, but talk to your doctor before you do since many medicated astringents are not suitable for use during pregnancy.

Q What changes in my skin and nails should I expect?

You're likely to have a pregnancy glow from about the middle of your second trimester. It's partly because your blood volume increases, which means nutrients are carried more efficiently to all your organs, including your skin. Plumped-up cells—the result of increased fluid levels in your blood—can smooth out wrinkles and blemishes, while increases in the hormone progesterone can cause pinkness, making you look rosy. Hormone changes can make your body produce more sebum, which can give your skin a sheen. In addition to making you look radiant, hormones can make your skin very dry and possibly itchy. Some

women sweat more, which can cause rashes. Make sure you drink plenty of water to keep hydrated and use an unperfumed moisturizer. Nails can become harder, more brittle, or softer.

25%
Up to a quarter of women have **itchy** or **sensitive skin** during pregnancy. Keep some calamine lotion on hand to soothe general rashes.

Q Are stretch marks inevitable? Why do we get them and is there anything I can do?

Stretch marks (or striae gravidarum) can appear on your abdomen, thighs, hips, arms, breasts, and buttocks. They tend to run in families, so if your mother, grandmother, or sisters had them, it's likely that you will too. There's very little you can do to prevent them, but you're not alone since 90 percent of women get them.

They're caused when the collagen—the connective tissue in your skin—weakens, stretches, and tears as your belly grows. Hormonal changes make the problem worse.

A diet that's rich in skin-supporting nutrients (found in nuts and seeds, and fresh fruits and vegetables, which contain high levels of antioxidants), and not "eating for two" (see p.59) can help to minimize the effects. Try to gain weight steadily throughout your pregnancy (see chart, p.126) so that your skin has time to stretch. If you stay fit you may be able to limit

the appearance of stretch marks. Keeping your skin supple with moisturizing creams will help it to ping back into shape after you've had your baby, but studies show that they have limited effect on stretch marks. This is because collagen works deep within the layers of your skin, so creams you put on top my not be enough.

Once you've had your baby, the stretch marks will gradually fade over time. In most women they will disappear altogether, or remain only as fine, silvery lines by the time a baby is six months old.

Q How common is it for skin pigmentation changes to occur and what exactly is the "butterfly mask?"

Chloasma, also known as the "butterfly mask" or melasma, gives you dark or pinkish patches over your cheeks, nose, eyes, and forehead—sometimes in a butterfly shape, hence the common name.

Butterfly effect Women with darker skin may be more susceptible than women with lighter skin.

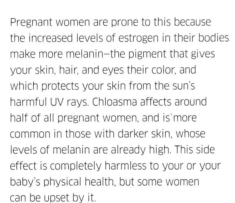

Pregnant women are prone to this because the increased levels of estrogen in their bodies make more melanin—the pigment that gives your skin, hair, and eyes their color, and which protects your skin from the sun's harmful UV rays. Chloasma affects around half of all pregnant women, and is more common in those with darker skin, whose levels of melanin are already high. This side effect is completely harmless to your or your baby's physical health, but some women can be upset by it.

Being in the sun can make it worse, so stay in the shade and use a high-SPF, broad-spectrum sunscreen that does not contain oxybenzone. You're probably already taking folic acid (see p.49), but if you aren't, or if you're past the 12 weeks' mark and have stopped taking it, talk to your doctor about a daily supplement; some studies show that being low in the mineral folate can make you more susceptible to chloasma. Finally, remember that it is almost always temporary; your skin should return to normal not long after you've given birth.

Cover up Exposure to the sun can make the mask more pronounced. Wear a hat to protect your face.

DARKENING SKIN

Increased levels of melanin in your skin are responsible for all kinds of skin changes that may occur in pregnancy. These can include:

» **A greater number of freckles** on your face.

» **Darkening in moles**, birthmarks, and scars.

» **The line that may appear** from your navel to your pubic bone, known as the "linea nigra."

» **Your ability to tan** more easily.

» **Darker areolae** around your nipples.

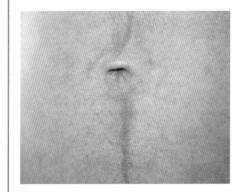

Linea nigra This is situated where the left and right vertical abdominal muscles meet. Your growing belly causes them to separate and darken.

Q **The palms of my hands are red and hot. Is this a recognized side effect of pregnancy?**

Around 30 percent of pregnant women get a condition called plantar erythema, which causes reddening in the palms, and in the fleshy pads underneath your thumbs and little fingers. It sometimes also appears on the soles of the feet. The condition is a result of higher estrogen levels, which increase the amount of blood in your circulatory system. This in turn raises your body temperature and how warm your extremities feel and how red they appear. The condition is nothing to worry about and will go away after you've had your baby. If the reddening is bothering you, though, simply do what you can to keep your hands cool.

Q **My hair is much thicker than it was before I got pregnant. Will it stay like this forever?**

No, it won't. All that thick, glossy hair isn't just the result of increased levels of sebum (your body's natural oil) over your scalp. Higher levels of progesterone in the second and third trimesters of pregnancy mean that you don't shed hair in the way that you did when you weren't pregnant. However, when your hormone levels fall dramatically after the baby is born, you shed all the excess hair over a much shorter period of time, so it can appear as if clumps of hair are falling out daily. So, unfortunately, the locks you love now aren't forever, but don't worry—after the birth, your hair is simply returning to its normal thickness.

Q **I have tiny red and blue lines on my face and neck. Will they go away?**

It's possible that you have some temporary "spider veins" appearing on your face, neck, shoulders and chest. They are simply where the very finest walls of your capillaries, close to the surface of your skin, have broken under the strain of the increased amount of blood in your circulation. They will usually disappear of their own accord once you've had the baby. Blue veins due to increased blood flow to breast tissue may become more noticeable.

Q **I've heard that pregnant women are prone to tooth decay. Why is this, and how can I prevent it?**

It's an old wives' tale that pregnancy rots your teeth. However, it is true that you're more susceptible to bleeding gums and gum disease, particularly if you had weakened gums before you got pregnant.

The weakening of the connective tissue that can lead to stretch marks can also make your gums softer and liable to tearing. Also, your saliva is now more acidic, which can exacerbate the effects. This can lead to infection and damaged teeth.

Reducing your sugar intake to protect your teeth and gums and good hygiene is essential. It's also a very good idea to keep up with your regular dental checkups and cleanings with the hygienist (which is typically every six months). If you do need essential dental work, it is fine to have a local anesthetic during the second trimester. There is no risk to your baby. Some dentists believe that because gum disease is linked with premature birth, it's better for the mother to have dental treatment when it's needed rather than waiting until after the baby's birth.

DENTAL CARE WHILE PREGNANT

The checklist below will ensure that you are clear about the things you need to do, what to tell your dentist and procedures that should be avoided.

» **Maintain good hygiene** using a soft toothbrush and floss regularly. Always brush after a meal, but be gentle, and use a nonalcohol-based mouthwash to help remove residual bacteria.

» **Tell your dentist that you are pregnant** when you schedule your appointment. You should inform your dentist about any medication your are taking since some might affect the development of your child's teeth.

» **Tell your dentist** if tenderness, bleeding, or gum swelling occurs at any time during your pregnancy.

» **Avoid dental treatment** during the first trimester and the second half of the third trimester (the last six to eight weeks), as these are key times in the baby's growth and development.

» **Avoid dental X-rays** during pregnancy. If an X-ray is absolutely essential, your dentist will be extra vigilant to keep your baby safe, and most dental X-rays don't affect the abdomen.

» **Postpone all elective**, nonessential dental procedures until after the delivery.

» **Avoid having an amalgam (silver) filling** removed or put in during pregnancy, as a precautionary measure.

Q Pregnancy seems to have me elated one minute and devastated the next. Is this normal?

During your first trimester, the hormonal changes in your body are rapid and raging. It's a primeval response that ensures you maintain your pregnancy. These surges, primarily in the hormones estrogen and progesterone, upset the chemical balance in your brain, causing neurotransmitters—your brain's chemical messengers—to switch on and off randomly. And that's what gives you the mood swings.

In many cases, your mood will settle down by week 12. However, some women continue to experience severe highs and lows and may be diagnosed with prenatal depression. This is as common as postpartum depression and can be just as serious. In addition to fluctuating hormones, there are other causes of prenatal depression such as anxiety about your pregnancy, feeling sick and tired, feeling low, previous depression, fear of something going wrong and isolation. If your mood swings are very extreme, or you suspect you may be suffering from depression (and almost 10 percent of women are thought to experience this during pregnancy), speak to your doctor, who will be able to get you the treatment you need.

Q What can I do to help myself manage my emotions?

There are many self-help techniques you can employ. Try some of these quick fixes when you feel a negative mood—sadness or irritation—taking hold:

» Walk around the block or through a park, even if it's just for 10 minutes. Fresh air and a change of scenery are sometimes all you need to clear your head.

» Have a healthy snack since sugar lows exacerbate negative feelings or irritation so keep your energy levels stable.

» Write a letter explaining how you are feeling. Even if you never send it, it can help to put things into perspective.

» Knead some dough, make cookies, or make something that involves using some elbow grease. Physical exertion can help you to work through what's troubling you and may provide an outlet for your pent-up adrenaline.

Q I am so forgetful. Is there really such a thing as "baby brain?"

Anecdotal evidence suggests that forgetfulness and lack of concentration are natural side effects of pregnancy. Scientists are still trying to find out if there is a physiological reason for this, with one recent study proposing that the emotional parts of the brain "plump up" during pregnancy and the more logical, functional parts wind down in order to maximize the mother's instinct for responding empathetically to her baby immediately after birth.

However, there are still questions about why physiological brain changes happen, if they do, with some studies pointing the blame at hormones. Experts tend to agree, though, that you are more tired, stressed, and distracted during pregnancy so the energy you have for clear thinking zooms in on important things (your health and that of your developing baby) rather than where you put the car keys. Just try to get as much rest as possible and be assured that there is no evidence to suggest that "baby brain"—physiological or anecdotal—lasts any longer than pregnancy itself, and the effects will reverse after birth.

Q My mood swings are causing spats with my partner. How can we learn to deal with them better?

First things first—get your partner on board. Learn about the hormonal changes of pregnancy together and try to rationalize your irrationality.

Your partner is less likely to take anything you throw at him personally if he knows what's happening in your body. Learning to support your mood swings, rather than dismissing or escalating them, is a key role for your partner, and should not be underestimated. Remember, too, that while the hormones are affecting your body, anxiety, nervousness, and excitement about impending parenthood are things that you both feel. Indeed, your partner may feel overwhelmed by the thought of an added responsibility.

Try counting to 10 when either of you is irritable and feels like snapping. It won't always work, but if enough seconds can elapse before you speak, your words are more likely to be constructive, conciliatory, or placatory.

Make time for physical contact such as holding hands as you walk down the street. Even giving each other a hug at the end of a tiring day will give you a surge of endorphins and oxytocin—feel-good hormones that help to stabilize your moods.

Find time to escape into your own personal space, if this suits the kind of person you are. Perhaps this happens naturally when you go to work, or maybe it means that one of you curls up with a book while the other takes a bath.

Make time for activities together that aren't related to the baby—give yourselves constant reminders of the good things about your relationship, so that when your mood swings you have a recent memory of why the two of you make a good team.

Q What happens to my amazing body during pregnancy?

Over the course of the nine months of your pregnancy, your body has to adapt and make space for your growing baby, to ensure your baby's growth and protection, and to prepare itself to give birth. Some of the changes you go through will be obvious—a growing abdomen and larger breasts, for example—but many will seem imperceptible to you, or you'll notice them only when they have a domino effect that makes you wonder what's going on. Here's an overview of all the amazing things your body is doing to adapt to pregnancy and nourish your baby.

NOSE
From early in your pregnancy you may notice that you have a heightened sense of smell. This may be due to more blood pumping round your body. However, some people believe it could be a protective mechanism—to keep you away from substances that could be harmful.

LUNGS
Your lungs move up and back as your pregnancy progresse. They are being pushed to their uppermost limits, which can make you breathless. Your air intake increases to help to supply you and your baby with enough oxygen.

DIAPHRAGM
The increasing size of your uterus during pregnancy means that your diaphragm—the flat wall of muscle that controls your breathing and lies beneath your lungs—is pushed upward, squashing your lungs in the process, but increasing your capacity for breathing deeply.

STOMACH
Your stomach may send signals to your brain for certain foods that you "must" have (cravings) and to avoid foods that make you feel sick (aversions). Some scientists believe that cravings encourage you to fill a nutritional gap, while aversions stop you from consuming substances that could be harmful to your pregnancy.

INTESTINE
Increases in progesterone during pregnancy inhibit the the action that moves food along your digestive tract. Although this can cause constipation and heartburn, the slowing down means you can get the maximum nutritional benefit from food as it passes through you.

Did you know?

Before you are pregnant, your uterus is roughly the size of a plum. By the time you have reached six weeks, although you may not feel pregnant, your uterus will have grown to the size of an apple. During your whole pregnancy, your uterus will expand to become between 500 and 1,000 times its normal size.

BEFORE PREGNANCY   SIX WEEKS

CERVIX
During your pregnancy it remains strong, and tight. In labor, following hormonal changes triggered by the pressure of your baby's head, the cervix thins and widens. The cervix lets go of its "plug" and when it is fully dilated your baby is ready to be born.

UTERUS
The lining of your uterus—the endometrium—thickens to receive the embryo, and its muscular wall grows to accommodate the baby and to give you the strength to push the baby out when the time comes. Once you reach your third trimester, your uterus will start to produce "practice" contractions, known as Braxton Hicks. No one is sure why we have these, but it's assumed it's to prepare the uterus for the job it has to do during birth.

BRAIN

Some research suggests that the more emotional parts of your brain become dominant during pregnancy. This may occur to begin the bonding process with your baby—making you more emotionally attuned to your baby's needs.

LIVER

Your baby's waste passes through your system, which means that your liver has to work harder than usual to detoxify your own body. To accommodate the extra workload, it will often increase in size.

BREASTS

Your breasts prepare to produce milk from as early as seven weeks pregnant and in the following weeks you will notice them begin to grow. You might also notice that your areolae are darker, and that little bumps have appeared around your nipples; these are known as Montgomery's tubercles and these will secrete fluid to help entice your baby to your nipple. Toward the end of your pregnancy, your body will create a highly sophisticated milk manufacturing and delivery system. Lobules within the breast get bigger and, even before you've had your baby, begin to make colostrum—a highly nutritious liquid that your baby drinks before your milk "comes in." Also, the delivery mechanism within your breast increases to make sure there are plenty of channels supplying milk to your nipples.

HEART

Your heart pumps harder throughout your pregnancy, increasing from around 65 beats per minute at the beginning of pregnancy to around 75 beats per minute by the time you are at full term. This is so that your body can meet your baby's increasing demands for nutrients and oxygen as she grows.

SPINE

As your pregnancy progresses, your center of gravity changes. As your belly grows forward, your center of gravity shifts forward, which means you have to "lean back" on your spine to correct your balance and stay upright. Your spine allows you to do this, but the unnatural posture may give you a backache.

PELVIS

This is key to your baby's safety during pregnancy and at birth. At the beginning, the pelvic bones provide protection for your developing uterus. Then, during birth, your pelvis expands and contracts to push your baby through into the birth canal, even forcing her to turn during her descent.

VEINS AND ARTERIES

Your blood volume will increase by up to 45 percent during your pregnancy and it gets better at clotting in preparation for when you give birth to your baby and when the placenta comes away from your uterus—the blood needs to clot quickly to minimize blood loss. Pregnancy hormones cause your blood vessels to dilate—that is, they open up to allow more blood to pass through them.

HIPS

Your body produces increasing amounts of the hormone relaxin, which loosens your ligaments. This can cause a few aches and pains during your pregnancy, but it allows your bones to move outward enough to enable your baby to pass through your pelvis during birth. Your hips may also become more rounded as your body stores extra fat during pregnancy. This provides fuel for making milk.

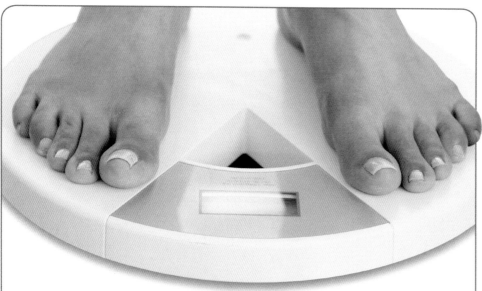

Q I was overweight before I became pregnant. Should I try not to gain weight now?

Never restrict your calorie intake during pregnancy: your baby and you need a basic level of nourishment in order to remain healthy.

This is true for whatever your weight was before you discovered you were pregnant. However, that basic level of nourishment can be slightly different depending upon your weight at the beginning of your pregnancy.

To find out if your prepregnancy weight is within normal range, calculate your body mass index (BMI). You can do this up until 8 weeks of pregnancy since you won't have put on a significant amount of weight by this time. Calculate by dividing your weight in kilograms by your height in meters, then divide it again

(or, use pounds and inches with an online BMI converter). You don't need to consume extra calories during the first and second trimesters—the recommended 2,000 per day is sufficient. In the third trimester you may need to eat 200–300 extra calories per day. Always discuss calorie intake and weight with your doctor before doing any "counting;" the most important thing is that you get enough calories and nutrients for your baby to grow properly. If you don't get enough, you can face a pregnancy that results in birth defects or other problems.

WEIGHT GAIN DURING PREGNANCY

The table below below shows the ideal weight gain during pregnancy for each of the four BMI categories—underweight, ideal weight, overweight, obese.

WEIGHT	BMI	WEIGHT GAIN	IDEAL WEEKLY WEIGHT GAIN
Underweight	less than 18.5	28–40 lb (14–17 kg)	approx 2¼–3 lb (1–1.2 kg) every two weeks in the second and third trimesters
Ideal weight	18.5 to 24.9	25–35 lb (11–16 kg)	approx 1¾–2¼ lb (800 g–1 kg) every two weeks in the second and third trimesters
Overweight	25 to 29.9	15–25 lb (7–11.5 kg)	approx 1–1¾ lb (500–800 g) every two weeks in the second and third trimesters
Obese	30 or higher	11–20 lb (4.5–9 kg)	approx ½–1¼ lb (300–600 g) every two weeks in the second and third trimesters

Q A few years ago I was bulimic. Is this significant now that I'm pregnant?

During pregnancy, your baby receives all its nourishment from you. If your reserves are depleted you can become malnourished and as a result risk having a baby with abnormally low birth weight and other possible problems. If you are suffering from an eating disorder such as bulimia or anorexia, or you are worried that a previous condition will return, you need to inform your doctor. He or she can help you by providing emotional support throughout your pregnancy and also put a plan in place, if you need it, to help you have a healthy pregnancy.

Q How long will it take me to get back to my prepregnancy weight after the birth?

That entirely depends on how much weight you gain during your pregnancy, whether you breast-feed, and how much of a concerted effort

Learn to love your **"mommy tummy."** Even when they lose their pregnancy weight, **some women never have the same figure** they had before they had their baby. Although this may cause wardrobe inconvenience, a different body shape—**curves** and angles in **different places**—it doesn't mean a body that is less attractive. In fact, it could be the start of a whole new image that you love even more than the last.

you make to lose weight after the birth. You'll feel extremely tired in the first few months of taking care of a newborn, and you may not feel up to doing much exercise other than taking your baby out for a walk in the stroller. But that's fine—gentle walking is wonderful exercise and there's no need to push yourself any harder than that. The most important thing is to try not to rush the process. Furthermore, making milk for your baby if you're breast-feeding uses a lot of energy, so you'll need to increase your calorie intake to keep going. In general terms, if getting back to your prepregnancy weight is a priority for you, think of your weight loss according to the old adage "nine months up, nine months down." Give yourself all that time to get back to where you want to be. Don't get frustrated if it takes you longer—some women take many years to regain their prepregnancy weight, often out of choice, waiting until they've completed their family so that they only have to think about weight loss once. Of course, some women also slip right back into their skinny jeans after birth. You're wonderfully lucky—and incredibly unusual—if that turns out to be the case for you.

Q How much of my weight gain is caused by my baby and how much of it is just me?

About a third of your pregnancy weight gain is your baby and the placenta, but that doesn't mean that two-thirds of it is you—or at least it's not "bad-for-you" you.

That two-thirds is made up of increased blood and fluid plumping up your cells; you also have more muscle around your uterus (it helps you to get the baby out), and the increase in progesterone and estrogen mean that your breasts grow larger and therefore heavier even before you start making milk. You also have increased fat reserves (usually around your hips) to prepare you for making milk and breast-feeding. All of these elements of your weight gain are positive, natural, and nothing to worry about. Try to welcome your curvier hips, larger breasts, and glorious skin. They are beautiful signs that your body is doing its job of nourishing your baby.

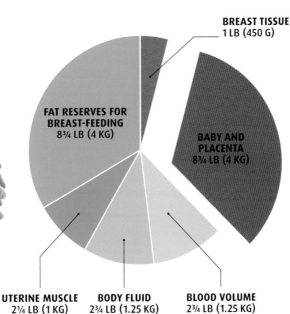

WHERE THE "PREGNANCY WEIGHT" GOES

A woman who gains 26½ lb (12 kg) in weight during her pregnancy will have that gain distributed roughly like this:

BREAST TISSUE
1 LB (450 G)

FAT RESERVES FOR BREAST-FEEDING
8¾ LB (4 KG)

BABY AND PLACENTA
8¾ LB (4 KG)

UTERINE MUSCLE
2¼ LB (1 KG)

BODY FLUID
2¾ LB (1.25 KG)

BLOOD VOLUME
2¾ LB (1.25 KG)

Key areas The increase in volume and weight supports and nourishes your growing baby.

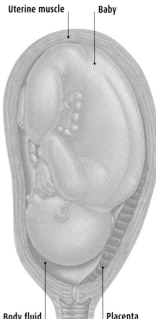

Uterine muscle   Baby

Body fluid   Placenta

Change over the trimesters
Your baby and its placenta will grow; however, the fluid around your baby will reduce.

Growing belly As it grows you will notice other parts of your body changing too. Try to enjoy this time.

Pregnancy is a time of **blooming** and beauty, when your body is doing the most amazing thing possible—**creating** another human being. However, it also means that **your body** undergoes changes to **facilitate** the **growth** of the **baby**, and these can sometimes be less than desirable for you.

Common complaints

Common complaints in pregnancy

The complaints on the following pages highlight side effects that some women experience while pregnant. The common complaints experienced during pregnancy can be grouped into seven main types.

1. General symptoms that are as simple as fatigue, difficulty in sleeping, protruding navel, nasal problems, blurred vision, swollen feet and ankles, fluid retention (edema), foot problems, and headaches.

2. Skin changes such as heat rash and extremely itchy skin.

3. Breast problems, including leaking fluid and clogged milk ducts.

4. Digestive problems such as nausea, vomiting, hyperemesis gravidarum, heartburn, indigestion, constipation, and increased flatulence.

5. Heart and circulation problems for example, dizziness, breathlessness, varicose veins, and hemorrhoids.

6. Aches and pains such as numbness in hands, lower abdominal pressure, abdominal pains, carpal tunnel syndrome, backpain, sciatica, and restless legs.

7. Urinary and vaginal problems which include yeast, vaginal discharge and bleeding, urinary tract infections, and the inability to urinate.

Dealing with common complaints

This section offers explanations and advice for dealing with the range of complaints you may or may not experience during pregnancy. Some are worse than others and some can be embraced as a sign of your belly getting bigger and your baby growing in size (protruding navel). Try to look at the issues you might be encountering as a positive sign that your pregnancy is progressing.

Illness and medications during pregnancy

When you're pregnant your immune system is suppressed slightly so that you don't reject the baby. This means that you might be more likely to get sick. If you are unwell during pregnancy it's important to know how to deal with an illness and which medications you can take. When you're pregnant, you should never take any type of medication on your own without consulting your doctor first—not even something that seems harmless enough, like acetaminophen or over-the-counter cold medication.

{Q What pregnancy complaints might I come across?

ou might be lucky and experience none or only some mild complaints during our pregnancy. Complaints can range from small things that are just plain nnoying such as yeast, to more debilitating conditions, such as severe morning ickness. Whatever you are experiencing, remember that it will soon pass. You ill quickly forget the heartburn or indigestion that pregnancy brings once you're olding your newborn. However, if you are experiencing a complaint that too difficult to deal with then ask your doctor for advice.

Headaches

What, when, and how often?
heavy, pounding head is common in pregnancy—specially if you were prone to headaches during your eriods. Headaches are most common in the early stages pregnancy and usually don't follow any particular pattern confine themselves to one part of the head. Later on ey can be related to anxiety about birth and parenthood.

What causes them?
ormonal changes in your body are probably responsible, though feelings of stress about your pregnancy and tigue can exacerbate the problem.

» What does it mean for my pregnancy?
Mild pregnancy headaches have no implications for your long-term health nor for the health of your baby: they're simply a side effect of what's going on in your changing body. However, if headaches are severe and long lasting, and/or occur later in pregnancy, they could be a sign of preeclampsia, and occasionally headaches in pregnancy indicate a stroke, so talk to your doctor if you're concerned.

» What can I do?
If your headache is bad, you may be able to take acetaminophen, but call your doctor to find out. Stay hydrated, get lots of rest, and limit your caffeine intake. If that doesn't resolve a headache, consult your doctor.

Low iron/anemia

» What, when, and how often?
Iron is the mineral that carries oxygen in your blood. It also helps to build and maintain muscles. The burden of pregnancy can cause your iron levels to drop in early pregnancy. When your iron levels are so low that you are deficient (measured as having less than 11 g of iron per liter of blood), you have anemia. This occurs in almost 22 percent of pregnancies in the US. Low iron levels make you feel lethargic and sometimes dizzy.

» What causes it?
A vegan or vegetarian diet can cause low iron levels, since meat and dairy products are the body's main sources. If you've had babies close together, your reserves will be depleted at the start of your second pregnancy. If you're carrying more than one baby, you're likely to suffer too.

» What does it mean for my pregnancy?
Your body will prioritize the baby's iron (oxygen) requirements over yours, so you'll feel the symptoms of low iron before there's any danger to your baby. You

have a slightly increased risk of having a low birth weight baby or going into labor early.

» What can I do?
Your doctor may prescribe supplements. However, don't take supplements without medical supervision, since having too much iron in your blood can be toxic. Otherwise, try to get plenty of rest and eat lots of iron-rich foods as well as foods rich in vitamin C, which helps your body absorb iron.

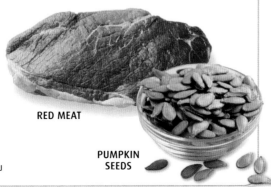

RED MEAT

PUMPKIN SEEDS

Dizziness and breathlessness

» What, when, and how often?
Dizziness, dizzy spells, and breathlessness can occur frequently for women during pregnancy. If you experience frequent dizziness, if you've fainted or had a blackout, or if symptoms are accompanied by swelling in the legs, then inform your doctor as soon as possible.

» What causes it?
In your first trimester dizziness can happen because there's not enough of a blood supply to fill your rapidly expanding circulatory system. In your second trimester it is likely to be caused by the pressure of your expanding uterus on your blood vessels. Dizziness can also be caused by low blood sugar, dehydration, or if you're feeling too hot. When you stand up too quickly it's caused by a quick change of blood flow away from the brain. Breathlessness is caused by your expanding uterus pushing everything upward, leaving your lungs with less room to expand when you take a deep breath. High levels of progesterone also increase your breathing rate.

» What does it mean for my pregnancy?
If you faint or feel dizzy on a regular basis then it might be a sign of anemia. Feeling dizzy every now and then isn't a cause for concern and won't affect your baby. It's completely normal to experience breathlessness and it doesn't harm you or your baby.

» What can I do?
Make sure you stay well-hydrated, get up slowly from lying down or a seated position, keep your blood sugar up, and avoid overheating. If you do feel like you're going to faint then try to increase the blood flow to your brain.

Overheating

» What, when, and how often?
Pregnant women often find they have hot hands and feet and are prone to their faces flushing.

» What causes it?
Increased blood supply to your skin and extremities, hormone changes, and the effort of carrying extra weight.

» What does it mean for my pregnancy?
Feeling hot is just part of being pregnant and isn't an indication of anything that can harm you or your baby.

» What can I do?
Wear loose cotton clothing, pop your feet or hands in a bowl of cold water, and try to keep your rooms cool.

Morning sickness

» What, when, and how often?

Appearing at around the fifth week of pregnancy, and usually at its worst around week 12, then disappearing by around week 20, nausea affects up to 80 percent of women. It can occur at any time of day and cause vomiting. Mild forms cause pervading feelings of nausea. Hyperemesis gravidarum is a stronger form of the condition, but is not common.

» What causes them?

Sudden increased production of pregnancy hormones that upset the gut, as well as a slowing down of the passage of food and waste material through it.

» What does it mean for my pregnancy?

Morning sickness is generally a good sign that your body is working hard to maintain your pregnancy. Hyperemesis gravidarum may, on rare occasions, lead to a baby having low birth weight due to it not getting enough nutrients from you, but overall, women who suffer with morning sickness are statistically less likely to have miscarriages or babies that are born prematurely.

» What can I do?

Snack little and often (see p.58), even if dry crackers are all you can keep down. Try not to have snacks that are high in refined sugar. Avoid strong-smelling and strong-tasting foods, and foods with a high fat content. Drink plenty of fluids and get plenty of rest. See your doctor if you're vomiting three or more times a day, or if you can't face eating anything at all.

Hyperemesis gravidarum

Hyperemesis gravidarum occurs in less than 2 percent of pregnant women. It's a severe form of morning sickness, characterized by frequent vomiting. If you are experiencing this condition and are unable to keep any food or drink down for more than 24 hours then you need to visit your doctor. You will most likely have your urine tested to make sure you don't have an infection. You might also be be given an ultrasound to rule out any issues with your pregnancy. You will be weighed and if you have lost more than 10 percent of your body weight then you are likely to experience complications with your pregnancy. Your doctor might send you to the hospital if you are very dehydrated and you will stay there until you are well enough to go home. In the hospital you will be given intravenous fluids, antinausea medicine, and possibly a vitamin supplement. The good news is that hyperemesis usually disappears when you are 13 weeks pregnant.

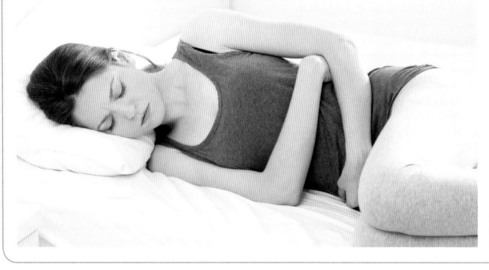

Nap time Try to take short naps or have periods of rest to help deal with the draining feeling that nausea and vomiting bring.

Heartburn and indigestion

» What, when, and how often?

Indigestion is the feeling that you have something permanently stuck in your windpipe, and may make you feel sick or as if you want to burp. Heartburn causes a burning sensation in your throat—it's usually a side effect of indigestion and often occurs after you've eaten. It is known medically as acid reflux. Around 80 percent of pregnant women suffer from indigestion during pregnancy, and it's more likely to occur if this is a second or subsequent pregnancy.

» What causes them?

Everything in your abdomen is squashed as your baby grows, which means that your intestines get pushed upward, making it harder for food to flow seamlessly through your system. This, along with the slowed-down action of your intestine (caused by increased progesterone), means that your stomach acid remains in contact with the lining of your stomach longer than it should, irritating it and causing the symptoms of indigestion. The relaxing of your muscles during pregnancy also relaxes a valve at the bottom of your esophagus, that normally prevents stomach acid from escaping back up to your throat.

» What does it mean for my pregnancy?

There is nothing sinister about indigestion during pregnancy and it poses no risks to you or your baby.

» What can I do?

Avoid spicy or highly flavored foods, and eat little and often so that your stomach has as little to deal with at a time as possible. If your indigestion is affecting your life (perhaps you constantly feel sick or you're burping), you may be able to take antacids to help settle things, but you will need to consult your doctor first.

Try propping yourself up with cushions at night or if you're having a nap during the day. This helps to prevent the acid in your stomach from coming up into your throat.

Flatulence

» What, when, and how often?

Unfortunately, pregnancy can increase the likelihood that you'll need to expel gas from your anus—flatulence. it affects almost all pregnant women at some time during their pregnancy.

» What causes it?

Certain foods, such as those high in fat or carbohydrate, are harder for your body to break down. During pregnancy they spend longer in your intestine than they would if you weren't pregnant and they create gas as they sit there. You expel this gas as flatulence.

» What does it mean for my pregnancy?

Flatulence poses no danger to your health or to that of your unborn baby, but it can be embarrassing and cause cramping. If you have cramping that doesn't feel like gas, contact your doctor.

» What can I do?

Try to avoid eating too many foods that are high in saturated fats and carbohydrates that are known for causing gas (brussels sprouts, prunes, cauliflower, asparagus, cabbage, artichokes, beans, and so on). A balanced diet should keep flatulence to a minimum. Eating little and often will help your gut keep up. Make sure you sit upright when you eat and slowly chew every mouthful of food.

Vaginal discharge

» What, when, and how often?

Known medically as leucorrhea, vaginal discharge is part of your body's natural cleansing system—and it's perfectly normal to have more of it during pregnancy.

» What causes it?

During pregnancy the layer of muscle in the vagina thickens and cells lining the vagina increase in response to rises in the pregnancy hormone estrogen. This helps the vagina to prepare for childbirth. The increase in cells mean a rise in volume of vaginal discharge.

» What does it mean for my pregnancy?

Healthy vaginal discharge is not an indicator of anything being wrong with your pregnancy. It's completely normal.

» What can I do?

If the discharge is so heavy that it could leak onto clothing, use sanitary pads to soak up excess. Consult your doctor if the discharge is foul smelling or tinged with blood. He or she will need to take a swab to see if you have an infection. Consult him or her if the discharge is persistent, which could indicate premature rupture of the membranes. Avoid the temptation to "wash it away" since you could upset your body's natural cleansing and antibacterial balance, and cause yeast.

Yeast

» What, when, and how often?

Yeast—or vaginal candidiasis to give it its medical name—is a fungal infection that causes a proliferation of candida albicans (a natural yeast) in the vaginal tract. It causes increased vaginal discharge (which can smell of yeast), sometimes pain during sexual intercourse, and some soreness and itchiness in the vagina.

» What causes it?

An increase in pregnancy hormones causes the body's natural sugars to increase around the vagina, which "feeds" candida. Sometimes the infection is sexually transmitted, but yeast often occurs while taking, or just after, a course of antibiotics.

» What does it mean for my pregnancy?

During pregnancy, yeast poses no risks to your baby, but the infection can pass to the baby during vaginal birth.

» What can I do?

Avoid using perfumed soaps and bubble baths, which can hamper the work of natural flora in your vagina at fighting the candida infection. See your doctor, who will confirm the infection using a vaginal swab and may then prescribe a topical cream or a suppository to kill the candida (don't use over-the-counter medicines and do not take oral medication for yeast). Usually one prescribed suppository will clear the problem. If you are at the beginning of your pregnancy, you'll probably have to wait until you are in your second trimester to have any treatment at all. Your partner will need to be treated too, since yeast can be passed back and forth between you.

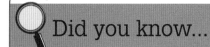

Did you know...

An alternative way to relieve the symptoms of yeast is to smear the area with live yogurt or wear a sanitary pad with live yogurt on the surface (for a short period of time). You can also try a warm bath with a few drops of vinegar added to the water. You should always wear cotton underwear since it allows your vagina to breathe. Do not wear tight jeans or pants that decrease the flow of air to this area and rub against it (if you already have yeast), making you more uncomfortable.

80% of women will experience nausea or vomiting in early pregnancy.

Constipation

» What, when, and how often?

Feeling that you need a bowel movement and either being unable to do so, or finding doing so painful or uncomfortable means that you are constipated. Stools, when they do pass, tend to be hard and dry, and may tear the delicate mucous lining of your bowel as they make their way out. This can cause some bleeding. Constipation can occur at any time during pregnancy, but is common in the first trimester.

» What causes it?

During pregnancy your intestines and bowel have slowed down because of the increase in progesterone in your system. This means that your stool spends longer in your colon, and water gets reabsorbed from it into your body, thus making the stool hard. The effects are compounded later in pregnancy because your bowel, like everything else in your abdomen, is squashed and has less room to do its job. Iron supplements (if you're taking them) can exacerbate constipation, so talk to your doctor about whether it's safe for you to stop.

» What does it mean for my pregnancy?

Constipation is uncomfortable for you and can cause embarrassing gas, but it doesn't pose any harm to your unborn baby.

» What can I do?

Keep yourself hydrated—drink at least eight glasses of water a day, as this will help to keep your stool soft. Make sure your diet contains plenty of fiber (see p.50), including dried fruit such as dried apricots and prunes, which can have a laxative effect on your bowel. Eat little and often so that your bowel doesn't have too much to deal with at any one time. Keep moving: doing regular, gentle exercise appropriate for your pregnancy will also give your bowel a helping hand.

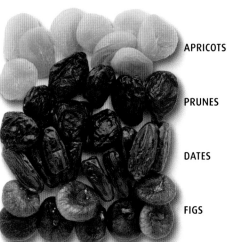

DRINK LOTS OF WATER

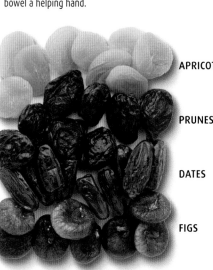

APRICOTS

PRUNES

DATES

FIGS

Urinary tract infection

» What, when, and how often?
A stinging sensation when you urinate is usually the first sign of a bacterial infection in your bladder, also known as cystitis. You may experience lower back pain (in your kidney region), and pain in your abdomen.

» What causes it?
Increased estrogen levels in your system can lead to increased levels of the E. coli bacteria in your gut, which makes you more prone to urinary tract infection. This is compounded by the slower transit of urine through your system as a result of pregnancy hormones, and the increased pressure of your uterus on your ureters—the tubes that carry urine from your kidneys.

» What does it mean for my pregnancy?
Urinary tract infections require treatment with antibiotics. If left untreated, they can lead to a more complicated kidney infection, which can increase the

Cranberries Research has been done into cranberry juice helping to prevent and alleviate the symptoms of urinary tract infections. The results are inconclusive, but it's worth a try.

amount of fluid in your circulation, putting pressure on your heart. About 2 percent of pregnant women in the US develop a kidney infection. This is also treated with antibiotics. You are at a small increased risk of preterm labor, and your baby may catch the infection during birth.

» What can I do?
Drink plenty of fluids throughout your pregnancy to keep flushing out your system. See your doctor right away if you suspect that you have a urinary tract infection.

Inability to urinate

» What, when, and how often?
This sounds like the opposite problem from the one most pregnant women complain about, but it is exactly as it sounds—you feel the need to go to the bathroom, but nothing comes out.

» What causes it?
As the baby grows, your bladder is pushed up inside your abdomen, and once it's out of the way, the baby is free to lie on the urethra—the tube that allows urine to run out of your bladder. If the tube is blocked or squashed, you can't urinate.

» What does it mean for my pregnancy?
You need to be able to drain urine from your body, otherwise toxins are reabsorbed back into your system, and you are at increased risk of getting a kidney infection.

» What can I do?
See your doctor immediately. Usually, your baby will shift position and naturally free up your urethra, but if that doesn't happen, you may need to have a catheter inserted in order to drain urine from your bladder.

Lower abdominal pressure and "PPGP"

» What, when, and how often?
A dull ache or stabbing pain low down in your pelvic region may cause lower abdominal pressure during your

pregnancy, particularly in the later stages. "PPGP" stands for pregnancy-related pelvic girdle pain. It was formerly known as symphysis pubic dysfunction and affects one in five pregnant women. It can be incredibly painful.

» What causes it?
As your uterus grows during your pregnancy, it presses on the various bones and ligaments of your pelvis. This effect is compounded when the baby grows into the space too. PPGP is caused by hormonal changes that affect the way the pelvic joint functions.

» What does it mean for my pregnancy?
There is no danger to you or the baby from this kind of

abdominal pressure—it's just a side effect of pregnancy. If, though, the pain is unbearable it could be a sign that something else is wrong. PPGP can continue for three to six months after the birth.

» What can I do?
For both conditions relax in warm bath water. For PPGP keep your legs together when getting out of bed and into bed or in and out of a car. Sleep on your left side with a pillow between your legs (see p.114). Ask your doctor for an elastic tubular bandage or a support belt.

Abdominal pains

» What, when, and how often?
Early on in your pregnancy, it's common to experience some cramping in your abdomen since your uterus prepares itself to provide a safe house for your developing fetus. By the second trimester, abdominal pain may move to the sides of your abdomen. Pain later in your pregnancy is more likely to be the result of indigestion than anything more sinister.

» What causes them?
Implantation and expansion in your uterus are the most common causes of cramping during early pregnancy. Then, when your body starts to loosen up as a result of increased progesterone and relaxin levels, you may feel as though you're getting pains at the sides of your abdomen—these are just signs that your ligaments are softening to allow room in your pelvis for your growing baby. Occasionally, you may have a small internal bleed in your uterus and this can give you abdominal pain.

» What does it mean for my pregnancy?
Early stage abdominal pains are normal, but mention them to your doctor so that you can be checked to ensure all is well. If you have any pain at any time in your pregnancy that is accompanied by bleeding, call your doctor

Hemorrhoids

» What, when, and how often?
Hemorrhoids are dilated blood vessels around the inside or edge of the anus.

» What causes them?
During pregnancy a woman is more likely to get hemorrhoids because the hormonal softening of the tissues around the anus. Also, the pressure from the baby's head on the blood vessels is another factor. Constipation can cause hemorrhoids to occur.

» What does it mean for my pregnancy?
Having hemorrhoids can be uncomfortable or even painful in more severe cases, but pose no risk to you or your baby.

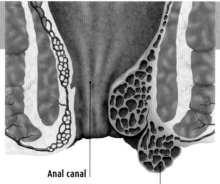

Anal canal

Hemorrhoid

» What can I do?
Avoid getting constipated or straining when you pass stool. Cold packs and creams can relieve the discomfort. A doctor might be able to reduce a hemorrhoid by pushing it gently back into place.

immediately. Cramping later in pregnancy that isn't accompanied by bleeding is probably nothing to worry about, but again mention it to your doctor.

» What can I do?
Most cramping is perfectly benign, but because very occasionally it is a symptom of something more significant it's always important to alert your doctor. Rest as much as you can. A warm bath can help to soothe aching, stretched, and displaced muscles and ligaments.

Restless legs

» What, when, and how often?
A tingling, creepy-crawly sensation in your legs, often when you're lying down or trying to sleep, restless legs affects up to 25 percent of pregnant women in the US and is most commonly reported in the third trimester of pregnancy. It's debilitating because it makes you feel like you want to move around all the time, even when you're trying to sleep.

» What causes it?
No one is really sure why pregnant women are more prone to restless leg syndrome, but it could be that there is increased circulation through the veins, pregnancy weight gain, low iron levels, or it may be a simple side effect of increased hormone levels. Studies indicate that it tends to run in families.

» What does it mean for my pregnancy?
As long as the condition is not related to an iron deficiency (see above), restless legs will pose no harm to you or your baby, aside from making you feel tired if it's hampering your sleep.

» What can I do?
Firstly, ask your doctor to check your iron levels. Do everything you can to encourage sleep—avoid eating too late at night, exercise gently (appropriately for your stage in pregnancy), and treat yourself to a soporific warm bath before bedtime. Walking around can cause temporary relief, as can giving your legs a quick rub.

Varicose veins and vulval varicosities

» What, when, and how often?
Varicose veins are enlarged veins that can develop in the legs and around the vulval area. They can look unsightly.

» What causes them?
During pregnancy the expanding uterus puts pressure on veins in the pelvis. This leads to increased pressure in the legs and vulval area, making varicose veins and vulval varicosities more likely to form (see p.120).

» What does it mean for my pregnancy?
Varicose veins can become uncomfortable and itchy in the later stages of pregnancy, but they aren't dangerous.

Back pain and sciatica

» What, when, and how often?
Most pregnant women experience some dull aching around their lower back during pregnancy. If that pain becomes sharp or shooting it may be sciatica—especially if it runs down the buttocks and backs of the legs, too (or more often down one leg). You are most likely to experience it during your third trimester, when your uterus is expanding into your abdomen and your baby is growing rapidly.

» What causes them?
Lower back pain is commonly caused by the shifting center of gravity as your baby grows and your uterus expands, causing you to stand and walk awkwardly in order to correct your balance. The loosening in your ligaments during pregnancy can also put strain on your back—all thanks to hormonal changes. Sciatica is a specific condition caused when there is compression on your sciatic nerve, which runs from your lower back down your legs. The compression may be the result of your shifting center of gravity, whereby other muscles in your lower back contract to keep you upright and in doing so squeeze the nerve. Or it may be specifically the baby's position in later pregnancy—when your baby's head descends into your pelvis it can press on the nerve. Weight gain and your expanding uterus are also common culprits.

» What does it mean for my pregnancy?
There is no specific danger to your baby from lower back pain or sciatica—the effects are really only on your own well-being and often your mood. Living in constant pain can be debilitating.

Sciatic nerve The main nerve leading to the legs and feet.

Sciatica This artwork shows the path of the nerve and the path of the pain resulting from compression of nerve at the pelvis.

» What can I do?
Kegel exercises (see p.67) and also swimming can help to strengthen and support your lower back, relieving the pain on the nerve. Although it's good not to let your lower back stiffen up, periods of rest when you've taken the weight off your feet will relieve pressure pain. You can try a hot compress on the sore part of your back. Ask your partner to give you a gentle lower back massage. Tell your doctor that you're suffering so that he or she can keep an eye on things. If you are in severe pain you might be referred to an obstetric physical therapist. Always consult your doctor before taking anything to ease your discomfort.

Varicosities in the vagina or vulval area won't rupture during birth or pose any other problems.

» What can I do?
Tell your doctor if you notice that you have developed a varicose vein. Wear pregnancy support hose or support underwear that a doctor can prescribe.

Foot problems

» What, when, and how often?
Many pregnant women suffer from aching arches and cramp in their feet. Swollen ankles and feet are another common pregnancy issue.

» What causes them?
Weight gain can put pressure on the arches of your feet, while using the muscles in your feet to correct your balance is also a cause of aching. Your extremities, including your

feet, are particularly prone to the problems associated with increased fluid in your system, which can cause edema, the medical name for fluid retention (see p.134).

» What does it mean for my pregnancy?
For the health of your baby nothing at all, but foot pain and swollen ankles can make walking around fairly debilitating. If your feet and ankles swell excessively or very suddenly, let your doctor know.

» What can I do?
Take the weight off your feet as much as you can, raising your feet above your hips to help disperse any excess fluid. Keep your feet moving, even when you are sitting. Turning your feet at the ankle, first in one direction and then in the other can help to relieve pain and swelling. Although it may seem counterintuitive, drinking plenty of fluid will help to flush excess from your system. Try to gain weight slowly and wear comfortable footwear with good support.

Edema

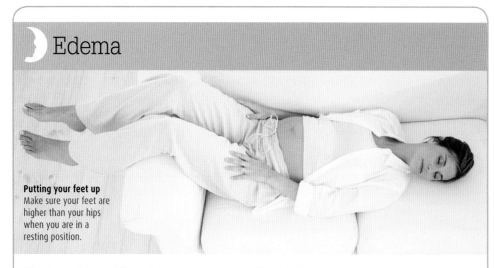

Putting your feet up
Make sure your feet are higher than your hips when you are in a resting position.

>> What, when, and how often?
Edema is otherwise known as water or fluid retention—and it causes swelling and puffiness in your cells. Edema can be partly responsible for a more flushed, plumped-up complexion on your face, but also for swollen ankles, feet, wrists, and fingers. Around half of all pregnant women suffer from edema at some stage in their pregnancy, particularly in the third trimester.

>> What causes it
In order to carry nutrients efficiently to your baby, your blood volume increases by up to one-third during pregnancy. However, not all this increase in volume is made up of extra red blood cells—a large proportion of it is fluid. When the fluid enters the cells in your body, it causes them to swell. Sometimes—especially when you've been stationary for a long period of time, or toward the end of the day, or if the weather is especially hot—the fluid pools in your cells, and this causes the excess swelling.

>> What does it mean for my pregnancy?
Most women will experience some normal swelling during the course of their pregnancy, usually in the extremities (fingers, hands, toes, feet, and ankles). If the swelling is excessive, consult your doctor.

>> What can I do?
Drink plenty of fluid since this helps to flush excess fluid from your body (although it may seem counterintuitive to do so). Eat a healthy diet and try to gain weight steadily throughout your pregnancy. Exercise regularly and appropriately for your pregnancy stage. If you notice that your extremities are swelling, keep them moving—make circles with your wrists and ankles and give your toes and fingers a stretch. Avoid too being stationary for long stretches of time—get up and walk around every 30 minutes or so to prevent fluid from pooling in your legs. When you rest, try to make sure your feet are higher than your hips.

Numbness in hands

>> What, when, and how often?
The very odd sensation of your hand going numb, along with pain in your thumb and first two fingers, may be the result of carpal tunnel syndrome. This condition can occur usually in the second or third trimester of pregnancy and affects around 50 percent of pregnant women. Carpal tunnel syndrome tends to run in families; and you're likely to get it again if you've had it in a previous pregnancy. It occurs most often in the dominant hand (so your right hand if you're right-handed).

>> What causes it?
Your pregnancy hormones increase the amount of fluid circulating in your system. When that fluid pools in your wrists (often at night when you're stationary), causing swelling, it can put pressure on your median nerve, which runs down your arm into your hand. This then leads to numbness and a pins-and-needles sensation in the fingers of your hand. You'll be more susceptible to the condition if you are overweight or are carrying more than one baby.

>> What does it mean for my pregnancy?
If carpal tunnel syndrome is the reason for your numbness, there are no harmful effects for your baby or your pregnancy, but you may find it hard to use your hand properly—in particular you'll probably find that you have a weak grip.

>> What can I do?
Aside from eating healthily and performing wrist exercises (somewhat like the ankle exercises you might try for swollen ankles), all you can do is wait it out. Most cases of carpal tunnel syndrome will pass within a few months of your baby's birth. If you find the numbness lingers, you may need to have surgery to relieve the pressure on your median nerve. Your doctor might give you a wrist support from to help support your hand.

Nasal problems

>> What, when, and how often?
Around one-third of all pregnant women experience nasal problems during pregnancy, commonly beginning around the middle of the second trimester and lasting until birth. Typically, the problems are frequent nosebleeds, increased nasal congestion, and snoring.

>> What causes them?
Nasal congestion and snoring is caused by increased estrogen in your system, which causes a proliferation of mucus in your nasal passages (you may also find you develop blocked ears). Nosebleeds become more frequent because the walls of the tiny capillaries in your nose thin out and are more liable to breaking.

>> What does it mean for my pregnancy?
Nosebleeds that don't stop need medical attention, because they could be a sign of a circulation problem; and very loud, very prolonged snoring may be a sign of gestational diabetes. Other than those circumstances, nasal problems are just a harmless side effect of pregnancy.

>> What can I do?
Talk to your doctor to make sure that what you're experiencing is normal. If there is cause for concern, your doctor will do more checks.

Blurred vision

>> What, when, and how often?
Eye problems are extremely common during pregnancy, most noticeably many women experience blurring in their vision. Dry eyes and temporary loss of peripheral vision may also occur.

>> What causes it?
The cells in your skin start to swell with increased fluid during pregnancy—and the same happens in your eyeballs. This causes the lens in your eye to thicken and distort, blurring your vision. It's possible that the effect is exacerbated because progesterone levels in your body, which cause your muscles to become more lax, may have the same softening effect on your cornea.

>> What does it mean for my pregnancy?
Blurred vision can be a sign of preeclampsia (flashes in your eyes, too), so it's very important that you let your doctor know if you experience any changes to your eyesight. Most of the time, though, it's just another side effect of pregnancy.

>> What can I do?
Keep up your fluid intake to try to minimize fluid retention in your cells. Your vision should return to normal after birth, but it may take several weeks. Some women experience permanent changes to their eyesight, so if you're still having sight problems six weeks after you've had your baby, visit your optician.

PUPPP/PEP skin rash

❱ What, when, and how often?

Pruritic urticarial papules and plaques of pregnancy (PUPPP) and polymorphic eruption of pregnancy (PEP)—is an itchy skin rash that usually appears on the abdomen (other than on the belly button) and then spreads to other parts of the body. It looks a bit like eczema, characterized by small, fluid-filled blisters. It's a condition of late pregnancy—usually occurring from around 35 weeks pregnant, but it occurs in fewer than half a percent of all pregnancies.

❱ What causes it?

No one is sure what causes PUPPP, but it is most common in women carrying boys (interestingly, a study found male DNA in skin biopsies of PUPPP rash) or multiples and in first pregnancies. It rarely occurs during second or subsequent pregnancies. Some people think it may be hereditary.

❱ What does it mean for my pregnancy?

The most significant effect is itchiness, usually worst in the first few days of the condition. It doesn't seem to have any effect on the unborn baby, though as a precaution many doctors recommend that the baby is induced at 39 weeks.

❱ What can I do?

Keep cool by wearing loose-fitting cotton clothing. You can talk to your doctor about topical treatments. The rash disappears of its own accord within a week of having the baby. In rare cases it may linger for a bit longer.

Heat rash

❱ What, when, and how often?

Also known as prickly heat, a heat rash is a raised red, itchy rash that affects parts of the skin where heat builds up—folds in the neck and abdomen, for example.

❱ What causes it?

During pregnancy you will probably feel hotter and sweatier than usual, which can cause a rash to develop where the air can't easily dry away the sweat.

❱ What does it mean for my pregnancy?

Nothing at all other than feeling irritated by your prickly skin. The rash is completely benign and has no side effects.

❱ What can I do?

Keep as cool as possible and wear loose-fitting cotton clothing. Cool and soothe your skin using a washcloth that has been soaked in cold water. Avoid highly scented soaps.

Clogged milk ducts

❱ What, when, and how often?

Many women don't realize that milk production begins during pregnancy. Part of this process means that the milk ducts in your breasts stretch and enlarge to accommodate the increase in fluid. Sometimes, in the second half of your pregnancy, the ducts can get clogged up, making your breasts feel lumpy and tender. The lumps may even look red compared with the rest of the skin on your breast.

❱ What causes it?

Your breasts are busy making milk, but until your baby is born, you don't have an outlet for it. The backup of milk can cause blockages in the ducts.

❱ What does it mean for my pregnancy?

A blocked duct is really a good sign that your body is making milk. It's really nothing to worry about, other than that it can cause some discomfort and tenderness. Note that if the lump isn't red or painful, it would be worth mentioning it to your doctor, just in case it's a breast lump that is unrelated to your milk production.

❱ What can I do?

A cool washcloth placed over the affected area on your breast can help to ease tenderness. Gently use your thumbs and fingers to massage around the blocked duct with the goal of freeing up the blockage. You may have some discharge from your nipple as you do this—that's fine.

Leaking milk

❱ What, when, and how often?

This can occur at any time from your second trimester, but is most likely to occur at the end of your pregnancy as your breasts become full. Usually you will leak colostrum rather than actual milk. Colostrum is a yellowish, thick secretion. It's more digestible and richer in nutrients than breast milk.

❱ What causes it?

Very simply, your breasts fill with milk but until the baby is born, there's no outlet for all the liquid. The result is that some of it gets squeezed out unintentionally from your breasts.

❱ What does it mean for my pregnancy?

Your body is gearing up to feed your baby once he is born. There is no relationship between leaky breasts and ability (or inability) to produce enough milk to nurse a baby.

❱ What can I do?

Use breast pads to soak up any fluid from your nipples. Change them regularly if you need to.

Bleeding

❱ What, when, and how often?

One third of pregnant women will experience some form of spotting or bleeding in their first trimester. It can be brown, pink, or bright red. Sometimes large blood clots are expelled. Bleeding or spotting can happen later on in pregnancy, too.

❱ What causes it?

In early pregnancy the increased levels of hormones make the surface of the cervix fragile and prone to spotting or bleeding. Later your cervix is softer and has increased blood flow to it. As a result it can bleed or become bruised.

❱ What does it mean for my pregnancy?

While worrying, bleeding is common in the first trimester. It doesn't neccessarily mean you have miscarried, though it should always be checked. Bleeding later in pregnancy should always be checked too, as it could be a sign of a low-lying placenta, placental abruption, or preterm labor.

❱ What can I do?

Speak to your doctor as soon as possible. You will probably be offered an ultrasound scan to put your mind at ease and check that nothing is wrong. Report any heavy bleeding immediately, especially if it is accompanied by any pain.

Protruding navel

❱ What, when, and how often?

During the third trimester of pregnancy, your abdomen will be heading toward full stretch and one of the results is that your belly button may appear to "pop out." This usually occurs after the 24th week of pregnancy and happens to almost all pregnant women.

❱ What causes it?

The simple matter of a growing abdomen (growing baby and growing uterus) is the cause of your popped-out belly button.

❱ What does it mean for my pregnancy?

A protruding navel is not the sign of anything sinister going on and its only effect is that it might look like a very low third nipple if you're wearing tight-fitting clothes.

❱ What can I do?

Absolutely nothing. Your belly button will stop protruding and sit neatly back in its original position as soon as you've had your baby.

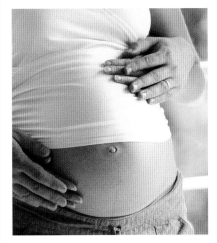

Standing proud If you are happy with your changing body, then show off your belly.

{Q} I don't feel very well. What medications are considered safe in pregnancy?

It's normal to get sick from time to time during pregnancy (especially since your immune system is suppressed), but the over-the-counter (OTC) medications you would naturally turn to if you weren't pregnant aren't necessarily safe. Be extra careful and always check with your doctor before taking any remedies.

Many minor ailments, such as common colds and diarrhoea, resolve themselves without medication. If you think you do need treatment, seek advice from a doctor—and always let him or her know you are pregnant. Before using an OTC remedy, check with the pharmacist that it's safe in pregnancy, take it at the lowest dose possible, and limit using it to the shortest amount of time possible. Many natural medicines—and particularly herbal remedies—can be unsafe for your developing baby.

It is best to avoid **over-the-counter medications** entirely—especially in the first trimester when your baby is most susceptible to risk.

Prevention is better than cure

You can be more susceptible to infections during pregnancy because your body is suppressing its immune system in order to maintain your pregnancy. You can boost your immunity and protect yourself against infection through good diet, moderate exercise, and sensible hygiene.

» **Wash your hands** before preparing or eating food, and practice safe toileting habits.

» **Drink plenty of water** and diluted juice, too, since fluids will help flush any infection from your system.

» **Boost your intake** of antioxidant foods (such as fruit and vegetables), which can support your immune system.

» **Get plenty of rest** since you're more likely to become sick if you feel tired and depleted.

» **Always talk to a doctor** before taking any natural remedy, even something as seemingly innocuous as an herbal tea.

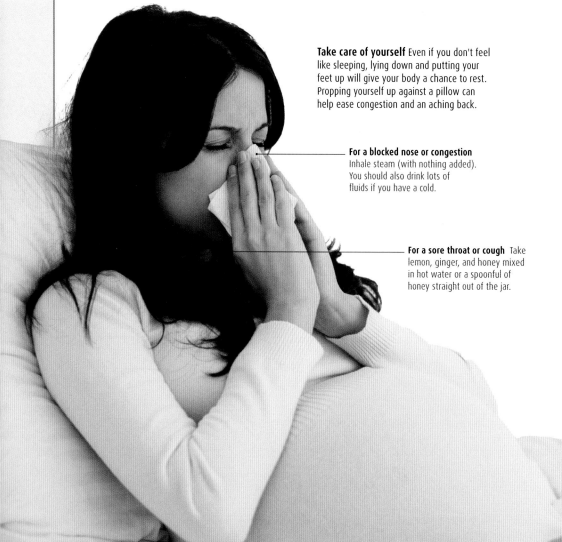

Take care of yourself Even if you don't feel like sleeping, lying down and putting your feet up will give your body a chance to rest. Propping yourself up against a pillow can help ease congestion and an aching back.

For a blocked nose or congestion Inhale steam (with nothing added). You should also drink lots of fluids if you have a cold.

For a sore throat or cough Take lemon, ginger, and honey mixed in hot water or a spoonful of honey straight out of the jar.

COMMON AILMENTS

No medication is 100 percent safe in pregnancy. Don't take any over-the-counter medication, dietary supplement or herbal remedy without checking first with your doctor about its safety during pregnancy.

AILMENT	WHAT DOES IT MEAN FOR MY PREGNANCY?	WHAT CAN I DO?
Flu and common colds	The common cold virus should not affect your baby, but severe flu may increase the risk of low birth weight. Flu can also lead to the more serious bronchitis, or even pneumonia. Colds are dehydrating so keep your fluid levels up.	Keep up your fluid intake, and use steam inhalation and hot, soothing beverages to relieve symptoms (see opposite). If you have a fever, ask your doctor if you can take acetaminophen. (This medication is preferable to ibuprofen or codeine). If you have flu symptoms, see your doctor, who may give you medicine to help shorten the duration of it.
Fever	A high temperature can affect your blood circulation so you should try to bring the fever down. Fever usually indicates a viral or bacterial infection.	Use a sponge dipped in cold water, cold compress, or ice bath to bring down your temperature. You can take acetaminophen if your doctor says it's okay—but do not exceed the maximum daily dosage stated on the box. Call your doctor if your temperature is more than 104° F (40° C).
Ear, throat, chest, or urinary tract infection	Severe bacterial infection can cross the placental barrier and affect your baby so it is important to see your doctor to get any infection treated.	Drink plenty of fluids, and see your doctor. Many antibiotics are safe in pregnancy, but they must be prescribed. He or she may do tests (saliva, or urine for example) to check which antibiotic would be most suitable. Take acetaminophen, if your doctor allows, to reduce the fever.
Diarrhea	Diarrhea will not harm your baby, but you must avoid dehydration. If your diarrhea is combined with vomiting or fever, speak to your doctor.	Diarrhea will usually stop on its own once your body has expelled the infection. Don't take diarrhea medication unless it is prescribed by your doctor. Rehydration solutions are safe to take, but consult your pharmacist first.
Food poisoning	The bacteria that cause food poisoning can be potentially harmful to your baby. The most dangerous of these is listeria, which can cause blood poisoning, meningitis, and pneumonia.	Let your doctor know if you suspect food poisoning and you will be advised on what, if anything, you can take to ease the symptoms. It is important to keep sipping water so that you don't become dehydrated. If you suspect listeriosis, seek help right away.
Pain	Backaches can be quite common in pregnancy, especially in the third trimester. Headache, muscular pain, and back pain will not affect your baby.	Ice and warm compresses can help muscular pain and sprains and back pain respectively, but see your doctor for persistent headaches. You can take acetaminophen if your doctor allows, but don't exceed the maximum daily dosage. Do not take ibuprofen or codeine.
Insomnia	Insomnia is quite common in pregnancy but can stem from a variety of causes. It should not affect your baby, but will be very tiring for you.	Consult your doctor to identify the causes and discuss steps you can take. Do not use any herbal remedies, aromatherapy, or medication to induce sleep without seeking advice first.
Hayfever	While hayfever does not affect your baby, treatment of it can. Always seek advice from your doctor before taking any form of antihistamine.	See your doctor. Some antihistamines are fine to use in pregnancy, but it is likely that you'll be advised to use them in the form of a nasal spray or eye drops rather than pills.
Fungal infections (such as athlete's foot)	Fungal infections such as athlete's foot or yeast have no effect on your unborn baby, but treatments for them can.	Keep the affected area clean, dry, and well-aired. Your doctor will want to see you to prescribe the right (pregnancy-friendly) medication for your situation. Not all OTC fungal treatments are safe in pregnancy. Speak to your doctor.
Itchy skin	Dry, itchy skin complaints can occur for a number of reasons, including eczema and pregnancy-induced pruritis gravidarum, which can be severe.	You can use emollients and water-based creams, which are available over the counter, but you should not use steroidal creams. Ask a pharmacist which are the safest options, or speak to your doctor.
Rashes	Rashes can be concentrated in one area (localized), or all over (generalized). Some rashes are harmless, but you should get them checked to find out the cause.	Ask your doctor to check your rash. If any rash (whether local or generalized) persists for more than 48 hours, see your doctor. You can use calamine lotion to relieve the symptoms of localized rashes, but not generalized ones. Cold water and ice can also help.
Cuts and scrapes	A minor cut or scrape will not harm your baby, but take the usual steps to keep the wound clean and free from infection.	Clean the wound using an antiseptic and keep it dry. Although antiseptics are not thought to be hazardous to pregnancy, check with your pharmacist for the safest options to use.
Head lice	Head lice are annoying for you, but luckily don't pose a threat to your unborn baby.	Tackle the problem first with a head-lice comb. Use the comb on wet hair; repeat every three days to keep clearing young lice as they hatch. You can get 4 percent dimethicone lotion over the counter, but always let the pharmacist know you are pregnant first.
Pinworms	Pinworm infection is not known to put your unborn baby at risk, but treatment for it can.	OTC treatments are not advised when you are pregnant, but strict hygiene measures can treat the pinworms (they have a life cycle of six weeks). See your doctor for advice.

Not every pregnancy is as straightforward as it could be. Complications don't happen to most women—**they are not the norm**—but if you experience a problem you will get **lots of support** from your doctor. With careful attention, the majority of complications have **good outcomes**.

Complications

Types of complication

A "complication" is a medical condition that could potentially compromise your health or that of your unborn baby. Many of the checkups you are given as part of your prenatal care (and in your preconception care when you plan a pregnancy) are designed to identify any complications that could occur as early as possible. In many situations, your doctor can manage problems to keep you and your baby as safe as possible.

There are a few broad types of complication. Some women have a long-term condition, such as asthma or congenital heart disease, that warrants special attention. Sometimes previous gynecological issues may have an effect on your pregnancy. Other complications can arise as a result of pregnancy—gestational diabetes and preeclampsia are examples of these. More rarely, some short-term infections can pose problems.

Plan pregnancy where possible

If you are able, it is a good idea to check your immunity to certain infectious diseases before trying to get pregnant. You can be vaccinated before conception, but not while you are pregnant because some vaccines can harm a fetus.

If you have a preexisting illness that requires medication and you are not already pregnant, you are strongly advised to put a preconception plan in place. Some medications aren't suitable for pregnancy, and some conditions need to be stabilized before you become pregnant. Giving yourself three to six months to get things planned and under control before conception can often mean the difference between a straightforward pregnancy and a difficult one.

When complications arise

If you experience a complication, your level of prenatal care might gear up with more tests, ultrasounds, and treatments. Throughout this process your doctor will explain what is going on in your body and its potential effects on your pregnancy, labor, birth, and baby.

Take someone with you to ultrasounds and appointments with specialists—they can listen if you are not able to take everything in. Sometimes you may need to make difficult decisions about whether or not to take medications that can help you, but potentially affect your baby. Sometimes, a complication might dictate where, when, and how you deliver your baby, forcing you to make unexpected decisions. It's natural to feel scared or nervous. There are support groups for people in the same situation as you—ask your doctor for information on these.

{ Q What happens if I get an infectious disease while I'm pregnant?

Treatment options are limited when you are pregnant, so some infections do present risks to your pregnancy. You should contact your doctor if you notice symptoms of serious infections.

Chicken pox

» What is it?
Also known as varicella, this viral infection causes fever and itchy red spots on the skin that turn into blisters.

» What does it mean for my pregnancy?
Complications from catching chicken pox are rare, but potentially serious. It can damage a fetus's eyes, brain, skin, limbs, bladder, or bowel. Risks to you include pneumonia, and inflammation in the brain and liver.

» What can I do?
If you have not had chicken pox before and come into contact with it, or if you develop symptoms, consult your doctor immediately. Antiviral therapy can help prevent any complications, although it can't cure the infection.

Measles

» What is it?
Measles causes flulike symptoms, spots in the mouth, and a red-brown rash that lasts for just over a week. Due to vaccination programs, measles is now rare in the US.

» What does it mean for my pregnancy?
Developing measles increases the risk of miscarriage, stillbirth, and premature birth, especially in the first trimester. The infection can also pass to your baby during birth.

» What can I do?
See your doctor immediately if you come into contact with the virus (it can take up to three weeks to develop) and you are not immune or vaccinated. You can be treated with human normal immunoglobin (HNIG), which lessens the symptoms and reduces (but doesn't eliminate) the risk to your baby.

Mumps

» What is it?
This viral infection causes fever and headache, and swelling of the cheeks and the salivary glands in the neck. Due to vaccination programs, mumps is now rare in the US.

» What does it mean for my pregnancy?
Mumps should not cause any birth defects in your unborn baby, but it can increase the risk of miscarriage through your fever and illness, especially in your first trimester. It can also develop into meningitis.

» What can I do?
If you lack immunity, consult your doctor as soon as you come into contact with anyone with mumps (symptoms may take two to three weeks to develop). Mumps cannot be treated but there are ways to ease the symptoms.

Rubella

» What is it?
Also called German measles, the rubella virus causes symptoms of headaches, fever, joint pain, sore throat, swollen glands, and a raised red-pink rash. Due to vaccination programs, rubella is now rare in the US.

» What does it mean for my pregnancy?
If you contract rubella before you are 18 weeks pregnant, it can cause serious birth defects and miscarriage. The later in pregnancy the disease affects you, the lower the risk. After 18 weeks, the risks to the baby are minimal.

» What can I do?
If you have not been vaccinated, try to avoid contact with rubella. If you think you could be infected, see your doctor immediately for diagnosis. There is no treatment for rubella, but your doctor will support you and advise options if the baby has congenital rubella syndrome (CRS).

Cytomegalovirus

» What is it?
A type of herpes, cytomegalovirus (CMV) is transmitted via saliva, urine, semen, or feces. It can lie dormant (without symptoms) and many people don't realize they have it.

» What does it mean for my pregnancy?
If you have CMV and it becomes active for the first time during your pregnancy (a primary infection), it can cause congenital disabilities and neurological problems in your baby. However, only about 1 in 750 babies in the US develops complications due to CMV.

» What can I do?
There is no cure for CMV, but you can try to prevent primary infection. Children under six are often carriers, so avoid contact with their feces, urine, or saliva (kiss them on the head rather than mouth or cheeks). Many adults don't know they have the virus, so use a condom if you have sex.

Lyme disease

» What is it?
This bacterial, tick-borne infection can go undetected for many years. Symptoms include fever, chills, joint or muscle pain, facial paralysis, and a red rash with an outer red ring.

» What does it mean for my pregnancy?
Lyme disease is potentially serious for you if untreated. It increases the risk of premature birth and miscarriage.

» What can I do?
Your doctor can give you a course of antibiotics—with treatment, the outcome for you and your baby is very good. You can get infected again after treatment, if bitten again, so take precautions to prevent tick bites.

Hepatitis

» What is it?
All forms of this blood-borne virus infect the liver. Symptoms can range from vomiting and stomach cramps, to mild, coldlike illness. Some people have no symptoms.

» What does it mean for my pregnancy?
Hepatitis can cause liver failure in a fetus. All women are offered hepatitis B (HBV) screening as part of prenatal care. Hepatitis C (HCV) is checked if you have risk factors.

» What can I do?
If you have HBV, your baby can be vaccinated against it at birth—this immunization has a 95 percent success rate. Passing HCV to a baby is more rare, but if your baby is infected he will be referred to a specialist for assessment.

If you are not sure whether you have **immunity** to chicken pox or whether you have been **vaccinated** against measles, mumps, or rubella, your doctor can do a **blood test** to check.

This section is a guide to some long-term (or chronic) conditions that can impact a pregnancy. Ideally, optimize your control of these conditions prepregnancy. Once pregnant, your care will be with an obstetrician. Most women with these conditions have healthy pregnancies and babies, though a home- or birth-center birth may not be recommended.

Asthma

» What is it?
This respiratory condition inflames and narrows the lung's airways, causing wheezing, coughing, chest tightness, and shortness of breath.

» Risks to your pregnancy, labor, and baby
Asthma is linked with placental problems, including low-lying placenta and placenta with poor function (reduced oxygen and nutrient supply), which slightly increases your risk of having a low birth weight baby and miscarriage.

» Medicines and tests
Asthma medication has no side effects on the unborn baby, so continue to take your medicines throughout your pregnancy. If you take oral steroids, you may need regular blood tests to check your glucose levels. Your pain relief choices may be limited during labor since diamorphine and other opioid analgesics can exacerbate asthma.

» Effects of pregnancy on your condition
If you have severe asthma at the beginning of pregnancy, it may become worse during pregnancy. Otherwise, asthma tends to stay the same or even improve in pregnancy, since increased levels of natural steroids can reduce attacks. Baby girls are statistically more likely to worsen asthma symptoms in the pregnant mother than baby boys.

Inflammatory bowel disease (IBD)

» What is it?
IBD describes inflammatory conditions of the digestive system, such as ulcerative colitis and Crohn's disease. It can cause pain, swelling, and cramps in the stomach, recurrent or bloody diarrhea, extreme fatigue, and weight loss. IBD does not include irritable bowel syndrome (IBS).

» Risks to your pregnancy, labor, and baby
Whether active or inactive, IBD can slightly raise the chance of a baby being "small for dates" and premature labor. If

you are at risk of needing bowel surgery in the future, your doctors may suggest a C-section to preserve the pelvic floor muscles that are crucial to bowel function. Your baby's chance of inheriting Crohn's Disease is small (5 percent) unless both you and your partner have it (36 percent).

» Medicines and tests
If you take methotrexate, stop taking it when you know you're pregnant (or ideally as part of your preconception care) because it can cause birth defects. You can continue with other medications, but see your gastroenterologist as soon as you can for a medication review, since managing your IBD is still a priority in pregnancy. Your doctor may advise increased dosage of folic acid because some IBD medicine can interfere with folate absorption. You may have a couple of extra appointments with your gastroenterologist during pregnancy to check that all is well. There is no reported ill effect if you have to have a colonoscopy or sigmoidoscopy to check the health of your bowel during your pregnancy.

» Effects of pregnancy on your condition
If your IBD is inactive at the time you become pregnant, and you continue your medication, the chances of a flare-up are no greater than if you were not pregnant, but you may have a flare-up after the birth. Active IBD might be more difficult to control while you are pregnant. If you have a stoma or pouch, it may become squashed as your abdomen grows, which may then increase your bowel frequency.

Hypertension

» What is it?
Hypertension (high blood pressure) is a higher than recommended pressure in your arteries. This condition puts you at increased risk of heart attack and stroke.

» Risks to your pregnancy, labor, and baby
You are more vulnerable to preeclampsia, placental abruption, stroke, and blood clots; your baby to premature birth, low birth weight, and a slight risk of stillbirth. You will usually be encouraged to have a natural birth, if this is what you want, unless there are specific reasons for advising a cesarean section.

» Medicines and tests
Continue to take your medication, but consult your doctor for a medication review since some blood-pressure lowering medicine may adversely affect your baby's development. If your blood pressure is raised, it will be monitored between your regular prenatal appointments. You may be advised to take a low dose of aspirin daily in order to thin your blood, if you don't already take one. You may also be given additional ultrasounds to check your baby's growth. Your labor may be induced early if your blood pressure remains high and needs controlling.

» Effects of pregnancy on your condition
Pregnancy hormones dilate your blood vessels, so you

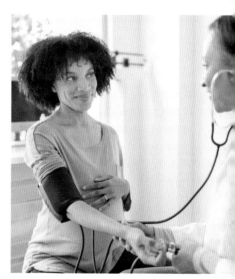

Regular monitoring is essential, whether you are managing your high blood pressure with lifestyle changes or with medication.

might find that your blood pressure decreases naturally for almost all of the nine months (rising again slightly at the end). In some cases, your doctor may even feel that you are able to stop taking blood-pressure lowering medicine during pregnancy.

Thyroid problems

What are they?
The thyroid gland regulates the body's metabolism. Disorders occur if it produces more thyroid hormones than the body needs, or not enough.

Risks to your pregnancy, labor, and baby
Untreated hyperthyroidism (overactive thyroid) or hypothyroidism (underactive thyroid) can pose serious problems in pregnancy. Thyroid hormones play a key role in developing your baby, so your doctors will try to keep your condition under control and avoid the risks of preeclampsia, heart failure, kidney failure, coma, premature labor, stillbirth, miscarriage. Preconception planning is very important to optimize your control of the condition as some studies suggest that a very underactive thyroid in the first trimester may affect a baby's IQ and increase the risk of learning difficulties.

Medicines and tests
Your doctor may review your medication and possibly advise increased dosage if you need it. Hypothyroidism is sometimes treated with the synthetic hormone thyroxine during pregnancy. Your thyroid function will be checked regularly throughout your pregnancy using blood tests. You will have additional ultrasounds to check the health your baby during your third trimester.

Effects of pregnancy on your condition
Women with an overactive thyroid that is stable may have a relapse since pregnancy hormones can increase the circulating levels of thyroid hormone in the blood. Pregnancy can cause swelling in the thyroid gland, called a goiter.

Rheumatoid arthritis

What is it?
This long-term inflammatory disease causes pain, swelling, and stiffness or immobility in the joints.

Risks to your pregnancy, labor, and baby
Other than a possibility of premature labor, rheumatoid arthritis (RA) doesn't usually directly affect your pregnancy or baby. If it affects your hips or pelvis, you may need to have a cesarean section.

Medicines and tests
Some RA medications are not safe for the baby. Others are safe, but can cause raised blood glucose or high blood pressure for you. Talk to your doctor as soon as you discover that you are pregnant (or planning a pregnancy) to discuss your medication.

Effects of pregnancy on your condition
Pregnancy can increase symptoms of fatigue, especially in the first trimester. In the second trimester, research suggests that in up to 70 percent of women with RA symptoms may improve, with these improvements lasting for the first few weeks after pregnancy. However, some women experience a flare-up after this period.

Diabetes

» What is it?
Diabetes is a condition in which the body is unable to control blood glucose levels, either because it produces too little insulin, or because it cannot use the insulin it produces (see box, right). Diabetes in pregnancy can be preexisting or can develop in pregnancy (gestational diabetes, see p.145). Here we discuss preexisting diabetes.

» Risks to your pregnancy, labor, and baby
Diabetes increases your risk of high blood pressure and preeclampsia (see p.144), and of having a baby with birth defects. It also increases your risk of miscarriage, stillbirth, and preterm labor. High glucose levels in your blood mean that glucose in your baby's blood also increases, and your baby may be large at birth. Babies born to diabetic mothers may also be small at birth.

» Medicines and tests
It is very important to optimize your control of diabetes prepregnancy to minimize the chances of birth defects. It is also essential to continue to manage glucose levels once pregnant. Talk to your doctor as soon as you know that you're pregnant for a referral to an an endocrinologist or a diabetes specialist. He or she will give you glucose targets to maintain in pregnancy. If you are on synthetic medicines you may switch to insulin injections, or you may continue with your oral medicine. You will need to follow a glucose-friendly diet; a dietician will work out a meal plan with you. Your doctor will encourage you to test your blood glucose levels at least four times a day to make sure they remain on target. As your pregnancy progresses, you'll probably have to increase the amount of insulin you inject to keep glucose levels stable. Make sure that your friends and family know how to use the testing kits, too, just in case you have a hypo or hyper episode (both of which can lead to unconsciousness) and aren't able to test for yourself. Throughout your pregnancy, you might be offered additional growth ultrasounds to make sure your baby is growing appropriately, remembering that a large baby may indicate that your blood glucose levels are too high.

» Effects of pregnancy on your condition
Pregnancy hormones increase insulin resistance; that is, they exacerbate your body's inability to use insulin to regulate blood glucose levels. As a result, you are at a greater risk of all the complications of diabetes—hypo- and hyperglycemia, eye problems, heart disease, and kidney disease, and you'll be monitored closely for these. If you suffer from vomiting, the concentration of acids called ketones may increase in your blood. Ketones are a by-product of burning fat reserves for energy, rather than glucose. Excessively high levels can lead to serious pregnancy complications, and may be life-threatening for you. This situation is extremely rare, and most women with diabetes have healthy pregnancies, but managing your glucose levels through your diet and insulin injections is of utmost importance.

DIABETES FACTS

Here are the important facts about preexisting diabetes and the signs to look for if haven't already been diagnosed.

» **Your body derives glucose** from the food you eat, in particular from carbohydrates, fats, and proteins in your diet.

» **The symptoms of diabetes** include having a dry mouth, frequently needing to urinate, fatigue, blurred vision, and yeast—almost all of which are also perfectly healthy symptoms of pregnancy!

» **Type I diabetes** occurs when your body makes too little of the hormone insulin, which it needs to take glucose from your bloodstream and turn it into energy.

» **Type II diabetes** occurs when your body makes enough insulin, but its cells become resistant to the hormone's attempts to draw glucose from them. It is often caused by obesity.

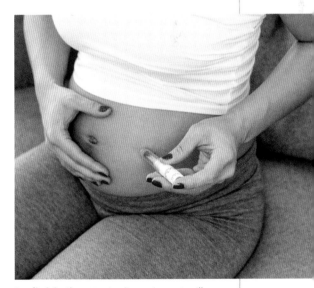

Insulin injections Your insulin requirements will change throughout your pregnancy. It's crucial that you keep your blood sugar under control.

Mental health problems

What are they?
Conditions as diverse as bipolar disease, depression, psychosis, neurosis, self harming, obsessive-compulsive disorder, addictions, and eating disorders.

Risks to your pregnancy, labor, and baby
Medications for mental health problems can affect the health of your unborn baby. You are also at increased risk of developing prenatal depression and postpartum depression. You may feel unable to take care of yourself and unwilling or unable to nurture your unborn baby; if you have an eating disorder, you may restrict your baby's access to important nutrients in utero. Studies show that babies born to women suffering from mental health problems are also at greater risk of developing depression-related conditions themselves in later life.

Medicines and tests
Do not change or stop taking your medication without first consulting your doctor. He or she will need to make a full assessment of your condition and will devise a medication maintenance program that you can use throughout your pregnancy to minimize the risks for your baby, while maintaining your health.

Effects of pregnancy on your condition
Scientific studies show that the anxiety associated with being pregnant, as well as the need to reduce medication can put women with a history of mental illness at greater risk of psychosis or depression during pregnancy. However, if your condition is under control before you're pregnant, there is evidence to suggest that with the right level of support and medicine, you are not at a significantly increased risk of a relapse.

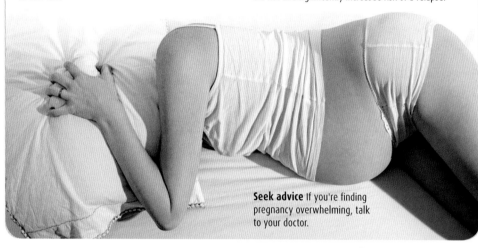

Seek advice If you're finding pregnancy overwhelming, talk to your doctor.

Epilepsy

What is it?
A disorder of the electrical signals in the brain, epilepsy causes repeated seizures.

Risks to your pregnancy, labor, and baby
You might experience nausea and vomiting, anemia, pregnancy-induced hypertension, or preeclampsia. Seizures don't harm your baby unless they're tonic clonic, clustered, or last for more than 30 minutes—all of which can starve a fetus of oxygen. Injuring yourself during a seizure could also harm the baby. Don't shower or bathe in pregnancy, or bathe your newborn, with the door locked or when there is no one in the house. There is a higher risk of premature or prolonged labor, and needing a C-section. After birth, your baby may have withdrawal from epilepsy medicines (AEDs) and may need an extra dose of vitamin K to help with blood clotting.

Medicines and tests
Take your medication unless your neurologist advises you not to. Some AEDs increase the risk of newborn congenital abnormalities, but 90 percent of women with epilepsy have healthy babies. The risks to your baby if you have a seizure are greater. A blood test can assess the levels of medicine in your body since increased blood volume in pregnancy means your usual dosage may be too diluted. Change your dosage only under medical advice. Talk to your doctor about increasing folic acid intake since some medicines inhibit its absorption (though folic acid can inhibit the efficacy of your medication). You may need a vitamin K supplement from week 36, since epilepsy medicines can affect blood clotting. You may need to avoid opioid analgesics in labor.

Effects of pregnancy on your condition
Most women with epilepsy find that there is no change in pregnancy. Sometimes symptoms improve; in other cases seizures increase, which may continue after birth. If seizures increase, ask your neurologist to review your medication.

Congenital/acquired heart disease

What are they?
Congenital heart disease (CHD) is a condition you're born with. Acquired heart disease (AHD) is usually caused by rheumatic fever, Kawasaki disease, or obesity.

Effects on your pregnancy, labor, and baby
Your baby is at a slightly increased risk of developing congenital heart defects (even if your own heart disease is acquired). There may be restricted oxygen to your baby, which can cause low birth weight, premature birth, or stillbirth. You are at increased risk of fluid on your lungs—see your doctor if you experience any chest pains or abnormally increased coughing. A recent study found that women with congenital heart disease were more likely to have a cesarean section and longer hospital stays. You'll be encouraged to give birth lying on your left-hand side, as this reduces the pressure on your major blood vessels. Your breathing during the final stage of labor will be carefully guided so that you don't hold your breath. Your baby will be attached to a fetal heart monitor throughout labor, and you will probably need your own continual ECG reading. You may need to have antibiotics during labor in order to reduce your risk of heart infection.

Medicines and tests
Your doctor may suggest increased blood pressure checks as a noninvasive measure of your circulation function. Anticoagulant medication can cross the placenta and cause your baby's blood to thin dangerously. Your doctor will advise you on keeping you and your baby healthy.

Effects of pregnancy on your condition
Your weight, diet, and exercise levels will be monitored over your pregnancy to ensure good nutrition and steady weight gain; excess weight during pregnancy can put strain on your heart. The opening of your blood vessels is a natural side effect of increased progesterone. This can help blood flow to your heart, but increased blood volume and any shortening of breath can strain your heart.

Systemic lupus erythematosus

What is it?
Sometimes known simply as "lupus," or SLE, this autoimmune disorder causes the immune system to attack healthy tissue in its own body by mistake.

Effects on your pregnancy, labor, and baby
You are at increased risk of preeclampsia, premature labor, miscarriage, and stillbirth. If SLE has affected your kidneys, you may be at increased risk of high blood pressure. If SLE antibodies cross the placenta, this can cause a harmless skin rash in the baby at birth, and more seriously, your baby

may have a heart arrhythmia, so if you have antibodies, your baby will be monitored in pregnancy. Babies may show signs of some liver or kidney disfunction at birth. In most cases this will right itself within six months and babies generally show no long-lasting effects.

≫ Medicines and tests

Throughout your pregnancy, your obstetrician, as well as your SLE doctor, will arrange additional visits to assess you and your baby. You'll need to see your rheumatologist at least once every three months throughout. Take your medication, unless your doctors advise you otherwise. There is a much better outcome for your pregnancy and baby if your lupus is under control.

≫ Effects of pregnancy on your condition

Pregnancy shouldn't cause any extra complications for sufferers of SLE as long as it's under control at conception.

Multiple sclerosis

≫ What is it?

Multiple sclerosis (MS) damages nerve cells in the brain and spinal cord, affecting muscle movement, balance, and vision.

≫ Effects on your pregnancy, labor, and baby

MS seems to have no secondary effects for your pregnancy or baby. If MS has affected your ability to feel contractions in the muscles of your pelvis, you may need to have an assisted birth or a C-section. There is only a very small increased risk that your baby will inherit MS. You do have an increased risk of a relapse in pregnancy and after the birth.

≫ Medicines and tests

Consult your doctor about your medication. Many women with MS can continue to take steroids, particularly after the first trimester. You may have additional prenatal visits.

≫ Effects of pregnancy on your condition

Hormone levels may help reduce the rate of MS relapse during pregnancy, particularly during the third trimester. You may experience exacerbated symptoms of fatigue, back pain, bowel dysfunction, and bladder weakness, as well as an impaired sense of balance as your baby grows and your center of gravity shifts forward. Your increased risk of falls may mean that you need increased support when moving.

Sickle-cell disease

≫ What is it?

A group of genetic blood disorders, such as sickle-cell anemia and thalassemia. Affected hemoglobin in the red blood cells means they are unable to carry oxygen efficiently around the body, causing lack of energy, sudden attacks of pain, or ongoing pain when the tissues are starved of oxygen, and damage to internal organs over time.

≫ Effects on your pregnancy, labor, and baby

You have an increased risk of premature labor and a low birth weight baby. Your baby will carry the sickle-cell gene (even if the baby's father has no sickle-cell gene); if the father is a carrier (without symptoms), your baby has a 50 percent chance of being born with sickle-cell disease (and a 50 percent chance of being a carrier). Your partner can be screened to figure out the risk of your baby inheriting the disease. You're at increased risk of preeclampsia, high blood pressure, stroke, breathing difficulties, and anemia. Your doctor may advise you to give birth in the hospital, where your baby will be attached to a fetal heart monitor during labor. During labor and delivery, you won't be offered every pain-relief medicine that other women are offered, but some analgesics should be fine.

≫ Medicines and tests

You will have lots of prenatal appointments, as well as regular visits to your hematologist. You may be advised to take extra folic acid and have a course of antibiotics to help protect you against infection. You may be advised to take a small daily dosage of aspirin after your first trimester to reduce the risk of high blood pressure. You will be offered an early ultrasound at between 7 and 9 weeks to assess the viability of your pregnancy, and then growth ultrasounds for your baby once a month in your last trimester.

≫ Effects of pregnancy on your condition

SCD symptoms may worsen during pregnancy. Sickness can exacerbate them—consult your doctor about the best way to minimize the effects.

Phenylketonuria

≫ What is it?

In this genetic condition, the body cannot break down phenylalanine, which can cause brain and nerve damage.

≫ Risks to your pregnancy, labor, and baby

High levels of phenylalanine can cross the placenta and cause serious defects and even fatality in your unborn baby. You will need to adhere strictly to a diet regimen in order to keep levels of blood phenylalanine within the range of 100–250 umol/L throughout the course of your pregnancy. Your baby could have low birth weight. Your baby will only inherit PKU if her father is a carrier, which in the US gives him about a 1 in 200 chance.

≫ Medicines and tests

You will need to have blood tests up to three times a week and you will see your PKU specialist up to once a month. You may be asked to go for additional growth ultrasounds.

≫ Effects of pregnancy on your condition

Your protein-controlled diet will be strict. As your baby grows he will use up protein, and later his liver may produce the enzymes you cannot. As a result, the amount of protein you eat to keep your blood phenylalanine at the correct levels will increase over the course of the pregnancy—all within the strict diet prescribed by your dietician in response to your blood tests.

Cystic fibrosis

≫ What is it?

Known as CF, this genetic condition causes thick mucus to build up in the lungs and digestive system, making it difficult to breathe and get nutrients from food.

≫ Effects on your pregnancy, labor, and baby

You will probably be advised that a lung function (FEV1) of 60 percent is necessary before you try to become pregnant. Pregnancy is best planned. The likelihood of having a healthy pregnancy and baby when you have CF is improving all the time. Your doctors can help you get a good outcome. You will pass the CF gene to your baby, who will become a carrier. He has a 50 percent chance of developing the disease only if his father is a carrier too. You have a higher risk of gestational diabetes, your baby may be small, and there is an increased risk of premature labor, miscarriage, and stillbirth.

≫ Medicines and tests

Most medicines used in CF, including antibiotics, are safe to use in pregnancy. You can continue any medication unless your CF specialist advises otherwise. You will see your doctor with your CF specialist. Both will monitor your nutrition and weight gain. In some cases you may need additional ultrasounds to check the development and growth of your baby. Check with your doctor if you can continue to take pain-relief medication. Consult your CF specialist before trying to conceive.

≫ Effects of pregnancy on your condition

The symptoms of CF might worsen. You might find that you have trouble with breathing as your uterus expands during your pregnancy. You may also experience malnutrition as your body struggles to absorb enough nutrients. Nasal tube feeding may be advised.

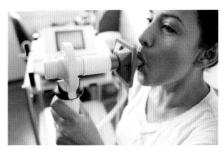

Good lung function This is a key factor in having a safe pregnancy and healthy baby. Your doctors will monitor your lung function throughout your pregnancy.

Pregnancy-induced complications are health issues that didn't exist before you were pregnant—and they will usually disappear after the birth of your baby. Throughout pregnancy, your doctor checks for signs of these complications. Some women have gynecological issues that can affect pregnancy, and sometimes problems arise with the placenta that is nourishing your baby.

Hypertension

》 What is it?
It means you develop abnormally high blood pressure in pregnancy.

》 What's the difference between pregnancy-induced hypertension and gestational hypertension?
There isn't a difference—both terms mean the same thing, that your high blood pressure in pregnancy is related. Your doctor took your blood pressure during your first appointment and will compare all subsequent blood-pressure readings to this one. In doing so she is making sure that over the course of your pregnancy there is no unexpected change—your blood pressure is expected to dip a little during pregnancy and then rise again to normal prepregnancy levels as you near full term. If at any point—and specifically after 20 weeks pregnant—it goes higher than 140/90 mmHg, you will be diagnosed with pregnancy-induced hypertension (PIH) or gestational hypertension (GH), depending upon the term your doctor chooses to use. The condition is subdivided into mild, moderate, and severe. If you have severe hypertension, this puts you at risk of a stroke, and you may have to have your blood pressure monitored up to four times a day.

Did you know...

》 5 percent of all pregnant women will develop some form of preeclampsia
》 2 percent of all pregnant women develop severe preeclampsia
》 85 percent of women with preeclampsia also have edema (fluid retention)
》 0.5 percent of women with preeclampsia go on to develop eclampsia

Preeclampsia

》 What is it?
Preeclampsia is a condition brought on by pregnancy. It's characterized by hypertension plus protein in urine. You have a slightly increased risk of developing the condition if you are 40 or over, you are a teenage mom, you are overweight, or have a preexisting condition such as diabetes.

》 My doctor says that I have pregnancy-induced hypertension. Does this mean I will get preeclampsia?
No, not necessarily. Although PIH can be a symptom of preeclampsia, it is not in itself a sign that preeclampsia is on its way. If you also have gestational proteinuric hypertension (protein in your urine), this is enough to diagnose mild preeclampsia, although other symptoms can lead to a diagnosis. If you also have one or more of the other symptoms, you are said to have moderate or severe preeclampsia. If you are diagnosed with any form of preeclampsia, your doctor will monitor your pregnancy very carefully over the remaining weeks, either with frequent office visits or at the hospital.

》 If I have preeclampsia will I have to spend the rest of my pregnancy in hospital?
That depends on how severe your preeclampsia is. If your preeclampsia is mild, you are likely to have to stay in the hospital for only a day or two while your blood pressure is monitored—usually up to four times a day. Often complete rest is all you need to get your blood pressure under control and you will be allowed to go home without further treatment. If you have moderate preeclampsia, your stay is likely to be longer and you are more likely to be given medication to bring down your blood pressure. You will probably also have a ultrasound to check that your baby is growing well. If your due date is still a while away, you may either be advised to stay in the hospital, or you will be closely managed as an outpatient, as long as your blood pressure has returned to normal and all seems well with your baby. If, however, you have severe early-onset

preeclampsia, you will probably have to stay in the hospital for the rest of your pregnancy so that you and your baby can be closely monitored. Your obstetrician may decide to deliver your baby early, although he or she will aim to deliver your baby no earlier than 37 weeks. If you develop preeclampsia of any severity after 37 weeks, you will usually be advised to have an early induction of labor.

》 Symptoms
> Frequent or permanent headache, usually above your eyes and over your brow.
> Blurred vision, or "lightning flashes" in front of your eyes.
> Pain in your abdomen or underneath your ribs.
> Vomiting or general feelings of being unwell.
> Reduced urination (called oliguria).
> Sudden swelling in the extremities or face.

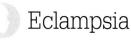

Eclampsia

》 What is it?
This is a serious condition, characterized by seizures as well as all the symptoms of preeclampsia. In severe cases, eclampsia can lead to unconsciousness.

》 Does having preeclampsia mean I will definitely develop eclampsia?
No. Only around one in every 200 women with preeclampsia will go on to develop full-blown eclampsia.

》 How will eclampsia affect my pregnancy?
If you develop eclampsia your doctor will advise you to have your baby immediately. You are also at increased risk of placental abruption, when the placenta comes away from the wall of the uterus, and HELLP syndrome (see below).

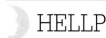

HELLP

》 What is it?
A severe form of preeclampsia, HELLP stands for Hemolysis (breaking down of red blood cells), Elevated Liver enzymes, and Low Platelet count.

》 What does it mean for my pregnancy?
HELLP puts both you and sometimes your baby in significant danger, so you will be encouraged to give birth to your baby as soon as possible, regardless of how far along you are in your pregnancy. HELLP is more likely to affect the health of the mother than the baby, so your baby has a good chance of a positive outcome unless she is very small. Very low birth weight babies will to be taken to the neonatal intensive care unit in order to give them the best possible chances of survival.

Gestational diabetes

» What is gestational diabetes? Does it mean I have diabetes, or my baby does?

There are two main types of diabetes, Type I and Type II (see p.141). However, if you do not usually suffer from either of these types of diabetes but you develop insulin resistance during your pregnancy, you have gestational diabetes mellitus—GDM. It's a condition that affects the mother, and potentially the baby's growth. GDM usually develops during the third trimester of pregnancy, after 24 weeks pregnant, and it will usually disappear once the baby has been born. However, if you have had gestational diabetes, you are more likely to go on to develop Type II diabetes in later life. Gestational diabetes occurs in between 2 and 5 percent of pregnancies worldwide.

» My mother has Type I diabetes, but I don't. Will I be screened for gestational diabetes?

Yes, you will be screened, but not specifically because of your family history. The US Preventive Services Task Force recommends that all pregnant women get screened for gestational diabetes after 24 weeks of pregnancy. Most doctors screen their patients between 24 and 28 weeks. The blood-glucose tolerance test can be done right in the doctor's office. Women of southern Asian, Afro-Caribbean, or African descent, women who have had a previous baby who weighed more than 9 lb (4.5 kg), who have had gestational diabetes in an earlier pregnancy, or who are obese are at greater risk for the condition.

» Will I have to have a C-section?

Not necessarily. Clinical guidelines state that gestational diabetes alone is not a good enough reason to recommend a C-section. However, one effect on the baby is to make her "large for dates." If this applies to your pregnancy, your obstetrician may recommend a C-section since your baby's size could make labor difficult or distressing for one or both of you (see below). You'll have ultrasounds throughout the final stages of pregnancy if you have gestational diabetes, so your baby's growth will be monitored carefully and you'll be able to make a fully informed decision about how you give birth, and to weigh your wishes against the advice of the doctors.

» Will I be allowed a home birth if I have gestational diabetes? What about an active birth?

It's unlikely. If your diabetes is severe, you will most likely need to be delivered on a labor ward because of the increased risks to you and your baby during labor and birth. You will also be attached to an IV of insulin and glucose, which will make moving around tricky.

Your doctor will meet with you at around 36 weeks pregnant to discuss the safest options for your baby's birth.

» How will gestational diabetes affect my baby? What about after birth?

GDM can cause a baby to become large for dates, but that is the only direct effect the condition has on the baby while she is in the uterus. This does increase the risk of labor complications, since the baby may be too large to pass through the pelvis, and has an increased risk of shoulder dystocia, when the head is delivered, but there is difficulty delivering the shoulders, so a planned C-section may be advised. There are other effects that can influence the baby's well-being. For example, gestational diabetes can cause too much amniotic fluid to be produced, which in turn can trigger premature labor, and there may be issues stabilizing the baby's blood sugar after birth. The condition also puts you at greater risk of preeclampsia, which can be dangerous for both you and your baby. Finally, studies show that babies born to mothers who had gestational diabetes are more prone to obesity in later life, with the domino effect of increasing their risk of developing Type II diabetes.

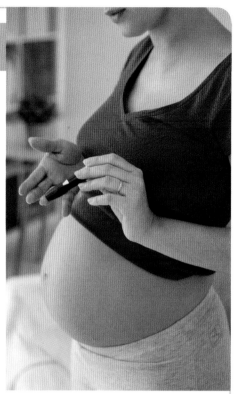

Blood glucose meter You'll be given a blood glucose meter. This allows you to check your glucose levels through a small pin-prick sample of blood.

If you had gestational diabetes in a previous pregnancy you have a **67 percent** chance of developing it subsequent pregnancies.

Diabetic treatments

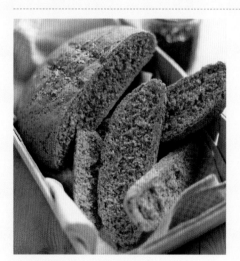

Food choices You will be advised to eat food that will help to keep your blood glucose as stable as possible. Whole-wheat bread and brown rice are both good for releasing energy gradually.

As a first step in your treatment, you'll be referred to a dietician, who will talk to you about how you can try to control your glucose levels through diet. Injecting yourself with insulin is something of a last resort.

» Food and drink

You will be given guidance on dietary changes and told specifically which foods and beverages you should consume.

» Exercise

Your doctor will talk to you about forms of exercise that are safe for you.

» Insulin

However, if you can't control your glucose using diet and exercise alone, you will need to lower the amount of glucose in your blood either by taking metformin orally, or through insulin injections. If you need injections, a specialist will talk you through this.

Tilted uterus

» What is it?

The uterus is normally in a straight, vertical position. A tilted uterus is one that tips backward toward the spine. It's also known as a retroverted uterus. Symptoms of tilted uterus usually include pain during sexual intercourse and pain during menstruation.

» What does this condition mean for my pregnancy? Will my uterus stay tilted after I've given birth?

The main implication for your pregnancy is that your baby may be hard to spot during an abdominal ultrasound. Some women with a tilted uterus have to have a vaginal ultrasound in order for the sonographer to be able to see the baby from all angles. This is simply because the baby is farther away from the front of the abdomen. Other than that, complications arising directly from your uterine anatomy are extremely rare—once you have completed 12 weeks of pregnancy, your uterus will expand out of your pelvis anyway and as it grows will fill the space in your abdomen. After birth, your uterus may or may not move back into its original position—it partly depends on the strength of the muscles and ligaments around your uterus. Whatever happens, the position of your uterus after you've had your baby is unlikely to affect your chances of conceiving again in the future, so try not to worry about it.

Endometriosis

» What is it?

In this condition, pieces of tissue that are normally part of the uterine lining (also called the endometrium) are found in the abdomen and pelvis, including on the ovaries, in the bowel, and around the bladder. The endometrium is the part of the uterus that sheds during your periods. This condition can result in heavy, painful menstruation and infertility, but the cause of it is not totally understood.

» I was diagnosed with endometriosis a couple of years ago. Could it affect my pregnancy?

Once pregnant, endometriosis is unlikely to affect your pregnancy, your baby, or increase any risk factors. (The main

Fibroids

» What are fibroids?

Fibroids are noncancerous growths in the uterus, affecting a quarter of all women at some point in their lives. The most common form grow within the muscular wall of the uterus (intramuscular fibroids), although they may also appear outside the muscle wall, growing into the pelvis (subserous fibroids); dangling from the lining of the uterus (pedunculated fibroids); embedded in the inner lining of the uterus (submucosal fibroids); or on the neck of your cervix (cervical fibroids). They may be small or large, and their exact cause is unknown, although excess estrogen makes them bigger. (This is why women who are overweight are more likely to have fibroids, because fat cells produce estrogen.)

» How will I know if I have fibroids and what effects will they have on my body and baby?

Fibroids may cause painful and/or heavy periods, pain during intercourse, abdominal bloating, or frequent urination (if the fibroid presses on the bladder). If fibroids are large or numerous, they can affect fertility because they make it harder for the embryo to implant in the uterine lining, and they may also make it more likely for you to miscarry if you do get pregnant. If you have had fibroid treatment prepregnancy, this can affect your delivery options once pregnant, so talk to your doctor about this. Many fibroids are asymptomatic—in other words, a large number of women don't even discover they have them until they have a routine pregnancy ultrasound, until the fibroids cause spotting during pregnancy, or until their doctor presses on their uterus to feel the position of the baby. Some fibroids restrict space in your uterus so that your baby doesn't have the space to grow properly. However, this is very rare. Also, as fibroids grow under the influence of pregnancy hormones, they can start to degenerate, usually in the

Fallopian tube

Subserous fibroid

Intramural fibroid

Submucosal fibroid
Grows under the lining

Ovary

Cervical fibroid
Grows within the cervix

Sizes Fibroids can range from as small as a bean, but can also be as large as a small melon. They can be seen on X-rays.

Where are they found?
Fibroids can grow in the inner, middle, and outer layers of the uterus. Polyps can form on the cervical or uterine lining.

second trimester, and this can cause pain and, rarely, premature labor.

» My fibroids are large and my doctor has said that I may have to have a C-section. Why?

There are several reasons why fibroids might mean that C-section is the safest way to deliver your baby. In pregnancy, a large fibroid may push your baby into an awkward position for delivery (called "malpresentation"), including the breech position and very occasionally presenting with a shoulder first. Cervical fibroids may block the entrance to your cervix, making it difficult for your baby to pass into the birth canal. If fibroids cause your placenta to come away slightly from your uterine lining (partial abruption; see opposite), your baby will continue to be well-nourished, but a preterm C-section, as soon as your baby is big enough to survive outside the uterus, will remove the risks to the baby if the placenta comes away completely. Finally, fibroids also put you at slightly increased risk of postpartum hemorrhage (excessive bleeding after the birth) and preterm delivery. Your doctor has a duty to ensure you are fully aware of any potential complications, but it's important to remember that fibroids only rarely cause any problems and all the situations given here are exceptional. Fibroids can be removed after pregnancy and if you do not want more children you can have a hysterectomy which means there is no risk of them reoccuring.

roblems of this condition are to do with conceiving).
uring your pregnancy, you may find that your symptoms of
ndometriosis improve or disappear, but it is likely that they
ill resume when your menstruation begins again after
egnancy and breast-feeding (if you are doing so) are over.

Uterus infection

What is it?
horioamnionitis is an infection in pregnancy of the membranes
urrounding the fetus. This is associated with prolonged
upture of the membranes (if there is a long period of time
etween your membranes rupturing and birth) and can
ffect mom and baby, so labor needs to be induced and
ou'll be given antibiotics. Chorioamnionitis makes a uterus
nfection after birth, known as endometritis, more likely.
ndometritis is also more likely if you have had a C-section
r a retained placenta. The infection causes pain in the
ower abdomen, and you may have a high temperature.
ntibiotics usually clear the infection.

I've had an infection in my uterus in the past
nd may have scarring. Will this make it harder
or me to carry a baby to term?
terine infection can cause scar tissue to develop in the
terine lining (endometrium). This, in turn, can make it
arder for a fertilized egg to implant, and if it does implant,
his may be less secure, increasing the risk of miscarriage.
ou're also at increased risk of placenta previa (see right)
nd placental abruption (see below). Inform your doctor
f your medical history. You will be given regular checkups
o monitor the progress of your pregnancy.

Cervical insufficiency

What is it?
ervical insufficiency is a cervix that is not rigid enough
o safely hold in the membranes surrounding your baby.
he cervix could open too early, in the second trimester.

How is this diagnosed, and what does it mean?
ervical insufficiency may be the result of a previous
regnancy that stretched the opening of the cervix too far,
r of previous cervical surgery. If undiagnosed, you are at
ncreased risk of late miscarriage, when your baby is heavy
nd the membranes are forced out of the cervix and
upture. However, most cases are picked up during prenatal
heckups, before becoming problematic. Your doctor may
end you for an ultrasound to look at your cervix (unless
ou've had a previous cervical insufficiency, in which case
n ultrasound isn't needed) and put a temporary stitch—a
erclage—into the cervix between weeks 12 and 16 to hold
hings in place. The stitch is removed before labor. You may
e given medicine if the cervix starts to open up and shorten.

Placenta previa

What is placenta previa?
More commonly known as "low-lying placenta,"
placenta previa occurs when the placenta's position
partially or completely covers your cervix—and thus
blocks your baby's exit to the birth canal. A diagnosis
of placenta previa is not certain until late pregnancy
because the placenta can move away from the internal
opening of the cervix (os) as the uterus grows and
stretches. The sonographer will check the position
of your placenta at your second ultrasound (the
anatomy scan). If your baby's placenta is noted to be
low-lying, you will have another ultrasound at between
32 and 34 weeks to see whether the placenta has
shifted upward. Around 90 percent of low-lying
placentas seen before 28 weeks will move to a better
position by the follow-up ultrasound. (This happens in
around 50 percent of cases if you have had a C-section
in the past.) Placenta previa can be the result of fibroids
or scar tissue preventing the placenta from attaching in
a good position, or it might happen by chance.

What impact does a diagnosis of placenta previa have on my pregnancy?
Most cases of placenta previa require a C-section
because a vaginal delivery isn't possible if the placenta
is ¾ in (2 cm) from the edge of the cervix or closer.
Your doctor will talk to you about the possibility of
an elective (planned) C-section in order to deliver
your baby safely. There could be some extra fetal
monitoring, too.

In addition to blocking the cervix, placenta previa can
cause painless, bright red bleeding. If you notice this

kind of bleeding, let your doctor know immediately.
Heavy bleeding can put both you and your baby at risk,
but most of the time it can be treated before there is
any danger. In severe cases, you might need a blood
transfusion. Your obstetrician might advise that you
abstain from intercourse to prevent the risk of bleeding,
or even advise bed rest or a hospital stay. If there is
profuse bleeding or risk of premature birth, your doctor
could recommend an emergency C-section.

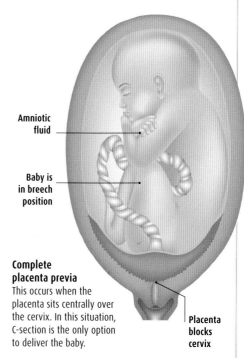

Amniotic fluid

Baby is in breech position

Complete placenta previa
This occurs when the
placenta sits centrally over
the cervix. In this situation,
C-section is the only option
to deliver the baby.

Placenta blocks cervix

**Although placenta previa often makes a cesarean section
necessary, the vast majority of women deliver healthy babies
and recover well from their surgery.**

Placental abruption

What is it?
Placental abruption, when part or all of the placenta
comes away from the wall of the uterus, is a serious
condition that significantly impacts your baby's ability to
receive nutrients and oxygen. Rarely, the entire placenta
may become detached. The first signs that it might be
happening are abdominal pain and bleeding. If you
experience any spotting during your pregnancy, call your
doctor. It is a potentially life-threatening condition, so
immediate attention is imperative.

My friend's baby was stillborn following a placental abruption. What can I do to stop this from happening to me?
Though you can't do anything specifically to stop a placental
abruption, it's possible to carry a baby to term as long
as the abruption is only mild—meaning that most of the
placenta remains attached to the uterus (enough to nourish
your baby). Severe or complete abruption is not treatable
and is more likely to result in premature birth, or stillbirth.
It is also dangerous for you, since it can result in significant
blood loss. If you smoke or take drugs—stop. These habits
are associated with an increased risk of placental abruption.
Preeclampsia and a small baby also increase the risk.

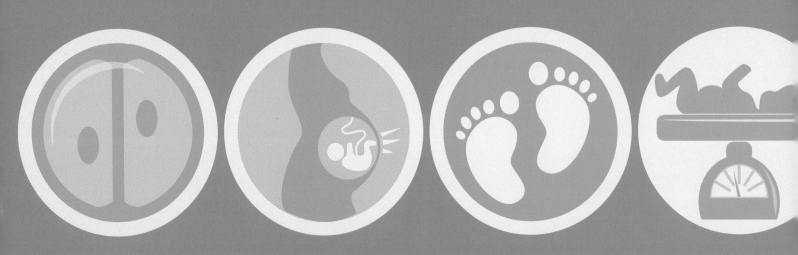

Your growing baby

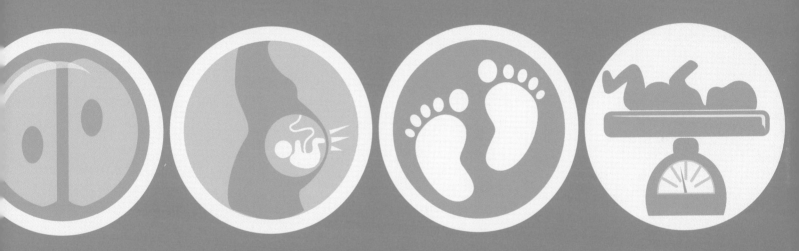

From feeling the first gentle movements to experiencing the fuller twists, **kicks, and hiccups**, you will marvel at the **magical changes** that are taking place inside you. As the tiny bundle of cells develops, you will become more and more aware of your baby **getting bigger and stronger** the closer you get to full term. Learn more about the placenta, your baby's developing organs, and his skeletal structure. Discover why your baby is so **unique and special**.

The biological and chemical processes that take us from a cell to a baby really are **absolutely incredible**. As soon as your pregnancy begins, your **amazing body** transforms so it can protect this **new life**, while the new life itself becomes a fully functioning human being, **one cell at a time** but at remarkable speed.

From cell to baby

The zygote of life

Your baby begins life as a single cell, created by a sperm fusing with an egg. This organism contains all the potential for new life—a full set of chromosomes (23 pairs, one in each pair from each parent). These carry your baby's unique blueprint encoded in genes. Although we often refer colloquially to this earliest stage of life as an embryo, in fact we're a few steps from an embryo yet. For the time being, your baby is a zygote. The zygote travels down the fallopian tube and as it travels, it is already subdividing and multiplying to make 16 cells. It's surrounded by a protective membrane called the zona pellucida, which has a very special function—it prevents the zygote from implanting in the fallopian tube, or anywhere that isn't your uterus.

Morula to blastocyst

During its journey down the fallopian tube to the uterus, the zygote becomes known as a morula (because the cells are grouped together and look like a mulberry, from the Latin morus). The morula is a hive of activity: its cells subdivide rapidly and eventually create a kind of bubble structure with an outer membrane (the trophoblast) containing a mass of cells (the endoderm) within a cavity. Amazingly, that bundle of cells sitting against the membrane wall will become the key to your baby's breathing and digestion, among other things. At this stage your baby becomes known as a blastocyst. The blastocyst floats around in the uterus for a while, then sends chemical messages that break down the zona pellucida. Now exposed, the "sticky" trophoblast latches onto and implants itself in the uterine wall. All this happens around seven to nine days after fertilization. Your baby has now doubled in size since fertilization and is made up of more than a hundred cells. Once implanted, the blastocyst is enveloped by the uterine lining (endometrium) and snuggles down deep within the cells of the lining. It can now receive nourishment directly from your uterus.

Embryo to fetus

At four weeks, the blastocyst can be called an embryo. The trophoblast has started to develop into the placenta (see p.154), and secretions from your uterus are nourishing the cells so that they divide and subdivide and begin to form your baby's organs, skeleton, and features. Crucially, the embryo is made up of three layers; each will develop into specific parts of your baby's body. Now that your baby is being nourished by your body, the business of becoming more "babylike" can begin. At about 10 weeks, when his facial features are in place and most of the major organs are on their way to being formed, your baby has become a fetus—the medical name he keeps until birth.

Q How are the fertilized cells nourished before there's a placenta?

The early embryo is fed by a "yolk sac," which develops from some of the cells of the blastocyst.

Despite being called a yolk sac, there's hardly any yolk in it, but what is there provides enough energy and nutrition to see your developing baby through until the fully formed placenta takes over at around 12 weeks. The placenta doesn't begin to form until you're about four weeks pregnant (which is about two weeks after conception, since pregnancy is dated from the first day of your last menstrual period).

The early embryo is just a disk of cells; on one side there is an amniotic sac, and on the other side is the yolk sac. A basic circulatory system draws nutrients from the yolk sac and delivers them into the developing embryo cells. As the embryo grows it is enveloped by the amniotic sac, while the yolk sac remains outside, but connected to the embryo. Part of the yolk sac then triggers cells in the blastocyst to begin making the placenta. The yolk sac slowly shrinks as the placenta becomes stronger, disappearing into the umbilical cord when the placenta is fully formed. It is while the embryo is dependent on the yolk sac that it is most vulnerable—this is one of the reasons why the risk of miscarriage is highest in the first trimester and becomes lower as the placenta begins to share the job of sustaining the baby.

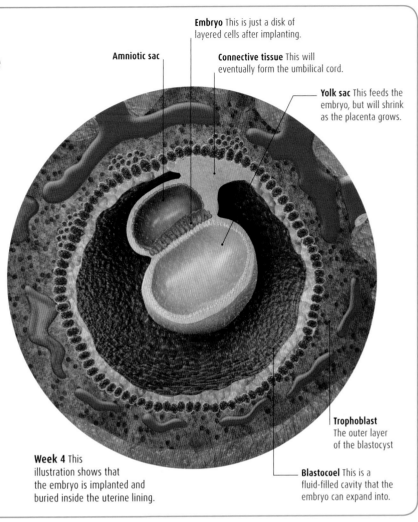

Embryo This is just a disk of layered cells after implanting.

Amniotic sac

Connective tissue This will eventually form the umbilical cord.

Yolk sac This feeds the embryo, but will shrink as the placenta grows.

Trophoblast The outer layer of the blastocyst

Blastocoel This is a fluid-filled cavity that the embryo can expand into.

Week 4 This illustration shows that the embryo is implanted and buried inside the uterine lining.

Q Does it matter where the cells implant in my uterus?

No and yes. The most important thing is that the bundle of cells finds a comfortable home in your uterine lining, rather than anywhere else, such as the fallopian tubes. (If this happens, your pregnancy is termed ectopic (see p.308), which can be life threatening for you.) Usually, your smart body draws the blastocyst toward the top (the superior wall) and back (the posterior wall) of your uterus. This is the best place for implantation because when the placenta grows, it's very unlikely to block your baby's eventual exit through your cervix. Sometimes, though, the blastocyst implants lower down in your uterus and the placenta forms too close to the cervix (this is called placenta previa; see p.147). This can happen if, for example, you have uterine fibroids (see p.146) or a scar from a previous surgery (such as a cesarean section) that make it difficult for

the blastocyst to implant. Although your baby can develop healthily wherever in the uterus the blastocyst makes its home, the place where it implants can have consequences for your labor and your experience of birth.

Q How does my baby develop from just layers of cells?

At five weeks, the embryo is made up of three layers of cells that develop into different parts of your baby's body. These layers undergo a complex process of three-dimensional folding to form the basic bodily structures. The ectoderm is the outermost layer of the embryo and will form, among other things, your baby's nervous system, his facial features (including his eyes, nose, mouth, and ears), and his skin, nails, and hair. It also becomes your baby's anal canal. The mesoderm is the middle layer, and, will become, among other things, your baby's circulatory

system, skeletal system (including bones, cartilage, muscles, and ligaments), blood cells and bone marrow, kidneys, and reproductive organs. The endoderm is the innermost layer of the embryo and will become your baby's respiratory system, digestive system, and bladder, as well as several important glands of his endocrine (hormone) system, including the thyroid, parathyroid, and thymus glands.

100–150

cells are present in the **blastocyst** (as a result of cell division) by the time it enters the uterine cavity, ready to implant.

Q How advanced is an embryo? Which parts of my baby's body develop first?

Even in the very earliest days, your baby is already developing some primitive, functional versions of the fully fledged vital organs she'll have when she's born. As a mass of cells, the embryo is not yet akin to how we might picture a developing baby, but it is brimming with potential.

During the first 10 weeks of pregnancy, your ball of potential undergoes a process called organogenesis—the creation of your baby's vital organs. Development of the organs is far more important than your embryo's growth, which is why she grows very little in length during the first 12 weeks compared with the second and third trimesters of pregnancy. All her cellular energy is diverted into creating her organs. This requires a process of rapid cell division

and the subdivision of groups of cells into their different functions: it's called differentiation.

By five weeks, your baby's thyroid, renal, adrenal, and gonadal organs (glands of her endocrine, or hormonal, system) are present in a primitive form. Cells that will form her brain, kidneys, heart, and nerves have appeared. She has a tube that will become her gastrointestinal tract. Her lungs and stomach have divided from a single tube within the embryo.

Over the course of the next five weeks, all the cells that have taken on these vital roles will keep dividing, folding, turning, and forming. By the time you're 10 weeks pregnant and probably looking forward to your first ultrasound, your baby will have a basic, functioning system of organs—a heart that beats, primitive kidneys that pass urine, and a brain that's beginning to send messages to other parts of the body.

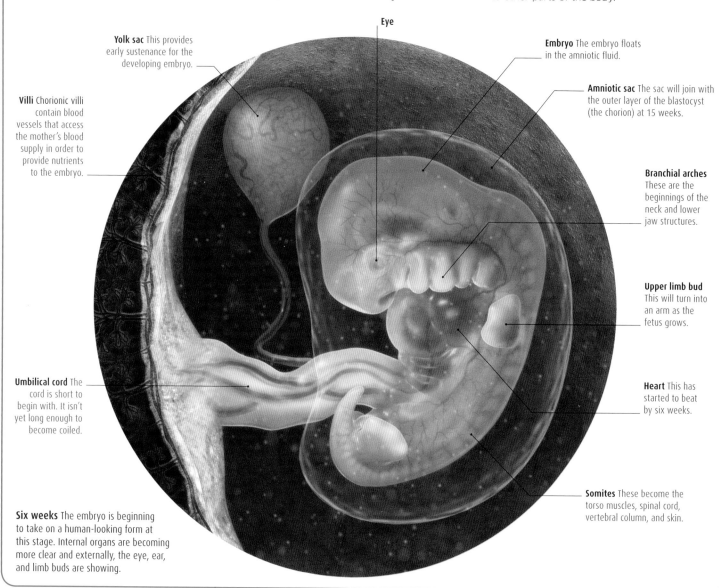

Eye

Yolk sac This provides early sustenance for the developing embryo.

Villi Chorionic villi contain blood vessels that access the mother's blood supply in order to provide nutrients to the embryo.

Umbilical cord The cord is short to begin with. It isn't yet long enough to become coiled.

Six weeks The embryo is beginning to take on a human-looking form at this stage. Internal organs are becoming more clear and externally, the eye, ear, and limb buds are showing.

Embryo The embryo floats in the amniotic fluid.

Amniotic sac The sac will join with the outer layer of the blastocyst (the chorion) at 15 weeks.

Branchial arches These are the beginnings of the neck and lower jaw structures.

Upper limb bud This will turn into an arm as the fetus grows.

Heart This has started to beat by six weeks.

Somites These become the torso muscles, spinal cord, vertebral column, and skin.

Q My baby's heart was beating on an early ultrasound! Has it formed yet?

At only six weeks pregnant, your baby has a simple heart that's beating, and is doing it at up to 160 times per minute.

Your baby needs a circulation system so that nutrients can pass into all her cells as they develop. At first, the yolk sac and placenta can diffuse nutrients and oxygen into her cells, but pretty soon the embryo is too large for this method and she needs a circulation system to help. That's why the heart is one of the first organs a baby develops—as early as 18 days after fertilization.

The heart begins life as two cords (the endocardial tubes) that fuse together, creating a "primitive heart tube." Once the heart tube has formed at around six weeks of pregnancy, it begins to pump blood cells. A mere three weeks later, this tiny, early heart has developed its chambers and valves.

Since your baby doesn't breathe in the uterus, she gets her oxygen from her mother through the placenta. Blood that leaves the body would normally go to the lungs to collect oxygen, but a fetus's heart has two extra connections that allow deoxygenated blood to bypass the lungs. Instead, fetal blood vessels pass out through the umbilical cord to the placenta to pick up oxygen. On the return journey, the rerouting sends oxgenated blood to the brain cells quickly. After birth, the two extra connections in the heart close.

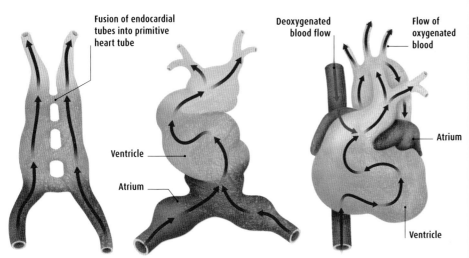

Fusion of endocardial tubes into primitive heart tube

Deoxygenated blood flow

Flow of oxygenated blood

Ventricle

Atrium

Atrium

Ventricle

1 Primitive heart tube The two cords merge from the base upward, forming a single primitive heart tube about 21 days after fertilization (five weeks pregnant).

2 Bending of the heart tube After forming, the heart tube begins to beat. It then elongates and loops to the right, forming a spiral and a basic circulation.

3 Final position of chambers The tube twists again to create four chambers. By nine weeks, the chambers are totally separate, and tiny valves have formed inside.

Q What is the neural tube, and how does it relate to my baby's brain and nervous system?

The neural tube is the structure that eventually becomes your baby's brain and nervous system. It develops when you are around four weeks pregnant and, at around five weeks of pregnancy, it separates to form cells that will become the outer layer of your baby's brain (the cerebellum) and other cells that will travel throughout your baby's developing body to become nerves. You may have heard of the neural tube in relation to "neural tube defects." These are conditions that can very rarely occur as a result of low maternal folic acid, among other reasons. You may be offered very accurate tests for these defects as part of your prenatal care (see p.97).

Q Why is my baby surrounded by amniotic fluid? What is it for?

Amniotic fluid protects your baby from trauma, aids lung development, helps maintain a constant temperature (slightly higher than your own), and gives your baby space to grow in. At the beginning of your pregnancy amniotic fluid is primarily made up of water and electrolytes. Around weeks 12–14 the fluid contains carbohydrates, proteins, lipids, phospholipids, and urea. As the kidneys start to function and produce urine, it passes into the amniotic fluid. By the end of your pregnancy your baby will swallow 1–2 pints (0.5–1 liters) of amniotic fluid a day and replace it as urine. The volume of amniotic fluid present in the amniotic sac decreases toward the end of the pregnancy as the fetal kidneys produce smaller amounts of more concentrated urine.

Q Is there anything I can do to encourage healthy organ development in my baby?

Yes, there are certain ways you can help. The first 10 weeks of pregnancy are the most vulnerable time for your baby's development, since it's when her organs are most susceptible to environmental harm. If your pregnancy is planned, you may already be taking folic acid (to encourage healthy nerve and brain development in your baby) and be avoiding toxins. But if that isn't the case for you, don't worry. As soon as you find out you're pregnant, start taking supplements of folic acid (400mcg) and vitamin D (10mcg) daily; cut out alcohol, nicotine, and any other recreational drugs if you take them (seek advice if need be); and avoid passive smoking. You can also steer clear of certain foods to lower the risk of getting harmful food poisoning (see pp.52–53).

Did you know...

The volume of amniotic fluid at 12 weeks is about 1 fl oz (30 ml), less than an egg cup full. By 32 weeks the amniotic fluid in the sac reaches its highest volume. This is usually 2 pints (1 liter), although this can be as much as 4.25 pints (2 liters).

What is the placenta and how does it work?

The placenta is your baby's life-support system. It's the means by which she receives oxygen and nutrients, it provides her with protection against disease, and it's where the waste she produces goes to be disposed of. The placenta is part of you and part of her at the same time. It's the link that enables you to nourish her while she grows inside you.

The placenta is formed

The placenta begins to form from cells in the embryo soon after the egg implants in the lining of the uterus. The embryo is surrounded by a chorionic membrane, which sends out tentacle-like projections that secure the embryo's place in the uterine wall. These projections are called "villi": they divide and branch out, and eventually fill with blood vessels from your baby's own circulatory system. Spaces around the villi fill with your blood. This whole structure—a mass of vessel-filled villi surrounded by maternal blood—is the placenta.

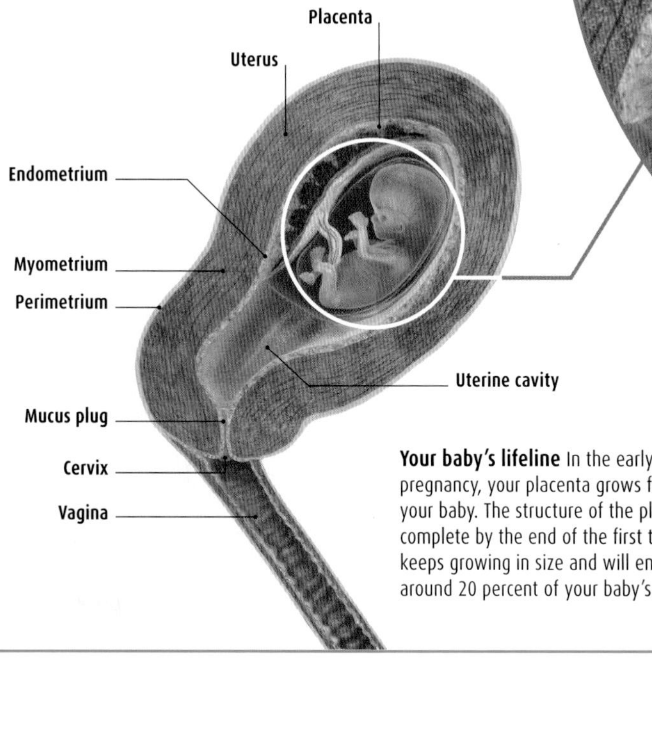

Villous chorion The frondlike texture of chorion creates a big surface area for gas exchange to take place

Placenta

At 12 weeks The maternal side of the placenta contains 15–20 lobes. These stop forming at this stage of gestation.

Placenta

Uterus

Endometrium

Myometrium

Perimetrium

Uterine cavity

Mucus plug

Cervix

Vagina

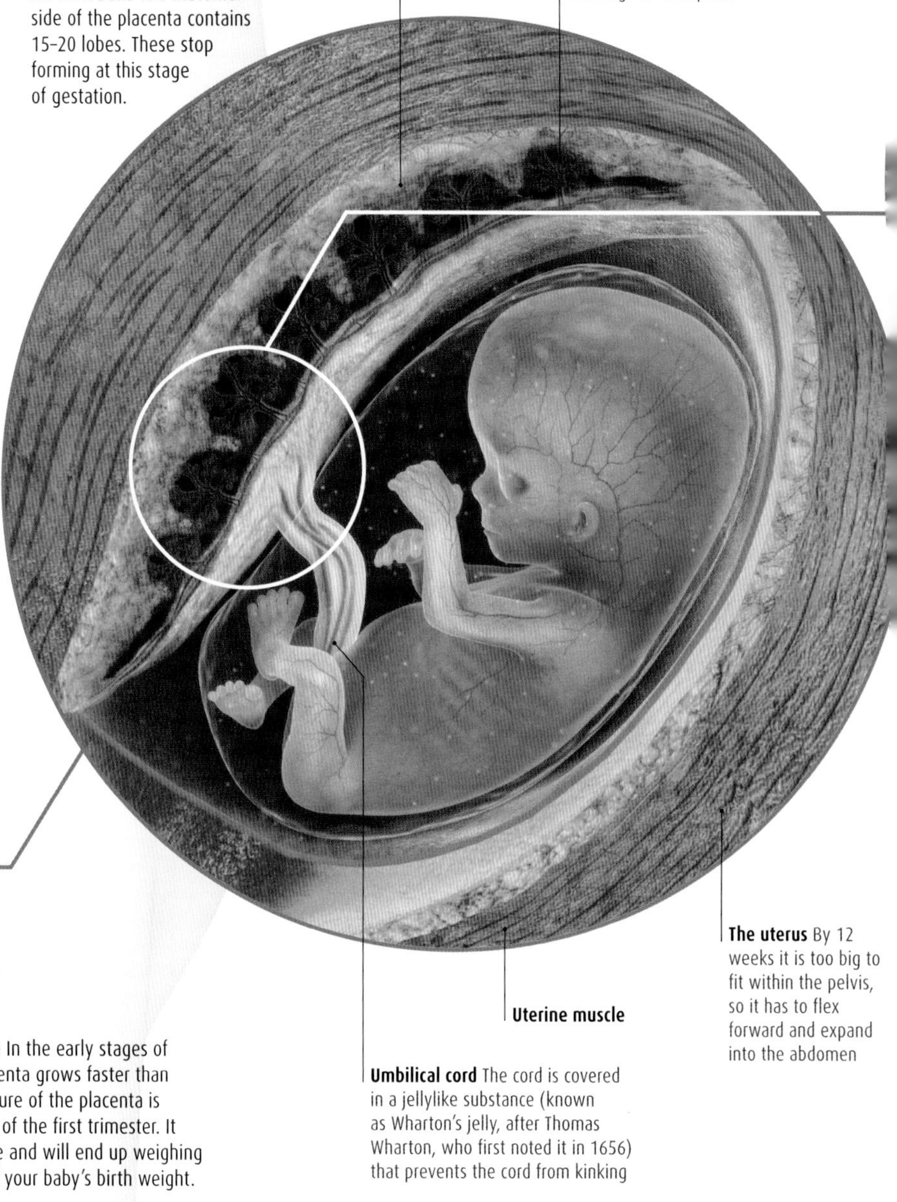

The uterus By 12 weeks it is too big to fit within the pelvis, so it has to flex forward and expand into the abdomen

Uterine muscle

Your baby's lifeline In the early stages of pregnancy, your placenta grows faster than your baby. The structure of the placenta is complete by the end of the first trimester. It keeps growing in size and will end up weighing around 20 percent of your baby's birth weight.

Umbilical cord The cord is covered in a jellylike substance (known as Wharton's jelly, after Thomas Wharton, who first noted it in 1656) that prevents the cord from kinking

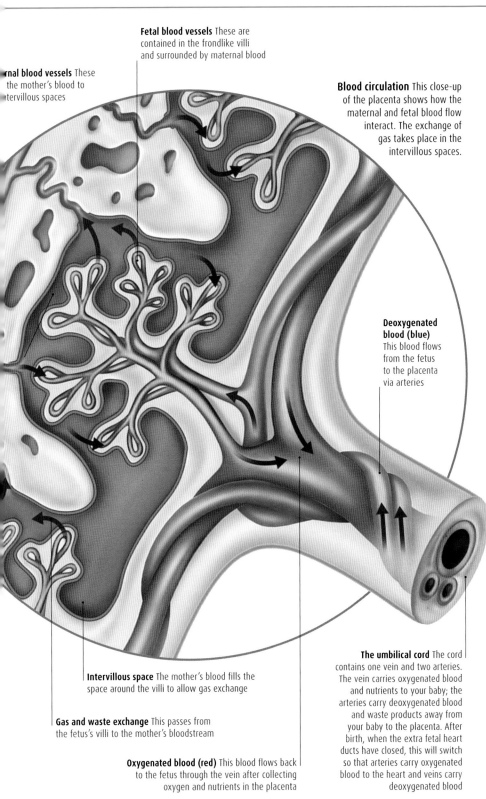

Fetal blood vessels These are contained in the frondlike villi and surrounded by maternal blood

rnal blood vessels These the mother's blood to tervillous spaces

Blood circulation This close-up of the placenta shows how the maternal and fetal blood flow interact. The exchange of gas takes place in the intervillous spaces.

Deoxygenated blood (blue) This blood flows from the fetus to the placenta via arteries

Intervillous space The mother's blood fills the space around the villi to allow gas exchange

Gas and waste exchange This passes from the fetus's villi to the mother's bloodstream

Oxygenated blood (red) This blood flows back to the fetus through the vein after collecting oxygen and nutrients in the placenta

The umbilical cord The cord contains one vein and two arteries. The vein carries oxygenated blood and nutrients to your baby; the arteries carry deoxygenated blood and waste products away from your baby to the placenta. After birth, when the extra fetal heart ducts have closed, this will switch so that arteries carry oxygenated blood to the heart and veins carry deoxygenated blood

THE PLACENTA'S ROLE

The placenta plays a vital role in your baby's survival. It has four key functions.

» Removing your baby's waste: there are two arteries in the umbilical cord as well as arterial vessels in the villi. These carry waste and carbon dioxide-filled blood from the baby. The waste gases travel through the walls of the villi into the mother's blood and are then processed as waste by the mother's liver and kidneys.

» Protecting your baby from disease: the cells of the villi are tightly packed. This means that organisms that are made up of large cells, such as bacteria and viruses that might be in the mother's blood, can't pass into the baby's blood through the villi walls. Not all organisms are too large though, which is why it's important to avoid contracting certain diseases (such as rubella or chicken pox) by being vaccinated against them. Toward the end of your pregnancy, antibodies from your blood will pass into your baby's circulation; these provide her with a basic level of immunity that lasts several weeks after she's born.

» Protecting your baby from chemicals: many chemicals (including toxins) are also made up of cells too large to cross the placenta. This is why you can continue taking certain medications while pregnant. Certain toxins, though, such as nicotine and alcohol, can pass through the villi walls.

» Producing hormones: the placenta serves as its own endocrine system. It's an important source of progesterone to help maintain your pregnancy and prevent premature labor, and of estrogen, to ensure your uterus expands to accommodate your growing baby and prepare your body for labor and, later, for breast-feeding. The placenta is also the source of the hormone hCG, which is the first signal your body receives that pregnancy has occurred. Growth hormones and relaxin (which softens the ligaments in your pelvis to make space for your baby and prepare your body for birth) are also produced in the placenta, along with several other hormones that optimize the transfer of nutrients and oxygen within the placenta itself.

The placenta expands in size from just a few cells to between **12 oz (350 g)** and **1½ lb (700 g)** in weight.

Q What's the difference between an embryo and a fetus, and what does it mean for my baby?

Your baby is called an embryo while his basic body structures and major organs form. From week 10 of your pregnancy (eight weeks after fertilization), this stage is complete and your baby becomes known as a fetus until he is born.

During the embryonic period your baby formed a face, limbs, fingers, and toes, and also rudimentary organs and body systems including the brain, heart, urinary tract, digestive tract, skin, bones, and muscles. By 10 weeks of pregnancy, the basic structures of all the major organs are present but they need further growth and development to gain the complexity of fully functioning systems that will support your baby after birth. The graduation to fetus status marks the next stage of your baby's development. The body and organs grow rapidly; by contrast, the growth of the head slows down relative to the rest of your baby's body. The shape of the head becomes more recognizably human, and the brain and nervous system link up. By the end of your second trimester your baby will double in weight and have emerging toenails and fingernails, the genitalia will be visible on an ultrasound, and you'll feel him move—he may even be very active. During the third trimester, fine-tuning takes place in your baby's brain and body systems. He will be able to see and hear in utero, and taste the amniotic fluid. His body will fill out with fat deposits under the skin to keep him insulated after birth. Finally, your baby's lungs are completed, having formed millions of air sacs that will allow him to take his first breath in the outside world.

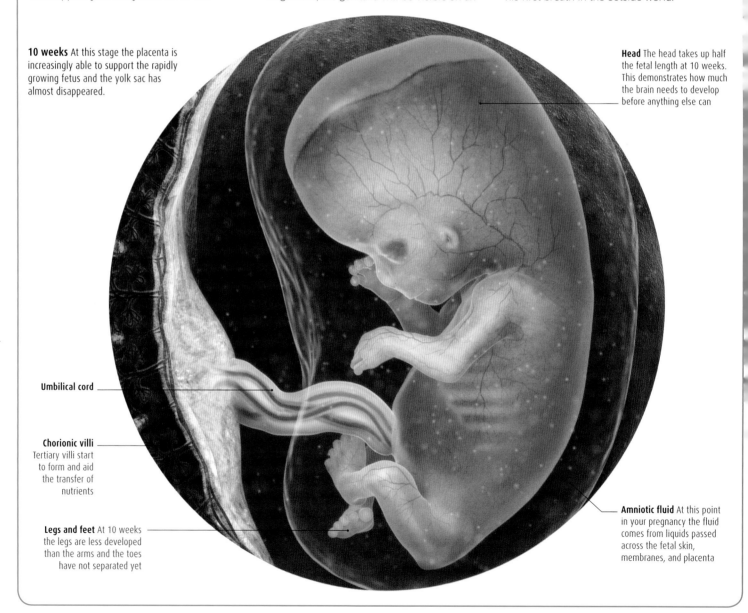

10 weeks At this stage the placenta is increasingly able to support the rapidly growing fetus and the yolk sac has almost disappeared.

Head The head takes up half the fetal length at 10 weeks. This demonstrates how much the brain needs to develop before anything else can

Umbilical cord

Chorionic villi Tertiary villi start to form and aid the transfer of nutrients

Legs and feet At 10 weeks the legs are less developed than the arms and the toes have not separated yet

Amniotic fluid At this point in your pregnancy the fluid comes from liquids passed across the fetal skin, membranes, and placenta

Q Is it true that my baby's entire digestive system begins as a simple tube?

The whole digestive system forms its structure by 12 weeks. By the time he is born, your tiny new baby will house an incredible 8 ft (2.5 m) of intestines.

Your baby's digestive system begins with a "gut tube" that forms from the endoderm layer of cells (the lower layer) and connects an opening at the top of the tube (which will connect to your baby's mouth) to an opening at the bottom (eventually your baby's anus). The gut tube then develops three sections—the foregut, midgut, and hindgut—and each of these forms specific organ buds. Between six and eight weeks pregnant, the foregut develops a bulge that will become your baby's stomach. All three sections of the gut tube continually lengthen so that by the time you are nine weeks pregnant, there's so much

bowel tissue (the bowel is the collective name for the small and large intestines) that there isn't room for it to fit inside the tiny embryo. Instead, it pushes out of a hole in your baby's abdomen so that it occupies some of the space in the umbilical cord. By 10 weeks pregnant, the baby's stomach will begin to produce digestive juices—a milestone in his transition from embryo to fetus. By the time you're 12 weeks pregnant, your baby's body is large enough for his bowel to come back inside his body and his umbilical cord is empty again, aside from the vessels that belong there.

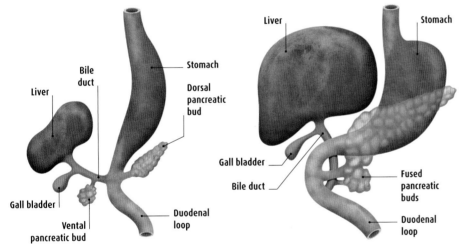

1 **At nine weeks** The main tube of the gut develops specialized structures that branch off from it. The early pancreas is made up of two separate buds.

Liver · Bile duct · Stomach · Dorsal pancreatic bud · Gall bladder · Vental pancreatic bud · Duodenal loop

2 **At 10 weeks** The pancreatic buds have fused. The liver and stomach are much larger, and the duodenum (part of the small intestine) is lengthening.

Liver · Stomach · Gall bladder · Bile duct · Fused pancreatic buds · Duodenal loop

Q Does my baby's bowel work in the uterus?

As soon as your baby's bowel is fully formed the process of making meconium—his first poop—begins. Meconium consists of waste products such as cells from the bowel lining, amniotic fluid, mucus, and bile. It builds up and is slowly forced into the large intestine—a process helped by the peristaltic motion of your baby's bowel from 20 weeks. At roughly the same time, the muscle around his anus—the anal sphincter—tightens up, keeping the meconium in so that he doesn't poop inside the uterus.

Q Does my baby have functioning kidneys? If so, where does the urine go?

By 13 weeks of pregnancy, your baby's urine can pass out of his newly forming kidneys, through his developing ureters, and into his tiny bladder. This urine is released into the amniotic fluid. Your baby learns to swallow at around the same time, so drinks the amniotic

fluid, swallows his urine, fills his bladder again, and so the process goes on. Although this might sound unappetizing, fetal urine is very diluted and most waste has already been filtered out of your baby's system via the placenta, which is then expelled by your waste system. The kidneys develop from 10 weeks onward, multiplying thousands of filtration cells. The ureters that collect the urine branch into the kidneys, a process that takes until 32 weeks, when there are around two million branchings.

0
Babies have no **kneecaps** when they are born. These will develop in infancy.

1
Only one organ, the **auditory ossicles** in the ear, is full size at birth.

33%
A new baby's **kidneys** are just a third of full adult size.

270
Babies have more **bones** than adults, who have 206. Many bones fuse as they grow.

30,000
The number of **taste buds** a baby is born with reduces to 10,000 by adulthood.

{Q How does my baby's skeleton develop while she's in the uterus?

What begins as a simple framework of cartilage to protect your baby's body hardens into bone through a gradual process of ossification that continues even after your baby is born.

Developing a supportive skeleton

Bones and muscles form early in pregnancy. At five weeks pregnant, your embryonic baby develops a sort of skeletal meshwork of connective tissue (collagen) that protects her rapidly developing organs. Over the next few weeks, this meshwork gets a blood supply, and bone cells called osteoblasts work to toughen it and form cartilage. At 10 weeks, your baby has a recognizable jaw, collarbone, shoulder blades, ribs, vertebrae, and arm and leg bones. Gradually, the osteoblast cells deposit calcium salts on the cartilage to harden, shape, and grow the bones. This process is called ossification and it continues throughout your baby's time in the uterus, and beyond until adulthood when her bones finally stop growing.

Your baby develops muscle tissue early, too: by 10 weeks she can make simple movements. By 20 to 24 weeks her nervous system is becoming connected and her musculoskeletal system has developed enough for her to bend and flex her limbs. In the third trimester of pregnancy, your baby uses 250–350 mg of calcium per day to continue developing her bones. Muscle mass increases rapidly, and your baby might double in weight in the last 10 weeks of your pregnancy.

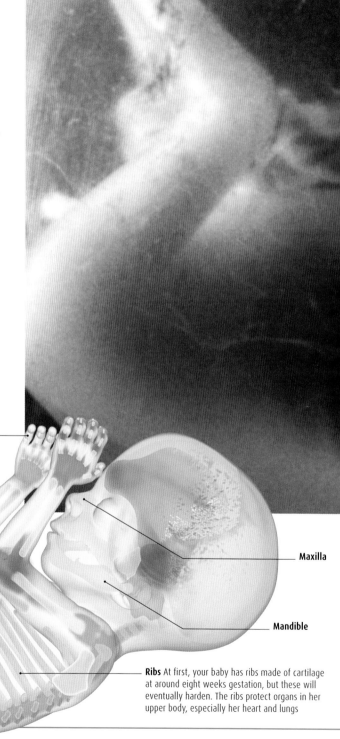

Body structure At 14 weeks, the fetal bones have begun to "ossify" from cartilage to bone, giving your baby enough strength to hold up and move her limbs.

Tendons and ligaments These connect bones to to muscles and cartilage

Metatarsal

Phalanges

Ulna

Radius

Tibia

Fibula

Maxilla

Mandible

Toes Your baby's toes separated into their individual digits at between 10 and 11 weeks of pregnancy. The small bones of her ankles have formed by the end of the first trimester

Skeleton at 14 weeks There are many recognizable bones present already. They will continue to form and reform through the process of ossification for many years yet.

Ilium

Ribs At first, your baby has ribs made of cartilage at around eight weeks gestation, but these will eventually harden. The ribs protect organs in her upper body, especially her heart and lungs

ARMS AND LEGS

"Limb buds" appear on the trunk of the embryo at around five weeks of pregnancy. Her limb buds extend so that by nine weeks, her arms and legs have grown in length. These are held in shape by the long bones that have formed within them. At 14 weeks gestation, your baby's arms will probably be long enough for her to bring her hands together in front of her face, but much of her skeletal structure is still cartilage. Her limb bones will ossify from the center outward, leaving the tips cartilaginous (and leaving room for growth) in childhood.

SKULL

The flat bones that make up the sides and top of your baby's skull skip the cartilage stage and ossify directly from the membrane that surrounds her brain. By 14 weeks, your baby has a nearly complete skull made up of the flat bones, the jaw, and the cartilage of the nose. The flat bones don't fuse properly, so that your baby's skull can mold to the shape of your pelvis during birth.

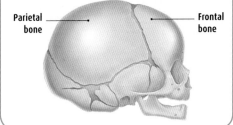

Parietal bone — Frontal bone

SPINAL COLUMN

This is the first part of your baby's skeleton to develop. At five weeks, a rudimentary spinal cord and structures called somites form down her back (see p.49). The vertebrae form when parts of the somites (sclerotomes), split in half to allow the nerves of the spinal cord to reach through them and attach to the emerging muscles. The skeletal muscles form from another portion of the somites (the myotomes) at around seven weeks; muscle groups form first at the spine, then extend to the torso and limbs.

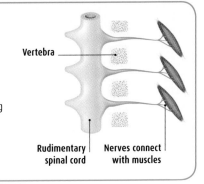

Vertebra

Rudimentary spinal cord

Nerves connect with muscles

Q When are my baby's lungs fully formed? How can his respiratory system work when there's no air?

By about 36 weeks, your baby's lungs are developed enough for fully independent breathing (this is why babies born from 37 weeks onward are considered full term), but his lungs can't inflate until there is contact with air, so "breathing" doesn't start until after birth.

Our respiratory system consists not only of our lungs, but also the nose, pharynx, larynx, and trachea. The whole respiratory tract begins life as a long tube—in fact, it's the same tube that also gives rise to most of the digestive system (see p.157). By 36 weeks, most babies' lungs are fully formed for birth, and they contain plenty of surfactant, a substance that will allow the lungs to expand and take in air without collapsing, which makes independent breathing possible. Premature babies are supported by artificial breathing apparatus, such as a ventilator, or their oxygen levels will be controlled in an incubator.

The diagrams show how the lungs start as buds that gradually branch out and complete their development at around 36 weeks of pregnancy.

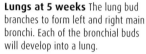

FORMATION OF THE LUNGS

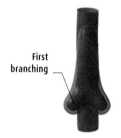

First branching

Lungs at 5 weeks The lung bud branches to form left and right main bronchi. Each of the bronchial buds will develop into a lung.

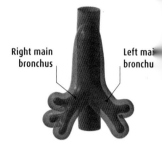

Right main bronchus **Left main bronchu**

Lungs at 6 weeks The two bronchi develop differently: the left bronchus branches into two buds, and the right bronchus branches into three.

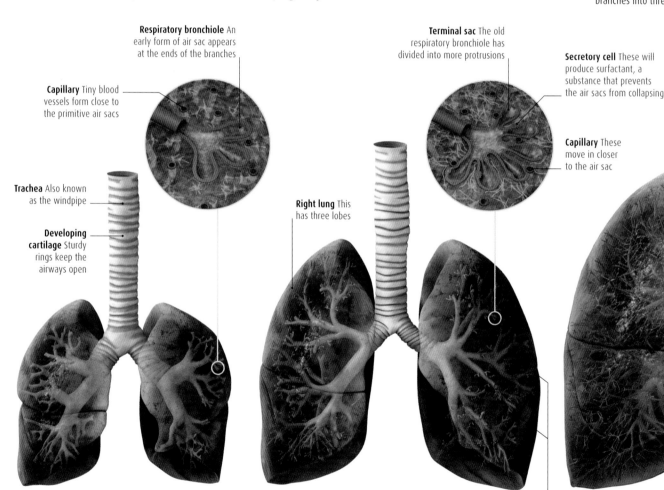

Respiratory bronchiole An early form of air sac appears at the ends of the branches

Capillary Tiny blood vessels form close to the primitive air sacs

Trachea Also known as the windpipe

Developing cartilage Sturdy rings keep the airways open

Terminal sac The old respiratory bronchiole has divided into more protrusions

Secretory cell These will produce surfactant, a substance that prevents the air sacs from collapsing

Capillary These move in closer to the air sac

Right lung This has three lobes

Left lung This only has two lobes, to make room for the heart.

Right main bronchus This is a a steeper angle and is larger than the left main bronchus

Lungs at 16 weeks There have been 20 subdivisions by this point, forming the bronchial airways. There are eight on the left and 10 on the right. The difference in number is because your baby's body is programmed to know that the left-hand lung should be smaller to leave room for his heart.

Lungs at 28 weeks There are now "terminal sacs" that will become alveoli—the air sacs where oxygen and carbon dioxide are exchanged. Until your baby takes his first breath, they're filled with amniotic fluid. The air sacs produce surfactant, a fluid that helps them to contract and expand, and prevents them from collapsing.

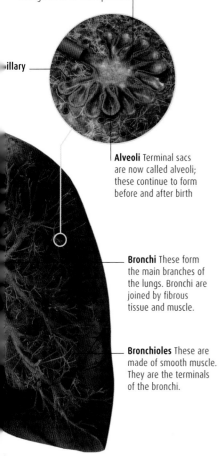

Lungs at 7 weeks The bronchial buds branch out into more buds. Secondary bronchial buds divide to form tertiary buds.

Blood-air barrier The alveoli walls are now so thin that gas can pass through them to the capillaries

Capillary

Alveoli Terminal sacs are now called alveoli; these continue to form before and after birth

Bronchi These form the main branches of the lungs. Bronchi are joined by fibrous tissue and muscle.

Bronchioles These are made of smooth muscle. They are the terminals of the bronchi.

Lungs at 36 weeks Development of the lungs is usually now complete. The terminal sacs have become thin-walled alveoli that allow gas exchange with the capillaries—a process that transfers oxygen and carbon dioxide between the lungs and bloodstream.

Q At my 20-week ultrasound it looked like my baby was breathing, but how can that be?

Your baby can make breathing-like movements as early as 10 weeks pregnant. These are the result of the involuntary contractions in the muscles that are forming around his lungs. The contractions serve to stimulate more muscle growth and the growth of lung tissue. He begins with short practice bursts that last about 10 seconds, and by week 38 of pregnancy these practice "breaths" are in a regular rhythmic pattern of 40 "breaths" per minute, just as he will breathe after he's been born. By the time you're 24 weeks pregnant, your baby will be able to synchronize these breathinglike movements with the rhythmic pumping of his heart, just as he will when he is born.

Q Why doesn't my baby drown in his amniotic fluid?

The simple answer is that a baby doesn't drown in amniotic fluid because he doesn't actually need to breathe when in utero. The important thing for living beings is that we can access oxygen and can remove carbon dioxide from our system, but this gas exchange doesn't have to occur through breathing—in your baby it happens entirely via the placenta. Your baby's circulation, which pumps blood around his developing body, actually bypasses his lungs and goes to the placenta for oxygen until the moment of birth. When your baby is exposed to the air after birth, temperature receptors in his skin trigger the absorption of amniotic fluid from the air sacs, the circulation to the placenta "switches off," and blood starts flowing to his lungs. Then, your baby takes his first breath (which will sound a bit like a gasp), and his lungs will take over the job of breathing. Before the system of bringing oxygen into his body via the lungs is up and running, it isn't possible for your baby to drown.

Q How soon is it possible to tell whether my baby is a boy or a girl?

Although your baby's gender was determined at the moment of conception, it will be at least 14 weeks before there are outward signs. In fact, male and female fetuses look outwardly identical for some weeks (known as the "indifferent" stage) because their genitals are formed from the same structure. This is called the labioscrotal swelling, and it consists of two ridges and a rounded bud. In boys, the ridges connect to form the scrotal sac and the bud elongates to become the penis; in girls, the ridges remain separate and become the labia majora, while the bud shrinks to form the clitoris. By 14 to 17 weeks, the genitals have become obviously differentiated, and have developed enough to be clearly visible.

Internally, the sex organs begin forming at about nine weeks. Depending on whether or not your baby has a Y chromosome (which makes him male), the sex cells create either testes, seminiferous tubules, and vas deferens in your son, or ovaries, uterus, and fallopian tubes in your daughter. The fetal ovaries contain millions of oocytes (immature egg cells)—all the eggs a female will ever have. These could become your future grandchildren. Both boys' and girls' sex organs descend from the abdomen to their correct positions after about 25 weeks. The testes have a long journey to make into the scrotal sac, which is why at birth about 1 percent of full-term, and 10 percent of premature male babies have an undescended testis.

At birth, your baby has in the region of **50–70 million alveoli** in his lungs, each one supplied with **hundreds** of tiny blood **capillaries** ready to exchange **oxygen** and **carbon dioxide**.

Q How many weeks does it take for my baby's face to form?

By the time you go for your ultrasound at around 12 weeks, all your baby's facial features will be clearly recognizable—her face has been developing since the early weeks after conception.

BABY'S FACIAL FEATURE DEVELOPMENT UP TO 12 WEEKS

The following table shows some of the major milestones in the development of her facial features up to the end of the first trimester:

WEEK	FEATURES
6	» Your embryo develops dark spots on each side of her head that will become her eyes. Firstly they form "optic cups" that link to her brain via an optic stalk. The cups eventually become her retinas (the "screens" at the backs of her eyes) and irises (the colored parts of each eye). » Minuscule indents on either side of her head are the beginnings of your baby's ears. Inner tubes that will transmit sound in your baby's ears begin to form.
7	» Her eyes start to form lenses; these are created when certain cells of the ectoderm layer fold over. Eyelids begin to form from folds of skin either side of each eye. » Skin at the sides of your baby's head begin to fold over, so that her ears begin to form. » Nostrils appear at the front of the face, and her nose starts to take shape.
8	» Changes in the ectoderm layer of your embryo mean that by eight weeks the two sides of her face have come together to shape her mouth. » Pigmentation (which gives your baby's eyes their color) starts to collect in the iris of her eyes (see p.168). » Your baby's tongue starts to form, initially above the plate that will become the roof of her mouth.
9	» Your baby's eyes can now move around in their sockets. » Her tongue has developed taste buds.
10	» Your baby's nose starts to protrude, giving her face a more human profile. » Her eyelids start to close over her eyeballs, protecting them from light coming through your abdominal wall. This light could damage the developing retinas. » Your baby's mouth and lips are now fully formed. » Your baby's outer ears now look exactly as they will at birth, but there's still some work to be done inside before she can actually hear.
11	» The roof of your baby's mouth—her palate—is complete. » Tooth buds begin to appear inside her mouth. These will become her milk and adult teeth when the two rows eventually separate.
12	» Your baby's eyes and ears have moved upward as her head has grown, and her eyes have also moved toward the front of her face and are now more or less in their final positions. Your baby can use her mouth, jaw, and tongue to swallow and yawn.

Q I've been singing to my baby, but can she actually hear me? And can she hear my partner singing, too?

Most doctors agree that by the time a fetus is 14 weeks old, she responds to familiar sounds with a quickening of her heart rate. Certainly by 16 weeks, the three bones that transmit sound in her inner ear and the auditory pathways that take sound to her brain are developed enough to suggest that she can hear what's going on inside your body. So she'll hear the swooshing of your blood, your heartbeat, and your tummy rumbles. By 24 weeks, studies show that she'll turn her head in response to a familiar sound—in particular the sound of your voice. Sounds outside the uterus are quieter and more muffled, so it's harder for her to make them out. But hearing a voice other than yours, even if it sounds as if it's being transmitted through water, is enough to make her familiar with it, so your partner's singing definitely isn't in vain.

Q If my baby is developing taste buds, does that mean she can taste the amniotic fluid?

Absolutely! At around the same time that she learns to swallow (roughly 16 weeks pregnant), she develops receptors on her tongue that mean her taste buds can start interpreting the flavors of the amniotic fluid. Contrary to what you might think, your amniotic fluid isn't neutral tasting: it's salty and is infused with flavors from whatever you've been eating, particularly strong flavors such as spices, onion, and garlic. Think of this as a good opportunity to get your baby used to some of your favorite foods—and to the healthy ones that you'll want her to eat when she's older!

Q When does my baby get her skin and what does it look like?

Skin begins to form from the moment a blastocyst becomes an embryo (see p.152), but until well into the second trimester, it's thin and translucent so that nutrients from the amniotic fluid can easily pass through its cells. By 15 weeks pregnant, this translucent covering is

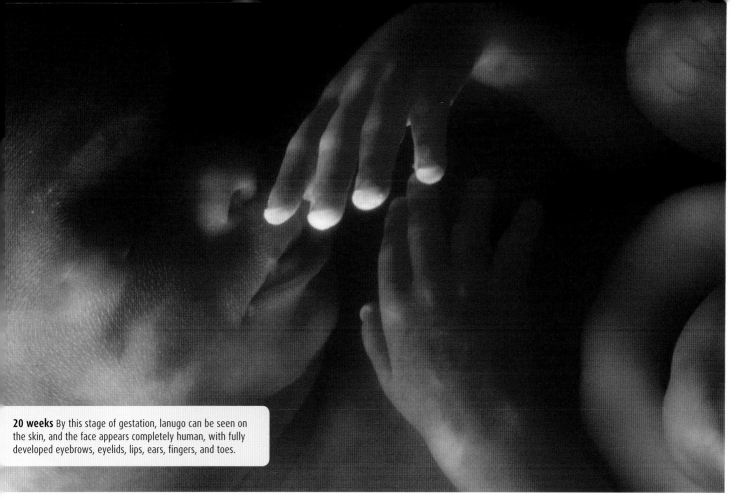

20 weeks By this stage of gestation, lanugo can be seen on the skin, and the face appears completely human, with fully developed eyebrows, eyelids, lips, ears, fingers, and toes.

made up of the three layers of skin we all have—the epidermis, which is the top layer, the dermis in the middle, and the hypodermis, the deepest layer. The skin doesn't become more "solid" looking or lose any of its permeability until you are 32 weeks pregnant. This is also when the babies' skin complexion starts to take on its pigmentation.

Lanugo is fine, soft, downy hair. It's the first hair to be produced by the fetal hair follicles, and it usually appears on the fetus at about 20 weeks of gestation. It is normally shed before birth, at around 28 or 32 weeks of pregnancy, but is sometimes still present at birth. It disappears within a few days or weeks of the birth. Lanugo keeps *vernix caeseosa* (a white, greasy substance) in place on your baby's skin. Vernix starts to appear at around 20 weeks and by 32 weeks it covers most of your baby's body. It's made up of skin cells, fetal skin oil, and lanugo. The Latin term *vernix caeseosa* translates as "cheesy varnish." Vernix helps to keep your baby's skin moist and protect it from exposure to amniotic fluid, which contains high levels of fetal urine (especially toward the end of your pregnancy). It is sometimes still present at birth and can act as a thick, slippery lubricator to encourage your baby's passage down the birth canal during labor.

Q Can my baby smell what's going on inside my uterus?

No one is sure. By 15 weeks pregnant, your fetus has all she needs for her sense of smell to work, but as aromas are passed through the air rather than through fluid, it's always been assumed that her sense of smell doesn't become functional until she's born and starts to breathe air. However, some research has thrown this in doubt and it's now proposed that because your baby is instantly attracted to the smell of your breast milk, she was exposed to the smell of something similar—and therefore familiar—while she was in your uterus.

Q Do my baby's eyes stay closed the whole time she's inside me?

No. Somewhere between 26 and 28 weeks pregnant, she'll close her eyelids in response to bright light and will start to blink. By this stage, her retinas are fully formed, so any risk of damage from bright light has passed. Not only that, but her eyebrows and eyelashes have formed, and they offer extra protection.

Q Can my baby cry tears when she is in the uterus?

Your baby has tear ducts—lacrimal glands— by the end of the first trimester. These are to ensure that her eyeballs are properly moistened throughout gestation, but whether or not they can create tears is still a mystery. Researchers believe that a fetus goes through the motions of crying (distress, frowning, and so on) in response to loud noises, but that's all we know.

Did you know...

» At 7½ weeks pregnant your baby has already developed her first sense—the sense of touch.

» At 18 weeks pregnant she has the ridges in her fingertips that will make her unique fingerprint.

» At 23 weeks pregnant she's covered in a soft, fine, downy hair called lanugo: this will probably almost entirely disappear by the time she's born.

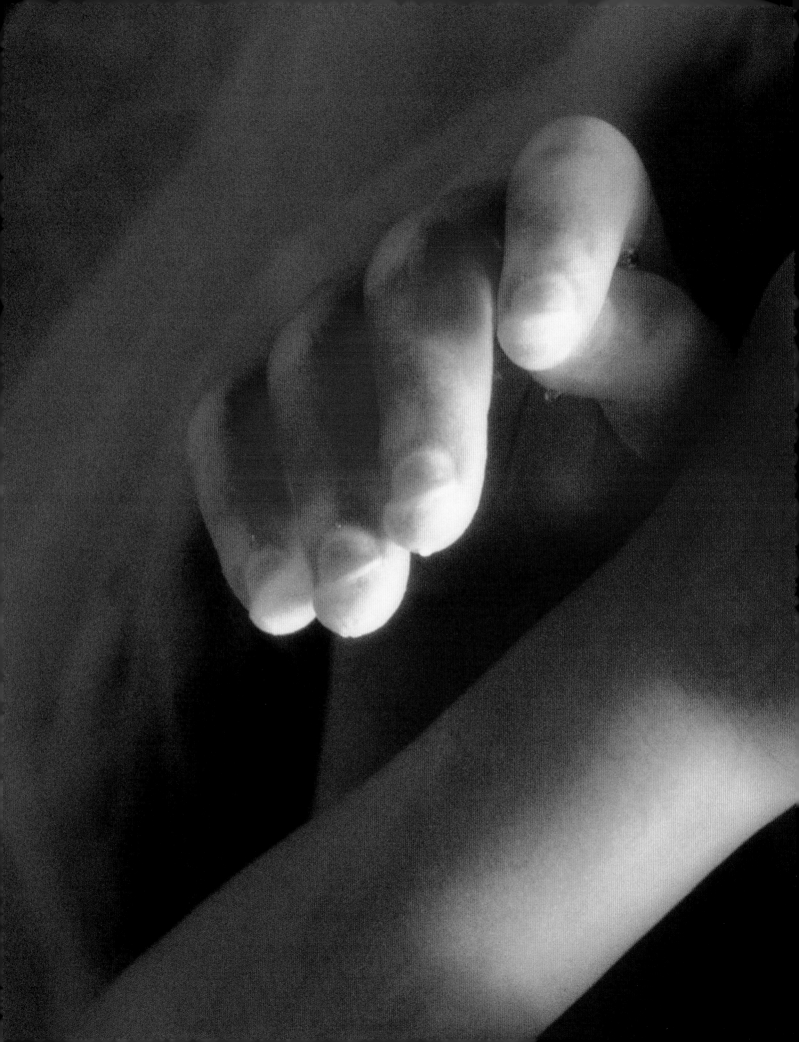

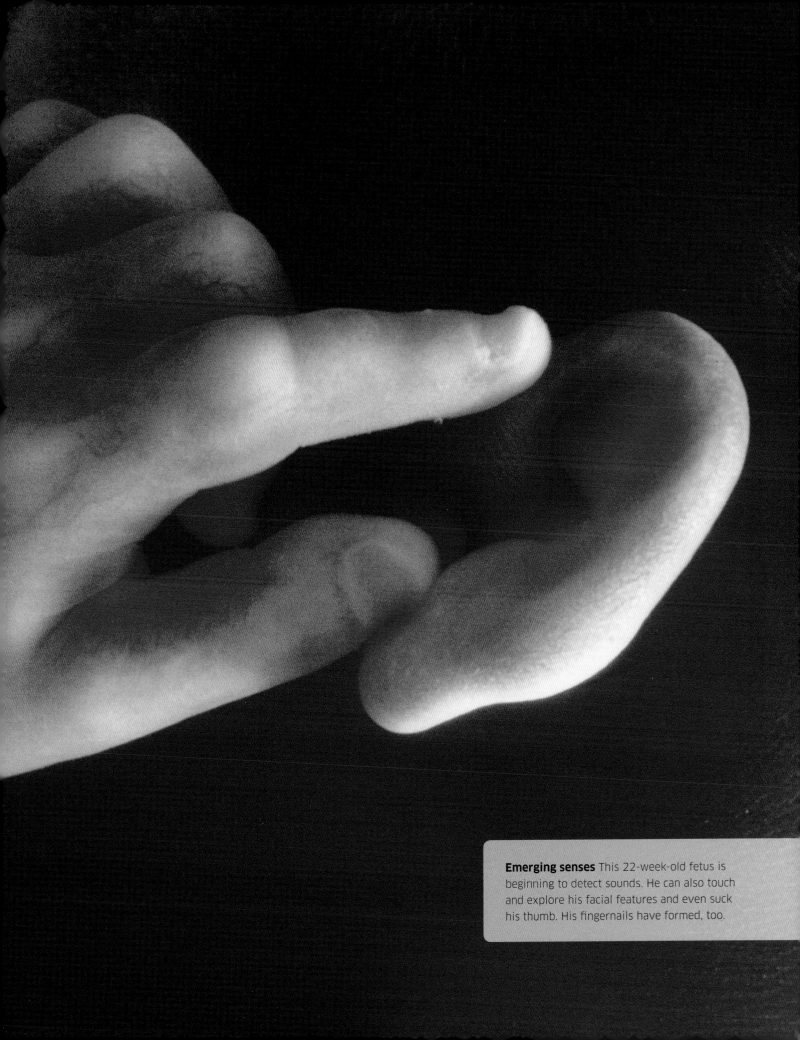

Emerging senses This 22-week-old fetus is beginning to detect sounds. He can also touch and explore his facial features and even suck his thumb. His fingernails have formed, too.

We can talk in general terms about the **development of a baby**—when organs grow, when features form, when she might be ready for birth—but the only certainty is that **your baby will be unique**. From the wave of her hair to her toe prints, she won't have a single **characteristic** that's exactly the same as any other living being.

My baby is unique

What makes babies unique?

Uniqueness comes from two main sources. Firstly, before your baby is born, the "soup" of chromosomes that she gets from each parent gives her a set of genes that might switch on or off, both in the uterus and after birth. Secondly, your baby's environment (for example, from where you live to your morals and values) molds her view and experience of the world. This leads to her responding to her environment in a conscious way–called learned behavior–but it also has physical effects in her body, mutating her genetic codes so that she can adapt to life. In primitive times, this was essential to survival.

Genes are the building blocks of DNA–the hereditary blueprint that's in every cell in your baby's body. Genes give her her eye and hair color, her fingerprints, her inherited character traits, and her inherited diseases and conditions. They're embedded in the chromosomes she receives from her parents. Current scientific thinking is that your baby (and every human being) has around 24,000 genes attached to 23 pairs of chromosomes. Aside from the chromosomes that determine gender, every chromosome has two copies of each gene. Every gene is also made up of variations of itself. Variations of the same gene are called alleles, and these can be recessive alleles or dominant ones. The dominant alleles "overpower" the recessive ones, producing a unique physical, mental, and emotional recipe for every human being.

The brain and the environment

Genes provide the raw ingredients, but other aspects of your baby's uniqueness–such as her personality, how she learns to do things, the way she responds to stimuli in her environment, how she displays her intellect, and the ways in which she forms relationships–are subject to her experience of the world around her.

From the moment of her birth, the information that your baby gets from her environment builds connections in her brain. At birth, brain imaging shows large sections of the brain waiting to form neural connections. These come with such speed that by 24 months, only small unconnected patches remain. By the age of three, your baby will have far more connections that she ever needs and a period of "synaptic pruning" begins. This eliminates and hones the connections so that brain efficiency rises.

The role of lifestyle and its influence on our genes is important when considering inherited illness. For example, we know that heart disease can also be inherited. However, while a baby might inherit a tendency toward it, her lifestyle choices can turn on or off the gene that causes the condition.

Q Which member of my family is my newborn baby going to look like most?

Your baby might have a range of features and characteristics from different members of each of your families—an aunt's hair, a cousin's sense of humor, or your mother's nose. How DNA and inheritance work can help to explain this.

Your baby shares half her DNA with you and half with your partner. In turn, you share half of your genes with each of your parents. This means that your baby shares a quarter of her genes with your parents—her grandparents.

Through each generation genes are shuffled and reshuffled. At conception, the embryo receives 23 chromosomes from the mother's egg and 23 chromosomes from the father's sperm. These pair up to make a total of 46 chromosomes. The chromosomes contain the genes that you inherit. When the sperm fertilizes the egg, chromosomes join together and randomly exchange genes.

Likewise, even though full siblings inherit genes from the same parents, these aren't necessarily the same genes, nor the same dominant alleles. Remember, you've each passed one of two copies of every gene you have to your baby, but because the two copies of each of your genes aren't identical (every copy has variations), you won't always pass the same version of each gene to each child. Mix this up for all the genes from both of you, and it turns out that the permutations are endless.

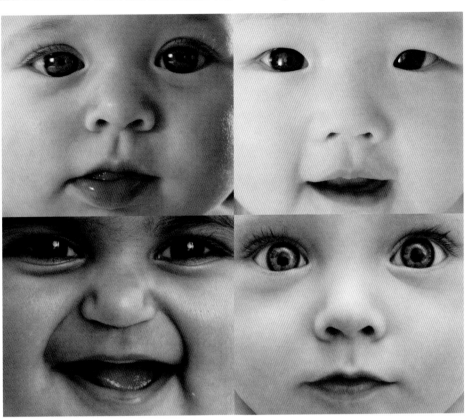

Blue eyes, brown eyes, different shaped eyes, and noses Humans are amazingly diverse. This is due to both genetic inheritance and variation in environmental factors.

Q What determines whether I have a boy or a girl?

Your baby's gender is determined by specific chromosomes—the tubelike structures that contain her unique genetic blueprint. Healthy human beings have 23 chromosome pairs; one chromosome in each pair is inherited from each parent. The 23rd pair of chromosomes is called the sex chromosome and it determines what sex a baby will be. A woman's egg always contains the female chromosome, known as X and a man's sperm contains either an X (female) or Y (male) chromosome. An embryo that has two X chromosomes will be female, whereas one with an XY combination will be male. It is therefore the man's sperm that determines whether a baby is male or female.

Q Can environmental factors influence how my children look if they are the same sex?

Children who grow up in the same household are never in the same environment at every moment. They could have different bedrooms, different teachers, and experience different emotions. Also, how tall each child grows is partly influenced by the food they eat. One child may have started solids with only carrots and pears, but your second is more likely to start with the foods that her big sister's now eating. What you eat plays its part, too. If your taste preferences have changed since the first pregnancy, the nutritional influence on each of your daughters will be different—and that can impact their physical characteristics.

Q Can my baby's genes determine whether or not she will be overweight later on in her life?

No, but they may predispose her to weight gain if it runs in the family. In this case, whether or not your baby turns out to be overweight will depend a lot on environmental factors. Her eating habits, stress levels, and enjoyment of sports, can all influence whether or not the genes for gaining excess weight switch on. How you eat in pregnancy can influence it as well. Your baby can taste what's in the amniotic fluid, so if she gets used to sweeter flavors, say, while she's inside you, it may be more difficult to encourage her to eat vegetables as she gets older.

Q What color will my baby's eyes be and what determines this?

You baby's eye color depends on how dominant and recessive alleles (variants of genes—see p.166) work.

Each person has two alleles for eye color (and other characteristics), one inherited from each of their parents. The brown allele (B) is dominant and the blue allele (b) is recessive, so when the two come together (Bb) brown dominates over blue and the result is brown eyes. In order to have blue eyes, a person must have two blue alleles (bb). Therefore, if your baby has blue eyes but both parents have brown eyes, both you and your partner must be Bb—each of you has one brown allele and one blue allele.

A Bb mother and a Bb father have a 25-percent chance of having a blue-eyed baby. It becomes a 50-percent chance if one of you is bb and the other Bb. If one or both of you is BB, the only possible outcome is a baby with brown eyes. Of course, if you both have blue eyes (you are both bb), your baby will have blue eyes, too.

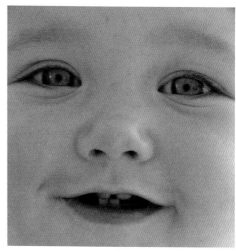

Blue eyes Many Caucasian babies' eyes look blue or gray when they are first born. It can take up to a year for the pigmentation to settle in and reveal the true eye color.

Blue and green are both recessive alleles. When blue and green are the only alleles present, they are actually codominant, so your baby's eye color could take on blue, green, or a mix of the two.

EYE COLOR

The diagram below illustrates how genes determine your baby's eye color. This principle

PARENTS' EYE COLOR AND GENE

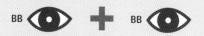
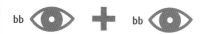
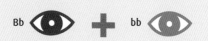
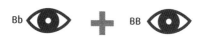
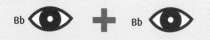

Q Why is it that not all brown eyes are the same shade of brown?

No one is really sure. While the overall color of your baby's eyes (brown, hazel, blue, or green) might be determined by one set of genes, the level of pigmentation in your baby's iris may be determined by another—perhaps many others. Pigmentation comes from melanin, which is present not only in the iris of the eye, but in hair and skin, too. So, if you have two babies and the first has dark brown eyes and the second has light brown eyes, both babies have

dominant brown alleles in the eye-color gene. However, certain other genes caused different amounts of melanin in the eyes of the two children—resulting in different shades of brown. The more melanin that's released, the darker the pigmentation in the eye.

Q Will our baby inherit his father's height? Can we tell at birth?

Both parents' genes have a role to play in a person's final height as an adult. The mid-parental height formula estimates a child's potential growth—you simply add both parents' height in inches together, divide by two, and then add an extra $2^{1}/_{2}$ inches for a boy or subtract $2^{1}/_{2}$ inches for a girl. For instance, if mom's height is 5'4" and dad's is 5'11", a son's potential height would be 5'10" and a daughter's would be 5'5". This formula only gives a rough estimate, however, and in reality your child's health, diet, and other environmental factors play a part in addition to genes. Your baby's

size at birth doesn't necessarily indicate what his adult height will be, either, especially if he is premature. Mom's health, weight, and diet in pregnancy are more likely to have an affect on your baby's birth weight than genes.

Q Could my baby have curly hair if mine is straight?

In Caucasians, curly hair is determined by a dominant allele, so the answer to this depends on what pair of alleles your baby inherits from both parents. If you have straight hair, but your partner has curly hair, your baby is 50 to 75 percent likely to have curly hair, depending upon whether your partner has two curly-hair alleles, or one curly and one straight. If you both have straight hair, then your baby's hair will probably be straight, too. If you both have curly hair, the chances are that your baby will have curly hair—although if you both are straight-hair carriers, there's still a 25-percent chance that your baby's hair will be straight.

Color blindness is a condition that is passed down from parent to child and is much **more common in men** than women.

eplicated for every possible trait, including
r color, skin tone, dimples, and so on.

BY'S POTENTIAL EYE COLOR AND GENE

 BB

 bb

 Bb bb

BB Bb

Bb bb

BB Bb

Q My baby's father is bald. Does this mean that if I have a boy, he will go bald, too?

The genetic inheritance of baldness is still not fully understood. For a long time it was thought that male pattern baldness (baldness that runs in families and begins with a receding hairline) was inherited from the mother's side. So, a baby boy was assumed to inherit baldness via his mother from his maternal grandfather rather than from his own father. However, anecdotal evidence shows that this isn't always the case, which has led researchers to look for a pattern that confirms heredity directly from father to son. Although there doesn't yet seem to be evidence that the faulty gene lies within the Y chromosome, there is some evidence that mutations in genes on chromosome 20 (which can come from a baby's mother or father) may increase the risk of a boy inheriting baldness. Environmental factors (including diet and stress levels) play a role, too. In short, while the percentages suggest that boys born to bald fathers are likely to go bald themselves, there are no certainties. As far as girls going bald is concerned, it's thought that high levels of female hormones make sure the baldness gene stays inactive.

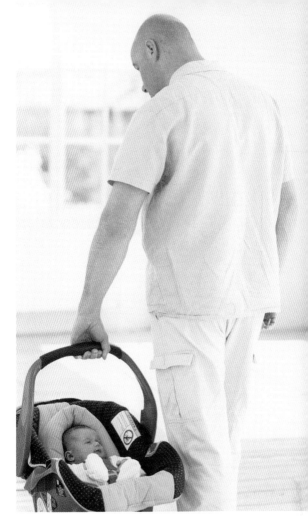

Male pattern baldness This is the most common type of hair loss in men. It is generally thought to be caused by hormones and a genetic predisposition.

Q What causes albinism?

This is a rare genetic condition, where the genes that control melanin production are faulty.

As a result the proteins in the genes don't get the message to trigger the release of melanin in the hair, eyes, and skin, which leads to lack of pigmentation. Those affected tend to be very pale in color, have pink or pale gray eyes, and white hair. It can cause sight problems and sensitivity to light, because eyes need melanin to make a healthy retina (the "screen" at the back of the eye). Albinism is inherited through autosomal recessive inheritance (in which both parents carry the faulty gene and the baby inherits it from both sides) and X-linked inheritance (in which the faulty gene is attached to the X chromosome in one parent).

X-LINKED INHERITANCE

An X-linked inheritance refers to conditions that occur as a result of a faulty gene within the X chromosome. The box below explains how this works.

MOTHER (XX)

A baby girl has a 50-percent chance of becoming a carrier of the faulty gene (and a 50-percent chance of not inheriting a faulty gene at all), but would not herself have the condition. This is because girls have two X chromosomes (XX)—in this case, one healthy and one carrying the faulty gene. The healthy X chromosome compensates for the carrier, and the baby girl appears healthy.

A baby boy has one X chromosome and one Y chromosome (XY), inherited from his mother and father, respectively, giving him a 50-percent chance that he will inherit the X chromosome from his mother that carries the faulty gene. If this happens he will develop albinism, because he has no healthy X chromosome to compensate.

FATHER (XY)

A baby girl will definitely become a carrier, because in order to become a girl (XX) she must inherit the damaged X chromosome from her father.

A baby boy does not become a carrier, because to become a boy he must inherit the Y chromosome from his father.

Q Will my baby's brain be fully formed when she is born or does it continue growing?

Your baby's brain grows faster than any other organ and, consequently, the head is still out of proportion with the rest of the body when she is born.

The brain continues growing and developing throughout childhood and into adulthood, but is at its most sensitive during certain periods in the early years. Between conception and about the age of three a young child's brain goes through an enormous amount of change. At birth, your baby will have around 100 billion brain cells (neurons) and that's roughly the number she has throughout her life. At this time, basic neural connections are in place, which help to control vital functions such as breathing, heart rate, digestion, and reflexes. The connections are formed at a very fast rate during the first few years and, as more links form, higher mental functions such as memory, increased attention span, language, intellect, and social skills develop. By adulthood, the neural network allows for reasoning, judgment, and original thought.

BRAIN FORMATION

During her time in the uterus, your growing baby's brain goes through an extraordinary amount of growth and development.

WEEK	ACTIVITY
5	The neural tube divides to create separate spaces for the development of her brain cells and nerve cells—effectively beginning the formation of her brain and central nervous system.
7	The two hemispheres of your baby's brain begin to separate. The right one will go on to govern her creativity, spatial awareness, and lateral thinking; the left will influence her logic and practical thinking.
8	The synapses, which open and close the pathways to send messages between neurons, start to form. Your baby is born with relatively few synapses; most of them form within the first two to three years of life as memories and her understanding of the world are laid down.
12	Your baby's cerebellum begins to form. At the same time, the two halves of her brain begin to communicate with each other and there's an enormous burst of neuron formation (called neurogenesis). Her hypothalamus and pituitary glands have formed.
14–16	Reflex responses in your baby's limbs and facial features suggest that she's now responding to stimuli in the uterus. This confirms that her brain's neurons are beginning to work, processing what she is experiencing. This coincides with maturing taste buds and the ability of the bones in her ear to transmit sound.
22–25	The formation of her brain matter is complete and her cerebral cortex starts to fold over on itself, creating her brain's typical ridged, wrinkled appearance. This increases her brain's surface area, which optimizes her chances for learning.
26–40	Your baby's nervous system is now fully developed. Her cerebral cortex begins to send out electrical impulses: researchers believe that memory has begun to develop because some of these impulses respond to the sound of familiar voices. Her cerebellum is three times bigger at 40 weeks than it was at 22 weeks, and her whole brain weighs approximately 12 oz (350 g).

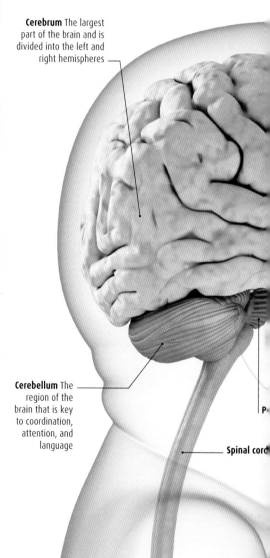

Forebrain prominence

Cranial nerves

Ear bud

Eye bud

Pharyngeal arches

At 5 weeks The neural tube forms the forebrain prominence.

At 9 weeks Swellings that will become different parts of the brain are growing and are beginning to fold into one another.

Cerebrum The largest part of the brain and is divided into the left and right hemispheres

Cerebellum The region of the brain that is key to coordination, attention, and language

P

Spinal cord

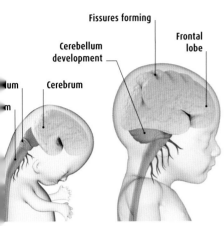

13 weeks Lobes have ~~ned~~. The connections ~~ween~~ the cells are ~~sent~~ and the hindbrain ~~des~~ into two parts: the ~~ebellum~~ and brain stem.

At 25 weeks The surface of the brain is still smooth. Folds are beginning to emerge as the number of cells begins to increase.

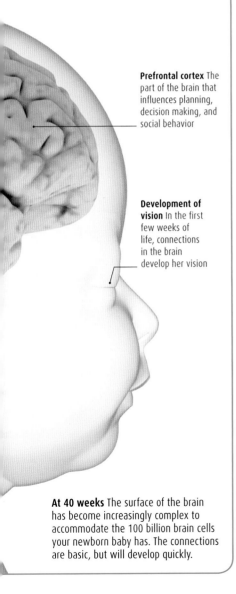

Prefrontal cortex The part of the brain that influences planning, decision making, and social behavior

Development of vision In the first few weeks of life, connections in the brain develop her vision

At 40 weeks The surface of the brain has become increasingly complex to accommodate the 100 billion brain cells your newborn baby has. The connections are basic, but will develop quickly.

Q I've heard that stress can affect my baby's brain development. Is this true?

Stress can affect a fetus, but it's also true that the majority of brain development happens after your baby is born. Research suggests that if you suffer from stress during pregnancy, it can have an affect on the way your baby deals with and responds to the world after she's born. However, it's not just your stress levels during pregnancy that make a difference. At birth, only a quarter of your baby's brain is "wired" with neural links; the rest are waiting to be formed by experience. So, how you teach your baby to deal with stress once she's born is very important, too, as is a consistent and loving approach to parenting.

Managing stress in pregnancy

If you are anxious or stressed, talk to others about how you are feeling–they may be able to help you find solutions. Your partner or family members may be able to take on more at home so you can rest, or your employer may offer some flexibility if you need it. Your doctor is also there to support and advise you. Make time to rest and relax; meditation and breathing techniques, massage, and gentle exercise such as walking and yoga are all helpful for managing your stress.

Q Are baby girls' and baby boys' brains the same?

Fundamentally, yes, though after birth, when the synapses start making their connections, the genders tend to wire themselves differently. We know that girls are more likely to stare intently at faces, even when they're tiny babies, while boys tend to look around, taking in everything that's going on. Although it sounds a cliché, boys have been shown to have greater spatial awareness than girls: the parts of the brain that orient us show more connections in a little boy's brain than in a little girl's. Girls, though, tend to have better wiring for language, empathy, and communication. Of course, there's a lot of debate about whether or not "girly" behavior and "boyish" behavior are influenced by environmental factors. They almost certainly are, although that's not the whole story–male and female hormones play a part, too. In the

end, though, the incredible plasticity of brain wiring means that our brains provide us with potential, but our genes and the environment of our upbringing decide how much potential we end up fulfilling.

Q Is something wrong if my baby doesn't follow the developmental milestones, such as smiling and walking?

Usually, it is likely that your baby is just learning at her own happy pace. Very occasionally, though, being a "late" developer (measured against averages that you might read about) may be a warning of something else. All babies develop at different rates. This is due to a combination of genetics and gender.

Despite the term, developmental milestones don't happen at set "miles"; they happen when your baby's ready and that's within a much broader time period than time lines generally suggest. All babies are unique and will develop in their own way. However, the order in which they acquire certain physical skills, also known as gross motor skills–strength in the head and neck, sitting up, smiling, waving, crawling, walking–is generally the same. Your baby's strength develops from the head downward over the first 18 months. If your baby shows little or no strength in her muscles, is unresponsive to stimuli, seems unable to coordinate her movements, or seems to deal with the world very differently from other babies her age, talk to your doctor for guidance. More often than not, you'll be reassured that everything's fine.

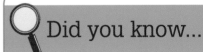

Did you know...

In order to help your baby learn to walk, it is crucial to play with your baby out of her carriage or crib for a little while every day. This will advance her overall mobility. Encouraging activities like "tummy time" will help development, strengthening the neck, head, and addominal muscles that she will need to use to be able to sit, crawl, and then walk.

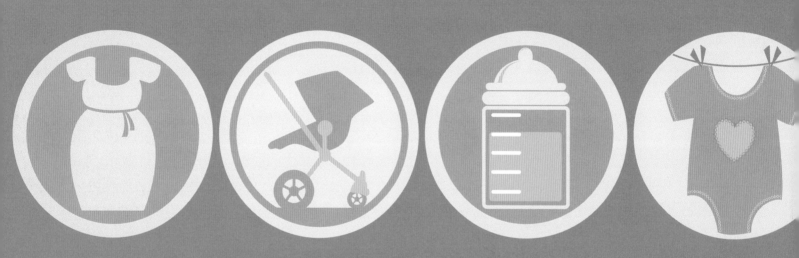

Practical preparations

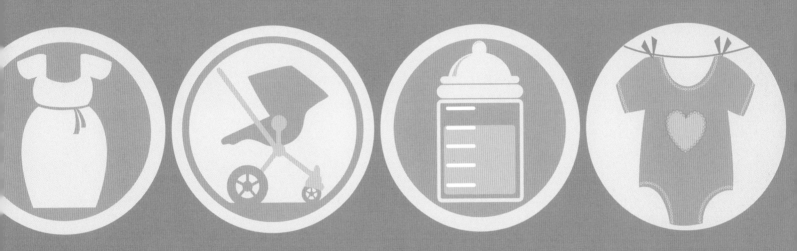

It's important to feel **ready and prepared** for labor, birth, and life with a newborn. Gain expert, practical advice on **what you will need** for you, your baby, and your home. It's best to borrow or buy a bassinet, car seat, feeding equipment, and a baby carriage or front-pack carrier in advance of your baby arriving. Find out exactly what you need to pack in your **hospital bag** and what your birth partner might need as well. This chapter also helps you think about other ways in which you can be prepared, especially if you're having a multiple birth.

As your body changes, you will want a comfortable **pregnancy wardrobe** that offers **flexibility** and **comfort aids** and props to help you to sleep and ease pregnancy complaints. You should also start buying **equipment** for **life after the birth**.

Practical tips for Mom

Do I need a maternity warbrobe?

Being comfortable is key during pregnancy. In the early months when your waistband first expands, you may get away with wearing normal clothes in a larger size or borrowing your partner's tops, but for most women this isn't a solution that will work for long. Clothes designed for pregnancy use fabrics and cuts that expand in the right places as you get bigger, whereas regular clothes may simply become tighter and uncomfortable. It can seem wasteful to splurge on maternity clothes that you will wear for a brief period only, but they will see a lot of use for five or six months and will get you through any future pregnancies, too, so it is worth a little investment. Happily, it is possible to assemble a decent maternity wardrobe on a budget by borrowing them or buying them secondhand.

Keeping in season

When you start to assemble your maternity wardrobe, think about what time of year it will be toward the end of your pregnancy. If your early pregnancy is in the summer months, you may not want to spend on maternity summer dresses or short-sleeved blouses that will see little use when you need bigger sizes. And likewise, you won't want a collection of long-sleeved, warm maternity tops if you are going to be heavily pregnant in the middle of the summer. You may be able to pick up some bargains in end-of-season sales that will be perfect in six months time.

A little support

Your growing belly can also cause pregnancy complaints such as backaches, which means that getting a good night's sleep becomes increasingly difficult. Even sitting can become uncomfortable in the latter stages of pregnancy. Props such as pillows and belly support bands can be invaluable now, and some support pillows double up as nursing pillows. You may also want to consider an exercise ball, which is useful before, during, and after the birth, and inflatable cushions and pillows that can make sitting easier if you're suffering with hemorrhoids—a common pregnancy complaints—or want to avoid putting pressure on any stitches you may have after the birth.

Q I want to wear my usual clothes for as long as possible. When will I need to start wearing maternity clothes?

It is usually around the start of the second trimester that women find their waistbands start to tighten. From this point onward, wearing your usual clothes becomes increasingly difficult and uncomfortable.

You may find early on in pregnancy that your bust size has gone up a little and your tops are fitting more snugly, but you can still wear your existing clothes. By 20 to 24 weeks, though, and perhaps earlier, your clothing choices may become restricted and you may feel that you need to start wearing real maternity wear. Invest in a few key pieces that make you feel and look good. Many women don't worry about trying to disguise their pregnancy and prefer to wear form-fitting clothes to flatter their new shape.

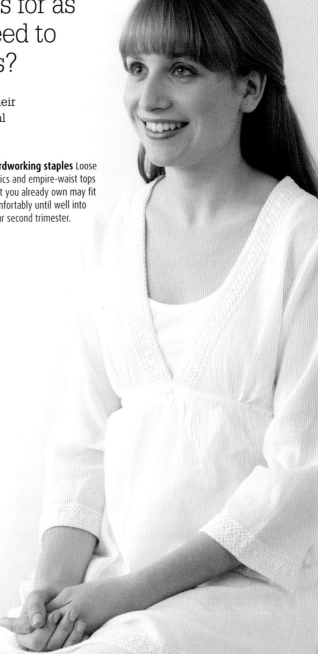

Hardworking staples Loose tunics and empire-waist tops that you already own may fit comfortably until well into your second trimester.

Extending the life of your clothes

A stretchy belly band is a great pregnancy innovation. Made in soft, breathable materials, the wide band is worn over your belly and the waistband of your clothes to cover any gaps that appear between your top and bottom garments. The effect is a seamless look of smart layering. The band's snug elastic fit helps to hold your pants up, too, so you can leave your zipper or buttons undone. After the birth, it can handily cover up post-delivery flab and reduce the amount of flesh you reveal if breast-feeding.

Other options

» Expand the waistband of your pants and jeans: thread an elastic hair band or sturdy rubber band through your pants button hole and loop each end around the pants button.

» Long tops will keep your emerging belly covered during your first trimester, since they won't ride up too much with your growing belly.

» Empire-waist tops, loose-fitting tops and tunics, and wrap-around tops and dresses are ideal during the transitional period when most of your clothes are too tight, but you're not big enough for maternity wear.

» Long t-shirt dresses and jersey skirts can stretch to accommodate your belly during the transitional period.

» Borrowing your partner's clothes can come in handy at the beginning of your second trimester. Check if any shirts or tops will work as casual wear for weekends and evenings.

Q Which fabrics will be most comfortable in pregnancy?

You may feel hotter than usual in pregnancy due to your increased blood circulation, so opt for lighter, breathable fabrics. It is a good idea to wear light layers that you can remove or add to easily to feel just the right temperature. Natural fabrics such as wool, silk, linen, and cotton are ideal, and there are organic versions of these fabrics if you want to avoid unwanted chemical exposure and prefer their softness. Newer fabrics such as bamboo and hemp are also soft and breathable. All these fabrics are hypoallergenic and will feel very comfortable against your skin. Many women experience itchiness as their skin stretches to accommodate the baby, so avoid synthetic fabrics such as polyester, viscose, and nylon, which may irritate your skin. Look out, too, for stretchy natural-fiber clothes containing lycra, such as cotton leggings, since they will be most comfortable to wear as your belly grows.

You may find that as your belly grows, you **prefer** to wear clothes that are designed to **flatter your new, curvier figure** and show off your belly rather than hide it.

Q What are the most useful items to buy for my pregnancy wardrobe?

Dressing a rapidly growing belly can seem tricky at first, but you can get great mileage from a small collection of key maternity items, especially if you mix and match with your existing accessories to suit the occasion.

You may want to build up your pregnancy wardrobe gradually, buying a few core pieces—perhaps one or two pairs of maternity pants or jeans, a dress, and a couple of tops—and then add one or two new items to suit your ever-changing shape. If you buy maternity clothes in neutral colors, it will be easy to mix and match them with floaty tunics or wrap-around tops, and existing clothes such as cardigans and jackets that you can continue wearing unbuttoned. Neutral pieces can also be styled with scarves or jewelry to give you a range of outfits.

A good pair of maternity jeans can be very versatile and work as both daytime and evening wear. They come in a variety of styles and waist options: some have a stretchy, expandable "bandeau-style" belly panel; some are designed with elastic side pieces that allow the waistband to stretch as you get bigger; and others have a low-rise waistband that sits beneath your belly. Look for stretchy cotton denim that is soft and comfortable to wear, even in the latter stages of pregnancy.

In addition to a pair of maternity jeans, you may want to invest in:

» **A pair of plain pants** to wear with a shirt or top and cardigan or jacket for work, or with a dressier top for evenings out.

» **A maternity dress or tunic.** Wrap-around styles are perfect, as you can let them out as you grow, or choose an empire-waist tunic, which is flattering and works well with stretchy leggings.

» **Tops such as T-shirts, tanks,** and long-sleeved tops, depending on the season.

» **Maternity tights** and leggings.

One of the most **hardworking** and **valuable** items in your pregnancy wardrobe is likely to be a pair of **maternity jeans**.

Sizing

Many maternity clothing lines advise you to stick with your prepregnancy size when buying maternity wear, but proportions are not necessarily the same across brands. If you can, try on some items first to check how true-to-size a brand's sizing is. Some stores have pillows in different sizes that replicate your growing belly—you can wear these when you try on clothes to see if the size is correct and works for you.

You might be tempted to buy regular clothes in bigger sizes, but beware the larger overall proportions they will have. It is likely they will fit poorly on the shoulders and arms and that hemlines will ride up at the front and won't hang properly over your belly.

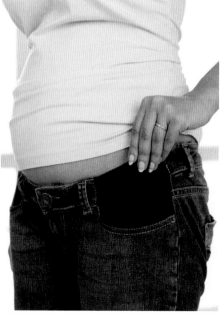

Maternity pants If you find a comfortable, well-fitting pair of maternity jeans, you should be able to wear them right up until the birth, and beyond.

Q I have a limited budget. Where can I find stylish but inexpensive maternity wear?

While your pregnancy is wonderful news, it does bring with it a financial cost, as you also need to factor in the nursery and travel equipment your baby will require. Fortunately, it's perfectly possible to be financially prudent and keep costs low when putting together your maternity wardrobe. Most box stores and department stores now stock good maternity clothes, which typically include many affordable basics that won't break the bank. If the timing works out and you plan ahead, you may be able to get some good deals in end-of-season sales that could be in the right season by the end of your pregnancy.

Be open, too, to any offers of maternity clothes from friends, sisters, and cousins who may be happy to pass on their entire maternity wardrobe, even if they are a slightly different size; many maternity items, particularly tops, can fit a range of sizes. You can always consider a clothing trade if that makes you feel easier about accepting the clothes.

Bargain hunting

Buying secondhand maternity clothes is well worth considering, since they are often in extremely good condition because many items are worn just a handful of times. Check out the local secondhand stores in your area that may sell maternity clothes, and also research consignment shop clothing stores, which can be a great place to hunt down some maternity bargains. Tag sales can be another great place to find clothes for a steal, and also take a look at maternity "bundles" on auction websites where new moms auction their maternity wardrobe in one lot.

Are your **shoes** feeling tight? You're not imagining things—some women find that their shoe **size increases** as **relaxin** loosens their foot ligaments. The new shoe size can be permanent.

Q Do I have to forego high heels completely?

There's no edict banning high heels in pregnancy, but most podiatrists advise against them once your belly starts to grow, so save them for special occasions.

High heels change your posture, increasing the strain on your knees and encouraging you to arch your back to compensate for the change in weight distribution. This effect is exacerbated in pregnancy due to your softened joints and ligaments (caused by the hormone relaxin) and your changing center of gravity, so wear high heels only occasionally to prevent aches and pains.

Comfort and support

During pregnancy, you will find low-heeled, wide-fitting, supportive shoes that preserve your foot arch much more comfortable for everyday wear. It's common for feet to swell in pregnancy, caused by extra fluids in the body (known as edema). Some women even find that their feet go up a half or whole size, again due to relaxin causing the ligaments in the feet to spread. Choose shoes with a slight, firm heel of 1 in (2.5 cm), to discourage you from leaning backward. Beware of completely flat shoes since they offer little in the way of cushioning and comfort as your weight increases.

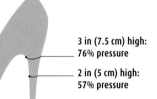

Higher heels It may not come as a surprise that the higher the heel, the more pressure you place on your forefeet. Choosing slightly lower heels, when you wear non-flat shoes, can help to reduce the strain on your feet, lower back, and knees.

3 in (7.5 cm) high: 76% pressure
2 in (5 cm) high: 57% pressure

WEARING HEELS IN PREGNANCY

When you're pregnant, wearing high heels is more of a balancing act than usual. Your growing belly throws your weight forward, forcing you to adjust your spine, knees, and leg alignment to maintain your balance.

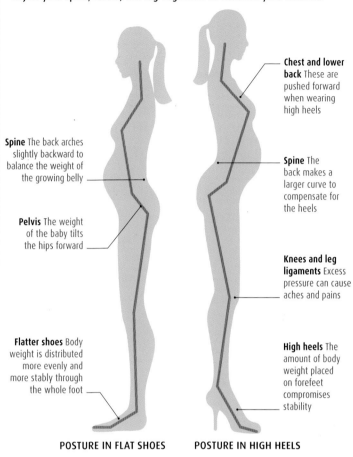

Chest and lower back These are pushed forward when wearing high heels

Spine The back makes a larger curve to compensate for the heels

Knees and leg ligaments Excess pressure can cause aches and pains

High heels The amount of body weight placed on forefeet compromises stability

Spine The back arches slightly backward to balance the weight of the growing belly

Pelvis The weight of the baby tilts the hips forward

Flatter shoes Body weight is distributed more evenly and more stably through the whole foot

POSTURE IN FLAT SHOES   POSTURE IN HIGH HEELS

Q Should I buy a special maternity swimsuit, or make do?

This depends on how much swimming you plan to do during pregnancy. If you want to swim regularly—swimming is a perfect pregnancy exercise, after all—it's worth investing in a pregnancy swimsuit specially designed to support your growing belly and bust and adapt with your changing body, while also providing comfort and ease of movement. However, if all you need a swimsuit for is a two-week vacation in the sun, then you may be able to get away with an existing stretchy swimsuit, or a bikini or tankini that fits under and over your belly.

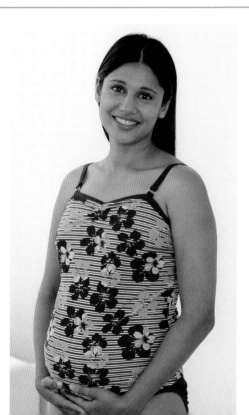

Pregnancy swimsuits If you are swimming regularly for exercise, a supportive maternity swimsuit is a worthwhile investment.

Q I will be heavily pregnant in the winter. Will I need to buy a maternity coat?

If you want to invest in a special maternity coat, by all means do so, but you may find that a winter coat will make you feel uncomfortably warm, even if the weather is cold. Before you shop for extra layers of maternity clothing, keep in mind that your natural body temperature will be higher toward the end of your pregnancy as your blood circulation increases. A maternity coat may not be necessary, and since a coat is quite a large investment, you may prefer to keep warm by wearing knit layers instead. You could put on a lighter waterproof raincoat, shawl, fleece, or scarf over these knit items so that you can remove one or more layers if you do get hot.

Q Why are maternity bras important? Won't my usual bras be OK to wear in pregnancy?

While a few women find that their breasts don't change size significantly during pregnancy, most women do go up around two to four cup sizes during these nine months as their breasts respond to hormonal changes and prepare for milk production.

It's not just your cup size that can increase in pregnancy: your rib cage also expands, sometimes by as much as 4 in (10 cm). The average woman goes up two band sizes in pregnancy. Additionally, your breasts can get heavier and feel tender. All of these changes mean it is important to make sure that your breasts are comfortable and well supported.

Soft and supportive

Wearing a well-fitting, supportive bra during pregnancy can help to prevent or reduce stretch marks, ensure good posture, and relieve tension on your shoulders and back. If your breasts don't change size during pregnancy, your usual bras may suffice, but it is still likely that your breasts will feel more tender than usual, and you will want to make sure that any bra you do wear is comfortable. Good maternity and nursing bras are made from soft materials, are usually nonwired, and offer extra support at the shoulders and back. Maternity bras also have enough stretch and flexibility to allow your breasts some room to continue growing.

Maternity and nursing bras are designed to offer **the right support** and are made of soft, breathable fabrics to provide **maximum comfort**.

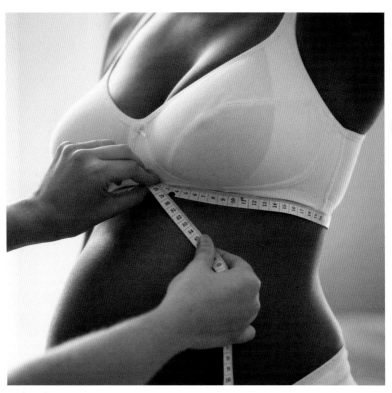

Go for a fitting Have a professional bra fitter check your size accurately. She will also take into account how your breasts may change through pregnancy.

Q Did you know...

Don't guess your new bra size! Many women end up with uncomfortable, poorly fitting bras when guessing—which is the last thing you want in pregnancy or after the birth. You can find professional bra fitters in certain lingerie stores and the lingerie departments of many department stores—and the service is usually free. The fitter will usually measure beneath your bust line and around the bust (over your clothes or with your bra on), ask you to try on a fit bra to gauge your correct cup size, or judge by eye which bra size you need.

Q When do I need to go and get fitted for a maternity bra?

This varies from woman to woman, but as soon as your normal bra starts to feel tight, it's time to get fitted for a maternity bra. If your bra leaves red marks on your skin, it is too tight. It is quite possible that you need to change your bra size two or three times during pregnancy since your breasts continue to grow.

Usually, the end of your first trimester is a good time to check how your bra is fitting, if you haven't already—some women start wearing maternity bras earlier if their bust is too tender to wear their usual bras. During the second trimester, your belly and rib cage start to expand too, so it's worth getting remeasured then as well.

Q I've heard that my breasts will get even bigger after the birth. When should I get a nursing bra?

It's a good idea to buy at least one nursing bra before your baby arrives so you don't have to go shopping right after the birth. Breasts usually stop growing by 36 weeks of pregnancy, so at this point a trained bra fitter can estimate what size your breasts will be after the birth. Your breasts will get bigger when your milk comes in (even if you don't intend to breast-feed), and you might need one or two larger nursing bras. Once your milk supply settles down, your breasts usually get a bit smaller again, so buy bras that you can tighten as your breasts change shape.

Q I'm almost 35 weeks and my maternity bra is feeling tight. Can I avoid getting a new bra now?

If your cup size still feels fine, but your bra is tight around your body, you could buy a bra extender. This cheap accessory is simply three or four extra sets of eyes that you attach to your existing bra strap so that you can let your bra out a few more inches as your rib cage expands. This saves you from buying a new maternity bra at this late stage.

Q What's the difference between a maternity bra and a nursing bra?

Nursing bras allow easy access during breast-feeding, usually via a clasp that allows you to pull the cup material down. This enables you to feed your baby without having to remove your bra. These bras are designed to avoid placing pressure on your breast tissue, which could lead to blocked ducts and problems with nursing. Maternity bras don't have an access system, but are stretchier and designed to adapt to growing breasts during pregnancy. Women who don't plan to breast-feed sometimes prefer maternity bras after the birth since they don't need accessible cups.

Q I prefer underwire bras. Can I continue wearing these?

It's generally recommended that you avoid wearing underwire bras during pregnancy and while nursing. As your breasts swell, the rigid underwire may dig into your skin and breast tissue, which is especially uncomfortable in pregnancy and can obstruct the blood flow to the breasts. Once you're breast-feeding, pressure from an underwired bra could lead to blocked milk ducts, obstructing the flow of milk, and even leading to mastitis (see p.274–75).

Most maternity and nursing bras are nonwired, but if you definitely prefer underwire bras (those with larger busts might find they offer more support), there are some underwire maternity bras that contain a more flexible wire made from a lightweight alloy. These mold more easily around the breast and avoid putting pressure on breast tissue.

Q My doctor suggested that I wear a bra at night, but that sounds rather uncomfortable. Is this really necessary?

If your breasts are very tender, you may find that a lightweight nonwire soft bra will help you to feel more comfortable at night. You can even buy a soft sleep bra that is designed for maximum comfort while you sleep, or you could try wearing a crop-top bra. After the birth, if you are leaking milk and using breast pads, then wearing a bra at night will make it easier to keep the pads in place (see p.275).

You may find that you start to outgrow your usual bra from as early as **8 to 10 weeks** into pregnancy. It's a good idea to be measured **every couple of months** by a professional bra fitter to check that your current bra still **fits** you **properly**.

Q What do I look for when choosing maternity and nursing bras?

Comfort and support are key. Don't be tempted to estimate your new bra size—it's definitely a good idea to ask a trained bra fitter to measure you and make sure that you buy styles of maternity and nursing bras that fit you perfectly.

Look for bras made of breathable cotton or cotton and lycra with some stretch in the cup. Wide adjustable shoulder straps will provide good support for your bigger breasts, but make sure the straps don't dig in. Likewise, the back strap should fit comfortably close to your body without being too tight, and should sit straight–if it rides up, the bra is too big.

A wide, curved underband at the front accommodates your growing belly. Choose maternity and nursing bras with four sets of hooks and eyes on the back panel so you can adjust the fit of your bra. Your rib cage expands in pregnancy and shrinks back after the birth, so when you're buying a bra early in pregnancy, make sure it fits on the tightest hook so you can let the strap out as your body changes; then when buying a nursing bra toward the end of pregnancy, choose one that fits on the loosest setting. Check that you can open and close the nursing bra cup easily with one hand.

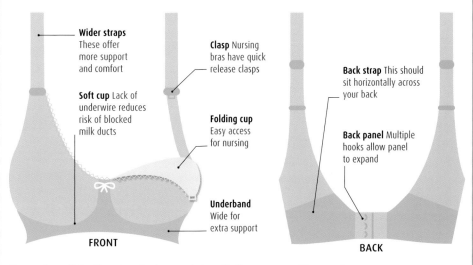

Wider straps These offer more support and comfort

Soft cup Lack of underwire reduces risk of blocked milk ducts

Clasp Nursing bras have quick release clasps

Folding cup Easy access for nursing

Underband Wide for extra support

FRONT

Back strap This should sit horizontally across your back

Back panel Multiple hooks allow panel to expand

BACK

Bra anatomy Maternity and nursing bras are designed in the same way, with supportive back and shoulder straps. Seamless bras are good if your nipples are tender. Nursing bras have fasteners on the shoulders or central panel that open and close each cup easily.

Q How much use is an exercise ball? Is it worthwhile to invest in one?

An exercise ball can be a valuable aid during labor, and it can help you perform exercises in pregnancy to prepare you for the birth. It also provides an alternative support if you find sitting uncomfortable or have poor posture.

Despite their name, exercise balls are also used as birthing balls, made of tough material—although some exercise balls have the advantage of a nonslip finish. It's worth buying an exercise ball early on if you do buy one, since it can be used for back support and as a base for both prenatal and postpartum exercise. If you choose to buy one, make sure you buy a ball that is at least 26 in (65 cm) in diameter, or 30 in (75 cm) if you are taller (5 ft 9 in/1.75 m or more).

Comfortable exercise

Sitting on the ball while you are pregnant can help with your posture, since you need to sit straight and upright to maintain your balance without curving your back, which in turn helps to strengthen the muscles in your back and prevent backaches. You can practice Kegel floor exercises (see p.67) while sitting on the ball, and perform gentle pelvis exercises (see below) during pregnancy and after the birth. Finding your balance on the ball can be tricky as first, so ask someone to help you sit down and get up until you feel confident doing this yourself. Use the ball on carpet rather than a smooth surface for stability.

In late pregnancy, when it can be difficult to sit comfortably, an exercise ball provides a supportive base that may be more comfortable than a chair. You may find that it is easier to get into a standing position from a ball than from a chair. You also naturally lean slightly forward when sitting on an exercise ball, which helps to move your baby into a good position before labor (see p.199).

During the first stage of labor, sitting on an exercise ball can help you stay upright and active (see p.210) and allow you to rock your pelvis, which can help to shift your baby into a good position for the delivery. After the birth, an exercise ball may be more comfortable to sit on if you have stitches, and can provide a good route back into a gentle exercise regimen.

EXERCISE BALL USES

An exercise ball can prove useful not just for labor, but throughout pregnancy and after the birth, too.

≫ **Sitting:** sit with your knees and feet apart so you feel balanced and stable. Keep your feet flat on the floor, your back straight, and your shoulders pulled back and down with your hands on your knees.

≫ **Pelvis exercises:** rotate your pelvis clockwise a few times, and then counterclockwise. Connect them by moving your pelvis in figure-eight movements. Then practice your Kegel exercises.

≫ **Labor:** gently rock your pelvis as you sit on the ball. If kneeling down feels easier during contractions, lean against the ball and wrap your arms around it for support.

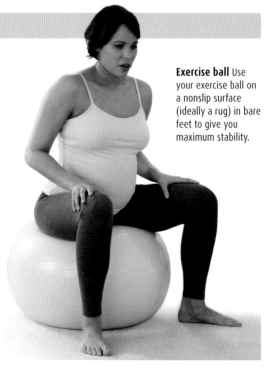

Exercise ball Use your exercise ball on a nonslip surface (ideally a rug) in bare feet to give you maximum stability.

Tips for backaches

≫ In addition to using support aids to relieve back pain, regular gentle exercise will keep you fit and supple and help to strengthen your back and muscles. Try swimming, pregnancy yoga, or simple strengthening exercises (see p.65).

≫ A firm mattress will provide important support while you sleep. If your mattress sags and you're not planning on buying a new one soon, try putting a hard board under it to make it firm.

≫ Try an exercise ball (see left), which will help you sit straight and ease back pain.

Q What can I use to support my back during the day? I'm getting some lower back pain as my belly grows.

There are a few support aids you can try, including a pregnancy belt and a lumbar support cushion. A soft, durable pregnancy belt helps to make your pelvic area more stable and support your abdomen and back. It is designed to be adjustable and fit under your belly, helping to lift and support your expanding uterus and, in turn, take the pressure off your back, relieving hip pain. Many women find these support belts helpful if they are on their feet or walking for any length of time.

Use a cushion to support your lower back when sitting in a chair or your car. Special lumbar support cushions mold to the shape of your lower back when you sit, improving your posture by stopping you from sinking into the seat, and relieving stress on your back ligaments.

A soft mattress can exacerbate your back pain. Use a firmer mattress if you can, or place a board under your soft mattress.

Back pain is up there with the most common complaints in pregnancy, with almost three quarters of women complaining of a backache at some point. See p.138 for more information on back pain while pregnant. Pregnancy-related pelvic girdle pain (PPGP) also causes pain in the lower back (see page 133 for advice). Let your doctor know about your back pain, too, since he or she may be able to refer you for obstetric physical therapy.

Q I'm planning to breast-feed. Is it a good idea to buy a nursing pillow?

A nursing pillow is usually a V-shaped or U-shaped cushion that supports your baby while she breast-feeds so you don't have to hold her continually, or you can use it to support your arms as you feed her so you don't get too tired or cramped.

Some women find these nursing pillows extremely useful, especially in the early weeks of breast-feeding when you and your baby are working on your technique and finding the most comfortable positions. The cushion sits around your waist and supports either your baby while she nurses, or your arms, depending on whether you want to cradle her as she nurses. Having this cushioned support under your baby or your arms stops you from craning forward during a nursing session, so your posture is improved and your milk flow isn't hampered. However, you can try using ordinary cushions to create a similar support if you feel a nursing pillow isn't worth it. If you do invest in a nursing pillow, it can double as a baby nest once your baby is a little older, acting as a support for her to lean against before she is able to sit up unaided.

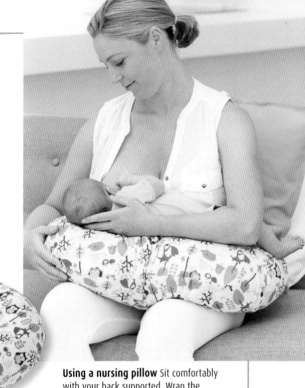

Baby bolster Cushions have a wide section on which to lay your baby.

NURSING PILLOW

Using a nursing pillow Sit comfortably with your back supported. Wrap the cushion around your waist and position your baby at the right angle to nurse.

Q It's getting harder to get a decent night's sleep as I grow bigger. Is there anything that can help?

Strategically placed pillows can help to bolster your belly and support your legs and back. As your abdomen grows, it can be hard to find a comfortable sleeping position. After around 16 weeks of pregnancy, lying on your back puts a strain on it and becomes more difficult. You should avoid this position anyway because it puts pressure on the major blood vessels—the aorta and the major vein called the inferior vena cava—and affects the blood circulation to you and your baby, making you feel faint. Don't worry, however, if during the night you turn onto your back—if your body feels unwell it will turn naturally to a more suitable position while you are asleep. Lying on your side, specifically your left side, is thought to optimize your circulation, and is usually the most comfortable position later in pregnancy. However, your abdomen can feel unsupported when you lie on your side, so many women find they need some support aids to be comfortable in this position (see pp.114–5).

Support pillows

You can try using one of the many pregnancy pillows available: there is a whole range of designs to choose from, and some are multipurpose, providing support during the daytime, too, and doubling as nursing pillows once your baby arrives. Compact wedge-shaped cushions slip under your belly when you lie on your side, and can also be used as a lower back support while sitting. For ultimate support, you can invest in a body-length pillow; these long pillows curl around your body supporting your belly, back, and legs while you sleep. After the birth, you can use them for supporting your baby's weight during nursing sessions. If you don't want to spend money on pregnancy pillows, you can use strategically placed bed pillows and cushions to create the extra support that you need.

Q Which inflatable cushions are most helpful for sitting down if I've had stitches after the delivery?

If you need stitches after a tear or episiotomy (see p.217) during the birth, an inflatable cushion can help to take the pressure off your perineal area when you sit down and bring temporary relief. You are likely to feel sore and tender in the perineal area as your incision heals, which can make sitting down uncomfortable. There are a few types to choose from:

» **C-shaped inflatable cushion** helps you avoid putting pressure on one particular area.
» **Valley-style cushion** is a uniquely designed cushion using a combination of foam and air, with two inflatable sides that you can adjust accordingly and a dip in the middle. You may be able to rent one of these cushions rather than buy it.
» **Doughnut-shaped inflatable cushions** with a hole in the center are also available. These cushions will enable you to avoid putting any pressure on your perineum when you sit down, although you should avoid sitting on these types of cushion for too long, since they can compress the area, which could become uncomfortable in itself.

Body-length pillows cradle your whole body while you sleep and are one of the most **popular** pregnancy accessories.

A CLOSER LOOK
Packing your bag

By the time you reach 36 weeks, prepare supplies for the birth itself, since you might go into labor at any point. Whether you intend to give birth in hospital or at a birthing center, you'll need a few essential items for labor, and the equivalent of an overnight bag with extras for you and your baby after the birth. Ask about any stipulations your hospital may have about what you can and can't bring with you, and consider packing items for your birth partner, too. Lastly, don't forget your birth plan!

Healthy snacks Most hospitals won't let you eat or drink when you check in and when you are in labor, but pack a stash of healthy snacks like fruit and cereal bars to keep your partner energized and hydrated during labor.

You will want a few toiletries for before and after the birth. Lips can get dry in labor, so a lip balm will be welcome, and a face spray or washcloth that you can wet will be refreshing and soothing during labor.

If you've had stitches, those first toilet trips can sting! Pack a small plastic pitcher, or an old plastic water bottle, so you can pour warm water over your perineal area as you urinate.

Comfort aids You might want a couple of home pillows for extra comfort, and an exercise ball if the hospital doesn't supply them. And remember to pack any other aids for labor, such as massage oil, a back massager or your favorite slippers.

Your things for after the birth You will need old underwear or disposable underwear and maternity sanitary pads for postpartum bleeding. A nursing bra, breast pads, burp cloths, and nipple cream will provide all you need to start breast-feeding. Pack some night wear, flip-flops, and some loose clothing for leaving the hospital.

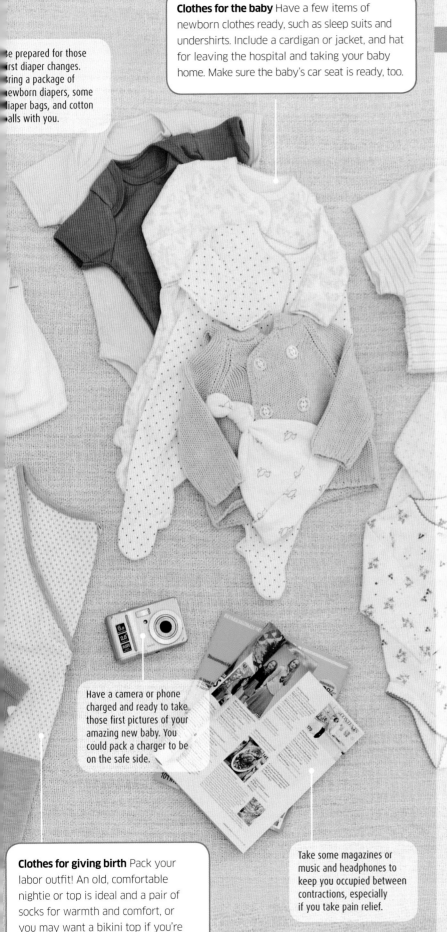

Clothes for the baby Have a few items of newborn clothes ready, such as sleep suits and undershirts. Include a cardigan or jacket, and hat for leaving the hospital and taking your baby home. Make sure the baby's car seat is ready, too.

...e prepared for those ...rst diaper changes. ...ring a package of ...ewborn diapers, some ...iaper bags, and cotton ...alls with you.

Have a camera or phone charged and ready to take those first pictures of your amazing new baby. You could pack a charger to be on the safe side.

Clothes for giving birth Pack your labor outfit! An old, comfortable nightie or top is ideal and a pair of socks for warmth and comfort, or you may want a bikini top if you're planning a water birth.

Take some magazines or music and headphones to keep you occupied between contractions, especially if you take pain relief.

It may be hard to believe some of these facts, but you'll soon find out from your own experience as a new parent.

12 diapers

This is the average number that a baby needs per day. She will urinate every 1–3 hours and will poop several times a day.

40 days

In some cultures around the world, this is the time frame that mother and baby are encouraged not to leave the house in order to fully recover from the birth.

3 outfits

Most babies will need three or more outfit changes a day. Make sure you have enough clothes ready for your newborn baby's wardrobe.

16 weeks

You might look about 16 weeks pregnant right after the birth. Your uterus still needs to go back to its prepregnancy size and you'll have weight from pregnancy that takes a while to lose.

5,850

This is the average number of diapers that a child will use in her lifetime.

Getting ready for your baby's arrival is truly exciting. This is an ideal time to start listing and **buying** what your **baby may need**. While you can, of course, still shop after the birth, you'll need a **core supply of basic items** ready from the beginning.

Preparing for your baby

Prioritize what you need

When you begin to feel secure in your pregnancy, it's a good idea to decide which essentials you and your baby will need. Then buy the equipment gradually so that once your baby is born you can focus on him, rest, and recover.

There are several larger items you need to have ready for your baby, including a stroller, a bassinet, a crib, and a car seat. Purchasing these things is likely to require the most consideration. For this reason, allow yourself enough time to browse and research. You may want to test out car seats and stroller before you buy, so plan a shopping trip before you get uncomfortably big. If budget is a consideration, think about what you could accept from friends and family if they have expressed an offer to buy an item, or what you can get secondhand.

Newborn baby clothes are adorable and it's easy to be tempted to buy items now that may actually see very little wear; many first-time parents don't realize just how quickly newborns grow. Buy some essentials now and then assess your baby's needs as he grows so that baby clothes don't go to waste.

Other worthwhile purchases to buy now are diaper bags, a thermometer (see p.292), and simple washing equipment. Breast-feeding requires little aside from a good nursing bra, but if you are planning to bottle-feed, buy a basic set of bottles and nipples. Don't panic if you think you want to breast-feed, but aren't sure how successful it will be; you can easily buy bottle-feeding equipment after the birth.

Longer-term purchases

Before you feel pressure to get a nursery ready, keep in mind that your baby will be best off in the same room as you for the first six months. And newborn babies don't need much in the way of toys for the first few weeks. Their new environment and time spent getting to know you and gazing at your face provide all the stimulation they need. If you would like to have a couple of play items on hand, look for age-appropriate toys. Babies love high-contrast patterns and looking at faces, so baby mirrors and soft books with black and white patterns or bright colors are all your little one will need at first.

Q What clothes will my baby need?

It's best to keep clothing simple for young babies. Your baby will be spending much of his first weeks feeding and napping indoors so you only need to buy a limited supply of items to keep him comfortable.

Layers Try dressing your baby in layers in the beginning so that you can remove or add items easily to regulate his body temperature.

Newborn babies cannot regulate their body temperature. As they get older, this improves. As a result, it is best to dress them in a onesie, adding more layers as and when required. To start with, buy no more than six cotton onesies with envelope-style necks and snaps around the diaper area, six to eight all-in-one sleep suits with snaps down the front—which are ideal for the first few months, a couple of light cardigans, a soft hat or wide-brimmed summer hat, a jacket or snowsuit, depending on the season, and some socks to keep his feet warm if they are uncovered. Front-closing outfits rather than items with ties and awkward zippers will be more comfortable for your baby, and make diaper changing much easier. In winter, add onesies under sleep suits, and a lightweight cardigan is useful when the temperature drops.

YOUR BABY'S FIRST WARDROBE

Choose baby clothes in soft, easy-care, machine-washable fabrics. Cotton is perfect for babies, since its natural fiber is gentle on your baby's sensitive skin, helps to keep him cool, is easy to wash, and is durable.

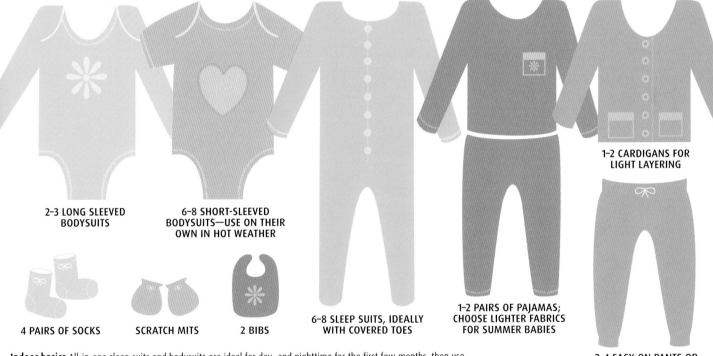

2–3 LONG SLEEVED BODYSUITS

6–8 SHORT-SLEEVED BODYSUITS—USE ON THEIR OWN IN HOT WEATHER

4 PAIRS OF SOCKS

SCRATCH MITS

2 BIBS

6–8 SLEEP SUITS, IDEALLY WITH COVERED TOES

1–2 PAIRS OF PAJAMAS; CHOOSE LIGHTER FABRICS FOR SUMMER BABIES

1–2 CARDIGANS FOR LIGHT LAYERING

2–4 EASY-ON PANTS OR LEGGINGS

Indoor basics All-in-one sleep suits and bodysuits are ideal for day- and nighttime for the first few months, then use pajamas at night and bodysuits and leggings during the day. Layer with a cardigan if your baby needs extra warmth.

Outdoor essentials On hot summer days, a short-sleeved T-shirt or undershirt may be all your baby needs, although do use a sun hat or bonnet and sunscreen too. Otherwise layer onesies with T-shirts, leggings, socks, and cardigans depending on the weather, and invest in a snowsuit or warm jacket, mittens, and a soft hat for winter.

2–3 ENVELOPE NECK T-SHIRTS

SUNHAT

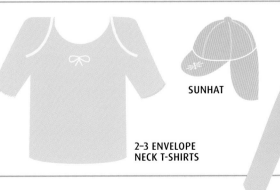

JACKET OR SNOWSUIT

2 HATS

MITTENS

Q What equipment will we need for washing our baby?

In the first few weeks of your baby's life, you will probably be combining regular bathing with sponge bathing (see p.284), where you clean your baby without immersing her in a tub of water.

There's no need to bathe your newborn every day, unless she loves having a bath and finds it soothing or enjoyable; she'll only need a bath two or three times a week on average. Carefully washing your baby's face, neck, hands, and bottom—known as sponge bathing—requires very little equipment, but does need to be done thoroughly every day that your baby doesn't have a bath. Whichever you do, get everything ready beforehand and make sure that the room and the water are warm.

SPONGE BATHING

You will need only basic equipment:

>> **Cotton balls.** Use a fresh piece for separate areas, including around the ears and eyes.

>> **Two bowls of water,** one for each end of the body to avoid cross infection.

WATER BOWL

BATHING

For bathing your baby you will need the following:

>> **Baby bath,** a sink, or a big bathtub. The advantage of a baby bath is that you can use it in any room. If your baby seems to dislike the water, try bathing together and soothing her as you do.

>> **Nonslip mat** only if you are planning to use a big bathtub.

>> **Bath thermometer** can be used to check the temperature of the water is 95–100° F (35–38° C), or you can test the bath temperature with your elbow, checking that it is warm, but not hot.

>> **A combined mild baby shampoo and bath product** used sparingly, although plain water is usually better for cleaning your baby at first.

>> **Soft washcloths or a sponge**

>> **2–3 hooded baby towels,** to wrap your baby up in after bathing and stop her from losing heat through her head.

>> **Olive oil or baby oil,** for rubbing into your baby's towel-dried skin.

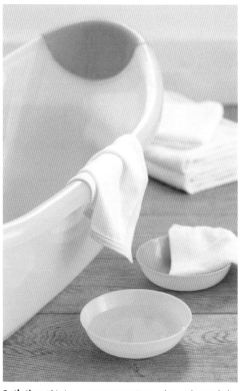

Bath time This is a great opportunity to play with your baby so have everything you need prepared around you.

Q I heard that you should wash baby clothes before they are worn. Is that really necessary?

Yes, it's a good idea to wash your baby's clothes before she first wears them. This simple precaution ensures that any residues of substances from the manufacturing process that could irritate your baby's sensitive skin are removed. Use nonbiological detergents to wash all your baby's clothes, bedding, and burp cloths, since these detergents don't contain enzymes, which can also prove an irritant.

Q Is it a good idea to buy a room thermometer? Where should we put it?

It is a good idea—making sure the room your baby sleeps in is the right temperature reduces the risk of sudden infant death syndrome (SIDS). The ideal room temperature for a baby is around 64°F (18°C). If you want to ensure your baby doesn't get too hot or cold, you may want to have several thermometers around the house. Options range from affordable strip thermometers stuck to laminated board to smart digital thermometers. Remember though that if the room temperature is right, your baby won't need more than a sleep sack.

Q How do I choose a good diaper bag and what should I put in it?

You can choose a diaper bag with a foldaway changing mat, although you don't have to buy a purpose-made diaper bag; you can use a bag of your choice and buy a separate fold-up changing mat. Have the following items ready as a diaper-changing kit in the bag for when you're away from the house:

>> **A few disposable diapers** and disposal bags.

>> **Travel-sized package** of unperfumed baby wipes (try to use sparingly, since they can be harsh on your newborn's delicate skin).

>> **A small container** or travel-sized container of diaper cream to prevent or ease diaper rash.

>> **Spare clothes** for your baby and for you. When you use any of these items to change your baby while you are out, remember to restock the supplies when you get home so the bag is all ready for your next trip out.

Q How many diapers and sizes do we stock up on before the birth?

Your baby will need diapers from the beginning, but it is sensible to exercise a little caution over how many you buy. While it is tempting to stock up on bargain deals at the supermarket, you don't yet know how big your baby will be.

If you have a newborn on the larger size, she may spend very little time in newborn diapers. It may also take a while to figure out which brand you prefer, and which fit your baby best.

During the first week, the number of wet diapers your baby has each day will be about six, which amounts to 42 diapers or so. After the first week the number will gradually build up, and you can expect to change at least 10 to 12 wet diapers a day. So you may want to start off buying a couple of packages of newborn diapers to see you through the first week or so, and then assess whether you need to continue with a newborn size or move to the next size up. Some newborn diapers have a cut-out section to accommodate the umbilical cord stump, but you don't necessarily need these—you can just turn the diaper down at the front.

Reusable cloth diapers

If you plan to use reusables, you need around 20 diapers from the beginning, as well as washable wraps if you are using two-piece diapers with a cloth diaper and outer waterproof layer. There is a larger initial financial outlay involved for cloth diapers, so unless you are sure you want your baby to wear reusables, you may prefer to wait until your daily routine has settled down and then look into the options.

12
Newborns need **12 daily** diaper changes—84 diapers a week.

6–8
Older babies need **6–8 daily** diaper changes—up to 56 diapers a week.

CLOTH OR DISPOSABLE?

If you are undecided about which type of diaper to buy, consider these pros and cons:

>> **Comfort:** disposables are more breathable, but their moisturizing, absorbing chemicals may irritate the skin. Cloth diapers may feel softer.

>> **Convenience:** disposables are more convenient when out, at day care, or traveling. Cloth diapers aren't as absorbent, so you may need to change a dirty diaper more frequently. Nowadays, changing a diaper, whether disposable or cloth, is quick and easy.

>> **Cost:** cloth diapers are usually cheaper than disposables unless you use a laundering service.

>> **Other:** disposables use resources such as trees and plastics in the manufacturing process, then collect in landfills. Washing cloth diapers uses clean water and energy, but produces only dirty water. Disposables, however, reduce the risk of infection in a group setting such as a day-care center.

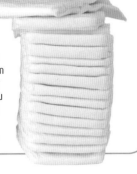

Disposable diapers Although these are an easy choice, consider all options before you make a decision; you may opt to use a combination of both.

Q Aside from diapers, what else will we need for diaper changing?

You will need a wipe-clean baby changing mat, cotton balls or baby wipes to clean your baby's bottom, and diaper cream. Ideally use moistened cotton balls rather than baby wipes at home to avoid skin irritations, and use a diaper cream such as zinc oxide or petrolatum to prevent or ease any diaper rash. You may also like a purpose-made diaper disposal for disposable diapers. Used diapers are folded then placed in the shute, which seals them as the diaper moves down into the container, locking away odors. However, this is not essential and is an extra cost to be aware of. If you are using cloth diapers, you will need a bucket to store dirty ones before washing. These are purpose-made, or you can buy a normal lidded bucket.

Q Are there any other items we need for our baby's everyday care?

There are a few more essentials that you'll need to help to make life easier with a newborn.
A supply of burp cloths is very useful for protecting your clothing during burping, and some women also like to use these to cover up a little more when breast-feeding. A soft baby brush or comb will help to gently untangle knots when your baby's hair starts to grow, and baby scissors will keep her nails trim.

If your baby is born in the summer, you will also need some sunscreen to protect her from the sun's harmful rays. The general advice used to be to avoid putting sunscreen on babies under six months because chemicals in the sunscreen could irritate their delicate skin, and to keep them out of direct sunlight instead,

especially between 10 am and 2 pm. However, it's now recommended that as well as keeping your baby well covered and avoiding direct sunlight, you should also apply small amounts of sunscreen to exposed areas of skin. Buy at least SPF 30 with a four- or five-star rating that protects against both UVA and UVB rays. Also make sure that you have a wide-brimmed sun hat for her. When your baby is a little older, if you are going to the beach, you may want to invest in a bathing suit that covers her arms and legs, offering effective protection against UV rays.

If you want peace of mind about your baby while she sleeps, a baby monitor is useful. You can buy audio devices, with a transmitter placed next to your sleeping baby and a speaker near you; audio with motion sensor pads, which sound an alarm if your baby doesn't move for a while; and video monitors that allow you to both hear and see your baby.

Q What should we buy for our baby to sleep in?

Your baby will need a bassinet or a crib for sleeping in. Another increasingly popular option is to opt for a co-sleeping crib which attaches to your bed, or you could try a "baby nest."

Although you can use a full-sized crib from the beginning, a newborn may feel cosier in a bassinet or crib for the first few weeks, since it more closely mimics the feeling of being cocooned in the uterus. A bassinet is also easy to use as a travel crib or move around from room to room so your baby can be in the same room as you for all his sleep time, both day and night.

Some cribs are designed to be gently rocked to soothe a baby; they last longer than bassinets because they are bigger and so a baby can sleep in them longer, but they are less transportable. A co-sleeping crib attached to your bed is great if you want to have your baby near you but not actually in your bed. The crib sits alongside your bed with a drop-down side so you can easily reach over to comfort your baby or get him for breast-feeding without having to get out of bed. Make sure there is no gap between the crib and your bed that your baby could fall into. Another option is a baby nest, a baby mattress with sturdy sides placed in your bed, that gives your baby his own dedicated sleeping space safe from hazards such as pillows or duvets. When you do come to choose a full-size crib, make sure it conforms to all health and safety standards (right).

A bassinet or crib closely mimics the feeling of being cocooned in the uterus, so is ideal in the first few weeks.

SLEEPING OPTIONS

It's personal preference as to which type of crib or crib you choose, but make sure they fit these criteria.

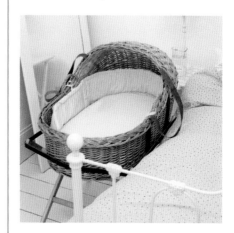

» Bassinet: choose one with a sturdy base and handles so that it's secure when you move it around. Babies can grow out of bassinets quite quickly, and you may find that at around two to three months your baby is looking a little cramped. She should be able to sleep with her arms out to the side, or flung up by her head, without touching the sides or top of the basket.

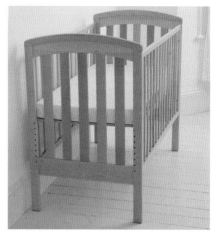

» Full-size crib: make sure the crib conforms to the US Consumer Product Safety Commission's federal requirements, as of June, 2011. Don't use a secondhand crib. Drop-side cribs are no longer sold or manufactured and crib slats are stronger to prevent breakage. Slats must be no more than 2⅜ inches apart, so babies can't get stuck. Some have an adjustable mattress that can be lowered as your baby grows.

Q Did you know...

Your newborn will be too young to play with toys, but he will be stimulated by his surroundings early on. Young babies can't focus far, but they enjoy looking at black-and-white patterns, high-contrast colors, and baby mirrors. Your baby will also enjoy watching a colorful mobile hung above his crib. Make sure this is secure and out of his reach. Some mobiles have a wind-up music box attached, which babies can find very soothing, or you could place a music box in the room. Young babies love to touch, so find a couple of first soft books with different textures for him to explore.

Q What bedding does my baby need in his bassinet or crib?

You need one or two mattress protectors if his diaper leaks at night and three or four sheets, so you have spare bedding as items are washed. Choose fitted cotton sheets because they stay in place. A lightweight baby sleep sack is better than a blanket for keeping your baby warm. Loose blankets aren't allowed, but a thin one is okay if you place your baby's feet at the crib's bottom. Tuck the blanket securely under the mattress's bottom and sides. Cover the baby only to chest height. Babies' hands and feet often feel colder than the rest of their body, so are not a reliable measure of their temperature. Feel the nape of his neck, or chest, to gauge his temperature as he sleeps, and adjust the bedding as necessary.

Q Are there any must-have items of furniture for the baby we should invest in other than a crib?

Since you will be spending a fair amount of time nursing, comforting, and perhaps reading to your baby, a chair is a worthwhile addition. Chairs marketed for feeding your baby are available, although these can be pricey. Whatever chair you choose, make sure it is comfortable for you with good back and arm support, and that you can place your feet flat on the floor. Dedicated changing tables are also handy and come in a variety of designs with shelves, drawers, and cupboard space though, again, these can be costly. Alternatively, a chest of drawers large enough to put a changing mat and some diapers on top is just as good, and good storage is essential in a nursery.

Keep the **color scheme** of the nursery fairly neutral and use pictures, accessories, and wall-hangings to **add color and fun**, since they are easiest to change as your baby grows.

Q We're starting to plan the nursery now. What do we need to think about first?

If you are planning to refurbish a room to turn it into a nursery, take the time now to research and buy appropriate lighting and chemical-free paints, since there is no immediate rush. The best and safest place for your baby to sleep for the first six months is in a bassinet or crib in the same room as you, to help reduce the risk of sudden infant death syndrome (SIDS) (see p.287). So you won't need a fully functioning nursery the moment your baby arrives home. Having said that, it's best to paint the room at least two to three months before your baby moves into it so you can air the room. Avoid using any paints that give off potentially harmful paint fumes and choose a brand that is free from harmful chemicals and toxins. Look for information that stipulates the paint has low, or zero, VOC levels. Volatile organic compounds, or VOCs, are gases found in products such as household paints that emit harmful chemicals.

Think, also, about the nursery lighting. A nightlight and/or dimmer switch will stop you and your partner from stumbling around in the dark during nighttime feedings, diaper changes, and midnight comforting sessions. And for many parents, blackout blinds are a must, ensuring that a baby isn't nudged out of sleep by early morning sunlight, especially in summer.

Q We have been offered a secondhand crib. Should we buy a new mattress?

A new mattress is best. This is because there is evidence that a mattress that isn't in the best condition can increase the potential risk of sudden infant death syndrome (SIDS), or crib

Q How do we make sure the nursery is a safe space?

You should think first about the layout of your baby's room and the most appropriate place to position the crib, and then arrange the rest of the furniture and equipment accordingly.

Avoid placing your baby's crib near a window or any area where it will get hit by direct sunlight, and make sure that it isn't next to any curtain cords or pulls that your baby could get tangled up in. And once your baby starts to pull himself up to standing, you will need to make sure that there are no pieces of furniture near his crib that he could climb onto, or shelves that he could pull things off. Make sure that all the furniture is sturdy, or well anchored to the wall, so your baby won't be able to pull anything on top of himself. A plain wood floor is ideal, since it is easy to keep clean and dust free.

NURSERY SAFETY ESSENTIALS

Run through these safety essentials to check that everything is in order before you move your baby into the room.

» Temperature: keep the room at an even temperature and make sure that it doesn't get too hot. Use a room thermometer to keep the temperature at a constant 64° F (18° C).

» Baby monitor: situate a baby monitor, if you use one, well out of your baby's reach, but close enough to his crib so that you can hear him immediately if he cries or seems to be distressed.

» Smoke alarm: you may also want to consider installing a carbon monoxide detector in or near your baby's room to prevent carbon monoxide poisoning, which has no outward signs.

» Hazards: make sure there are no cords, pulls, toys, or decorations such as a hanging mobile so close to the crib that your baby could get tangled in them. Secure any rugs to the floor with double-sided tape so that no one can slip on them.

You can make it easier to control your baby's **temperature** as he sleeps by choosing **cotton sheets** and **lightweight cotton baby blankets** for his bedding so you can **add or remove layers** if he is too hot or cold.

death, which usually occurs during sleep. When choosing a new mattress, look for firmness and breathable covers that can be removed and washed. The least expensive are foam mattresses, which may come with a waterproof covering, but have the least longevity and lose their shape most quickly. Coiled spring interior mattresses are better since they have inner springs sandwiched between layers of felt or foam to offer sturdy support. Coir (coconut fiber) or other natural fiber mattresses are the firmest, most durable, and more expensive. Hypoallergenic mattresses have a removable quilted top layer that can be washed at a high temperature to remove any dust mites. Also, importantly, be sure the crib was manufactured after June 28, 2011, so it conforms to current safety standards.

Q I'm planning to breast-feed my baby. Is there anything I can do now to prepare?

One of the best things you can do to prepare for breast-feeding is to go to a breast-feeding class during pregnancy. These are usually short sessions of a couple of hours long, and may be available free in some hospitals, or you can pay for a private one. It's best to go to a class in your last trimester so that all the information is fresh in your mind when your baby arrives. You will either be shown a DVD of breast-feeding, or an experienced mom may come in to demonstrate how it's done. Experts will talk about how to latch your baby on, which positions you can try, and how to get a good milk supply established. The class leader may also discuss potential pitfalls and issues such as how to avoid nipple confusion by not introducing a bottle or pacifier too early, and how to prevent and treat sore nipples. Look for classes run by an accredited lactation counselor or consultant. You may also want to read up on the subject before you give birth so you feel fully prepared. See pages 266–77 for more information on breast-feeding.

Q I've heard of breast-feeding pillows. Is it worth buying one?

Breast-feeding can be a wonderful experience for mother and baby and it is vital that you are comfortable so that you can enjoy your time together. However it is not always easy. When nursing, it is important that you bring your baby up to nipple height rather than lean toward him. In the early weeks when your baby is very small, a good, supportive pillow will allow you to do this without having to take his weight in your arms. There are specially designed breast-feeding pillows and these can be more supportive than a normal pillow.

Similarly, most normal chairs are too high for breast-feeding so many recommend a nursing chair. These should be low and supportive in the right places for you to maintain good feeding positions. You may need to place pillows behind your back for extra support. Your lap should be flat or slightly raised so that your baby tips toward and not away from you. A nursing chair and pillow may reduce the chances of breast-feeding problems.

Q Is there anything I need to buy for breast-feeding?

One of the many benefits of breast-feeding is that it is very economical, but there are a few items you can buy that will support your breast-feeding experience and add to your comfort.

A nursing bra is essential, so it's worth buying two or three comfortable nursing bras. Make sure that the bras you buy have a clasp that you can release with one hand (see p.179), since your arms will be full with a newborn once you start to breast-feed. The bra cups should also open completely so that nothing presses on your breast tissue and leads to blocked ducts or mastitis. Even if you want to decide about whether or not to breast-feed once your baby arrives, you should buy at least one bra before the birth, since it's not so easy to go shopping once your newborn has arrived. Breast pads, nipple cream, and burp cloths are all additional, but affordable, items.

Breast pumps

You may want to wait to see if you need a breast pump once you're in a routine with breast-feeding, but a manual or electric pump can prove invaluable if you have to bottle-feed your baby at some point.

Buy at least one **nursing bra** before the birth, since it will be more difficult to go shopping after.

WHAT YOU NEED TO BUY

With the exception of a breast pump, buy everything before the birth and pack them in your bag for the birth so you can start using them right away.

» A professionally fitted, supportive nursing bra will be your main purchase. You can get fitted for a bra from about 36 weeks of pregnancy, when a bra fitter will be able to predict what size you will need after the birth (see p.178). You may also want to buy a soft nighttime bra to hold your breast pads in place too.

» Disposable or washable breast pads help to collect milk that leaks when you're not feeding. Slim and discreet pads are available that are extremely absorbent; those without a plastic lining are less likely to irritate your skin and nipples.

» Nipple cream helps to protect and treat sore nipples. Look for pure, hypoallergenic, lanolin-based creams that are paraben free.

» Burp cloths are useful for draping over your shoulder after nursing to mop up any milk your baby spits up. They can also provide some cover if you want when you're breast-feeding in public, or you can use a shawl or scarf.

» Breast pumps enable you to express your milk (see p.272). Manual pumps have a suction cup or shield attached to a bottle, and a pump handle that you operate manually, while electric pumps operate essentially in the same way, but there is an electric motor that operates the pump action to make it a much faster process.

» Front-opening nightie or pajamas to enable you to nurse easily at night. There are breast-feeding tops that are designed to make breast-feeding easier too.

Q There are a lot of bottles and nipples to choose from for bottle-feeding. What should we look for?

All bottles and nipples can be used with both formula and with breast milk if you have expressed using a pump. There is no right or wrong choice. All of the items will be easy to buy once your baby arrives, so you shouldn't need to stockpile too many supplies before the birth.

Standard baby bottles are popular. These are usually available in a small or large size (around 4oz/125ml and 9oz/260ml), and with these you can tailor feeds depending on your baby's age and stage. Standard bottles usually come with nipples and lids, are easy to clean, and are compatible with most sanitizing systems (see p.279) and bottle coolers. Some bottles are designed to help ease colic by limiting the amount of air your baby swallows with her milk, so these are worth trying for babies who often seem to be unsettled after being fed and have uncomfortable gas. Colic bottles tend to be more expensive, and those that have a valve or tube to adapt the milk flow can be trickier to keep clean. If you have a microwave, consider a self-sanitizing bottle, which can be sanitized in a microwave. Again, these are a bit pricier, but can be convenient. Ready-sanitized disposable bottles are also available; you just add the formula and discard the bottle after use. While useful for traveling, these are expensive and wasteful if used regularly. Glass bottles, made of toughened glass, are favored by parents who worry about chemicals used in the manufacture of plastic bottles. These are more expensive, and breakable, but more environmentally friendly.

Bottle nipples

Nipples can be silicone or latex and have different flow speeds. Latex nipples tend to be more flexible and softer, but are less durable then silicone. Slow-flow nipples are designed to release the milk more slowly, and are usually best for newborns and young babies. Traditionally, nipples are bell-shaped; wider nipples are available that are thought to resemble the shape of a human nipple more closely, so manufacturers recommend these if you are combining breast and bottle, or trying to move a breast-fed baby over to bottle-feeding. However, it's unlikely a bottle nipple can truly mimic the human nipple and the unique sucking action required, and there's no evidence that these are easier to use.

WHAT YOU NEED

Keep an eye on the condition of your equipment, especially the nipples, and replace them when they become damaged or worn.

» 6–8 bottles in a combination of large and small sizes.

» 6–8 nipples appropriate for newborns.

» Formula powder.

» A sanitizing system—either a cold-water sanitizing system or a steam sanitizer. You can also boil bottle-feeding equipment. See p.279 for how different sanitizing systems work.

» Bottle- and nipple-cleaning brushes.

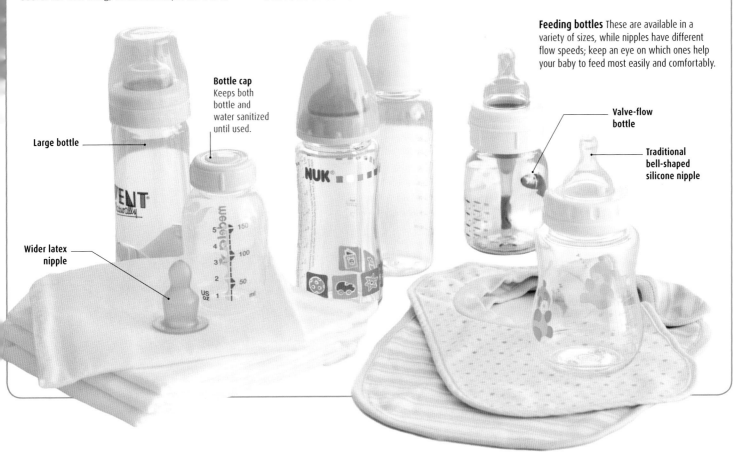

Feeding bottles These are available in a variety of sizes, while nipples have different flow speeds; keep an eye on which ones help your baby to feed most easily and comfortably.

Large bottle

Bottle cap
Keeps both bottle and water sanitized until used.

Wider latex nipple

Valve-flow bottle

Traditional bell-shaped silicone nipple

Q The range of strollers and carriages is incredible. How on earth do we choose?

When thinking about what to buy, the best starting point is to focus on your specific needs: what will suit your lifestyle, your budget, and work well for both your baby and you and your partner.

If you use public transportation often or travel up and down steps regularly, you may find that a lightweight, easily foldable stroller, or a more compact carriage, meets your needs well. If you drive regularly, consider a travel system where you can alternate a chair or car seat on a base, making it easy to move your baby from home to car to stroller without disturbing him too much. Sturdy models with swivel wheels are easy to maneuver and great for walking in cities and towns; if you walk on rough terrain, a fixed wheel is best, making it easier to push the carriage over uneven ground.

Comfort is key

Your baby will spend an extraordinary amount of time in his stroller or travel system. Some carriages have adjustable seats that start off fully reclined and can be adjusted into a more upright mode as your baby grows. Check that the stroller is well padded and has a sturdy back support, and decide whether you want your baby to face inward toward you, or outward. Some models have a reversible seat so you can keep an eye on and make eye contact with your newborn, and turn the seat out when your baby is older. Double check that the handle is high enough for you so you don't have to lean over and strain your back. If you and your partner are significantly different heights, you may want to choose a model with an adjustable handle.

> Make sure you **try out** the model in the store **before you purchase** and practice using it before the birth.

HOW TO DETERMINE WHICH TRAVEL SYSTEM IS RIGHT FOR YOUR FAMILY

The following summary looks at the range of options, explaining key features and highlighting the pros and cons of different models.

RANGE	DESCRIPTION
Convertables 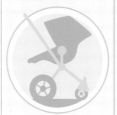	These allow your newborn to lie flat and are more traditional looking than strollers. Your baby has an enclosed, cosy environment, and can see you as you push him along. Later, these can convert to accommodate a seated baby.
Carriages 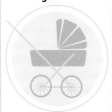	These allow your newborn to lie flat and are more traditional looking than strollers. Your baby has an enclosed, cosy environment, and can see you as you push him along. Models with detachable carrying cribs double as travel cribs for the first few months.
Travel systems 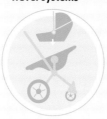	Stroller frames that can snap on your baby's infant car seat are suitable from birth and are easiest for you to bring your baby anywhere you go—for a walk, for a drive—without needing to rouse or disturb him when it's time to put on a seat belt. This option likely won't last through your baby's first year; he's likely to outgrow the car seat when he's 9 to 12 months, depending on his size and the manufacturer's requirements.
Strollers 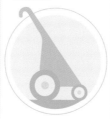	Strollers are lightweight and easy to use and usually fit easily into a car trunk, so are great for travel and shopping. While some strollers are only for older, sitting babies, some models recline fully to accommodate newborns. Strollers can't be used as part of a travel system with car seats or as a carry crib.
Double strollers 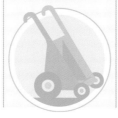	If you have twins or a toddler who needs to be pushed around with your newborn, you will need a double stroller. These can be side-by-side or tandem strollers, where one seat is positioned behind or under the main seat. Side-by-side strollers allow your babies to see each other and have an unobstructed view. Tandem strollers mean that one child has a restricted view and can be difficult to manage on steps, but can be easier to get through tight spaces such as doors. You can also buy single stroller models that can be upgraded into a double stroller when required.

Q Do I need to buy extra stroller accessories or are they really a waste of money?

There are a few useful extra items that are worth considering if you want to buy, especially if you intend to be out in all weathers. Transparent rain covers, which attach directly onto the carriage or stroller, can give your baby complete protection from wind and rain. Air passes beneath and through side air vents so your baby can breathe easily even while the cover remains fixed in place. Foot muffs are cosy for chilly days. Some manufacturers include this as part of the model, or you can buy a foot muff separately. On sunny days, a parasol or shade attachment will help to keep your baby protected from the sun. Very small babies often need a head support, or head hugger, that fits around their head, stopping lolling to the side; these can be used in car seats as well as strollers.

Q I like the idea of carrying my baby in a sling and being hands-free. Which ones give enough support for newborns?

Front carriers and baby slings will support a newborn baby, although you need to take more care if using a sling. Front carriers hold your baby upright against your body, have safety restraints, and are suitable for newborns weighing at least 7½lb (3.5kg). Your baby can either face inward toward you, and then when older, can face outward. Choose fabrics that can be easily cleaned and look for styles that provide good support for your baby, have broad, comfortable shoulder straps, and if possible a hip strap, so that your baby's weight is evenly distributed across your back.

Baby slings and baby wraps are made from soft, flexible fabric. Some can be worn over your shoulder in a cradle hold; others can be adapted to hold your baby in different positions. There have been safety concerns around baby slings, that babies can suffocate if carried incorrectly. Make sure you can see your baby's face at all times, he is held as high up on your chest as possible, he is held securely against your body, and his chin isn't touching his chest, as this could hamper his breathing; and his back and neck are well supported.

Q We don't drive much. Is a car seat essential for newborns and babies?

Even if you rarely make car trips, the law states that your baby must be in a properly installed car seat for all car trips, even if this is just in the taxi on the way home from the hospital.

It's recommended that your baby's car seat is rear facing until your baby reaches the correct weight for the type of car seat you are using—see the guideline table (right). In the event of a collision your baby's head and spine will be better protected; if he is in a forward-facing seat, any sudden forward movement could seriously damage his weak neck muscles and ligaments.

A baby shouldn't spend more than a couple of hours at a time sitting in a car seat, since the semi-upright position can compress a young baby's chest, which can lead to breathing difficulties and damage his developing spine.

Safety standards

When purchasing a new car seat, look for a good rating from the National Highway Traffic Safety Administration (NHTSA). Choose a seat with a five-point safety harness, which offers optimum safety, and follow the manufacturer's instructions when installing and using it.

Your baby may outgrow your infant car seat, for height and weight, at around 9 to 12 months. He still needs to sit in a rear-facing seat. For his next car seat, purchase a convertible or all-in-one car seat, which has higher height and weight limits. Your baby can use this seat for a couple of years, and eventually, the seat can be turned around so it's forward facing. The NHTSA recommends keeping babies rear facing for as long as possible—until three years old—for safety's sake.

INFANT CAR SEAT GUIDELINES

Car seats are classified into groups based on your baby's weight. Your child will move into the next car seat group when he has reached the weight limit for his seat, or his eye line is level with the top of the seat.

SEAT	DESCRIPTION
Infant car seat	This is the ideal car seat to bring with you to the hospital. It should last you until your baby is about nine months old, give or take.
Convertible car seat	Babies stay rear facing until they're at least two years old, based on weight limits. Then seats can be turned around.
All-in-one car seat	These seats are intended to be used for every stage of your baby's childhood. They can accommodate babies as small as 4 lb (1.8 kg) and can be used for children as old as 10 years.

Car seat This is an essential piece of equipment, and because of strict safety regulations it should be bought new.

{Q What can I do now so that the first few weeks go as smoothly as possible?

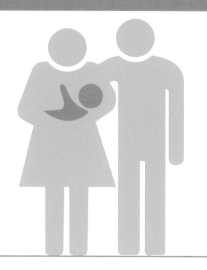

There are plenty of practical ways in which you can prepare for the arrival of your baby (see below). By getting things in order now, you'll feel more at ease and ready for the first few weeks.

Get ahead of the game

With all eyes on the main event, it can be easy to overlook the more practical considerations of how you will manage once your baby has made his appearance. However, it's most definitely worth putting some preparation and thought in now so you can make life as easy as possible after the birth, when you will find that taking care of your new baby takes up a surprising amount of your time with little opportunity to deal with other matters.

ORGANIZE YOUR HOME LIFE

If you find yourself having sudden urges to clean the house, for example, go with it—it's all part of your nesting instinct. But don't forget to take some time for yourself now, too, and consider practical and emotional support from family and friends once your baby arrives.

Line up support

Many new parents find support and help from family and friends invaluable in the early weeks after the birth. You will probably be exhausted and interrupted nights can come as a bit of a shock. Anything that can lighten the load will be appreciated. If you expect twins, or you have a planned C-section, you will need additional help such as having a close relative to stay, using a maternity nurse or a doula. Discuss whether your partner can take time off.

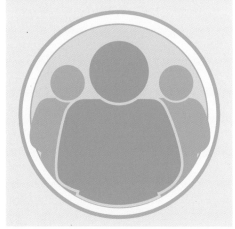

Meet friends

Another important source of support after the birth will be other new parents—and a crucial mental boost at a time when you are adjusting to an entirely different routine. If you belong to a childbirth group, make sure you have contact details for the other mothers. Once your babies arrive, you will be very busy and it can be easier to stick to prearranged dates. Meeting up can help you feel connected and supported.

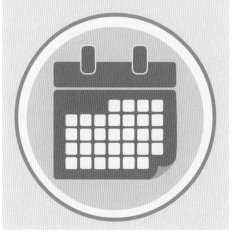

Rest & relax

It may not feel like getting organized for your baby's arrival, but taking a little time for a treat now can help you relax, increase your sense of well-being, and generally put you in a good place mentally and physically for your new baby. Whether it's lunch with friends, a relaxing pedicure or massage, or a movie date with your partner, make the most of your free time now. Schedule a little treat for yourself, especially if it's something that will require much more organizing after the birth.

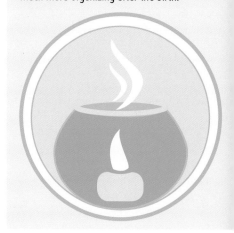

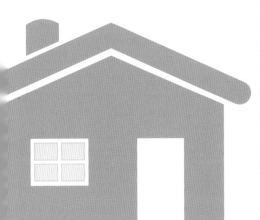

If you find toward the end of pregnancy that you have a sudden **burst of energy** to scrub the house thoroughly from top to bottom, put this down to a **primal nesting instinct** thought to stem from a need to **prepare for** and **protect** your new arrival.

Tidy your home

A well-documented phenomenon, the desire to clean, organize, and "nest" can take hold of many an expectant mother. It's fine to deal with the house now; cleaning thoroughly will be one less thing to worry about when your baby arrives, and should make your environment more relaxing and enjoyable. Use eco-friendly cleaning products where you can so you don't inhale hazardous fumes. You may also want to store clothes you won't wear until the next season to create more room in your closet, or file paperwork, for example. However, be sensible and don't overdo it. And if you don't get everything organized just so, try not to worry.

Get cooking

Spend some time rustling up a few nutritious home-cooked meals for the freezer to enjoy in the weeks after the birth. First-time parents are often surprised by just how much time a new baby takes up; you may be too exhausted to spend time cooking. This will reduce the temptation to resort to unhealthy convenience foods, and help to ensure you eat a nutritious diet while breast-feeding. Label and date items so you can keep track of what needs to be eaten when. Take a look in your freezer and pantry too, and stock up on supplies. Consider setting up an online food shopping account if you don't have one already.

A QUICK CHECKLIST

Make your own checklist to refer to and check off the tasks as they are done. You might want to include some of the following:

CLOTHES AND EQUIPMENT
» Look through everything you have bought and check that it is all there.
» Wash new clothes, burp cloths, and bed linen using nonbiological detergent.
» Pack some baby clothes in your hospital bag along with your own supplies.
» Make sure you know how the bottle sanitizing unit works.
» Test out the stroller.
» Install the car seat.

GOING TO THE HOSPITAL
» Make sure you are familiar with the route.
» Check that you have the money for parking, if needed.
» Ask if you need a pass when you arrive.
» Check that your hospital bag is packed and ready to go.
» Make sure you have contact details of friends and family.

HOME LIFE
» Make a list of chores that will need to be done.
» Discuss with your partner how to split tasks when your baby has arrived.
» If you have other children, make a plan for what will happen to them when you go to the hospital.
» Stock the freezer and pantry with nutritious food.
» Buy files to store bills and mail that require a response.
» Get up to date on bills.

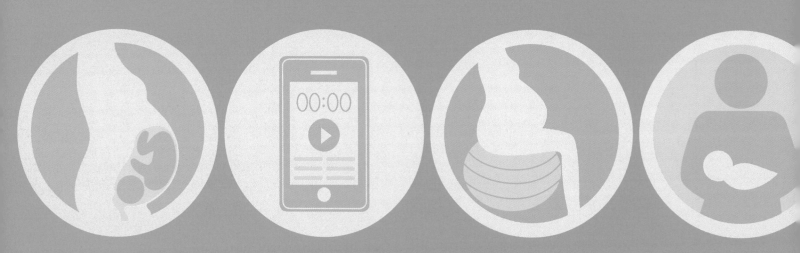

⟫ In this chapter...

Labor
and birth

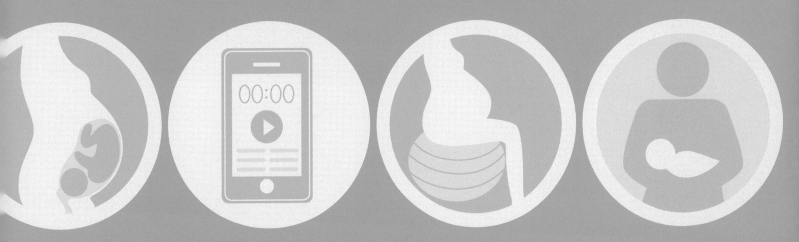

As labor and birth draw nearer, so does the day that you will finally meet your baby. It's natural to feel nervous, but the information in this chapter will help give you the **confidence to feel empowered** for what lies ahead. Find out about the early signs of labor, the different **stages of labor**, the best positions for each stage, and the role of a birth partner. Learn about **pain relief** and how to have a natural birth, or what to expect if you have a C-section or assisted delivery.

By the time you reach around 36 weeks of pregnancy, the prospect of **meeting your baby is tantalizingly close**. Your doctor will begin to note how she is positioned in your uterus, whether or not her **head is engaged**, and find out your preferences for your labor. Your body could also start to give you signs that your baby will soon be here

Before labor begins

Time and space

During the last four weeks of your pregnancy, your baby grows rapidly—at a rate of about 8 oz (225 g) per week. The space within your uterus becomes restricted and you may feel that your baby is now squirming around rather than kicking. Keep note of the movements, and if your baby "sleeps" for longer than you would expect, or her movements are weaker or less frequent than is normal for her, call the doctor immediately. Your doctor will pay special attention to the size of your belly over these last few weeks, to check whether your baby has plenty of amniotic fluid surrounding her and to make final predictions on the baby's size at birth.

The doctor will also figure out, by palpating your abdomen, what position your baby is in. The presses may seem firm and even cause you discomfort at this stage, but don't worry since they don't harm your baby. Your doctor may be trying to nudge her into a better position, or to establish whether or not her head has engaged (see p.202), and if it has, how deeply engaged it is.

Talking about labor

During these last few weeks, you'll find that conversations with your doctor will turn to labor. You'll have the opportunity to go over your birth plan (see p.88–89),

and to raise any remaining questions. If your baby is in a breech position, or positioned across your abdomen, your doctor will talk through the implications for your labor and you'll be encouraged to discuss these with your birth partner. Remember that labor is a constantly evolving situation, so the more information you can gather now, the more confident you'll be about any decision you might have to make while you're in the delivery room.

Watching and waiting

Many women spend the last few weeks of their pregnancy eagerly watching for signs that labor might be imminent and even trying myriad old wives' tales to get the process started. Your remarkable, pregnant body is responsive to all sorts of chemical changes right now—and these can have quite surprising effects on your behavior, mood, and well-being. Try to keep yourself distracted—engage in nonstrenuous activities that require your concentration. Read the book that you've been meaning to try; teach yourself to knit, sew, or crochet; plant some herbs in pots; spend an afternoon watching movies. Don't overexert yourself, but do try to keep busy and keep your mind off the looming question of "When?" And ignore all comments in the vein of "Still no sign, then?" Just smile and change the subject.

Q My doctor has told me what position my baby is in, but what does this mean and why is it important?

The skeleton of your pelvic region is remarkably flexible, but your baby's position can influence how easy it is for her to get through the pelvic bones and under the pubic arch when the time comes. In an ideal world, your baby's position will allow the smallest point of her head to come out first, and with enough space to bend her neck, and fold in her shoulders.

PRESENTATION POSITIONS

Your baby could be lying in the uterus vertically (known as longitudinal), horizontally (transverse), or diagonally (oblique). If lying vertically, the part the baby "presents" toward your cervix can vary.

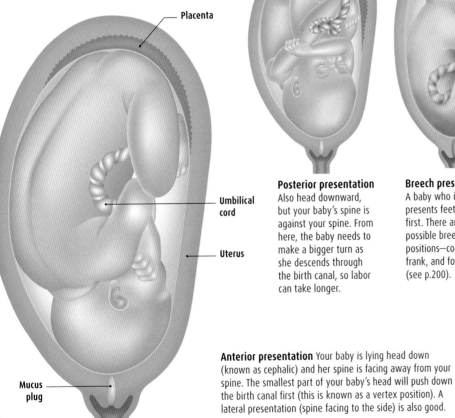

Placenta

Umbilical cord

Uterus

Mucus plug

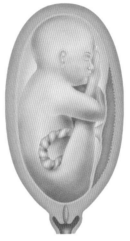

Posterior presentation Also head downward, but your baby's spine is against your spine. From here, the baby needs to make a bigger turn as she descends through the birth canal, so labor can take longer.

Breech presentation A baby who is breech presents feet or bottom first. There are three possible breech positions—complete, frank, and footling (see p.200).

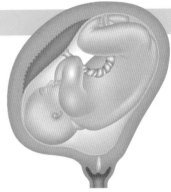

Oblique lie If a baby is lying diagonally across the uterus, the position is called oblique. It's highly unusual for a baby to remain in this position right up until labor. Only one percent of babies will be transverse or oblique.

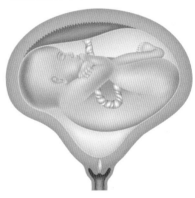

Anterior presentation Your baby is lying head down (known as cephalic) and her spine is facing away from your spine. The smallest part of your baby's head will push down the birth canal first (this is known as a vertex position). A lateral presentation (spine facing to the side) is also good.

Transverse lie In the transverse position, your baby is lying straight across your uterus horizontally. The angle means the baby's body doesn't present toward the cervix.

Q How does the position of the baby affect my experience of labor?

Your baby must both descend and rotate through the birth canal to be born (see pp.214–15). In anterior or lateral cephalic presentation (vertex positions), the smallest part of the head leads the way and the baby can maneuver quite easily, helping to keep your labor relatively short and trouble-free. In the posterior position, a wider part of the head presents first and the baby needs to

rotate more to make her descent, making labor progress more slowly. More rarely, it may mean that the baby gets stuck. Labor isn't necessarily more painful in these circumstances, but for your baby it can become distressing. If your doctor feels that labor is taking too long and the baby shows signs of stress, he or she may decide to change the course of your birth plan. Depending upon the circumstances, you may be offered an assisted delivery or, if necessary, a cesarean section. Babies in the transverse and oblique positions during labor are quite likely to need a cesarean section.

37 weeks

Your baby is considered **full-term** at 37 weeks. If you reach 41 to 42 weeks, you are likely to be offered induction to start your labor.

Q I'm 36 weeks pregnant and my baby is breech. Should I worry?

There's still time for your baby to turn—some babies change position up until days before birth—but your doctor will discuss your options with you.

Most babies have turned into a head-down, vertex position by 34 weeks pregnant, but it's also perfectly normal for a baby to move and swing around a few days before birth, and even during labor itself. It's an evolving process. If the baby hasn't turned by 36 weeks, your doctor will offer to try manually turning your baby with a technique called external cephalic version (ECV).

If successful, this can help avoid a cesarean section. Your doctor should spend time with you to discuss the pros and cons of vaginal delivery versus cesarean section so that you can make a fully informed decision in the event that your baby stays in a breech position. Not every situation will be the same, partly because there are three possible breech positions (shown below).

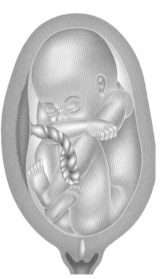 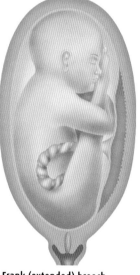 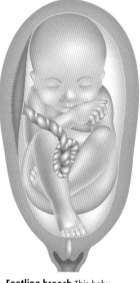

Complete (flexed) breech In this bottom-downward position the baby's legs are flexed and he is curled up, knees and chin to chest, and with ankles crossed.

Frank (extended) breech Both the baby's legs are extended so that his feet stick upward, and his bottom presents first. He might be hugging his knees.

Footling breech This baby presents his foot first: both knees are bent, but one foot is extended downward, pressing against the cervix.

Q Can I turn a breech baby myself, or will a doctor have to do it?

If you are past 36 weeks pregnant, you should be offered an external cephalic version (ECV). This noninvasive technique involves a doctor pressing hard on your abdomen to try to push the baby round into the cephalic (head-down) position. It's a perfectly safe procedure for both of you, and works in around half of all cases, but it may feel a bit uncomfortable at the time. If it works, ECV greatly lowers the risk of cesarean section. If you want to help things along at home, some moms report that adopting

certain positions to "tip" the baby out of the pelvis can help give it more room to move. You could try either kneeling forward on the floor with one cheek resting on the floor and your bottom in the air, or lying on your back with a pillow beneath your hips to raise them, knees bent, feet flat on the floor. While there is no research evidence to suggest that these techniques will necessarily work, they won't harm your baby either. Just be careful you don't hurt your back or neck in the process. You can also try moxibustion, which advocates of traditional Chinese medicine believe can turn the baby. Acupuncture is also a popular therapy to try.

Q If my baby isn't lying head down, will I definitely have to have a cesarean section?

Although cesarean sections are often considered the safest option for breech babies, sometimes a vaginal birth is possible. If your baby presents bottom first, is of average size, and you have an average-sized pelvis, your doctor may be happy to allow a vaginal delivery, if that is your preference. If the baby presents with foot or knee first, cesarean section is usually advised as the safer option.

Only around 3.5 percent of births are breech (bottom downward). Your doctor may try to turn your baby into a vertical position using ECV (see below, left), during the last few weeks of your pregnancy if he himself isn't showing signs of making the turn. If your baby is transverse (lying across your uterus), however, unless the baby can be turned manually, you will probably need to have a cesarean section.

Q Will I be able to have a normal experience of labor if my baby is in a breech position?

Yes. The early stage of labor is more or less the same for both vertex and breech births, but you're likely to be monitored more frequently if your baby is breech. You can still move around, but your doctor may need you to remain attached to a fetal heart monitor, which would limit your movements a bit. Ask if there are any portable methods for monitoring the baby, and make a decision based on your doctor's advice. Keep emptying your bladder during your labor—every two hours or so—in order to give your baby as much space as possible to move into a good position for birth.

Remember to **monitor your baby's movements** in the uterus. Reporting changes in the **pattern of behavior** to your doctor immediately could prevent a stillbirth.

Q I'm so huge I feel like I must be close now. Are there signs that can tell me if my labor could start before too long?

Even before you experience the symptoms of actually going into labor, if you know what to look for, you could notice your body signaling that labor is only weeks or days away.

This table describes some of the most reliable indications that your labor is approaching. The signs are organized from the very earliest possible indications at the top, to those symptoms that you should call your doctor about at the bottom. Remember that it's impossible to be prescriptive about the character of every woman's labor, and even signs that seem genuine may stop and start, while others may not appear at all. Listen to your body, but reassure yourself that labor is impossible to miss—you'll know when it's happening! If you're at all worried or unsure, never hesitate to call your doctor, who can offer you reassurance and guidance as necessary.

EARLY SIGNS OF APPROACHING LABOR

SIGN OF LABOR	SYMPTOMS	HOW SOON WILL I MEET MY BABY?	ACTION
Nesting	An uncontrollable urge to clean, tidy, shop, make; a burst of energy; an overwhelming urge to protect your belly and other family members.	Could be days or weeks.	Try not to overdo it, and make sure that every energy burst is followed with quality rest; eat little and often, and drink plenty; keep an eye out for other labor signs.
Lightening	A feeling of being able to breathe more deeply yet increased pressure on your bladder and/or pelvic pressure.	Could be days or weeks.	Let your doctor know about this feeling at your next prenatal appointment; he or she will assess your baby's position.
Sleeplessness	Difficulty sleeping despite being tired; waking in the night; alarming dreams.	Could be days or weeks.	See pages 114–15 for advice on getting more and better-quality sleep.
Practice contractions/ Braxton Hicks	Erratic tightening across the abdomen; belly feels rigid when you touch it; discomfort but not pain.	More numerous practice contractions, or Braxton Hicks contractions, as you approach your due date can certainly indicate that your body is preparing for labor, but there's no need to assume that labor might be imminent.	If you're worried, unsure, or have any bright-red bleeding or abdominal pain, or if you think your water has broken (see p.206), call your doctor. Don't be anxious about possibly raising a false alarm.
Lower back pain	A dull, persistent ache across the lower portion of your back.	Lower back pain close to your due date can be a sign that your cervix is beginning to dilate; labor may be a few days away, or perhaps less.	Call the doctor if back pain is accompanied by abdominal pain or cramping, or a bloody show (see p.206); ask your doctor if you can take acetaminophen for pain relief; distract yourself with a warm bath or other calming activity.
Diarrhea or feeling sick	Loose or runny stools, and persistent urge to go to the bathroom; waves of nausea or even vomiting.	No one is sure why—perhaps it is due to a hormone surge or your baby pressing against the bowel—but many women feel sick or have loose stools in the days before they go into active labor. Make sure you have everything ready, but your baby may still be a few days away.	Keep hydrated and eat little and often; call your doctor if you have diarrhea or vomiting that persists for more than 24 hours.

Q My belly keeps getting hard and I get a tightening sensation. Is this a contraction?

You could be experiencing "practice" contractions, also known as Braxton Hicks (after the English doctor who first noted them). If the tightening sensations are short-lived and last no longer than a minute, if they come and go without any clear pattern, but are perhaps particularly strong after you've done something strenuous, if they are uncomfortable, but not really painful and if you have no other signs of labor (see p.206), the chances are you're having "practice" contractions, rather than those of active labor. These are thought to be present throughout pregnancy, getting gradually more noticeable and more frequent as you reach full term. You'll probably really start to notice them in the last three or four weeks. Although they are popularly thought to help the uterus tone up for real contractions, some researchers believe that in later pregnancy they begin the process of effacement—when your cervix begins to open and draw upward, becoming part of the smooth muscle of the wall of your uterus.

Q Are there any natural ways to bring on labor?

Anecdotally, there are various "natural" ways to induce labor. However, there is not enough scientific evidence to confirm that they are genuinely effective at starting birth. Still, as long as your pregnancy has been complication-free, you are full term, and you have no reason to believe your baby could become distressed, they can be worth a try. Tell your doctor if you intend to try any of these methods.

» Meditation and hypnosis: when you're stressed or anxious, your body releases adrenalin, which signals to your brain that now would not be a good time to give birth. In turn, this inhibits the release of oxytocin, the hormone that starts your labor. Meditation and hypnosis can help you relax, in turn removing the neurological barriers to oxytocin release.

» Having sex: it's said that the contractions of the uterus during an orgasm can act as a catalyst for bringing on labor contractions, while the intimacy of sex itself, and of being close to someone you love and trust, releases the hormone oxytocin. Furthermore, some say that the prostaglandins (chemical messengers) in semen can soften the cervix to trigger the start of labor. Don't have sex if your water has broken, though, since you are at increased risk of infection.

» Nipple massage: gently rubbing your nipples and rolling them between your thumb and forefinger can release oxytocin. The goal is to simulate the action of a baby sucking on your breast, so you'll need to be methodical if you are to use this approach. Just as a breast-feeding baby would feed from one breast for 20 minutes or so, and then the other, and every few hours, for the best effects you

need to do the same. It can take up to 72 hours to have the necessary effect on your body to induce labor–so you will need to be dedicated to the cause to make this worthwhile!

» Acupuncture: in this form of traditional Chinese medicine a qualified acupuncturist inserts tiny needles into your body along "meridians"–energy lines that interconnect to trigger certain effects throughout the physical body. Some women swear by acupuncture for induction of labor, but there is no rigorous scientific evidence that says it works. If you want to give it a try, aim to find a practitioner who is experienced in treating pregnant women, and talk to your doctor first.

» Homeopathy: there is no firm evidence that homeopathy works for inducing labor. If you want to try a homeopathic remedy, though, make sure you consult a registered homeopath with experience of treating pregnant women. You should always talk to your doctor first.

» Spicy foods: some curry and chili-pepper dishes stimulate your digestion and create "heat" in your body. Many women claim that the activity in the intestine and bowel has helped to bring on labor. There's no harm in giving it a try (aside, perhaps, from an increased risk of heartburn and indigestion!).

» Fresh pineapple: pineapple stimulates your digestion (this time because it contains a digestive enzyme called bromelain), which some claim can help stimulate the uterus to begin contracting. However, it takes a lot of pineapple to raise the levels of bromelain in your system for any effect–several whole pineapples–so you are probably more likely to end up with an upset stomach in the next 24 hours than delivering your baby.

» Herbal remedies: there are some herbs that are said to help bring on labor. These include black cohosh and evening primrose oil. Remember, though, never to use any herbal remedy without getting the go-ahead from your doctor, since it may have harmful effects on you or your baby.

» Raspberry leaf tea: while evidence does suggest that raspberry leaf stimulates the action of the uterus, medically it is discouraged for the induction of labor because overstimulating the uterus can cause distress for the baby.

Q What does it mean for the baby's head to "engage"?

Known colloquially as "dropping," a baby engages when the widest part of her head has descended into the cavity in your pelvic bones (the pelvic inlet).

Engagement isn't something that happens in a single moment, but over time–usually starting between 34 and 36 weeks pregnant. It can take several weeks for a baby slowly and methodically to move herself into position. Other times, the baby will wait until labor has actually begun, allowing your contractions to provide the push she needs finally to make the move down into the pelvic

cavity. A large baby, multiple babies, fibroids in your uterus, or a badly placed placenta are all reasons why engagement might take longer. How soon or late the baby's head engages doesn't indicate when you'll go into labor or how quick your labor will be. A baby who engages at 32 weeks is no more likely to make a speedy entry into the world than one who waits until labor has started.

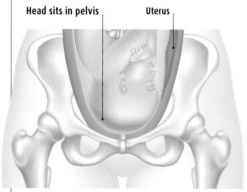

Head sits in pelvis   Uterus

Before engagement Your baby's head hovers freely above your pelvis and she is able to turn and swing around.

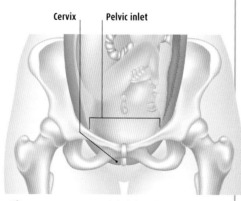

Cervix   Pelvic inlet

After engagement Your baby's head lies within the cavity of your pelvic bones, which can offer relief for your lungs, but you may feel your baby bearing down on your pubic bones.

Q I have reached my due date and my doctor is talking about inducing my labor. What does this mean?

Induction means artificially kick-starting labor, and if your baby is late it will be offered at 41 weeks. After 42 weeks the placenta becomes less efficient and the risk of stillbirth increases, so induction is often recommended before that point.

Your doctor will explain to you why it is appropriate to consider induction in your case, and the options available. Even if you are 41 or 42 weeks pregnant, you can request to "wait it out," but the associated risks will be discussed so that you can make an informed decision about what's best for you. If you decide you're happy for intervention to get your labor started, she will begin by suggesting a cervical "sweep." Your doctor can perform the sweep at a normal prenatal appointment; she will insert her index finger into your vagina and make a circular, sweeping motion beyond your cervix, around the wall of your uterus, with the goal of separating the two membranes that surround the baby. This can provide the hormonal stimulation your body needs for your cervix to start softening and labor to start naturally within the next week or so. About half of all women who have a sweep will go into labor within two days. The procedure may be repeated if you haven't gone into labor within a week. If a cervical sweep is unsuccessful, medical induction will be suggested.

MEDICAL INDUCTION METHODS

If a sweep didn't work to start your labor, your doctor will explain the medical methods available and the reasons why they are appropriate for you (or not, as the case may be).

	WHAT IS IT?	WHEN AND HOW?	SUCCESS
Prostaglandin	Prostaglandin is a naturally occurring hormone that triggers the softening of the cervix. A gel or suppository containing the hormone is inserted the vagina, or you may be offered it in tablet form.	A doctor will administer the gel, suppository, or tablet at the hospital. You will be asked to stay there to be monitored, because some women have strong contractions after a short period of time, while others may need more than one dose. Be sure to bring along your packed hospital bag if your doctor tells you that you're going to be induced.	Studies show that if your cervix was already softening, a prostaglandin induction can start labor within 24 hours of treatment.
Membrane rupture	Also known as ARM (artificial rupture of membranes) and amniotomy, this technique involves a doctor deliberately breaking your water to kick-start the labor process.	You'll be offered this if you have not had a successful prostaglandin attempt. You will usually need to be in hospital because rupturing your membranes increases the risk of infection. Your doctor will use a special hook, called an amniohook, to puncture the amniotic sac in two places, in the lower part and in the upper part.	There is no guarantee of success. However, used with oxytocin, studies show that women will generally go into labor within 24 hours of membrane rupture.
Oxytocin	This is the hormone that your body produces when it feels your baby pressing down on your cervix, and it starts labor.	Oxytocin is the most common form of labor induction used in the US today. It's most likely that it will be administered intravenously. Your doctor will suggest oxytocin if prostaglandin gels haven't been successful.	If this last step in the induction process hasn't worked you will be asked to consider a cesarean section.

Q I can suddenly breathe more easily—has my baby moved position? Is that a bad sign?

If you're approaching your due date, it's more likely to be a good sign. To prepare for birth, your baby makes a descent into the lowest part of your pelvis—this is called "lightening" (or sometimes "dropping") because it "lightens" the pressure in your abdomen. The effect of your baby dropping into position is that your lungs suddenly have more space to expand, which means you can breathe more easily again.

On the flip side, you might find that the new position puts more pressure on your bladder, and you need the bathroom more often.

Q I've heard an induced labor can be more painful. Is this true?

When you go into natural labor, signals to your brain mean that your body releases endorphins, hormonal painkillers that help you to cope with labor and birth. In an induced labor, your body hasn't had the natural gearing up that makes sure you have good levels of circulating endorphins from the earliest, imperceptible beginnings of labor. As a result, many women report that an induced labor is more painful than one that occurs naturally. However, try not to worry—being induced doesn't place any restrictions on the pain relief that is available to you, so ask your doctor about the options if you feel things are getting to be too much for you. Statistics show that women having an induced labor are more likely to ask for an epidural. Your baby is also slightly more likely (about 15 percent more likely) to need an assisted birth (see p.222).

Labor is a process, a series of changes that will finally bring your baby into your arms. Although clinically there are signs, phases, and markers, **each woman's labor is different** from another's. If this is your second or subsequent baby, the experience will be unlike your previous ones—it's **unique and remarkable**.

Being in labor

Understanding the big event

Your doctor and doctors will refer to labor as having three stages. The first stage is usually the longest, beginning with the first contractions and sometimes a "bloody show" (see p.206) that indicates that your cervix has started to open, and lasting until your cervix is fully dilated. The second stage is characterized by the act of pushing your baby down the birth canal and out into the world. The third stage refers to the delivery of the placenta and membranes. It's always helpful to be aware of the terms your doctor will use, but in practice labor is really just a single event that begins with a few small signs and ends with the emergence of your baby.

Listen to your body

Referring to labor in clinical terms—stages, centimeters, and time spans—while helpful for a medical staff, isn't really what labor is about for you. This is a magical time: the start or expanding of a family, the beginning of new life, and a time when your body performs the most

natural, fundamental, and significant event. Many women worry about labor—how they will "deal" with it, will they be "good" at it, will labor follow the clinical patterns they have read so much about? It's helpful to remember that clinical markers are not "rules" and there isn't one set way to give birth—try not to focus on what stage you're in, whether you are 2 cm or 9 cm dilated, or how many hours your baby has shown signs of coming. Instead, concentrate on listening to your body, responding to its signals (don't worry—they will be obvious), and focusing on the baby that you will soon be able to hold. Remain as calm as you can and stay warm. Stress inhibits the release of oxytocin, which is the hormone that triggers your contractions. Walk around if it makes you feel more at ease, or sit or stand, or lean over an exercise ball. There is no rule that says you must lie in a bed.

If you need to be hooked up to a monitor for medical reasons, you can still stand or sit on a chair or ball and let gravity lend you a helping hand. Make this an event that feels right for you.

Q What can I expect to happen during labor? How long is it likely to last?

As your body enters into labor and prepares to give birth to your baby, it will go through a sequence of events and stages. While no two labors are the same, this progress of labor does follow a pattern that helps the doctor and nurses monitor you, and encourages you that your baby is on his way.

Leaning over an exercise ball This can help you feel more at ease and comfortable during labor.

Understanding **how labor works** helps you gauge when to stay at home and when to **call the doctor**.

ENGAGEMENT

Toward the end of pregnancy, your baby's head drops down into the lowest part of the pelvis, or engages (see p.202), to prepare for labor and delivery. Engagement tends to happen earlier in first pregnancies, when uterine muscles that have never been stretched before can exert greater pressure to push the baby down into the pelvis.

Time it takes This sign of approaching labor can happen any time, from several weeks before labor in first pregnancies to just as labor starts in subsequent pregnancies.

Action Your doctor will palpate your abdomen at your prenatal appointments to find out whether your baby's head is engaged.

1ST STAGE—ACTIVE LABOR AND TRANSITION

The second part of the first stage is known as "active labor." You will know it by frequent, strong contractions that are impossible to ignore. The cervix opens more quickly and at 7–9 cm dilation, the active phase moves into transition, when contractions become more intense and you feel the urge to push. The first stage ends once the cervix is fully dilated, at 10 cm.

Time it takes In an average first labor, the cervix dilates about 1 cm an hour. Active labor can progress much quicker in subsequent labors.

Action Call your doctor when you reach active labor. You will probably be advised to time the contractions and rest at home until the contractions are closer together, about every five minutes and lasting 60 seconds.

3RD STAGE

The third stage marks the delivery of the placenta and membranes after your baby is born. In other countries this final stage may be "actively" managed, when an injection of oxytocin speeds up delivery of the placenta. This is uncommon in the US but If the idea appeals to you, ask your doctor if she gives patients oxytocin injections.

Time it takes A natural third stage takes 20–30 minutes, and this time guide is the same for first and subsequent deliveries.

Action You may need to push a little more to deliver the placenta.

1ST STAGE—LATENT LABOR

The first stage of labor opens the cervix. Early labor, known as the "latent" phase, is marked by relatively mild, irregular contractions that start to thin and draw up the cervix, a process known as effacement. Then the cervix begins to dilate and will reach around 3–4 cm dilation. The pain is strong but bearable, with periodlike cramping.

Time it takes This longest phase can account for as much as two-thirds of the total time of labor. It can last from several hours to a few days in a first labor; it is often much shorter in subsequent labors.

Action You'll usually be encouraged to stay at home during the latent phase. Try to get comfortable, but keep the contractions going.

2ND STAGE

The second stage of labor begins when the cervix is fully dilated and ends with the birth of your baby. This stage is marked by a strong urge to bear down as contractions push your baby against the pelvic floor. Your doctor will support and guide you, encouraging you to push with your contractions.

Time it takes The active, pushing part of delivering your baby takes roughly 1–2 hours for a first labor, with the total second stage taking up to 3 hours. The second stage in subsequent labors often takes 2 hours or less, with 30 minutes to 1 hour needed for pushing.

Action The end is nearly in sight. Draw encouragement from your birth partner and let your doctor guide you.

Q Will I know when I'm about to go into labor? Are there signs, and what should I do if I experience them?

When you are very close to true first stage labor, there are three signs that could appear. It's not guaranteed that you will see them all—some women skip them entirely—but if you do, you should inform your doctor.

It is natural to be concerned about recognizing the signs of early labor–unsurprisingly, it is a common worry among pregnant women–but the truth is your experience can be quite different from the next woman's. While the symptoms described below do indicate that labor is imminent, for some women active labor (see p.205) could still be a couple of days away, especially if this is their first pregnancy. Getting a "bloody show" or the first labor contractions indicates that your cervix has started to soften and thin (known as "effacement") in order to open and allow your baby to pass through the birth canal. The length of time this takes can vary greatly, so listen to your body and time your contractions. If your water breaks, it mostly does so once contractions have started; if it happens beforehand for you, call your doctor.

SIGNS OF IMMINENT LABOR

	SYMPTOMS	HOW SOON WILL I MEET MY BABY?	ACTION
A "bloody show" (dislodging of the cervical mucus plug)	A brownish or yellowish vaginal discharge, your mucus plug has a jellylike consistency and may look like congealed, yellowed phlegm, or be tinged dark brown with blood. It may come away in one "blob" or several. Some women never have a show; others pass the plug without noticing while going to the bathroom.	Even though the dislodging of the mucus plug is a sure sign that your cervix is opening, active labor could still be a few days away, or even weeks if this is your first baby.	Call your doctor. You will probably be advised to have a relaxing bath or otherwise try to distract yourself, and to look out for first contractions. However, if you have any bright red bleeding, you are feeling unwell, or the baby has not been moving, call your doctor right away.
Labor contractions	Painful, periodlike cramps that begin in the upper portion of your abdomen and spread downward. Contractions may be irregular and spaced fairly far apart at first, becoming more regularly spaced and lasting for one to two minutes each.	These "latent-phase" contractions could indicate that "active labor" is only a few hours (or less) away, but in some cases contractions will be slow and last a few days (at most).	Call your doctor. If you're going to a hospital to give birth, they will probably ask you to stay at home as long as you feel you can. If you experience any bleeding or your water breaks, call your doctor and go to the hospital.
Water breaking (rupture of membranes)	This may happen as a gush or a trickle–amniotic fluid looks a lot like pale urine, so you may think you have stress incontinence.	Your baby's arrival may still be a few days away, but now that the amniotic sac has broken, your baby is at risk of infection, so will need to be delivered sooner rather than later.	Call your doctor immediately for advice. Since your baby is now at risk of infection, you will need to be carefully monitored. You should not lie in a bath, in case of infection. If the amniotic fluid is greenish in color, go to the hospital right away (it could be meconium, a fetal bowel movement).

Q I have a "bloody show." Does this mean I'm in the first stage of labor?

If the show is accompanied by irregular contractions, yes, you are probably in the first "latent" stage. However, by itself, losing your mucus plug is not an indication that the first stage of labor has started, it's simply a sign that things are moving in the right direction. It's definitely time to start watching out for more certain labor signs, especially contractions that build in intensity over time.

Q I think I'm in early labor and I feel sick. Should I eat?

Eating is discouraged even in the beginning stages of labor. Though some doctors may allow women to eat light snacks in the first stage of labor, the American College of Obstetricians and Gynecologists (ACOG) recommends that you do not eat at all while in labor. Women laboring in hospitals are usually offered only ice chips to suck on instead of water to drink and no food all. Recently, however, the guidelines from the ACOG changed a bit. Instead of only ice chips, it's now believed to be OK for moms-to-be, who are having uncomplicated labors, to drink small amounts of clear liquids such as water, fruit juices without pulp (though the acidity of orange juice may upset your stomach), carbonated beverages, clear tea, black coffee, sports drinks, and clear broth.

The restriction on eating during labor comes from the theory that food could be breathed in (aspirated) during an emergency surgery in the unlikely event you would need to have general anesthesia.

WHEN TO GO TO THE HOSPITAL OR STAY AT HOME

Timing contractions and helping decide when to go to the hospital is a key part of your role.

Your partner may be increasingly preoccupied, which means you may need to judge when to leave for the hospital. If contractions are irregular (albeit painful), and she can talk through them, it's best to stay at home. Once contractions are five minutes apart, intense, and last for around 60 seconds, head in. It may sound obvious, but factor in your distance from the hospital, and leave earlier if it's far away.

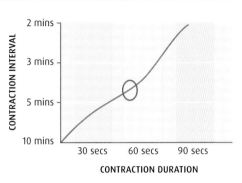

CONTRACTION INTERVAL

2 mins
3 mins
5 mins
10 mins

30 secs   60 secs   90 secs

CONTRACTION DURATION

SUDDEN BIRTH

Very occasionally, labor moves so quickly that there isn't enough time to get to the hospital. If you are with your partner and she feels an overwhelming urge to push, you will need to take an active role.

» Help your partner stay calm. Call your doctor or 911 so that paramedics can be sent to you.

» Turn up the heat, if it's cold, and ask your partner which room she would like to be in. Gather about four clean towels and two or three blankets. Fold two towels and place them beneath your partner's bottom. Find a plastic bag or container that doesn't have any holes in it for the placenta to be placed in.

The birth itself

» Call 911 again and the operator will stay on the line and advise you. (Speakerphone is useful, since you'll need your hands free.) If you can see the baby's head, support it as it crowns. Check the cord, and if this is compressed around the baby before he is born, untangle it if it is loose enough to do so; if it isn't loose enough to free easily, leave it as it is and unwrap it once the baby is completely out.

» Encourage your partner to push gently with each contraction. Once the head, shoulders, and finally the body are delivered, place the baby on your partner's belly. Leave the cord intact—it should be long enough for you to put the baby on your partner's abdomen. Dry the baby, then keep him warm with a towel and blanket. Don't pull on the cord and don't try to cut it or clamp it in any way. The cord will continue to pump blood into the baby for 10 minutes or so after the birth, then it will stop pulsating. You can leave it attached even then.

» Your partner will have one or more contractions to deliver the placenta and membranes. This should come out in one piece with the cord and the membranes of the amniotic sac attached. There'll be some bleeding, which is normal. Put the placenta in a plastic bag for the doctor to check. Keep your baby warm, listen to the paramedics, and stay calm.

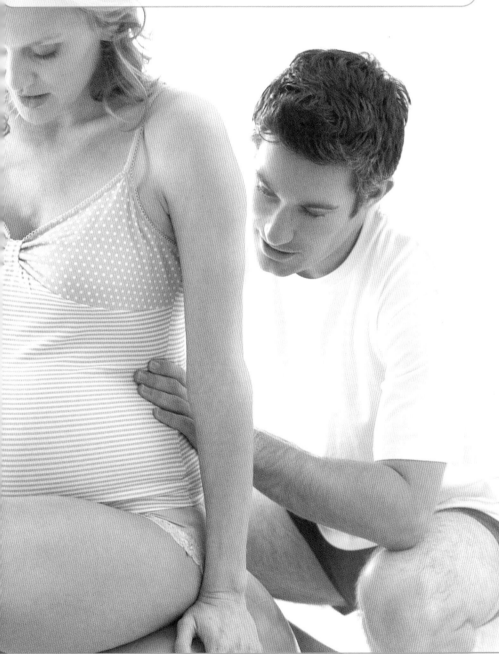

Soothing touch A lower back massage can be relaxing in the early stages of labor, and may be especially welcome if contractions are causing lower back pain.

Q What are the best birthing positions to adopt during first stage labor?

A combination of active and restful positions help you to get through first stage labor. Active positions are thought to encourage the progression of labor, and restful, supported positions allow you to have vital respite between contractions.

Follow your **instincts** and decide yourself how you want to **move, sit, or stand** during first stage labor.

Standing upright in labor encourages your baby to move down, deep into your pelvis, and to press against your cervix. This has the effect of sending messages to your brain to release more of the hormone oxytocin, which stimulates further contractions. These become more frequent, longer, and more effective than in other birthing positions, which makes labor shorter than if you were lying down. Walking around also helps your baby to move lower into your pelvis, so labor progresses more quickly. Studies show that staying active in the first stage makes you less likely to ask for pain relief or to need a C-section, and your baby is less likely to become distressed. However, lying down and sitting positions allow you to recover from contractions, but don't stay still for too long since it will slow down your labor.

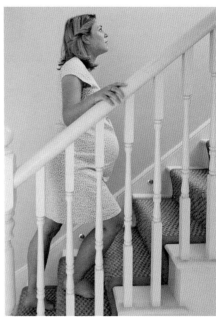

Walking up and down stairs If you have stairs near you, use them to keep active. Remember to hold on to the bannister for support.

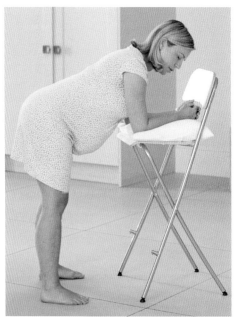

Standing, leaning on a tall chair or stool Use a chair to support your body weight. Place a cushion under your arms for extra comfort.

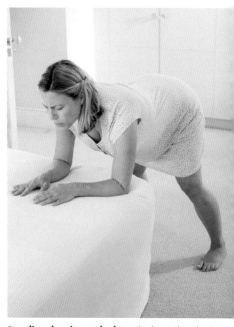

Standing, leaning on bed Ease back pain by adopting this pose. This particularly helps when your baby is lying with her back against your spine.

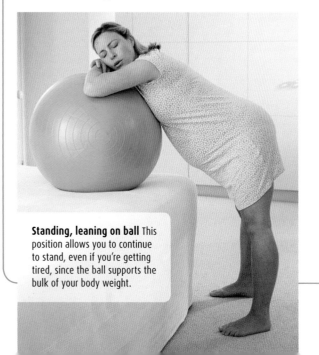

Standing, leaning on ball This position allows you to continue to stand, even if you're getting tired, since the ball supports the bulk of your body weight.

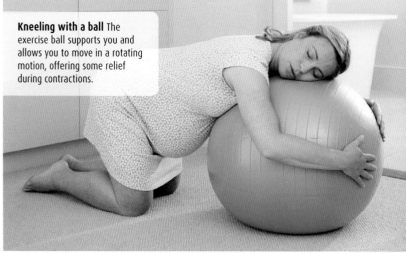

Kneeling with a ball The exercise ball supports you and allows you to move in a rotating motion, offering some relief during contractions.

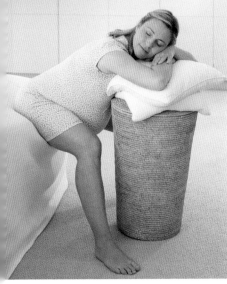

Sitting, leaning on a laundry basket or stool Rest your body in this position, allowing yourself to build up your strength for the next wave of contractions.

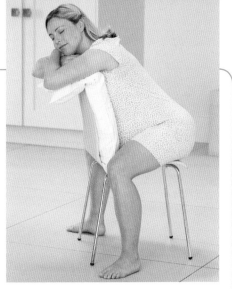

Straddling a chair This will help open your pelvis while allowing you a rest so that you can save energy to deal with the next contraction.

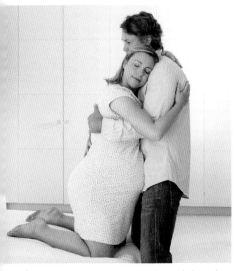

Kneeling, partner support Gain comfort and physical support by kneeling on a bed and embracing your partner.

Standing, leaning forward on partner This position can make you feel close to each other and help you to relax. Your partner can support your body weight.

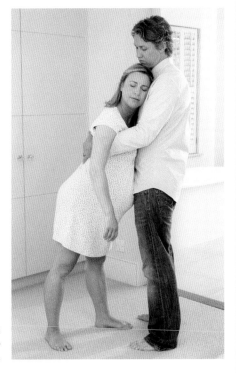

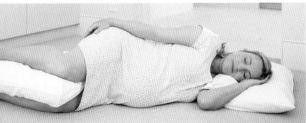

Side lying Lying on your right or left side can help soothe the pain and help alter your baby's position slightly if your baby is lying back to back.

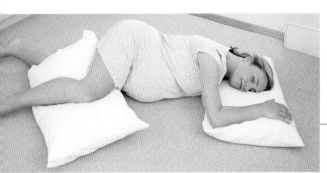

Semi-prone, fetal back toward the ceiling If you know that your baby is facing right with its back against yours, you can lie on your left side for short periods. Gravity may pull the baby into a more comfortable position.

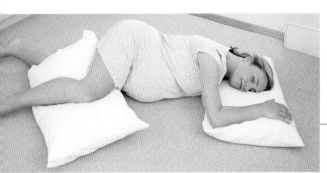

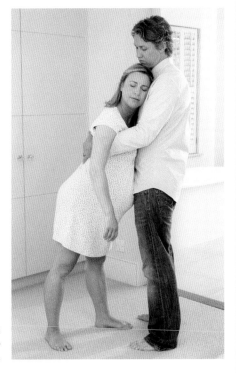

Q What are the benefits of laboring in water, and are there risks?

Women who labor in water make fewer requests for pain relief. It's thought that this has to do with the calming effect of being in water, because the measured amplitude (intensity) of contractions in fact remains the same in and out of the water. Women who labor in water also find it easier to change position since they are supported by the buoyancy of the water, and are less likely to need an episiotomy. There are no risks that specifically relate to going through your labor in water. Your doctor can monitor the baby's heart rate using a waterproof handheld heart monitor to make sure your baby shows no signs of distress, and will take appropriate action if she does.

Q When should I get into my birthing pool?

Some experts believe that being in water during the early stages of labor can slow contractions and prolong labor. They advocate getting into the water only once you are 7 cm dilated. Others believe that being in water eases pain and promotes relaxation, improving labor. If you are using a pool at a hospital or birthing center, you will need to follow their protocol. At home, you can decide when to get in and out of the pool. Always make sure the water temperature is never over 99.5°F (37.5°C).

Q I want to lie on a bed, but will this make my labor more painful?

Lying down pushes the lower part of your spine against the baby's head. The added pressure when the baby tries to move past this part of your back and deeper into your pelvis can make labor more painful. Lying on your back also narrows the space that you have for your pelvic bones to separate to allow the baby through, which can increase the pain. Contractions when lying down can be more painful and less effective, lengthening your labor. If you need to lie down, don't lay flat on your back but on your left side. Lying down can be the position that is most useful for your doctor, because he or she can easily examine you. Your baby can be monitored if you are in a sitting position.

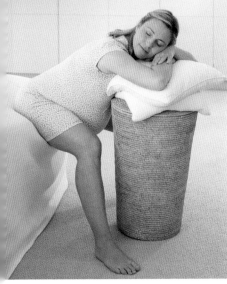

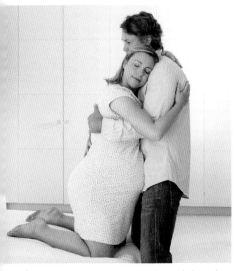

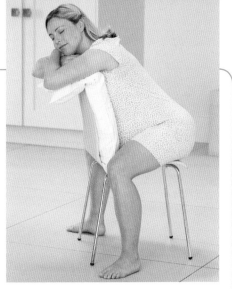

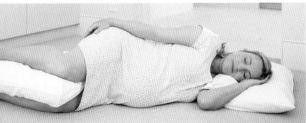

Q What does cervical dilation mean and how does it affect my labor?

In pregnancy, the cervix forms a closed, thick muscular base for the uterus. In early labor, it starts to soften, draw up, and thin (efface) and then open (dilate) so that your baby can pass into the vagina to be born.

Your doctor assesses how far and how quickly your labor is progressing by looking to see how much your cervix has thinned, or effaced, and how wide it has opened, or dilated. The width of the dilation is measured in centimeters. These changes begin in early (or latent) labor, but they can happen slowly because the contractions that act on the cervix are irregular at this point. You may feel as if your labor isn't progressing if the cervical width isn't increasing, but the cervix could still be thinning before opening wider. Dilation can cause the mucus plug to come away from the cervix. Once the cervix has reached 3–4 cm dilation, it marks your passage from the latent to the active phase of first stage labor. In active labor, contractions become stronger, longer, and more frequent and start to open up, or dilate, the cervix more rapidly. Once the cervix is 10 cm dilated, you are fully dilated and at this point you will feel an urge to push, or bear down.

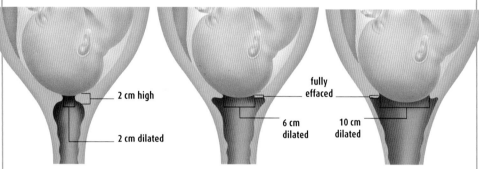

2 cm high

2 cm dilated

fully effaced

6 cm dilated

10 cm dilated

At around 2 cm dilation The cervix is just beginning to open. This is the early (or latent) part of labor and it's likely that your contractions are still fairly irregular.

At 6 cm dilation You are well established in active labor. Your contractions are now strong and regular and increasingly painful, and you may want pain relief now.

At 10 cm dilation Your cervix is fully open and, once your doctor gives you the okay, you can start to push. It may feel like contractions are coming continuously now.

Q At what point should I call my doctor?

You can call your doctor as soon as strong, painful contractions begin. Your doctor will ask you questions about your contractions and how you are feeling to assess how your labor is progressing. He or she will also gauge how you are doing from the tone of your voice and how you are responding to contractions. If your contractions are painful but irregular, and you're planning to have your baby at the hospital or in a birthing center, you will probably be encouraged to labor at home for as long as you possibly can. In this case your partner should make sure you stay well-hydrated, give you back rubs and run a warm bath to help you manage the pain. Studies show that labor progresses better when women are in comfortable and familiar surroundings, where relaxation and rest support the release of oxytocin, which in turn encourages longer and more frequent contractions. Once your contractions are occurring around every five minutes and lasting at least 60 seconds, it is time to call the doctor again to let him know you are heading in. If you're having your baby at home, your doctor will probably ask you to call again when your contractions are closer together (say, around 10 to 15 minutes apart) and lasting between 30 and 45 seconds each. Wherever you're having your baby, call your doctor (or hospital) immediately if your water breaks, or if you have any bleeding. And call at any time if you are worried, even if you've already been told to wait. Doctors are very used to reassuring and guiding women in this way the early stage of labor.

Q What happens if my early labor is very slow or it starts and stops?

Labor is never an exact science, and what can be a relatively quick experience lasting only a few hours for one mother can take days for another. It's normal for early labor to start and stop over several days, especially if this is your first baby. The timing of your contractions, and their strength and length, are the key to knowing when you've moved from the latent phase of first stage labor to a more active phase

Q What if my baby comes quickly and I don't have time to get to the hospital?

It is very unusual for this to happen with a first baby. If you do think labor is progressing too quickly for you to move to the hospital, try to remain calm. First call your doctor, then either your hospital emergency number or 911 for an ambulance, then your birth partner. If you are by yourself and have a friend or family member nearby, get them to come over. Gather clean towels, blankets, and a plastic bag, and choose a warm, draft-free room. If you feel the urge to push, you can try to slow things down by adopting a knee-to-chest position to take pressure off the perineum: get down on all fours, rest your forearms on the floor and raise your bottom in the air. If you still feel an urge to push, go with this. Reach down to see if you can feel the baby's head, and once your baby is born, put her immediately onto your belly for warmth, dry her with a clean towel and lay another towel and blanket over her. Leave the cord intact until help arrives. When you feel another urge to push, go with this to deliver the placenta, which you can place in a plastic bag.

Q What will happen when I arrive at the hospital?

Once you get to the hospital, you will check in to the maternity ward. Then depending on whether you appear to be in active labor, either you will be given a labor room, or you will wait in an assessment bed so that a nurse can come and check on your progress (see opposite). If your nurse assesses that you are still in early labor, you may be sent home and told when to return.

Q How will my doctor be able to tell how my labor is progressing?

Soon after you arrive at the hospital's labor and delivery ward or the birthing center, if you are planning to use one, you will be given a checkup that will look for several signs that indicate where you are in your labor journey and your general health. Your nurse will take your temperature and blood pressure (and he or she will continue to check these signs every four hours throughout your labor), and you might be asked to give the nurse a urine sample. Between your contractions, your nurse will give you an abdominal examination to make sure your baby's head is engaged, and to assess his position, known as the "presentation" (see p.199) which indicates how your baby is likely to be born. If your nurse thinks that you are in active labor, he or she will do a vaginal examination to confirm this and to see how far your cervix has dilated (see box, opposite). You will be given a vaginal examination about every four hours during your labor to see how your labor is progressing.

Q Will my baby be monitored during labor?

Your baby's heart rate will be monitored throughout labor to assess her well-being. Usually, your baby will be monitored intermittently. The doctor will use a handheld Doppler device, which he or she will place against your abdomen to pick up your baby's heartbeat. If there are any concerns during your labor, you will be advised to have continuous monitoring, using a cardiotocograph (CTG) machine. This machine measures both your baby's heartbeat and the frequency of your contractions. Two devices will be attached to your abdomen using straps, which means you will need to stay close to the monitoring machine. The results are printed out on a graph. If at any point your baby appears to be distressed, your doctor may suggest you have internal monitoring, whereby an electrode attached to a wire is passed through the cervix and placed on your baby's scalp (this doesn't hurt the baby). This is not a routine procedure and your doctor will always discuss with you first the reasons why it is being recommended to you.

Q Can I start pushing as soon as I feel the urge?

It is important that you wait for your doctor to give you the okay to push before you start to bear down. Toward the end of the first stage, when the cervix is around 7–9cm dilated, you move into the transition phase (see box, below). You may feel a strong urge to push now, but if you do so before you are fully dilated, the cervix could swell as the baby's head bears down on it before it's ready to give way to let the baby pass through, which can make labor much more difficult. If your doctor thinks it's not yet time to push, you may be asked to take little panting breaths followed by a long, slow exhale, which can relieve your urge to bear down. Or, you may be asked to sit and draw your knees up to your chest, another way to ease the need for pushing. Pain relief, such as an epidural, can also slow things down, but your doctor will judge whether this is a good idea now, or if it is better to keep moving forward as you are.

Q I've heard of the stages of labor, but what is "transition"?

The term "transition" describes the end of first stage labor, as your cervix moves toward full dilation, which marks the beginning of second stage labor.

Physiologically, during transition you may feel a strong downward, aching pressure in your lower back, and a heaviness in your perineum as your baby bears down on your cervix. This releases more hormones that cause your cervix to open that final bit—from around 7cm to 9–10cm dilated. However, rather than being a stage that is mapped by distinct physiological changes, you (and particularly your birth partner and doctor) will know that you have moved into the transition phase of labor because you will undergo some particular behavioral changes, which are listed below.

HOW YOU MIGHT ACT

» **You may start to panic** or become suddenly anxious or fearful.

» **You may appear** disorientated or confused.

» **You may start yelling** or snapping at your birth partner and his or her attempts to calm you.

» **You might demand pain relief** when previously you've been confident that you wanted to have a natural birth.

» **You may say** that you can't go on.

» **You can move "inward,"** becoming uncommunicative and perhaps dropping in and out of sleepiness (this is sometimes called the "rest and be thankful" stage).

HOW YOU MIGHT BE FEELING

» **You may feel nauseous** or weak.

» **You may feel shivery.**

» **It may feel like your contractions** are coming more frequently or there is no pause between them.

» **You may feel an urge** to push or bear down.

» **There may be** bloody discharge.

Your birth partner could **learn about the behavioral changes** at this stage so that he or she understands your change in attitude!

Q I know that "second stage labor" is when my baby is born, but what actually happens during this stage?

While intense, this is possibly the most exciting part of labor since you finally get to meet your baby. Although this stage can be tiring, many women feel encouraged that they can actively start to push their baby out now and that the end is in sight.

The second stage of labor begins when you are fully dilated at 10cm, and ends with the birth of your baby. As the characteristics of transition (see p.213) pass, this signals that the second stage of labor has begun. Along with the waves of contractions, you will feel an unrelenting urge to "bear down" into your perineum (the section of muscle and skin between your anus and your vagina) as your contractions push your baby against the pelvic floor. This bearing down, known as the "Ferguson reflex," means that

your baby has reached the muscles of your pelvic floor. As the baby presses against nerve receptors there, messages flood your brain to let you know that it's time to push the baby out. Once your doctor confirms that you are fully dilated, you can do so. Your uterine muscles get some help from your diaphragm and abdominal muscles now, too: the messages to your brain lower your diaphragm and force your abdominal muscles to contract. Your whole amazing body is working to help your baby through your pelvis.

Twists and turns

Your baby's journey through the birth canal and out into the world involves a series of maneuvers that are known as "the mechanism of labor." Rather than a straightforward descent down the birth canal and out, in fact, your baby has to make several twists and turns to be able to pass safely through your skeleton. This means that the time it takes for the second stage of your labor to progress is affected both by your baby's position in the birth canal and just how easy it is for her to turn in the space

THE BIRTH

As your contractions push your baby downward, her body rotates to enable her to emerge through the pelvic opening and out through your vagina.

1 **Your baby's body moves down** through your pelvis gradually as your uterus contracts. Your baby's head is tilted down slightly, toward her chest, and her arms and legs are folded inward, helping her journey through the birth canal.

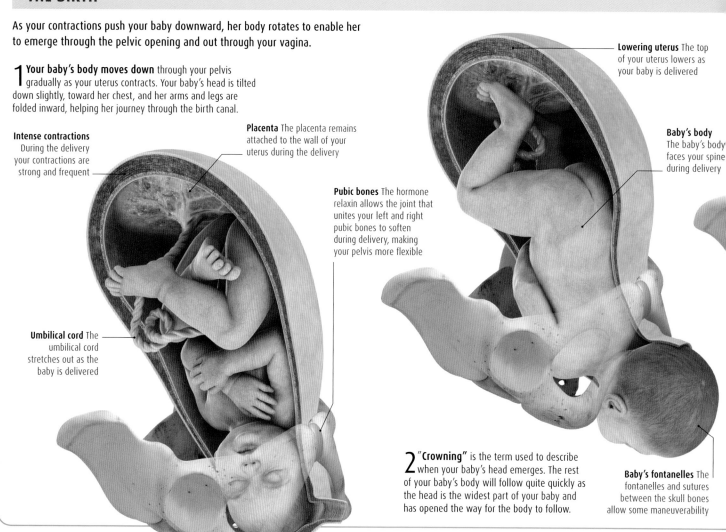

Intense contractions During the delivery your contractions are strong and frequent

Umbilical cord The umbilical cord stretches out as the baby is delivered

Placenta The placenta remains attached to the wall of your uterus during the delivery

Pubic bones The hormone relaxin allows the joint that unites your left and right pubic bones to soften during delivery, making your pelvis more flexible

Lowering uterus The top of your uterus lowers as your baby is delivered

Baby's body The baby's body faces your spine during delivery

2 **"Crowning"** is the term used to describe when your baby's head emerges. The rest of your baby's body will follow quite quickly as the head is the widest part of your baby and has opened the way for the body to follow.

Baby's fontanelles The fontanelles and sutures between the skull bones allow some maneuverability

your pelvis provides. You will feel a sense of satisfaction with every push—you are getting closer to meeting your baby.

Crowning and birth

As labor progresses and your baby's head presses against the pelvic floor, she rotates by about 45 degrees so that her face looks toward your spine. This position enables her to fit her head through your "pubic arch"—a pair of pelvic bones that form an arch. When her head makes it through these bones, your baby "crowns"—her head is out. Crowning can prompt a burning feeling, known as the "ring of fire." At this point, she turns another 45 degrees so that she can fit her shoulders through your pelvis; her head will turn too. Once the shoulders have made the turn, they, too, emerge into the world, quickly followed by the rest of your baby's body.

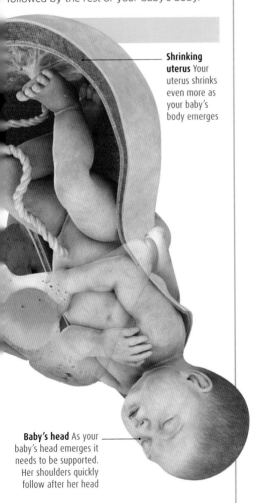

Shrinking uterus Your uterus shrinks even more as your baby's body emerges

Baby's head As your baby's head emerges it needs to be supported. Her shoulders quickly follow after her head

3 The rest of your baby's body comes out soon after the head. Her shoulders will come out one after the other, followed quickly by the rest of her body.

Q Are there positions that make it easier for me to give birth?

Some positions naturally open up your pelvis so are more efficient for delivery. Ultimately, the position you choose should be the one you find most comfortable.

The more upright you are in the second stage of labor, the more you have gravity on your side to help with the descent of your baby. One of the most efficient positions to give birth is in the squatting position. This has all the benefits of standing up (see p.211), but also opens out your pelvic bones, creating space for your baby to pass through more easily. Some researchers believe that a woman who labors standing up and gives birth squatting can reduce her labor by up to an hour. If you want to squat during the final stages of your labor, you will need to have strong thighs! Ask your birthing partner to hold you under your armpits to ease the strain on your muscles. Other positions that have the same beneficial effects are resting on all-fours and the kneeling pose. For kneeling, you will need physical support since it requires good balance. If your baby is being monitored, you might have to be in a bed, but follow the guidance from your nurse.

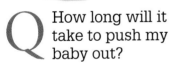

Supported squat
Your partner can support you from behind, or you can face him, putting your arms around his neck while he holds you firmly under your arms.

Kneeling on all fours You can try doing this on top of a bed or on the floor. In this position, your birth partner can give support and gently massage your back.

Q How long will it take to push my baby out?

This partly depends upon whether or not this is your first baby. First babies may take up to three hours from the start of the second stage of labor to be born, whereas second babies can take up to two hours or less. The position of your baby within your pelvis will also affect how long she takes to be born. Your doctor will stay with you during this stage, so listen to guidance on what's happening and when to push. The doctor will monitor your progress now by looking and feeling, and will also check your baby's heart rate for about one minute every five minutes or so. Some women worry that this frequent checking means something is wrong, but it's quite normal.

Try to remember that the second stage of labor is not measured by the length of time it takes, but by forward progress—as long as your labor is progressing, even if it seems slow, you and your baby are doing fine.

Q Is there anything I can do to speed up the delivery of my baby?

An upright position can make labor quicker, but bear in mind that speed is not always best. A controlled, well-managed labor allows your perineum to stretch, minimizing damage to the pelvic floor muscles and the likelihood of tears or episiotomy (see p.217). Work with the messages your body is sending you. Breathe into a push, easing the baby down the birth canal; holding your breath makes you pull up rather than bear down. Release the push as each contraction subsides. Your baby moves back a bit, but each push makes gentle progress.

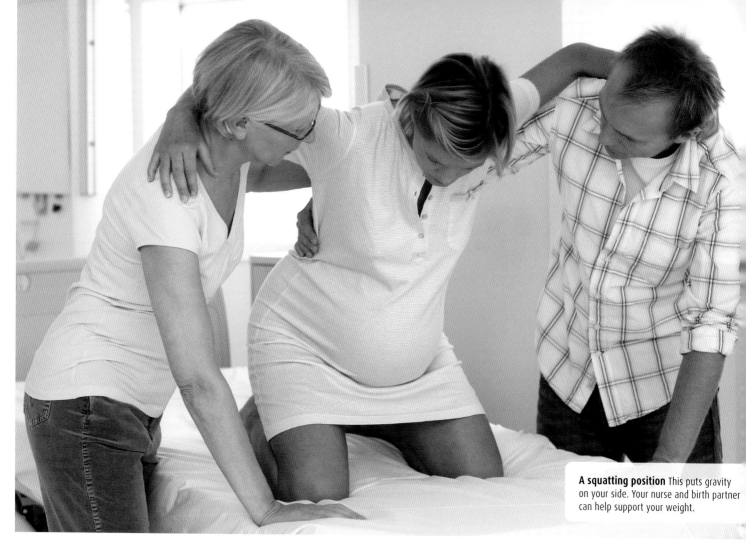

A squatting position This puts gravity on your side. Your nurse and birth partner can help support your weight.

Your birth partner's **support and encouragement** are hugely beneficial now, giving you strength to bear down and push.

Q If giving birth in a squatting position is helpful, why are women often shown lying down on their back?

There have been times in our history during which women were encouraged to lie on their backs on a bed to give birth. It is now more usual for doctors and hospitals to encourage women to do what feels right for them. It is generally acknowledged that lying "supine" is not necessarily the most comfortable or effective position to deliver a baby. There are other positions that can be more effective such as side lying, squatting, and resting on all fours. With more upright positions, gravity can give you a helping hand to keep your labor progressing. In this way, upright positions could reduce the chances of your needing an episiotomy or an assisted birth, although

they don't improve the risk of tearing. Birthing chairs and stools (see box, above right) provide similar benefits.

Lying down can be restful, but without gravity on your side labor may be slower. You will also need to be propped up so that you don't put too much pressure on your blood vessels, which could restrict the blood flow to both you and your baby. Lying down may make it easier for a doctor to give you an internal examination and to monitor the health of your baby because you can be hooked up to a stationary heart monitor. However, the latter can be done from a sitting position, too.

An advantage of giving birth in a bed is that as soon as your baby is born, a nurse can place him on your belly without you having to maneuver yourself into a comfortable and safe position, which can be especially tricky if you feel a bit unsteady after the effort of birth.

Q I'm considering a water birth. Is it safe to birth in the water or should I get out when pushing?

Yes, it is perfectly safe. Although many parents-to-be worry that a water birth poses a danger of drowning for the baby, in fact there is no known increased risk–for drowning or any other complication–compared with babies who are born out of the water. As your baby emerges into the pool, he will continue to be "fed" by the umbilical cord, giving your doctor plenty of time to lift him from the water before the breathing reflex kicks in. If you're worried, you can get out of the water to give birth.

Q I'd like to give birth lying down on my side. Is this possible?

Yes, this is completely possible. In fact, if you don't like the idea of expending effort to retain a squatting, lunging, or standing position during the second stage of labor, lying on your side s the next best thing. Studies show that giving birth in this position reduces the risk of episiotomy, assisted birth, and lowered heart rate in your baby when compared with lying on your back. Lying on your side also helps to open your pelvis (as with squatting), which makes it easier for your baby to pass through.

Q If I am attached to a heart monitor, must I lie down or can I sit up?

As long as your position doesn't interfere with the electrodes and wires that are attached to your belly, you can sit up if you prefer. You can even kneel on all fours, or kneel upright leaning on your birth partner's shoulders as he or she stands by the bed. Being on a bed doesn't necessarily mean you have to lie down.

Q Will having an epidural mean that I have to give birth lying down?

You will probably need to stay in bed if you have an epidural because you will lose the sensation in your body from the waist down. Some hospitals will carefully monitor the administration of the epidural drug, and as you near the pushing stage they will allow it to wear off, with your consent. This will help you to be guided by your own body during the moments your baby is being born. Your doctor will advise you as to which positions you may be able to manage safely with support.

Q Does every woman tear, and will I need stitches if I do?

Around 85 percent of women will have some perineal trauma (injury) during birth, accounting for both tears and episiotomies (see below). Tears are graded according to the amount of trauma they cause.

» A first-degree tear is a superficial wound to your vagina, damaging only a small area of the vagina's skin and fat layer and it probably won't require any stitching.

» A second-degree tear is deeper, extending into the muscle of your perineum. Your doctor will probably stitch the tear and you may need pain medicine to ease the soreness for a few days.

» A third-degree tear extends into the anal sphincter, causing significant trauma. This type of tear needs to be repaired by a doctor in an operating room, usually under epidural or spinal anesthesia. The wound can take several weeks to heal, and you may experience some fecal incontinence while everything knits back together, but rest assured that this should only be a temporary effect.

» A fourth-degree tear is uncommon and extends into not only the anal sphincter, but also the muscular wall of your anal canal. Usually this kind of tear requires stitching in an operating room. Again, the wound can take weeks to heal and you may suffer some temporary fecal incontinence. Your doctor and a physical therapist will talk to you about how you can help the damage to heal and strengthen any damaged muscles so that your recovery is as quick as possible. If at any point the soreness seems to get worse or the area around the stitches becomes inflamed, let your doctor know in case it has become infected.

Q What is an episiotomy and why might I need one?

An episiotomy is a surgical incision that opens the perineum, allowing your baby an easier passage, and you will be given one only if there is a sound clinical reason.

An episiotomy enables the doctor to control your baby's exit, but this will not be done routinely, and you will need to give your verbal consent before an incision. Your doctor will explain the reasons why the procedure is being recommended. Among those reasons are that your perineum is too rigid to stretch to allow your baby through, putting you at increased risk of a third- or fourth-degree tear (see above); to ease the delivery if you have a medical condition that makes the effort of giving birth dangerous for you, for example, if you have a heart condition or high blood pressure; if your baby is showing signs of distress (a rapid or a weak heartbeat); or if your baby is stuck and you need an assisted birth (see p.222).

The cut itself is about 3–4cm long and made with round-ended surgical scissors or with a scalpel as your baby descends into the perineum. You will have a local anaesthetic to numb the area both while the cut is being made and later when you're being stitched. The stitching will usually be done within an hour of the end of the delivery of your baby. Once the anesthetic has worn off, you are likely to feel sore for about a week while the incision heals, and you may have a stinging sensation when you urinate. Pouring warm water over the area while you urinate can help to reduce the stinging sensation.

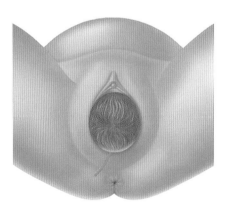

A diagonal episiotomy The cut is usually made from the back of the vagina, then out to one side. Dissolvable stitches are used to repair it.

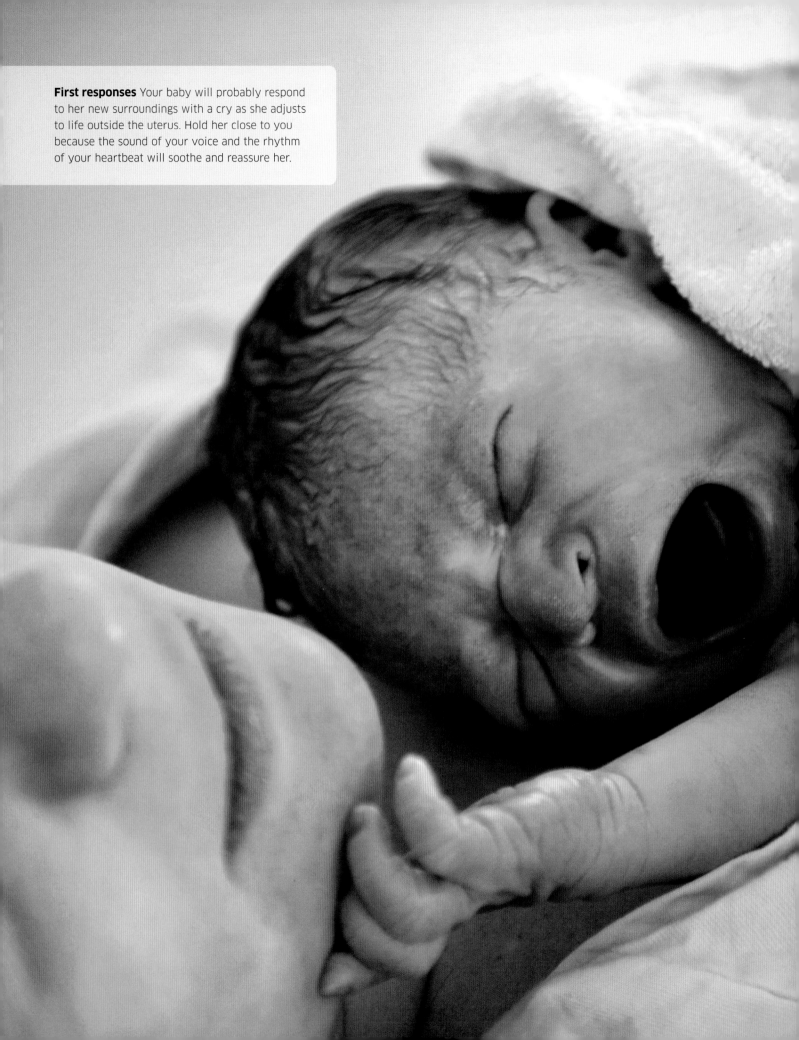

First responses Your baby will probably respond to her new surroundings with a cry as she adjusts to life outside the uterus. Hold her close to you because the sound of your voice and the rhythm of your heartbeat will soothe and reassure her.

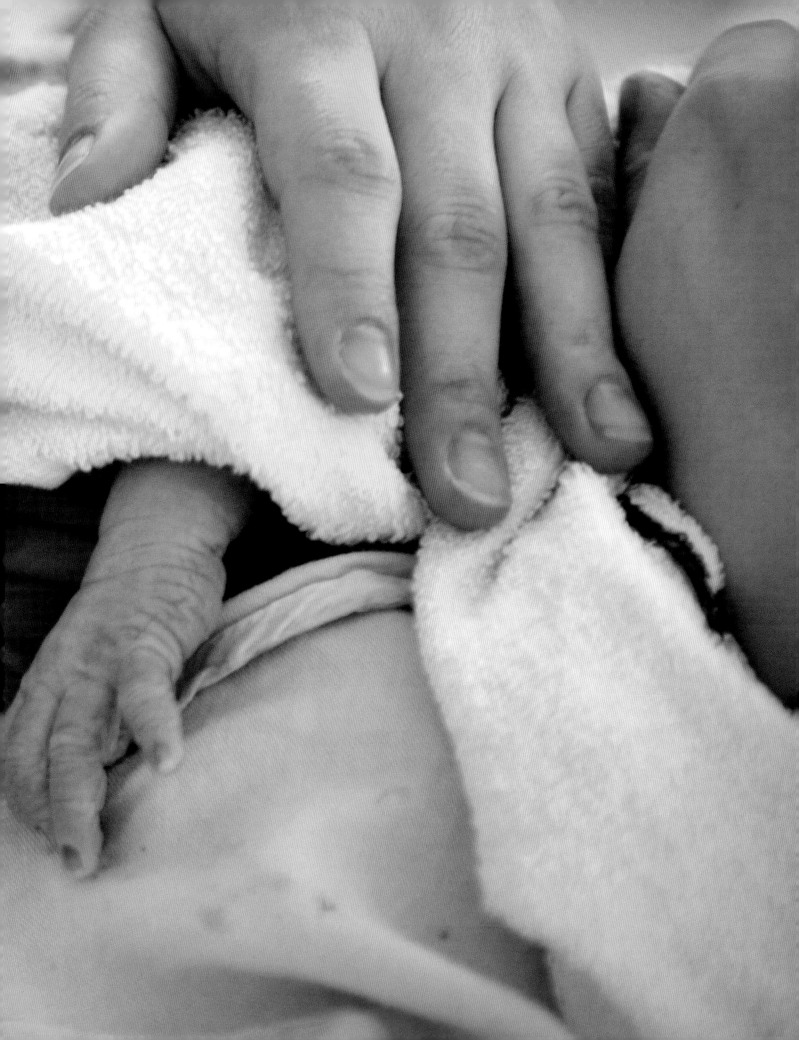

Q What is the "third stage" of labor and what will I need to do during this stage?

Your baby has arrived, but labor is not quite over. Once you've enjoyed a first embrace, there will be a few more contractions to deliver the placenta and membranes.

Although arguably the most exciting part of labor is over, there is still the business of giving birth to the placenta and membranes that have nourished and protected your baby during pregnancy. Your placenta, which begins to come away from your uterus lining as soon as your

baby's body is out, bears down on your perineum, just as your baby had, triggering the release of more of the hormone oxytocin, which keeps your contractions coming. Your doctor will guide you through these contractions and in most cases only a few pushes are needed to get the placenta and membranes out. Compared to the delivery of your baby, you may not feel the delivery of your placenta very much or at all. There will be some bleeding as the placenta comes away from the wall of the uterus.

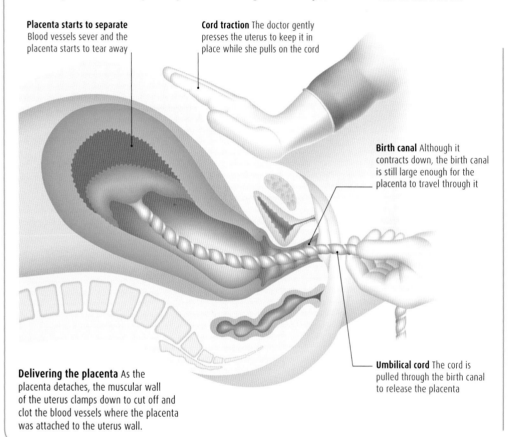

Placenta starts to separate Blood vessels sever and the placenta starts to tear away

Cord traction The doctor gently presses the uterus to keep it in place while she pulls on the cord

Birth canal Although it contracts down, the birth canal is still large enough for the placenta to travel through it

Delivering the placenta As the placenta detaches, the muscular wall of the uterus clamps down to cut off and clot the blood vessels where the placenta was attached to the uterus wall.

Umbilical cord The cord is pulled through the birth canal to release the placenta

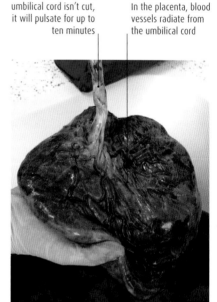

Umbilical cord If the umbilical cord isn't cut, it will pulsate for up to ten minutes

Network of vessels In the placenta, blood vessels radiate from the umbilical cord

A healthy placenta The average full-term placenta weighs around 1 lb 2 oz (500 g) and is 8–10 in (20–25 cm) in diameter. The membranes also need to come out of the uterus to avoid the risk of infection and serious bleeding.

Q I just want to get to know my new baby. How long will the third stage take?

This depends on whether you opt to deliver the placenta naturally, or to have medical assistance to deliver it. Without medical intervention, third stage labor usually takes 20–30 minutes, but it can take up to an hour. With medical intervention, this stage may take only around 15 minutes or less. For many women who decide to deliver the placenta naturally, it's just a matter of three pushes and

the placenta comes out. If the process takes longer than an hour, you are at an increased risk of excessive bleeding and your doctor will talk to you about active management to deliver your placenta (see below).

Q What is an "active" third stage of labor? Should I opt for it?

An active third stage is one that is managed medically by speeding up the delivery of the placenta. There is evidence that an active third

stage reduces the risk of serious bleeding after the birth, known as postpartum hemorrhage. An active delivery is uncommon in the US, and it's unlikely that your doctor will offer you the procedure if you don't mention it. If your doctor agrees to manage the delivery of your placenta actively, you'll receive an injection of synthetic oxytocin hormone—which triggers contractions that help release the placenta—in your thigh around the time of your baby's birth. Your doctor will pull gently on the umbilical cord, drawing the placenta away from the uterine lining and out of your vagina, with the attached membranes following behind.

Q I'm eager to deliver the placenta as quickly as possible. Are there any ways to do this?

As with the delivery of your baby, if you stand or sit, gravity will help to push out the placenta and membranes. Be careful if you stand; make sure your birth partner is there to support you, since you will probably feel wobbly after the exertion of giving birth. In addition, holding your baby "skin-to-skin" or starting to breast-feed will increase your body's release of oxytocin, which can speed up the process. Delivering your placenta naturally shouldn't affect your ability to get to know your baby—usually the cord is long enough for you to hold (and even feed) your baby while he is attached.

Q Can we keep the placenta?

If you're having your baby in a hospital or birthing center, you'll need to check the policy on whether or not you'll be allowed to keep your placenta. Even when it's fine to do so, you'll probably have had to seek permission in advance. Hospitals won't have any containers for you to take the placenta away in, so make sure you've packed one in your hospital bag—a plastic container with a secure lid should do.

Q I always thought the umbilical cord was cut immediately, but my doctor said it probably won't be. Why?

When your baby is born, blood flow between him and his placenta continues through the cord for about ten minutes or so after birth. For this reason the clamping of the umbilical cord may be deferred for one to five minutes to allow the extra blood to boost your baby's iron reserves. Adequate iron is important for your baby's early neurological development. Once the cord has stopped pulsating (pushing the remaining blood into your baby's body), your doctor will let you know that it's time to clamp and cut it. She will ask if your birth partner would like to cut the cord, or you may have already requested this in your birth plan. Deferred cord clamping can be carried out for both active and natural third stage labors and C-sections.

Q I'm worried that if my partner doesn't cut the cord properly the baby will have a funny belly button. Is this the case?

The look of your baby's belly button has entirely to do with the way the umbilical cord was attached to the baby in the uterus and has nothing to do with the way it is cut after birth. If your partner wants to take an active role and cut the cord, encourage him or her to do so. Some dads feel this is a good way to play a significant role in the first moments of their new baby's life, setting the baby free in the world. If your birth partner is eager to do the honors, make a note of it in your birth plan and mention it to your doctor.

Did you know...

Some people eat the placenta. This practice is called placentophagy. While many view the placenta as a waste product of birth, others believe it can benefit the mother, delivering an iron boost and helping to ward off postpartum depression. There are references to eating it in various cultures, and while in the West the placenta has traditionally been incinerated, there is a growing trend in eating it. Evidence on the benefits is anecdotal, but there is no doubt that it is rich in nutrients and hormones.

Q What is the procedure for cutting the cord?

Cutting the umbilical cord is a significant moment when your baby makes the full transition from life in the uterus to an independent existence in the outside world.

Shortly after the birth of your baby, the doctor or your partner will cut the umbilical cord to release your baby from the placenta. First the cord will need to be clamped to prevent bleeding from the baby or the placenta. The cord is clamped in two places. A plastic clip is placed 1½-2 inches (3-4 cm) from your baby's belly button, then a second clip is placed at the other end of the cord near the placenta. The cord is then cut between the two clamps. This procedure isn't at all painful for your baby since there are no nerves in the umbilical cord. Your baby will be left with a stump where the cord was, which will gradually blacken and fall off naturally around 5 to 15 days after the birth.

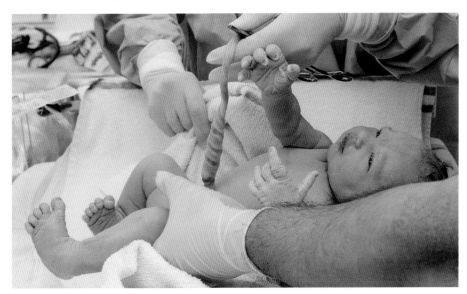

Cutting the cord This procedure is a straightforward one that can be done by your doctor or birth partner if he or she would like.

Q What does it mean when a delivery is assisted and how is this done?

An assisted, or instrumental, delivery is when an obstetrician uses a specially designed instrument, either forceps or a vacuum extractor, to help birth your baby vaginally, avoiding the need for a cesarean section.

Forceps These are tongs, usually made of metal, that open and close like scissors and are curved to fit the shape of your baby's head. The doctor will carefully position the tongs either side of your baby's head, then will gently pull during a contraction to guide your baby out.

Vacuum extractor This is a device with a plastic or metal cup at one end that is placed on your baby's head. A vacuum is created by the suction cup, making it stick to the head, then, during your contraction, the doctor will pull on the cup to help deliver your baby.

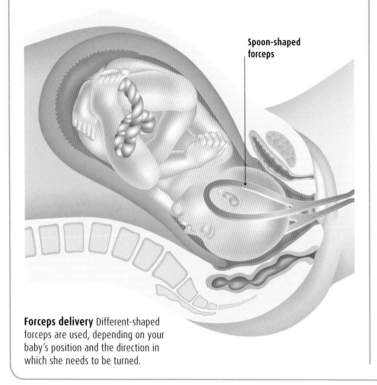

Spoon-shaped forceps

Forceps delivery Different-shaped forceps are used, depending on your baby's position and the direction in which she needs to be turned.

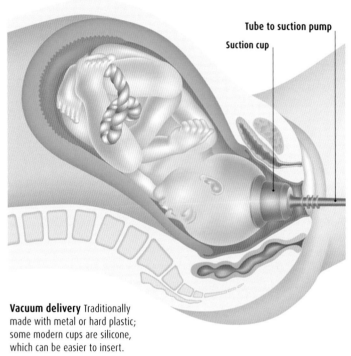

Tube to suction pump

Suction cup

Vacuum delivery Traditionally made with metal or hard plastic; some modern cups are silicone, which can be easier to insert.

Q What reasons could there be for me to need an assisted delivery?

An assisted delivery is only done when there is concern for the well-being of either you or your baby in the second stage of labor. For example, if your baby shows signs of distress; if you have a heart condition or high blood pressure that makes the effort of natural birth dangerous for you; if your labor has been protracted and you're exhausted; or if you've had an epidural that has affected the ability of your pelvic muscles to turn your baby so that she can emerge safely. The goal is for you to have a vaginal delivery while minimizing the risks to you and your baby, and the procedure is only done if it is considered the safest option.

Q If I do need an assisted delivery, will they just launch in with the instruments?

Before the procedure takes place, you will be asked for your consent. This can be given verbally if the procedure is being done in the delivery room, or you will need to give written consent if you are moving to an operating room. First, you will need to be in the best position for the procedure to be performed. The doctor will ask you to sit, leaning back slightly, with your knees drawn up, and thighs open. You could be asked to place your feet in footrests, which eases the strain on your back. You will have a catheter inserted to empty your bladder before the procedure can begin; and you may need to

have an episiotomy (see p.217) to make the opening of your vagina wide enough to allow the forceps or vacuum extractor through to wrap around your baby's head. To relieve the discomfort of the procedure, you will be given either a local anesthetic inside the vagina, known as a pudendal block, or sometimes an epidural, which may be recommended if your baby needs help rotating in your pelvis. If you do have an epidural, this makes the transition to a cesarean section easier should the assisted delivery be unsuccessful. Your doctor will explain what is happening and why, and will encourage you to ask as many questions as you need. Your birth partner can play an important role in this situation by asking questions to help make sure you are both fully informed.

11.5% One in eight first-born babies in the US are born using assisted delivery.

Q Who will perform the assisted delivery if it becomes necessary?

The procedure will be done by your own doctor, possibly with help from a nurse who has had specialized training in assisted deliveries. During the procedure, the delivery room may feel quite busy since you will have your doctor and some nurses present, plus a pediatrician, who will be there just in case your baby needs attention after the birth. The presence of the pediatrician is often precautionary, but if you're concerned, ask your doctor to explain everyone's role, which he or she will be happy to do.

Q Which is better, forceps or vacuum extractor, and will I have a choice?

Both types of delivery are considered safe and effective, but the choice of which type depends on the medical circumstances; thus it is best to be guided by your doctor. For example, vacuum extractor is the preferred method if your baby needs to rotate to move down the birth canal. This method is less likely to cause injury to your vagina and/or perineum. On the other hand, forceps are gentler for the baby, but can increase the risk of trauma to you. But if your baby is in difficulty, your doctor's priority is to act quickly and forceps will provide the faster delivery. If your doctor begins with the vacuum extractor and the attempt is unsuccessful, he or she may decide to try again using forceps. However, if a forceps delivery is unsuccessful, whether this is used first or after a vacuum extractor attempt, you will usually need to have a cesarean section.

Q How long will the assisted delivery procedure take?

Once you have been prepared for the procedure and the forceps or vacuum extractor is attached to your baby's head, you will usually be guided through a maximum of three pushes to deliver.

If your baby isn't born after three pushes, your doctor will decide whether to try again, to switch to a forceps delivery (if you started with vacuum extractor), or to send you for an emergency cesarean section. Your doctor will be with you the whole time, explaining what is happening at each step. If you are having an assisted delivery because an epidural has made it hard for your baby to rotate, your doctor will tell you exactly when to push to help deliver the baby.

Q Are there risks for me if I have an assisted delivery?

You may have some vaginal or anal tearing, or need an episiotomy, which will be stitched after the birth. If there is bleeding during delivery there will be an increased risk of developing a blood clot (as with any birth where bleeding occurs). Approximately a third of women who have had an assisted delivery have some urinary incontinence afterward, so talk to your doctor about Kegel exercises to help speed your recovery. Occasionally, there may be trauma to the anal sphincter (the circular muscle around your anus), which can lead to temporary fecal incontinence.

Q How can I avoid an assisted delivery in the first place?

Being well-supported throughout labor, by both a doctor and a birth partner who remains with you, can help you to avoid an assisted delivery. Staying upright during labor or lying on your side can help with your baby's position and descent in the birth canal, reducing the need for an assisted delivery. Stay calm and be guided by your doctor about when to push to help prevent you from becoming exhausted. Avoiding an epidural also reduces the chances that you will need help with the delivery.

Q How will my baby be affected by an assisted delivery?

An assisted delivery often leaves a mark on your baby. Swelling, bruising, and cuts are all common, but these effects soon disappear after the birth.

It's common for a baby's head to look elongated after a vacuum extractor delivery due to the effects of the suction cup. Referred to as a "chignon," this swelling doesn't cause any damage to your baby's skull or brain, and your baby's head will return to its regular shape within 24–48 hours of the birth. Your baby may also have a small bruise, called a cephalic hematoma, where the suction was strongest, which again should disappear quickly. The stress of a vacuum extractor birth is thought to be the reason that vacuum extractor babies have lower than average apgar scores (see p.238) at five minutes after birth; however, these return to normal by 10 minutes. After a forceps birth, it's common for babies to have small marks on their face, and there may be cuts on the face and head, which heal and disappear quickly after the birth.

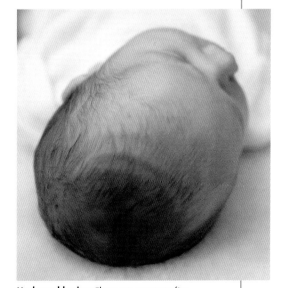

Marks and bruises These are common after an assisted delivery, but these side effects are superficial and will soon disappear.

Q I'm carrying twins and hoping to have a natural birth. How will my labor differ from having a single baby?

Many twin births have no complications, but your doctor will keep a close eye on you.

Length of labor

The dilation of the cervix (first stage) takes about the same length of time whether you are having one baby or more. Birthing the babies (second stage) may take longer, because your body has to do the job twice, but the babies are typically smaller than singletons, and can pass through the pelvis more quickly. The overall length of labor is not very different from a singleton birth.

Close monitoring

The heart rates of your babies will be more carefully monitored than if you were giving birth to only one baby. You may initially be able to walk around, especially if your babies are being monitored with handheld devices or unpluggable electrodes on your belly. As your labor progresses closer to the second stage, and usually once your water has broken, you may have continual monitoring that requires you to be stationary. Discuss your hospital's policy on monitoring labor for multiples well in advance of your due date so that you can manage your own expectations of the amount of freedom you're likely to have.

Birthing two babies

If both your babies are positioned head down, or one is head down and the other breech or transverse, it may be possible to deliver first one twin and then the other vaginally. The first baby opens up the birth canal as it is born, and the second baby often turns, or can be turned by palpating your abdomen, after the first is delivered. When your first twin is born you'll be encouraged to bring him to your breast and allow him to nurse (even if you don't intend to breast-feed later on), since this stimulates

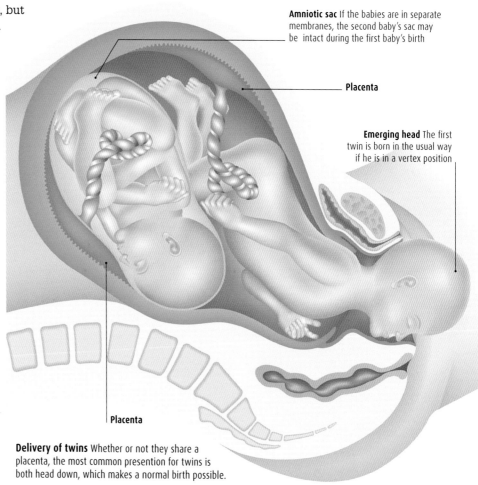

Amniotic sac If the babies are in separate membranes, the second baby's sac may be intact during the first baby's birth

Placenta

Emerging head The first twin is born in the usual way if he is in a vertex position

Placenta

Delivery of twins Whether or not they share a placenta, the most common presentation for twins is both head down, which makes a normal birth possible.

your body's natural release of the hormone oxytocin and triggers your uterus to contract again, continuing your second stage labor. Your doctor will try to ensure that your second twin is born within 30 minutes or so of his sibling. If your labor slows down, you may be offered an injection of oxytocin to restart the second stage for the second twin. A long delay between the two births can increase the risk of placental abruption—when your placenta comes away from the uterus lining—for the second baby, which would cut off his blood supply.

Possibility of intervention

On rare occasions—for fewer than five percent of twin births—it is possible that you could need a C-section for the second baby, even if you didn't need one for the first baby. This is more likely if your second twin can't be nudged into a good position for birth, or gets into difficulty, or you become exhausted.

If you ask for pain relief, you are likely to be offered an epidural—not because labor is necessarily more painful with twins, but because analgesics can slow down the babies' heart rates and your medical team won't advise any treatment that could be high risk for multiple births. In addition to this, an epidural works as anesthesia if you suddenly need assisted delivery or a C-section.

In almost **50 percent of twin births** both babies present with their head downward—sometimes the first baby is head down, and **the second turns once the first is born.**

25%

About 25 percent of twin births in the US happen vaginally. But mothers expecting triplets or more are usually encouraged to opt for a cesarean section to minimize risk.

Q Will I have to have my labor induced if I'm carrying multiples?

The majority of multiples arrive prematurely, but if yours don't, your doctor will recommend that you be induced or scheduled for cesarean section before 40 weeks. In all pregnancies there is a risk of stillbirth if the baby remains in utero too long, and for multiples that risk happens earlier. For twins this means early induction (see p.203) at around 37 to 38 weeks. For greater multiples, it will mean an early cesarean section, usually at 34 weeks for triplets, and at 32 weeks for quads or more.

Q My doctor says that there might be quite a throng in my delivery room. Why?

Multiple births are more complicated than singletons, so when you go into labor there may be a team of clinicians for each baby. Teams may be made up of your doctor, an anesthesiologist, nurses, and pediatricians. This means that if you are having twins there will be twice as many people in the room as for a single baby; if you're having triplets there will be three times as many, and so on. The number of resuscitators (the bedlike trolleys that have oxygen equipment for newborns; see p.86) and other items of equipment in the room will also increase. This can all seem pretty overwhelming, but stay focused on your birth partner and your babies, be reassured that so many people are there to help you, and always feel free to ask what someone's role is if it's not immediately obvious.

Q Is delivering the placenta(s) and membranes different for twin births?

Usually, after a vaginal twin birth you will be encouraged to have an oxytocin injection in order to speed along the third stage of labor. A managed third stage labor can help stem postpartum bleeding: you are at greater risk of excessive bleeding after a twin birth. The doctor will check that the placenta or placentas are intact, the same as for a single birth.

If your twins are the same sex and have a placenta each and you are not sure whether they are identical or nonidentical, your doctor will examine the placentas and membranes to see if it's possible to figure it out. If it isn't possible, you can opt for private DNA testing if you want to find out definitively. Of course, with many identical twins, identicality becomes fairly obvious within a few years.

Q Will my babies go to the neonatal intensive care unit? Will this hamper the bonding process?

If one or all of your babies are very tiny because they are born early, they may need to spend a little time in the neonatal intensive care unit (NICU) after birth to help them thrive and make sure they are continually monitored. Try not to worry. As long as it's medically safe to do so, you'll be able to hold them first. Remember that bonding with your babies began while they were in the uterus, so you already have a good start. Take photographs of each baby and of the babies together so when they aren't with you looking at the photographs will help to trigger some of the bonding hormones that you'd have if you were holding them. It can also help trigger the let-down reflex that enables you to express your own milk for your babies to drink. It will help you adjust to the idea of parenthood, too.

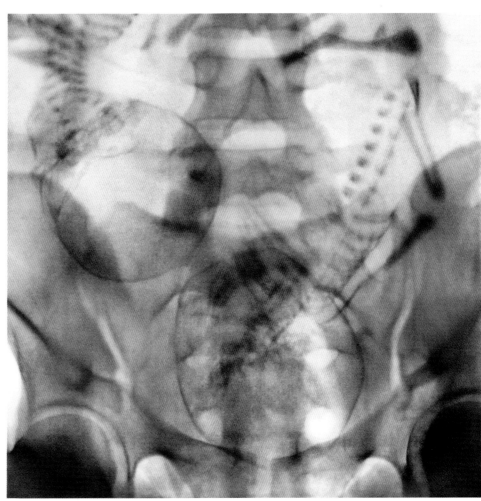

Full-term twins in the uterus Both babies are head down—their skulls point to their mother's pelvis, and their spines are seen curving upward. On the right, the baby's head is engaged in the pelvis, ready for birth.

It's impossible to know in advance **how you will experience** the pain of labor, and certainly levels of pain **can vary greatly** between women. Your approach to labor, though, can have a big impact on how you fare: being informed about labor and what can help with the pain will **reduce tension and fear**; that in itself, will help you cope

Pain relief in labor

Your experience of pain

The pain of labor is different from almost all other types of pain you will ever experience. Unlike pain that acts as a warning sign that something is amiss and you should stop what you're doing, labor pain is a sign that something is very right: your baby is about to be born.

The levels of pain, or perceptions of pain, women report in labor vary greatly. Some experience only moderate discomfort through much of labor, while for others the pain feels overwhelming. The nature of the pain, though, is characteristic of different stages of labor. The cramping feeling in the first stage occurs as the uterus contracts to push the baby into the pelvis. It's widespread and longlasting: you'll feel it in your abdomen, perhaps in your lower back, and sometimes even through your buttocks and down your thighs. In the second stage, pain is more localized as the muscles and tissues of the birth canal are stretched as your baby makes her way through the vagina.

The psychology of pain

Many women worry that they won't be able to deal with the pain of labor, and that if they need medical pain relief they will somehow have "failed" in this rite of passage. Studies show that women are able to manage better if they are informed about labor pain, which helps them feel more empowered and relaxed. Understanding where labor pain comes from, exploring the options for pain relief, and making decisions about which forms you would like to have and which, if any, you would rather avoid are all important ways to take control of your labor. And in itself feeling in control of what's happening and the choices you're making will help you deal with labor pain. Modern methods of pain relief don't harm your baby; the fear of pain, on the other hand, can make birth traumatic, not just for you, but for your baby, too. Thinking about labor pain as "positive" pain that helps you achieve something incredible can motivate you to prepare for this event, just as you would for, say, running a marathon.

Types of pain relief

Pain relief during labor is either natural or medical. Natural forms of pain relief (see p.228-29) include breathing and relaxation techniques and water births; and medical pain relief includes the use of certain opioid analgesics and some tranquilizers, as well as spinal blocks and epidurals. There is no right or wrong approach to pain relief in labor. If you start out thinking you'll be able to manage using breathing techniques alone, but then decide you need an epidural—ask for one. The most important thing is that your labor is as calm and as positive as possible.

Q What different types of pain relief are available, and when can I use them?

Some women manage using mainly natural methods of pain relief, such as breathing, for much of labor. For others, effective methods of pain relief may change as labor progresses and intensifies, and many women choose to supplement natural techniques with medical forms of pain relief.

WHAT PAIN RELIEF YOU MIGHT USE

The table below charts how different types of pain relief are commonly used during labor. The delivery of the placenta in the third stage is commonly managed without pain relief.

STAGE	HOW THE PAIN MIGHT FEEL	NATURAL PAIN RELIEF OPTIONS	MEDICAL PAIN RELIEF OPTIONS
1st stage of labor— latent phase	Contractions may stop and start, and can feel like severe menstrual pain, and there may be lower back pain. Pain is usually bearable, such that you can continue to move around and talk during contractions. Contractions gradually get closer together and stronger.	» **Breathing:** this helps you focus during contractions. » **Meditation:** can keep you calm and focused. » **Water:** warm water is soothing and relaxing early on. » **Massage:** can ease backache and promote relaxation. » **TENS:** takes the edge off contractions and relieves backache. » **Acupuncture:** this can help you relax in early labor.	» **Analgesics:** Occasionally, opioid analgesics may be used to help manage your stronger contractions now..
1st stage of labor— active phase	Contractions are regular, frequent, and intense: you're unable to talk or move through them. There may be nausea, strong pressure in the back, and pain may radiate down the legs.	» **Rhythmic breathing:** controlled breathing helps you focus and maximizes oxygen flow to the muscles. » **Meditation/massage:** these continue to be helpful. » **Water:** supportive and relieves pressure on back and pelvis.	» **Opioid analgesics:** These drugs can dull the pain to help you deal with contractions. » **Epidural:** this may be requested and set up now if pain feels unmanageable.
Transition phase	Contractions can be extremely intense now, with little rest time in between. Pressure in the lower back and rectum is strong, and you may be exhausted, overwhelmed, and nauseous. You may vomit.	» **Controlled breathing:** breathing techniques can be used if you feel panicky and out of control: use a combination of more shallow in-breaths and longer exhalations. » **Water:** you can remain in a birthing pool now if you want to give birth in water.	» **Opioid analgesics:** These are not an option now; they're avoided close to delivery since they can affect the baby's breathing. » **Epidural:** can be topped off; you may be encouraged to avoid setting one up now.
2nd stage of labor	Strong, long-lasting contractions and an urge to push down. Strong pressure in the rectum and stinging or burning as the head crowns.	» **Breathing:** slow and focused exhalations can help you bear down. Panting as the head crowns is important. Pain can feel productive as you push your baby out.	» **Epidural:** You may still feel the effects of your epidural now.

Q Can I use more than one type of pain relief?

Yes. Most types of natural pain relief can be used alongside medical pain relief. And some types of medical relief can be used together. You may ask for an opioid analgesic at first, then feel that you need an epidural later. That's fine to do. Your doctor should allow you to have opioid analgesics any time up until the point at which you need to start pushing; because the drug crosses into the baby's system and can slow down his breathing, it's better that they aren't administered too close to when the baby is born. If you feel anxious and need a tranquilizer, that can be given with other drugs, but not too close to when the baby will be born, because it also can affect breathing.

Q What kinds of medical pain relief will I be able to have for a home birth?

Women who choose a home birth often want to escape the trappings of a traditional hospital birth: the institutional environment. Maybe they want to sit in a birthing pool at home for pain relief. Maybe they have practiced hypnobirthing or another method that they are comfortable with. Keep in mind that home births are opposed by the American College of Gynecologists and Obstetricians because of the potential for complications, even in low-risk pregnancies. (To be considered for one, you must have a low-risk pregnancy and no preexisting medical conditions.) You can have a medication-free delivery in a hospital, too.

Q Did you know...

Although home birth limits your access to analgesics, studies show that women who have had a home birth feel more positive about their experience of labor pain. Whether this is because they have little expectation of being able to have pain relief (so have already reached a certain level of acceptance about the pain), because they are more relaxed in their environment, or a combination of the two is unknown. At home and in a hospital, the support of a doctor and a birth partner is beneficial.

Q Can breathing techniques really help me to cope in labor?

When we feel anxious or worried, we tend to hold our breath, which reduces the oxygen circulating in our blood, and we tense up, tightening muscles and restricting blood flow. In this state of hyperarousal, the perception of pain is greater, and labor becomes harder work. Conversely, calm and steady breathing lowers the heart rate, reduces anxiety, and maximizes the oxygen flow to you and your baby. If you learn breathing techniques (see p.72) before labor, you can use these to help you breathe purposefully through your contractions, focusing in particular on breathing out (releasing) as the contraction peaks, so you remain as relaxed as possible. Techniques such as Hypnobirthing (see p.73), an increasingly popular practice that anecdotally has positive results, use breathing techniques to help you focus during contractions and breathe through the pain, rather than try to resist it.

Q My midwife asked if I was interested in using a birthing pool. How does water help labor?

Getting into a warm bath is a well-known relaxation aid. Similarly, being immersed in warm water in labor can be instantly soothing. As your muscles relax, levels of endorphins, the feel-good hormones that provide natural pain relief, increase; and it's thought that the warm water blocks pain messages from getting to your brain, reducing your perception of pain. Being in water also makes it easier to move around since the water supports your belly, so you can rely on your own sense of balance and buoyancy to change position, rather than the strength of your birth partner or midwife. If you are using a birthing pool at home, it's up to you when you get in, but some experts believe that it's best to wait until labor is established since it's thought that warm water may slow contractions early on. The water shouldn't be above 99.5°F (37.5°C) since higher than this can raise your core temperature and distress your baby. You can stay in the pool as long as you like, and, if you have a midwife trained in water birth, you can give birth in it, too. If you don't have a birthing pool, you can benefit from the soothing effects of water by lying in a warm bath.

You'll need to have someone with you while you are in water to make sure you don't become so drowsy that you fall asleep and slip under the surface, and to help you to get in and out.

Q I've heard about women using meditation in labor. How does this work?

Techniques such as meditation attempt to redirect your focus away from the pain of labor to help raise your pain threshold. Meditation is simply the act of stilling the mind so that you can remain detached from the physical sensations in your body. The idea is that if you train your mind to believe that you will be able to deal with the pain of labor, you are far more likely to manipulate your experience to that end, whereas if you tell yourself labor is going to be unbearably painful, you'll almost certainly experience the full force of your pain.

Choosing a visualization or affirmation to focus on during meditation can help:
» Visualize a stream that tumbles over stones—can you see the light on the water? How fast does the water move? What sounds does it make? Does it splash or foam as it flows? The more detail you can conjure up, the more focus you have away from your pain.
» Visualize a candle flame. To keep the outbreath long and slow through a contraction, close your eyes and imagine blowing it so gently that the flame flickers, but doesn't go out.

Monitoring your baby In a birthing pool your baby's heartbeat will be monitored with a waterproof handheld device.

» As a contraction starts, repeat a word or phrase (in your mind or out loud), such as "love," or "calm," or your baby's name if you've chosen it. Or choose a phrase such as "I feel powerful and strong." Imagine the letters or words in front of you as you say the affirmation.

Q I'm planning to use a TENS machine for as long as possible. What do I need to know?

TENS is an acronym for Transcutaneous Electrical Nerve Stimulation. A TENS machine is a portable unit that emits low-voltage electrical impulses to your nerves via electrode pads secured on either side of your spine. When you have a contraction, you push a button to send impulses to your body, which are thought to stimulate the release of endorphins and to block your pain receptors. TENS is noninvasive, has no known harmful effects on you or your baby, and allows you to move around and feel in control of your pain relief. The only place it's not possible to use your TENS machine is in water.

It can take up to an hour for endorphins to build up in your body, so as soon as you feel contractions, ask your birth partner to hook you up to the machine (it's a good idea to practice before labor starts). You'll be able to adjust the voltage of the electrical impulses to a comfortable level, increasing the frequency of the impulses as the pain gets more intense.

TENS machines are common in the UK, but they're rarely used in the US, so you may have to shop online for a unit or have one shipped from abroad to get your hands on one.

Q Is acupuncture safe to use during labor, and will I be able to move?

Acupuncture is becoming increasingly common and popular as a form of pain relief during labor. This practice of inserting tiny needles at specific sites on the body is used to reduce pain sensitivity and encourage the release of endorphins. Acupuncture is safe to use during labor, but does require a trained acupuncturist. You will need to arrange to have an him or her there during labor. You might want to try a few sessions in pregnancy first. In labor, the acupuncturist is likely to work on points such as the ear, so that your movement isn't restricted.

Q I've always found massage soothing. Will it help me in labor?

Massage during labor can help you to relax between contractions, release held-in tension, and alleviate lower back pain. Touch can be also calming and increase your confidence in your ability to deal with the pain of labor.

A study published in 2013 showed that women who were given a lower back massage for 30 minutes during established first stage labor reported significantly less pain than those who weren't. The average lengths of the labors were roughly the same in both the massage and the control groups, and the physical therapists who performed the massage visited every woman in the control group for 30 minutes, too, but made no physical contact with them. The researchers concluded that massage has a measurably positive effect on the perception of pain.

If physical contact is something you find supportive and reassuring in everyday life, encourage your birth partner to come to the massage sessions of your childbirth classes, or find an prenatal massage class that you can both attend. Practice the techniques during your pregnancy to get a good understanding of what feels best for you (both in terms of technique and pressure levels), so your birth partner is well-prepared to put the techniques into practice during your labor.

Some women find that when in labor they don't want to be touched. It's impossible to know how you'll feel on the day, but discuss this possibility with your birth partner in advance so that he doesn't take offence if you decide you don't want to be touched at all.

SOOTHING MASSAGE

Experiment with the following techniques so you can ascertain which strokes you feel comfortable with and the ones you think might be helpful during labor.

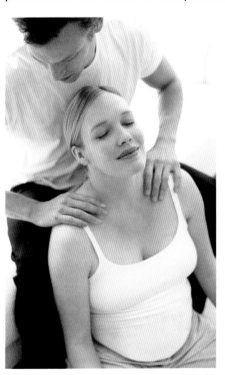

Relaxing massage Both you and your partner should be in comfortable, supported positions during a massage session so that you can both relax fully.

» **Back sweep:** sit on a birthing stool or fold yourself over an exercise ball to expose your back. Ask your partner to run his hands from the outer sides of your shoulders inward, across your shoulder blades and down each side of your spine in one swooping, stroking motion. Repeat several times.

» **Tension release:** sit in a chair, on a stool, or on the edge of a bed and ask your partner to gently knead and squeeze the muscles of your shoulders and neck.

» **Relaxing head massage:** ask your partner to massage the top of your head, applying firm pressure with just the tips of his fingers, almost as if he is washing your hair.

» **Soothing touch:** if you don't like the idea of being stroked in labor, ask your partner to hold your palm between his two palms, gently squeezing and releasing your hand. Many women find this simple contact deeply reassuring and nurturing.

» **Foot massage:** ask your partner to use firm thumb pressure all over the soles of your feet, rubbing, pressing, and making small circles to release knots and tension.

Q What if I am too anxious and nervous about labor and delivery to do anything?

It's possible for your doctor to prescribe tranquilizers to help you endure labor and delivery, if you really are very anxious. Tranquilizers make it easier for some pregnant women who are very anxious to more fully participate in the labor and delivery process. Each woman's reaction to these drugs is different. Some women find that they are able to cope more easily with labor and delivery with the help of the gentle drowsiness that tranquilizers afford. Other women feel like the drugs make them feel out of control during an extremely important moment in their lives, and too sleepy to participate fully in the events at hand. Tranquilizers don't relieve labor pain, but they can work in combination with your opioid analgesics to help you feel more comfortable than you would with the pain medications alone. Because tranquilizers can affect the breathing of your baby, they are given well before you will need to begin to push.

Q What is a walking epidural? Is it right for me?

Many women are intrigued by the idea of a walking epidural, because they'd like to walk around the hospital during labor with reduced pain. But it's common for women who have this procedure to stay in bed after it's been done. Walking epidurals aren't available at all hospitals, and they don't offer as much pain relief as a regular epidural. If you're interested in having this procedure done, check with your doctor before your delivery to see if the anesthesiologists at the hospital where you'll be delivering are trained to perform walking epidurals.

More than **60%** of American women choose to have an epidural for pain relief during their labor.

Q What is an epidural, and how does it work?

An epidural is a procedure that injects painkilling drugs directly into the epidural space around your spinal cord through a fine tube. It works by numbing feeling below the waist, so is a very effective form of pain relief.

An anesthesiologist first gives you a local anesthetic injection to numb the section of your mid-to-low-back where the epidural goes in. He or she then inserts a long, hollow needle carrying a thin tube, or catheter, into the epidural space. (You may be asked to curl up on your side, or to sit up and bend forward for this part, since it opens the space between your vertebrae.) The anesthesiologist removes the needle, leaving the catheter in place. The painkiller (a mixture of anesthetic and narcotic) is either injected into your spine through the catheter, or pumped in intravenously, to block the nerve pathways that run from your uterus to your brain. Although epidurals traditionally caused complete numbness, many now allow sensation without pain, which means you can feel to push when the time comes.

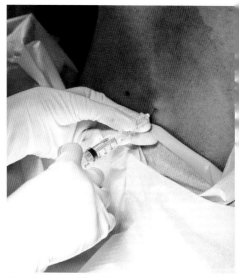

Top offs The painkilling drugs can be topped off by injecting through the small catheter placed in the spine.

Q What should I expect if I want to ask for opioid analgesics?

Opioid analgesics are derived from the seeds of the opium poppy, which gives us morphine. They offer limited relief from labor pain that can last for between two and four hours per dosage. They block the pain as it travels down your spinal column by "switching off" the cells in your pain receptors. The drug doesn't have any effect on your contractions; it dulls the sensation while letting your body go about its important work. Dosages are administered by your doctor usually via an injection in your thigh or buttocks, although they may also be given intravenously. (The pain relief will be quicker intravenously—becoming active within two or three minutes, compared with 20–30 minutes by injection.) Depending on how long your labor lasts, you can be given additional injections after the pain relief begins to wear off (within two to four hours). Some are likely to have more significant side effects on your baby's alertness, breathing, and feeding—it can take several days after birth for the effects of the drug to wear off in a newborn, depending upon how soon after your last dose the baby was born. For this reason, doctors don't like to give the drug when it looks like your baby will be born during the next two or three hours. Depending on the drug and your reaction to it, you may feel nauseous or even vomit. Note that none of the analgesics will give you a pain-free labor, and for some women they simply don't work. These drugs can be useful if your first stage labor is lasting a long time and you need some sleep, since they can help you to relax.

Q Can I have opioid analgesics if I want a water birth?

Yes, although you will need to have had the drug in your system for at least two hours before you get into the pool. This is just to make sure that you don't feel overly drowsy in the water. Of course, the water itself will help with pain relief.

INSERTING INTO THE EPIDURAL SPACE

The epidural space lies around your spinal cord, up and down its whole length. When you are given an epidural, a fine catheter is inserted directly into this space in order to administer drugs.

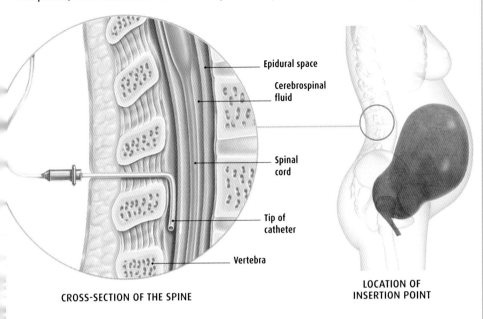

Epidural space
Cerebrospinal fluid
Spinal cord
Tip of catheter
Vertebra

CROSS-SECTION OF THE SPINE

LOCATION OF INSERTION POINT

A mixture of **anesthetic** and **narcotic** injected into the spine **blocks the pain messages** from the uterus to the brain.

Q How long does an epidural take and how long does it last?

An epidural takes around 10 minutes to set up and around 15-20 minutes to become fully effective, and will last for as long as the anesthetic is topped off. Some hospitals have pump systems that allow you to control how much anesthetic you receive and when, leaving you to judge how much of your labor you want to be able to feel and when. Once you stop receiving the anesthetic, the effects should wear off and you should regain the feeling in your legs within around two hours.

Q I'm worried that an epidural might damage my spine. What are the risks and side effects?

Permanent damage to your spine following an epidural is very rare—occurring in between 1 in 80,000 and 1 in 320,000 cases, depending upon the source of the statistics.

If you experience any significant discomfort or pain in your epidural site when the needle is going in or immediately after it has been withdrawn, let your anesthesiologist know so that he or she can reposition the catheter if necessary. It is normal to feel a little achy in your back after an epidural, but if you have severe pain, tell your doctor.

Between 1 and 5 percent of epidurals may lead to a "dural tap" in which the epidural needle makes a small puncture causing cerebrospinal fluid to leak from around your spinal cord. The first symptom is often a bad headache. However, just like a nick anywhere else on your body, the wound will heal and the leak will stop on its own—all you will need to do is rest. Occasionally your anesthesiologist may want to plug the hole with a little of your own blood- almost like creating a scab to give the tissues beneath time to heal.

Other complications of an epidural include feelings of nausea and itchy skin, both of which are easily treated and will pass, and low blood pressure (you will probably be given medication intravenously to help prevent this side effect).

Q A pain-free labor sounds perfect! Are there any drawbacks to having an epidural?

There are several reasons why you might decide against an epidural for your labor.

» Restricted mobility: you will be limited in your ability to move around because you won't have any strength in your legs and because you will need to be attached to a fetal heart monitor. Even so-called mobile epidurals are still limiting—talk to your doctor about what's available in your hospital and how much freedom you'll be able to have.

» Longer labor: you may experience a slower labor because the pain medication can make the muscles of your pelvis weaker and so less effective at turning your baby into a good position for birth. This also slightly increases your chances of needing an assisted (instrumental) delivery (see p.222).

» Increased odds of intervention: there is a slightly increased risk of assisted delivery for women who have an epidural. Your doctor is likely to delay your pushing in second stage labor by up to an hour to reduce the risk of your needing an assisted delivery. However, you will need to deliver your baby within four hours of the start of the second stage, otherwise your doctor will recommend a C-section.

» Limited effectiveness: even if it has been effective for the first stage of labor, an epidural doesn't always work against the pain of the second stage of labor, when there is localized sharp pain as the baby emerges.

» Risk of complications: while most doctors agree there are no risks to your baby, epidural carries certain risks for you (see left).

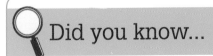 Did you know...

If you choose to have an opioid analgesic you will probably also be given an antiemetic—a drug that limits the side effects of nausea associated with these methods of pain relief.

You may already know that your baby will arrive **via cesarean section** (C-section), or you may be wondering what would happen if you were told during labor that you could need surgery. Knowing what C-sections involve will **help you prepare mentally** and practically for **what lies ahead** for both you and your baby.

Cesarean section

The decision to operate

Around a third of all babies in the US and a quarter of all babies in the UK are born surgically. The vast majority of C-sections are done for medical reasons, of which many are known in advance, such as placenta previa, a multiple birth, or a breech position. In these cases, you will have an "elective," or planned, C-section.

Roughly one in eight births in the UK is an "emergency," or unplanned, C-section. Some vaginal births can develop complications that mean this is the safest option for you and your baby. However, not all situations are life threatening: a long, slow labor is the most common reason given for unplanned surgical delivery. Your medical team will always talk through the reasons why a C-section is being recommended. These discussions are open to your partner, too, but it is for you to decide and consent to. For some women, a C-section may come as a relief, whereas others may feel a sense of disappointment or failure at not having a vaginal birth. These are normal responses; asking questions about the risks and benefits will help you to make a decision you are happy with.

You can request a C-section without a medical reason if you want, and this should be set out in your birth plan (see pp.88–9), but it is important to be fully aware of the risks and recovery implications, which are greater on

balance than those for a vaginal birth. Your doctor will explain the pros and cons so that you can make a fully informed decision.

What to expect from a cesarean section

Although having a C-section is major surgery, it can be a life-saving one. Like any surgery, it can carry risks. For the mother this may mean increased blood loss (both during and after surgery), cardiac arrest, infection of the uterus or uterine lining, bladder damage, complications for future pregnancies, greater risk of future hysterectomy, and a longer hospital stay.

Your baby may experience more stress, because you won't have the benefit of the labor hormones that calm the baby. She may be born with residual fluid in the lungs and nasal passages that make independent breathing more difficult. There is a small risk (about 2 percent) of your baby receiving a nick or cut, but this will heal within a few days. There is a possibility that your baby could be admitted to the neonatal intensive care unit (see p.310).

Before you are discharged, you'll be able to discuss the surgery and ask any further questions about aftercare or possible complications. Your recovery will take about six weeks so it may be a good idea to get help taking care of your baby at first if you can.

85%

of C-sections are performed for **one of four reasons**: previous C-sections, lack of progress in labor, fetal distress, or breech birth.

Q What happens before surgery? Do I need to prepare myself?

For both planned and emergency C-sections, there is a set of procedures to follow.

» Written consent: you will need to sign a consent form to say that you agree to the surgery, understand the risks, and allow the doctors to act in your best medical interests.

» Meeting the anesthesiologist: If there's time, the consultant who will administer the drugs will explain what form of anesthetic you will have and what its effects will be, both during and after the surgery.

» Preparing yourself: you'll need to remove any jewelry, makeup, nail polish, and fake nails (so that the anesthesiologist can monitor your skin and nail color to check oxygen levels).

» Being prepared by the medical team: a nurse will shave your pubic hair around the intended incision site. For a planned C-section, you will be given a blood test for anemia (which increases risk of blood loss) and blood type, in case a transfusion is necessary during surgery. You'll be attached to an arm cuff and chest electrodes to measure your blood pressure and heart rate throughout. You'll be given antibiotics to reduce the risk of postoperative infection, and low blood pressure medication if you need it. For general anesthesia you will be given antacids and medication to prevent nausea and vomiting.

» Immediately before surgery: finally, you will be given your anesthesia, and a catheter will be inserted into your ureter, to provide bladder control during surgery.

Q Why might I need a cesarean section?

There are many reasons for a cesarean section, but usually they are used to prevent or solve health risks to you or your baby. Nearly half are elective, planned in advance for known medical problems or by request. The remainder are advised when issues arise during labor and a quick delivery is needed.

REASONS FOR PLANNED CESAREAN SECTION

» Repeat C-section could be proposed by your obstetrician if your medical history presents risk factors, such as complications with the previous procedure or a high chance of old scars tearing in a vaginal birth.

» Breech presentation or transverse lie (when your baby is in a bottom down or sideways position in the uterus) might need a C-section if the baby can't be turned manually using external cephalic version.

» Preeclampsia, a condition that can develop during pregnancy, could make the strain of vaginal birth dangerous for you.

» Low-lying placenta can block the passage of your baby or make heavy bleeding likely.

» Twins or multiples often require a C-section, although vaginal delivery is possible in twins if the first baby is positioned head down.

» Some heart conditions make vaginal birth unsafe for the mother.

» Maternal requests for a C-section are sometimes made if a previous birth was difficult.

REASONS FOR UNPLANNED CESAREAN SECTION

» Lack of progress in labor can happen if your cervix hasn't opened enough after a long, slow labor, or contractions are too weak. Although not life threatening, this is the most common reason for unplanned C-sections.

» Fetal distress is sometimes detected during labor. Doctors monitor the baby's heart rate as standard practice for all births.

» Unsuccessful assisted delivery (using forceps or vacuum) can be followed by a C-section.

» Placental abruption is when the placenta comes away from the wall of the uterus either before or during labor. It is a rare occurrence but necessitates an emergency C-section.

» Uterine rupture occurs if a scar from a previous C-section tears during labor. It happens in less than 1 percent of women with prior C-sections. Your doctor will assess the risk of rupture before planning a vaginal birth.

» Umbilical cord prolapse is another very rare event. If the umbilical cord slips down the cervix ahead of your baby, it can get compressed and affect the baby's oxygen supply.

Q Can I stay awake during a C-section?

In most cases, you can stay awake because you will be given either spinal anesthesia or an epidural; both numb the lower body without making you unconscious. Spinal anesthesia (or spinal block) is a single injection that is used only in the event of surgery. With these forms of anesthetic, you won't feel any pain during surgery, but you might feel a bit of pushing and pulling in your abdomen. It helps to focus on music—arrange to take some music of your choice to be played in the operating room. However, if a quick delivery is vital, your doctor might use general anesthesia, which is faster to administer, but means that you will be fully asleep. General anesthesia is only used if the benefits outweigh the risks—it can cross the placenta and make your baby drowsy, but studies show there are no long-lasting effects on the baby. The surgery usually takes 40–50 minutes; maybe longer if you've had a C-section before.

Q Will I be able to see my baby being born during the surgery?

In order to spare you unnecessary trauma, nurses will construct a screen between you and your belly so that you can't see your doctor cut through your skin and into your uterus. However, you can usually ask for the screen to be lowered enough so that you can see your baby lifted out. The screen will be removed as soon as you've been stitched up.

Q Will my doctor be in the O.R. with me? Who else will be there?

Yes, your doctor will perform your C-section and be present with you throughout the procedure. Also expect to have an anesthesiologist present, as well as a labor and delivery nurse, who can offer reassurance to both you and your birth partner and answer questions as they may arise. There may also be a technician present to assist the doctor. And there should be a pediatrician or neonatologist for the baby—or one doctor for each baby, if you're having multiples. All in all, the operating room can get quite busy!

Q Can my birth partner come into the operating room (OR) with me?

One birth partner is usually allowed into the operating room as long as you are having a spinal anesthetic or an epidural. He or she will need to wear a surgical gown and a surgical mask, but will be allowed to sit beside you as you have your surgery. If you have general anesthesia, you will usually not be permitted to have anyone in OR with you (you'll be completely asleep). Your birth partner will be able to wait just outside the operating room.

Q I am HIV positive. Will I have to have a C-section?

No. The most recent guidelines from the US National Institutes of Health (NIH) recommend that women who are HIV positive and on medication that is controlling the effects of the virus are given the option of having a vaginal delivery. Overall, studies show that there is no increased risk to the baby of contracting the virus by vaginal rather than C-section. Your doctor will be able to advise you in your specific circumstances.

Q If the only reason for having a C-section is because my labor is taking a long time, can I refuse?

Yes, although your doctor gives his or her advice with your best interests in mind, so you should ask why he or she is suggesting the procedure, what it involves, and what would happen if you don't opt for it. Consider the risks carefully before you decide. If you choose to refuse medical intervention, your doctor will respect your wishes. They will continue to work to ensure the best outcome for you and your baby in any circumstances.

Q Who will take care of my baby if I have to have general anesthesia?

Assuming all is well with your baby after birth, that's really a decision for you—let your doctor know your preference before you go into surgery, if possible. As a default, your birth partner will be encouraged to hold and cuddle with your baby until you wake up, to have skin-to-skin contact if that is you want, and to bottle feed her if necessary.

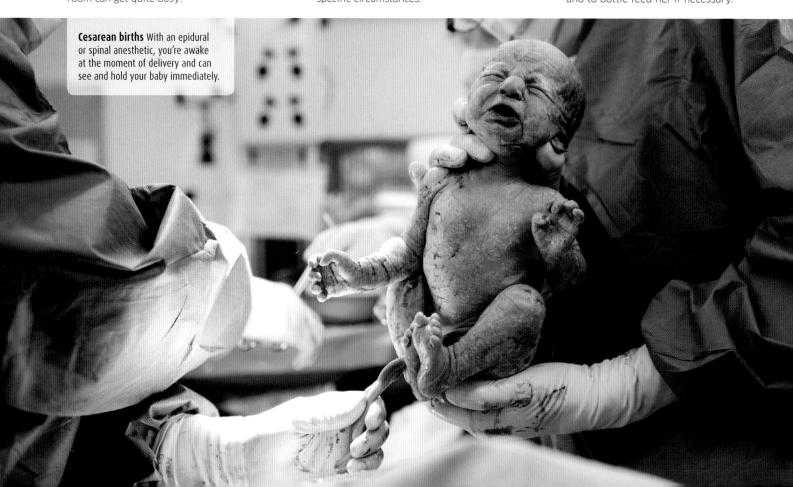

Cesarean births With an epidural or spinal anesthetic, you're awake at the moment of delivery and can see and hold your baby immediately.

Q How quickly will I be given a C-section if it is decided during labor that I need one?

That depends on the level of emergency for your C-section. The procedure will be performed as quickly as the clinical need, and your baby should be delivered within 30 minutes or up to 75 minutes of a C-section being decided upon. Most hospitals use a two-level grading system. If either you or your baby is considered to be in danger, you'll have a Category 1 C-section, done as speedily as possible. When neither you nor your baby is in a life-threatening situation (for example, if you're too tired to keep going, or if your baby is awkwardly positioned), your C-section will be a Category 2 and there will be a little more time to prepare for surgery.

Q How is the placenta delivered when I've had a C-section? Will it have to be cut away from my uterus lining?

No, once your baby is out, your doctor will deliver the placenta in a very similar way that he or she would do if it had been a vaginal birth. Your doctor will gently pull on the umbilical cord to separate the placenta fully and draw it out through the incision in your abdomen. Once the entire placenta and the membranes have been removed from your uterus, your doctor can begin to put everything back into place in your abdomen to get you ready to be stitched up.

Q Will I be able to go right to a postpartum ward with my baby after the surgery?

Usually you will spend a few hours in a recovery room adjacent to the operating room, with your baby if possible. The doctor or nurse will check your blood pressure and heart rate regularly, and make sure you have no signs of complications relating to the surgery. You will be given some pain medication and your doctor will make sure you feel able to eat and drink normally. If all is well and you are awake and alert, you can usually then move onto the postpartum ward.

Q What will happen during the cesarean section?

After giving the anasthetic, the anesthesiologist will make sure you cannot feel anything. You may feel some pushing and pulling, but it should not be painful.

You will have a catheter tube inserted through your urethra to drain your bladder during the surgery and once your abdomen is swabbed with antiseptic solution the surgery can begin. An incision is made just below the top of your pubic hair. The obstetrican divides the layers of fat and fibrous muscle tissue before making an incision in the lower part of your uterus. If the membranes surrounding your baby have not ruptured, this will be done now. Whatever part of your baby's body is below the incision will be delivered first. Your baby is normally delivered in the first ten minutes once surgery is underway. After the delivery, the cord is clamped and your baby can be handed to you for her first embrace.

The low horizontal incision (known as transverse) made in your abdomen is usually 6–8in (15–20cm) long–this is the cut seen on your skin. It leaves a modest scar that fades over time. The incision made in the uterus underneath is only 2¼–2¾in (5–7cm) long, to keep scarring on your uterus to a minimum. This helps to reduce the risk of gynecological problems later and increases your chance of having a safe vaginal birth if you go on to have another pregnancy. In unusual and very specific circumstances, a vertical (longitudinal) cut may be done. Try not to worry about scarring too much–it is just one of many changes that will take place in your body.

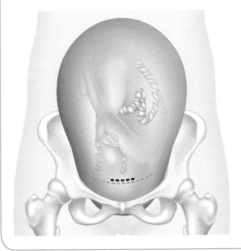

KEY
- - - - - 2¼–2¾ in (5–7 cm) incision in uterus
- - - - - 6–8 in (15–20 cm) incision in abdomen

Transverse incision This is the most common incision and is associated with fewer risks and a better chance of subsequent vaginal births. It leaves a discreet scar along your bikini line.

Q How soon will I be able to leave the hospital? Will I have to go back to have stitches out?

You can usually leave the hospital between three and four days after your C-section. Sometimes you can leave as quickly as 24 hours later (your catheter will come out around 12 hours after the surgery), if your baby is well and you have made a fast initial recovery. It's very unlikely you will need to go back to hospital to have stitches taken out. The stitches in your uterus will be dissolvable. You may also have dissolvable stitches at your abdominal incision. If you have surgical sutures or staples in your abdomen, these will be removed around five days after the surgery. This may be done in the hospital if you are there, or your doctor can remove them if you have gone home. If you had a longitudinal (vertical) incision, you may need to have your stitches in for a little longer.

Q How quickly can I get out of bed and resume normal activities?

You'll be encouraged to walk around and eat and drink normally as soon as possible after your C-section, as long as the anesthesia has worn off and you aren't feeling dizzy or unwell. Movement will also decrease your chances of blood clots (an injection to prevent thrombosis is often given as well). Activities such as lifting and driving will take longer. See page 260 for some of the commonly asked questions about recovering from a cesarean section.

Your labor is done: you have your newborn **baby in your arms**, and you are ready to get to know this tiny new person, and to start your life as a family. The doctor has a **few more checks** to make, and this **care you receive** immediately after the birth is sometimes referred to as the fourth stage of labor.

Right after birth

Your baby's first moments
Just after your baby is born, and provided all is well, the doctor will place him on your chest to enjoy a first embrace. Your baby will be rubbed and patted dry and have a clean towel placed over him while you hold him skin to skin. Meanwhile, the cord will be clamped and cut by the doctor, or by your partner if so planned.

Your baby will be given an initial checkup (see pp.238-39), which may be done while you are holding him, then he may be weighed. Whether at home or in a hospital or birthing center, your doctor will try to do the necessary checkup as unobtrusively as possible, so as not to interfere with these first moments when you and your partner begin bonding with your baby. If you or your baby needs medical attention after the birth, the medical team will try to reunite you as soon as they can.

If you have decided to breast-feed it is important to offer this to your baby within the first hour. Your nurse will help you to get your baby to latch on. His sucking and rooting reflexes (see p.267) are strong at this time.

Taking care of you
Before you leave the delivery room, or before your doctor leaves you if you're at home, she or he will check that your body is beginning to show signs of recovery from the birth. Your nurse will take your blood pressure and temperature, feel your belly to make sure your uterus has begun to contract, assess your blood loss, and examine your placenta and membranes to ensure they are complete. Your doctor will also ask to assess your perineum to check for any injury—primarily this means checking whether or not you suffered a tear as your baby was born, and if so whether or not this needs stitches.

Your doctor will explain what he or she is doing as the checkup is being done, and you should be able to continue to hold your baby while you're given the once-over. In fact, your baby can provide the perfect distraction from this final stage in the delivery room.

Your emotions right after birth
Unsurprisingly, you're likely to feel emotional when you've given birth: not only do you have raised hormone levels, but also the relief and excitement of meeting your baby can be overwhelming. Don't worry if you feel like crying—doctors and nurses are used to all kinds of emotions in the delivery room and will offer support, encouragement, reassurance, or quietude as your mood dictates.

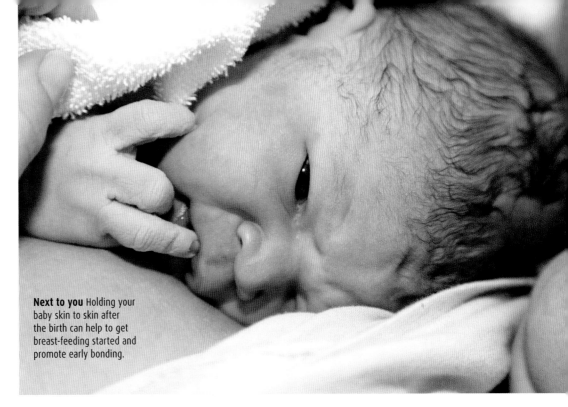

Next to you Holding your baby skin to skin after the birth can help to get breast-feeding started and promote early bonding.

Q What will be my baby's first reactions after being born?

Your baby's first reaction will be to cry—this is a positive sign that he is able to breathe successfully on his own. Sometimes, babies need assistance and can be given oxygen in the delivery room. Some babies splutter slightly and may need help to clear mucus out of the airways. Your baby will be observed in the first minutes after birth to check his responses.

When first holding your baby, you may notice him turning toward your nipple very soon after birth, displaying the strong instinct newborns have to seek out food immediately.

Q Will I need to have stitches if I tear during the delivery?

This depends on the severity of the tear (see p.217). A first-degree, or superficial, tear will usually be left to heal by itself. A second-degree tear can be stitched by your doctor in the delivery room under a local anesthetic while you hold your baby. A third- or fourth-degree tear needs to be repaired in an operating room. If you've had an epidural this can be topped off before surgery, otherwise you will be given either a spinal block or a local anesthetic. Very rarely, general anesthesia is given. Your birth partner and your baby may be able to stay with you while you are being stitched.

The stitches are almost always dissolvable so will disappear on their own, within two weeks or so for superficial stitches, and three months for deeper stitches. There is usually no need for a doctor to check them unless you have concerns.

🔍 Did you know...

On average, women lose around 12 lb (5.5 kg) immediately after the birth, as they shed the combined weight of the baby, placenta, and amniotic fluid. However, you will still appear pregnant after your baby is born since your uterus takes time to shrink back down and it takes several days or weeks to lose the excess fluid you carried during pregnancy.

Q I've heard there is some bleeding after birth—how much is usual?

There will be some bleeding right after the delivery of your baby when the placenta comes away from the wall of the uterus, exposing the blood vessels it was connected to. Normal levels of blood loss can be up to about 2 cups (600ml) of blood in the first 24 hours. Once the placenta is delivered, the uterus continues to contract, which helps to close the blood vessels and stem the bleeding. If you have an episiotomy or a tear, that may also cause some bleeding.

Postpartum hemorrhage (PPH) is when you have more bleeding than normal. Heavy bleeding within 24 hours of birth is known as primary PPH, and it affects 5 percent of women. The main reason for primary PPH is that the uterus isn't contracting efficiently, which can lead to heavy blood loss.

You will also get a bloody discharge known as lochia after delivery as the uterine lining renews itself (see p.259).

Q What if the bleeding is so heavy that it doesn't stop?

Unless bleeding is obviously profuse, your doctor will first try to stem the flow. He or she may massage the uterus, and/or give you anticoagulant drugs to encourage your blood to clot, or an injection of synthetic oxytocin (see p.220). If your placenta is incomplete, or the bleeding has no obvious cause, you will probably be taken into an operating room, where, under general anesthesia, an obstetric surgeon will remove the remainder of the placenta surgically, or investigate why you're still bleeding and treat you as necessary. If you have lost a lot of blood, you may be given a blood transfusion.

Q Will I be able to take a shower shortly after the delivery?

Yes. If all is well, you'll be encouraged to wash. You may feel a bit wobbly, so have someone with you. Your birth partner and baby can come with you (you can wheel your baby in the hospital crib). After an epidural, you will be given a sponge bath, then once you can walk safely, you can shower or take a bath.

Q I'm anxious about going to the bathroom after the birth. Will this hurt?

Your doctor will want to know that you are urinating before discharging you from the hospital, so you'll need to brave the bathroom. If you had a tear or episiotomy, urinating may sting; pouring lukewarm water over the area as you urinate can be soothing. To make sure first stools are soft and easy to pass, drink plenty of water and eat lots of fiber over the first few days.

How will I know that my newborn baby is healthy?

Your baby's first cries will be a wonderful sound but, understandably, you will want to know she is in perfect health. It is reassuring to know that she will be thoroughly checked immediately after the birth, and have more checkups before leaving the hospital. These are noninvasive and effective in highlighting possible health problems.

The APGAR test

In the early 1950s, American obstetric anesthesiologist Virginia Apgar developed a simple five-measure test to assess the health of a baby minutes after birth. The test has been criticized for being too simple, but it remains one of the first assessments your baby will have–at one minute after birth, and then again at five minutes after birth.

Hands The doctor will place a finger in your baby's palm to check that she grasps it

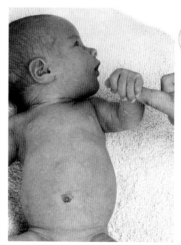

Grasp reflex You may be surprised by the strength of your newborn's grip. This is due to the grasp reflex; she will instinctively grasp something that is placed in her palm.

Back Spinal checks are very important since abnormalities can indicate spina bifida

THE APGAR SCORE

Virginia Apgar's surname is used as an acronym for the five measures in this test, which is done immediately after the birth. This is why you will sometimes see it written as APGAR:

>> **Appearance:** Skin and lip color indicate whether your baby is getting enough oxygen.
>> **Pulse:** Your baby's heart rate is measured with a stethoscope.
>> **Grimace:** Your baby's response to stimuli, such as light or touch, will be checked.
>> **Activity:** Arm and leg movements give an indication of muscle tone.
>> **Respiration:** The rhythm and effort of your baby's breathing is checked.

After both the one-minute and five-minute check, a combined score of seven or more indicates that all is well. Between five and seven can mean the baby needs help breathing, but probably no more than a rub on the chest to kickstart her reflexes. A score of under five can indicate more help is needed, and a pediatrician will be called to examine the baby.

SCORE	0	1	2
Appearance Skin and lip color	Completely blue skin all over	Pink body with white or blue extremities	Completely pink skin all over
Pulse	No heartbeat	Slow heartbeat	Fast heartbeat
Grimace	Unresponsive	Reacts to stimulation	Crying spontaneously
Activity	Inactive, limp	Slow movements to extend and retract arms and legs	Lots of activity in the arms and legs
Respiration	No breathing	Slow, weak, or very uneven breathing	Strong breaths and crying

Instant health checkup

Your doctor will do the Apgar test so quickly that you are unlikely to notice it is being done. Another top-to-toe check (see right) in the delivery room will highlight if there are any health concerns. If the doctor's checkups do highlight any problems, these will be explained to you, and your baby will be given the appropriate care. In some circumstances, the doctor may request that a pediatrician gives a second opinion.

Assuming all is well with your baby, you will be able to take her to the postpartum ward. Within 72 hours of the birth, your baby will be examined again (see p.246), either in the hospital or at home. If at any point you are concerned about your baby's health, inform your doctor immediately.

Feet Your baby's feet will be checked to ensure she has five toes and that there is no webbed skin

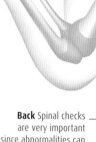

YOUR BABY'S TOP-TO-TOE EXAMINATION

1 Head: Are the soft spots on your baby's skull (the fontanelles), the head shape, head circumference, and hair texture normal?

2 Facial expression: As your baby scrunches up her face in response to a stimulus, is her expression symmetrical? This is a sign of overall well-being.

3 Eyes
» Do the pupils dilate with changes in light?
» Is there "red-eye," indicating cataracts?

4 Nose: Is there any mucus blocking the nasal passages, affecting baby's breathing?

5 Cheeks: Does your baby turn to the side when her cheek is stroked? This indicates her response to touch and tests for the "rooting reflex."

6 Mouth
» Is the roof of your baby's mouth fully formed?
» Does her tongue move freely, and is it a good color and size?
» Does your baby suck when the doctor puts his or her little finger inside your baby's mouth?

7 Lips: Does your baby "root for food" when a finger is brushed across the top of her lip?

8 Ears
» Does your baby turn her head to a sound?
» Are her ears symmetrical?
» Are there any skin tags?
» Do the ears fold forward and backward?
» When the earlobes are gently pinched, does blood flow back quickly to show healthy circulation?

9 Neck: When the neck is manipulated, does your baby's head bend forward, backward, and from side to side?

10 Collarbone: Was there any injury to the collarbone during birth?

11 Chest:
» Do your baby's lungs sound clear?
» Are the heart position and heartbeat correct?

12 Skin
» Does your baby's skin color show she is getting a healthy level of oxygen?
» Is there any sign of jaundice (see p.249)?
» Is your baby's temperature normal?

13 Arms
» Are the arms proportionate to the baby's size?
» Does she throw her arms back in the "startle reflex" (also known as the Moro reflex)? If it doesn't happen spontaneously, the doctor will cup your baby's head and safely allow it to seem to fall; this should trigger the reflex.

14 Hands and wrists
» Does your baby open her fingers as if to hold something when the back of her hand is brushed?
» Does she grasp the doctor's finger and hold on when it is placed on her palm? She or he will pull her hand upward, raising your baby slightly, to test grip.
» Are all your baby's fingers there and of the expected length compared with one another?
» Are there any creases in your baby's palms? Some creases can be a sign of Down syndrome, but there will be other signs with this condition.
» Do the wrists give the full range of movements?

15 Back
» Do your baby's shoulder blades look symmetrical?
» Are there tufts of hair or fat deposits along your baby's spine line? These can indicate spina bifida.
» Are all the vertebrae there and properly aligned with no unusual kinks or curves?
» Does gently pressing on the spine seem to cause your baby any pain?

16 Abdomen
» Are the size and symmetry of the abdomen normal?
» Do the organs feel normal? For example, it would be normal to be able to feel the edges of the liver, but unexpected to feel the spleen or kidneys.
» Is the cord stump infected or bleeding?

17 Hips: Is there an appropriate range of movement around the hip joints?

18 Genitals
» Has your baby passed any meconium, showing that the anus is open?
» Do genitals look normal and healthy, and have the testicles descended in a boy baby?

19 Legs
» Are the legs the same length as each other?
» Do the knees and ankles have full movement?

20 Feet
» Is the position of the feet at rest normal and are the ankles and the arches of the feet flexible?
» Is there the correct number of toes and are they of the expected length compared to each other?
» Is there any webbing between the toes?

Mouth The roof of the mouth is checked to ensure it is fully formed

Skin The color of your baby's skin can be checked in an instant. If it is pink all over, that is a sign of good health

Legs The doctor will manipulate your baby's legs to ensure her knee joints have the correct range of movement

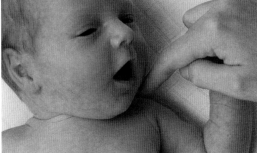

Rooting If anything strokes your baby's cheek, she'll turn her head to root for the object. This reflex ensures successful breast-feeding.

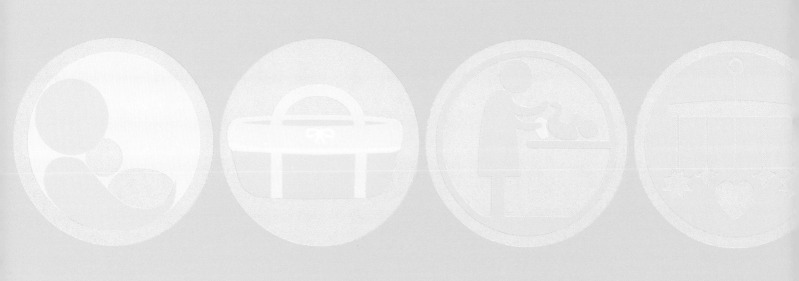

» In this chapter...

The postpartum period

The first few hours, days, and weeks with a newborn can be **challenging, but delightful** at the same time. This chapter will prepare you for what to expect. Read up on **breast-feeding and bottle-feeding** so you're ready to go as soon as your baby is. Once you finally have your **beautiful new baby** to cuddle and love, information on practical baby care will help you get the best out of your precious time together.

A CLOSER LOOK
The first 12 weeks

We talk about babies being fully formed at birth, but of course there are still myriad phases of growth for them to go through, physically, mentally, and emotionally. When you look back in three months at photographs of your baby on the day he was born, you'll barely be able to believe how that tiny, wrinkled, curled-up bundle could become the bouncing, smiling, laughing, grasping, and inquisitive little person you hold now.

1 WEEK OLD Your baby will spend time curled up as he adjusts to life outside the uterus. His fists will remain clenched for much of the time.
What you can do: Get your baby to look in a mirror—he loves looking at faces and will seek out yours immediately after birth.

2 WEEKS OLD Your baby may now be able to hold his head up for a few seconds when held to your shoulder.
What you can do: Make faces at your baby and stick out your tongue. He will try to mimic you.

3 WEEKS OLD You may notice that your baby movements are less jerky and more control He is gaining control of his muscles. Some of his more primitive reflexes are beginning to fade.
What you can do: Although your days and nights are still a blur, you can help your baby to start to differentiate them by darkening his room at nigh to help him identify nighttime.

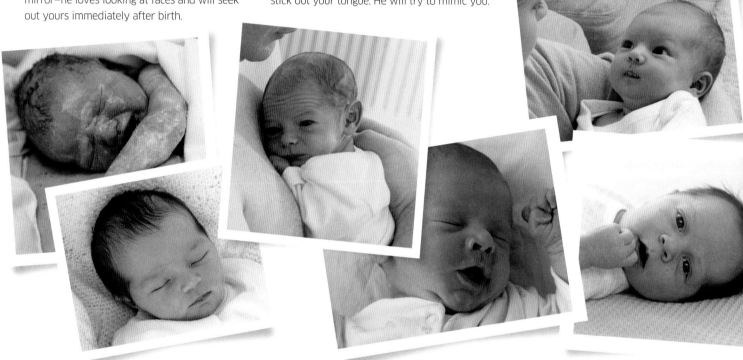

4 WEEKS OLD At four weeks, your baby's neck muscles are growing stronger and you may notice him holding his head up a little longer when he is supported on you.
What you can do: Place your baby on his tummy; he will try to lift his head up from the surface. This helps him build more strength in his back and neck.

5 WEEKS OLD Your baby can now focus both eyes and is working his eye muscles hard to focus on objects near and far. He can track a moving object from the side of his vision until it is in front of him.
What you can do: Young babies love black-and-white patterns. Try placing some where your baby can look at them while he is lying down.

6 WEEKS OLD At around six weeks you will see something that makes all the hard work worthwhile: your baby's first smile. He is becoming more socially aware and responds to your voice, holding your gaze when you speak.
What you can do: Talk to your baby, it will help him develop his language skills even though he can't respond with words. You may even get a few throaty noises in reply.

FASCINATING FACTS

8–10 in
(20–25 cm) is the distance your baby can focus on at two weeks old.

4 weeks
At four weeks your baby will be less curled up than after birth.

10 days
The umbilical cord usually comes off naturally 10 days after birth.

7 WEEKS OLD Your baby is beginning to discover his hands, you may notice him gazing at them and moving his fingers. This is the start of hand-eye coordination. He may bring his hands toward his mouth to explore them. His eye muscles have developed enough so that his eyes can now move in unison. Cooing and gurgling can start around now, as your baby realizes that he has a voice!

What you can do: Try dangling objects over him—just within swiping reach—as he lies on his back.

8 WEEKS OLD Your baby's back and neck muscles are now strong enough for him to hold his head in the midline of his body when he is lying on his back. Try holding your baby under his armpits and letting him bat his feet against the floor. Some babies are able to bear a little weight on their legs at this stage.

What you can do: Give your baby plenty of space to move, stretch out, and build strength in those growing muscles.

9 WEEKS OLD Your baby is becoming more social. He recognizes his parents and responds to your attention. He is beginning to associate people with fun and playtime.

What you can do: Your baby already loves your voice, but try using varied tones and interesting facial expressions. Copy your baby's coos to help him learn that the art of conversation is better with two!

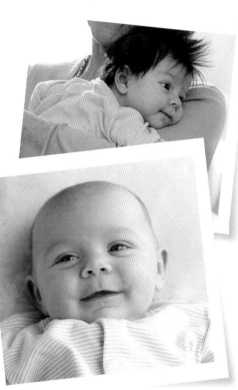

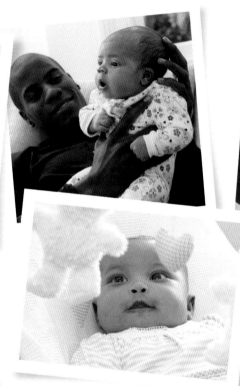

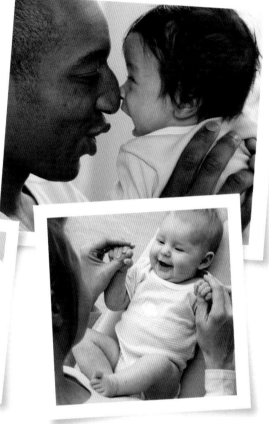

10 WEEKS OLD The ability to calm and soothe himself is an important skill for your baby to learn and it may be developing by around 10 weeks. You may notice that your baby can cope with higher levels of stimulation. He may have figured out how to bring his hands together in front of his face or body.

What you can do: Sing nursery rhymes to your baby. He'll be transfixed by the rhythm and the stanzas will help him begin to understand the complexities of language and speech.

11 WEEKS OLD Your baby is beginning to recognize objects, such as his bottle or the movements you make to prepare for breast-feeding, and will show signs of eagerness to feed. He is also able to connect sounds with the object that makes them.

What you can do: Try making a sensory box filled with items of different colors and textures that can make different sounds, such as crinkly paper, rustling foil, and rattles. Put them in your baby's hands so that he can explore them.

12 WEEKS OLD By now, your baby is really starting to communicate with you. You may hear coos, squeals, and even a little babbling. Your baby may start reaching out to grab things with intent, rather than simply grasping what's handed to him. Your baby's digestive system is fully matured now. Your baby's giggles begin around now—a sure sign that he thinks you're funny!

What you can do: Try incorporating gentle movement with nursery rhymes.

14–18
The number of hours that your baby will sleep during a 24-hour period.

6 million
There are some six million cells on every square centimeter of a newborn's skin.

4 reflexes
Your newborn baby has four natural reflexes at birth: startle, rooting, grasping, and stepping.

Congratulations on **your wonderful new baby!** Nothing can prepare you for how it feels to become a parent. You are likely to experience a tumult of emotions—joy may be mixed with a sense of **unreality and wonder** as you marvel at this new addition to your family. Enjoy this precious time getting to know this incredible little person.

The first 12 weeks

A new family

In addition to bonding with your baby, as a new mother it is crucial that you take care of yourself and get plenty of rest. On the following pages, you will find a snapshot of what to expect in the first 12 weeks.

If you gave birth in a hospital, you will be transferred to a ward with your new baby. If you have opted to breast-feed and haven't yet in the delivery room, you will be encouraged to do this now with support from a nurse. Rest assured that it can take time to establish feeding–both you and your baby are learning–so don't worry if you have some difficulty at first.

Once you are alone with your new baby, the reality that she is actually here may hit you, bringing with it a wide range of emotions. Your baby is likely to be asleep and you may simply spend much of the time staring at her in wonderment. Try to hold her close, preferably skin to skin, and talk to her. You are the one familiar person in this new world, the person whose voice and smell are instantly recognizable to her. If you have had a cesarean section and find it difficult to hold her, ask your partner to hold her skin to skin instead.

While you will want to share the news of your new arrival with family and friends, contact the key people and then consider turning off your phone. These first hours with your newborn baby are best enjoyed with little interruption. Although you will be allowed visitors to the hospital, it is a good idea to keep the number of people who come to a minimum. There will be plenty of time for everyone to meet the new arrival in the weeks to come.

Going home

Depending on your circumstances, you may be discharged from the hospital two days after your baby is born (if you had a vaginal delivery) or four days later (if you had a C-section). Use the time you are in hospital to ask questions about your baby's care, from diaper-changing and bathing to feeding and sleeping.

Having responsibility for this little person may feel overwhelming, but try to relax and remember you are the best person to take care of her. Rest assured that you will visit your baby's new pediatrician within just a couple of days to check your baby's process and offer advice and support. If you're having trouble breast-feeding, you can get back in touch with the lactation consultant at the hospital for help or use an independent lactation consultant.

Q Do most people instantly fall in love with their baby?

Some people feel a rush of love, and some don't. If this feeling doesn't hit you right away, don't worry. For some bonding is a much more gradual process, but the relationship that develops in the end is just as strong and secure.

In the past, experts believed that there was a critical window for bonding shortly after birth, but we now understand bonding as a much more subtle, complex, and long-term process that develops in the days, weeks, and months following your baby's arrival. The deep attachment that comes with a strong and lasting bond is something that happens gradually over time. Holding your baby and taking care of her day to day will create a secure attachment, a sense of trust, and a growing mutual love that becomes immeasurable and profound. You may even be unaware that a bond is developing—for many parents, the first time they experience that heart-jumping jolt is the first time their baby smiles several weeks after the birth.

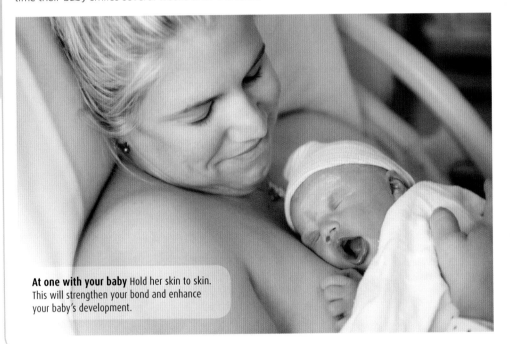

At one with your baby Hold her skin to skin. This will strengthen your bond and enhance your baby's development.

Bonding tips

» **Hold your baby close:** eventually your baby will need to learn to self-soothe and fall asleep alone, but in these early days and weeks cuddle with her as much as you want to.

» **Interact:** spend as much time as you can with your baby when she's awake: make eye contact; sing to her; talk to her. She can see you and hear you and this communication will only serve to strengthen the growing bond between you.

» **Make her your priority:** forget the chores and don't be afraid to accept help from others around you. These early weeks are precious so devote as much time as you can to your baby.

» **Limit visitors:** relatives and friends are bound to want to meet your new arrival, but in these early weeks try to stagger visitors. It's important to have time to spend together as a new family.

» **Give yourself time:** don't put pressure on yourself to feel or behave in a certain way. Try to relax and allow the relationship between you and your new baby to develop. If after several weeks you still feel detached, speak to your doctor.

Q It's a boy! I was sure I was having a girl. How should I adjust to this surprise?

Whether you have had a boy or girl, this is a time of enormous change. The first few days and weeks following childbirth are all about adjusting to the reality of having a small, fragile baby to take care of. In addition to this, your baby may look and behave differently from how you might have expected. You will also be experiencing a whirlwind of emotions due to hormone changes, exhaustion from the birth, and the hospital environment. Try to focus on bonding and getting to know your new baby.

This can take time, but as the days and weeks roll on, you will develop your own unique relationship, regardless of gender.

Q I am finding the first feedings difficult. Is this normal?

Rest assured that this is normal. Newborn babies are born with reserves and may not require much feeding during this time. Like you, your baby is probably exhausted from labor and birth and will sleep a lot. As a result she may be hard to feed. It may take time for both of you to get the hang of breast-feeding.

However, if you want to breast-feed, it is best to get this going as soon as possible. Enjoy skin-to-skin contact and put your baby to your breast every few hours, which will aid the production of breast-feeding hormones. If you are struggling, make sure to ask for guidance from a nurse or a lactation consultant.

On average, newborn babies tend to feed around **8 to 12 times a day**, or more, in the first weeks after birth.

Q What tests will my baby have while she's in the hospital nursery?

This thorough head-to-toe checkup is given within three days of the birth, and its goal is to identify abnormalities or certain conditions that were missed during prenatal screening.

Your baby will be thoroughly examined immediately after the birth (see p.239), but will be checked again, usually by the staff pediatrician at the hospital before you are discharged. If the pediatrician that you will be seeing in private practice is making rounds at the hospital to see his or her patients, there's a chance that the doctor will see his brand-new patient before your baby leaves the hospital.

Detecting any health problems this early means that babies can be referred promptly for treatment if needed, which usually leads to better long-term outcomes.

> A newborn baby's **heart rate is usually around 110–160 beats per minute.** To begin with, the heart is large in relation to the chest wall.

NEWBORN BABY CHECKUP

The checks below are done to confirm that your newborn baby is in good health. The pediatrician may also test your baby's reflexes again at this examination.

» **Skin:** the overall skin color and any birthmarks are observed.

» **Heart and lungs:** a stethoscope is used to make sure heart sounds and breathing patterns are normal. The pulse is checked.

» **Head and face:** the fontanelles (soft spots) on the head that allowed the bony plates to squeeze through the birth canal, are checked. Your baby's facial features are checked for symmetry.

» **Eyes:** a special light called an ophthalmoscope is used to check for "red reflex" to makes sure there are no cataracts.

» **Mouth:** the roof of the mouth is examined to ensure there is no split, or cleft, in the palate.

» **Mouth:** the tongue is checked for tongue-tie, since restrictions can interfere with breast-feeding.

» **Hips:** the legs are gently bent upward and rotated at the hips, to check that hip joints are not malformed (see p.324).

» **Genitals:** in boys, the position of the testes and the penis is checked. You'll be asked if your baby has urinated and pooped.

» **Back:** the spine is examined to ensure it is properly formed.

» **Hands and feet:** the fingers and toes are examined and the creases on the palms of the hands and the resting position of the feet and ankles are checked.

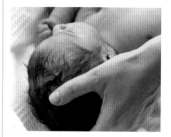

Head The soft spots on your baby's head are examined. Any effects from an assisted delivery will also be checked.

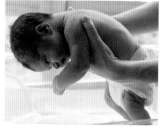

Spine The spine and back are examined to ensure they are straight and free of any abnormalities.

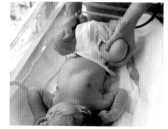

Hips Any signs of dislocation will be found when the pediatrician rotates the baby's hips.

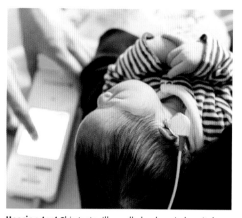

Hearing test This test will usually be done in hospital before you and your baby leave, or alternatively it may be done at the pediatrician's office during your baby's first week of life.

Q Why does my newborn baby need to have a hearing test in the first 24 hours after the birth?

Around 1 in 900 babies is born with some degree of hearing loss. Being aware of this early on is important for a baby's development since it means he can be given the right support and assistance and have the best chance of developing speech and language skills.

A small earpiece placed in your baby's outer ear transmits clicking sounds down the ear canal; these are received by the inner ear, which responds with an echo. It is a quick and painless procedure, which can be done while he's asleep.

Q What is vitamin K? Why does my baby need it after the birth?

Vitamin K plays an essential role in blood clotting. Some babies are born with inadequate amounts of vitamin K since it doesn't cross the placenta easily, and breast milk contains very little. This puts them at risk of a rare, but potentially fatal, condition—vitamin K deficiency bleeding of the newborn (VKDB), where bleeding can occur in the nose, mouth, and sometimes in the brain. The American Academy of Pediatrics recommends that every newborn baby receive a single vitamin K intramuscular injection, especially for those that are breast-fed.

Q My baby sleeps all the time. Should I wake him every 3 hours to be fed?

Rest assured that your baby won't starve himself. After your baby's initial alertness following the birth you may be surprised at how much he sleeps and you may worry that he isn't getting enough to eat. In the first few days, your baby only needs small amounts of the pre-milk colostrum. A teaspoon's worth of this thick and creamy, antibody-rich substance that your breasts produce is perfect for his very small tummy. However, it is fairly good practice to put your baby to the breast every two to three hours at first. This is not to get him into a feeding schedule–it's far too early for this–but to help you both develop your technique, and to stimulate your breasts to produce milk. While your first breast milk arrives on average about three to five days after the birth, the more your baby nurses, the faster your milk is likely to "come in."

Q Why does my baby breathe so noisily when he sleeps?

Your baby breathes in and out through his nose only, which means he can breathe comfortably during a long feeding. However it also means that if mucus is blocking his nasal passage, he may snuffle and snort to clear it, or make a wheezing, whistling sound while he breathes. He may gurgle if the mucus makes its way to the back of his throat. Since his air passages are still very small, it's easy for them to get blocked.

Babies also spend about half their sleep time in "active" sleep, when dreams occur, so they tend to be more restless and noisy. Young babies may also have periods during sleep when they stop breathing altogether for a few breaths, which can be for as long as 10 seconds, then revert to shallow and rapid breathing before resuming normal breathing. This "periodic" breathing is especially common in babies born prematurely, but can also occur in full-term babies, and is a passing phase. Noisy breathing that is intermittent is nothing to worry about, but if your baby is persistently noisy, or his breathing seems very labored and fast, he flares his nostrils, makes a barking or rasping sound, his breathing pauses for longer than 10 seconds, or he has a blue tinge to his skin, seek medical guidance.

Q My baby has had his first poop and it was black! Is this normal?

It can be a bit of a shock when you peek inside your newborn's diaper to discover a greenish-black stool. Don't worry—it's a sign of good health.

This greenish-black, tarlike substance is called meconium. It is made up of dead skin cells, lanugo, bilirubin, mucus, and bile that accumulated in your baby's intestines while he was in the uterus and which your baby passes in the first 24 hours.

Although meconium looks a little alarming and is difficult to clean, this first sticky bowel movement is quite normal, and its appearance is a welcome sign that your baby's bowels are in good working order. Your baby's stool will change over the first week or so as he settles into feeding. If you are concerned at all speak to your pediatrician.

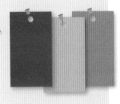

Bowel movements When you change your baby's diaper it is normal to find stools of differing colors.

WHAT DOES A NORMAL DIAPER LOOK LIKE?

It's often news to first-time parents that baby stools come in a whole range of colors and textures. So knowing what's normal (most of it), and what isn't quite right will stop you from worrying each time you look in your baby's diaper. Here's what you can expect:

» In the first couple of days, your baby will pass meconium, the thick, green-black, tarlike substance that accumulated in his bowels while in the uterus.

» From days three to five, stools gradually change, turning from dark green through to yellow and light brown.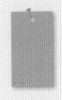

» Your breast-fed baby's stools will be a mustardlike color and may be seedy and watery. They are also surprisingly sweet smelling.

» Your formula-fed baby's stools tend to be more formed and a slightly darker yellow-tan color. Some formula can lend a greenish color to stools.

 » In the first few days, your baby may poop frequently, sometimes after each feeding. After about day four, your baby will usually pass around two stools a day for the next few weeks. Breast-fed babies sometimes pass stools less often, and may occasionally go several days without a bowel movement. As long as the stools are soft and not uncomfortable for your baby to pass, this isn't a concern.

Q My baby looks nothing like the pictures in magazines. Why is this?

First-time parents can be surprised at the appearance of their newborn. The bundle of joy you are handed after birth may not be the picture-perfect vision you had in mind. It is good to understand why and to remember that even though each baby is unique, they all share some physical characteristics at this time.

Whether your baby has been pushed, squashed, and squeezed down the birth canal following a vaginal delivery or has been delivered by cesarean section, she has been through an enormous event. Added to this, her appearance bears testimony to the nine months she has spent curled up in your uterus, floating in the amniotic fluid. Given this, it is not surprising that she emerges swollen, bruised, and bloody. Rest assured that many of her newborn features—a larger head in comparison to the rest of her body, swollen facial features, skin covered in a strange coating and enlarged genitals—will settle down after a day or so as she recovers from the birth. Try to enjoy her newborn looks while you can, since they won't last long!

HEAD

Your baby's head is a quarter of her body length. The skull bones are soft and flexible and have gaps between them. These "soft spots" are called the fontanelles—handle these areas gently after birth. They will disappear completely by 18 months old. During labor, the skull bones move and mold the head to help it pass through the birth canal. This can give newborns a cone-shaped head. If you had an assisted delivery, there may be bruising where the forceps were positioned or a swelling where the vacuum extractor was placed; this goes down in 24-48 hours. Your baby's head will gradually round out and any marks will disappear.

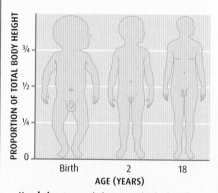

Head size As your baby grows, his body will become more in proportion with his head.

HAIR

Your baby may be virtually bald or have an impressive shock of hair. This hair is often shed in the first few months, and the new hair that replaces it may bear no resemblance to the newborn crop, but look more like the hair you would expect her to have.

SKIN

Your baby is likely to emerge covered in blood, amniotic fluid, and a creamy, waxy substance called vernix caseosa—this coated her skin in the uterus, ensuring that she didn't become waterlogged. If she is born after 41 weeks, she may have shed some of the vernix already, and her skin might be a little dry. Your baby may also have patches of fine, downy hair called lanugo. This would have kept the vernix in place.

While the skin may look purplish at first, once your baby starts to breathe on her own, her color will settle down. Her skin will also look quite fine, and you may be able to see tiny blood vessels under the surface in certain areas. Because the circulation is immature, the hands and feet may appear blue for a day or so.

EYES AND NOSE

Your baby's nose may be quite squashed after a vaginal birth, and that cute, turned up appearance enables your little one to breathe easily while feeding. Your baby's eyes may be swollen and puffy and the whites of the eye may be bloodshot from the pressure of squeezing through the birth canal.

WHEN YOUR BABY HAS JAUNDICE

Jaundice in newborns is so common that it's more unusual if your baby doesn't develop this condition.

It is caused by a buildup in the blood of a yellow substance called bilirubin, which causes the skin and the whites of the eyes to turn pale yellow. All newborn babies can tolerate mild jaundice and monitoring is all that is needed. It tends to clear up naturally within two weeks, and just 1 in 20 babies needs treatment (see p.322).

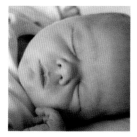

Jaundiced babies Jaundice improves quickly and often babies don't need treatment.

SPOTS AND RASHES

Your baby may be born with a cluster of tiny, white spots over her nose, cheeks, eyes, and forehead, or these may develop in the early weeks. These are known as milia, and are thought to be caused by underdeveloped glands in the skin. They are harmless and will disappear within a few weeks.

GENITALS

A surge in maternal hormones just before the birth means that both girls and boys may be born with swollen breasts and genitals from the hormones crossing over the placenta. Girls may have a vaginal discharge, which may even have a little blood in it, and there may be a white discharge from the breasts. All of this is normal, and the swelling will die down in the first few days.

BIRTHMARKS

Marks on the skin at birth are common and are usually nothing to worry about. Birthmarks fall into two categories: vascular or pigmented. Vascular birthmarks include:

BIRTHMARK	LOOKS LIKE	DESCRIPTION
Stork marks		Stork marks are also called salmon patches or nevus simplus. These light pink marks can appear on the forehead, the nose, around the mouth, on the eyelids, or the nape of the neck. These usually fade over time until they are hardly noticeable.
Strawberry hemangiomas		These are harmless, raised red marks formed by a concentration of immature blood vessels. They can grow quickly in the first few months, then start to shrink back and disappear. Depending on their size and position, they sometimes require treatment.
Port-wine stains		Port-wine stains, also called nevus flammeus, are flat, red or purple marks caused by a concentration of dilated blood vessels. They darken over time and are permanent. They can appear anywhere on the body, but are usually on the face, neck, or the limbs.

PIGMENTED BIRTHMARKS

Café au lait spots		These coffee-colored patches can appear anywhere on the body. They may be present at birth, and more may appear over the first years of life. While usually harmless, if your child has several, it's worth asking the doctor to have a quick look.
Mongolian blue spots	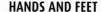	Mongolian spots are more common on darker-skinned babies. These blue-gray patches of skin typically appear on the back or buttocks, and usually fade on their own in the first few years.
Moles		Known as congenital nevi, these are brown or black, and can be flat or raised. These marks are usually harmless, but should be monitored since they carry a risk of becoming malignant later in life.

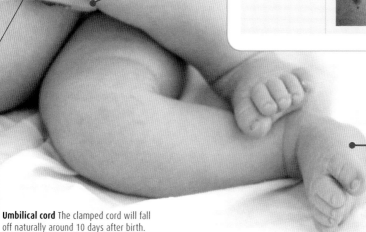

Umbilical cord The clamped cord will fall off naturally around 10 days after birth.

HANDS AND FEET

Your baby's legs may be "bowed" and her feet curved inward, reflecting the curled up position she adopted in the uterus. Her limbs and feet will straighten out over time. If your baby was full term, her toes and fingernails may be quite long, and she may even have managed to scratch herself. The nails will be soft, so you can peel them off very carefully or clip them with baby scissors.

Q What checkups will my baby have when I leave the hospital, and in the early weeks?

You'll visit your baby's new pediatrician at his office during the first few days that your baby goes home.

During the appointment, your pediatrician will want to know how feeding is progressing, especially if you are breast-feeding. He'll also examine all aspects of your baby's health and well-being at this first appointment, including the hearing, vision, and hip-joint tests that she had at the hospital. Pediatricians provide an invaluable resource for help and advice and are there to help you in this early period. If you need help to establish breast-feeding, the pediatrician is an excellent person to ask for help. If you have questions about your baby's sleeping patterns and whether she's sleeping too much or too little between feedings, your pediatrician will have advice. The doctor will also weigh your baby. Your baby will be weighed at regular intervals throughout her first year of life. The pediatrician will also plot your baby's height, weight, and head circumference on charts, allowing for growth patterns to be observed over a period of time.

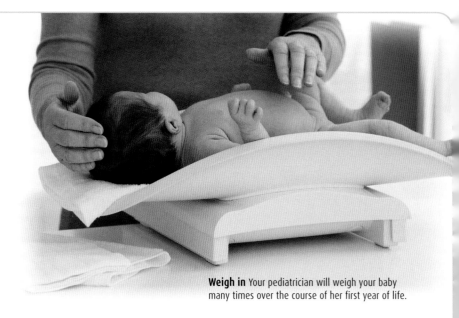

Weigh in Your pediatrician will weigh your baby many times over the course of her first year of life.

The average newborn weight is **7 lb 8 oz (3.4 kg) for boys** and **7 lb 4 oz (3.3 kg) for girls.** It is normal for babies to lose some of their birth weight in the first week and then regain it.

Q The doctor said she will do a heel-prick test on my baby in the first week. What exactly is it?

This quick procedure, also known as the "blood spot" or Guthrie test, checks for a number of conditions. This test is not compulsory, but it is recommended since the benefits of early screening are enormous. Early treatment can improve the health of your baby and prevent severe disability. You should be given information about this test and the diseases it screens for in advance so you can make an informed decision for your baby.

The test is done two or three days after the birth. The doctor will prick your baby's heel to collect a blood sample on a card, which is then sent off for analysis. Your baby may feel a little discomfort during this test, which can be upsetting for parents, too. Holding and cuddling your baby and feeding him while the test is being done is thought to minimize any discomfort your baby feels. The heel-prick test screens for nine conditions: the genetic blood disorder sickle-cell disease; cystic fibrosis, an inherited condition; congenital hypothyroidism, a condition that affects growth and mental development; and six inherited metabolic diseases such as MCADD and phenylketonuria (PKU).

You should receive the results by the time your baby is about eight weeks old. If any of the screens are positive, it means your baby is more likely to have one of these conditions and he will be referred for further testing.

Q My baby is hardly gaining weight. Should I be worried?

It's easy to worry if you think your baby isn't piling on the pounds. Watching a baby's weight steadily creep up is a reassuring sign for parents that they are getting it right. However, some babies are just naturally slower at gaining weight. If your baby is happy, alert, responsive, and reaching milestones, he is probably fine. If you feel uneasy, talk to your pediatrician who can check your baby's growth chart. If your baby has gone down two percentiles, or has dropped below the third percentile for growth, more checks and investigations may be recommended.

A failure to gain weight usually happens when a baby isn't getting the calories he needs, or his body isn't absorbing or using nutrients properly. There is often a simple explanation. If your baby has been sick, he may have lost weight and it can take a couple of weeks for his feeding to get back on track. Alternatively, he may not be latching on (see pp.268–69) properly and this can affect his milk intake. If this is the case, seek guidance from your doctor or a breast-feeding consultant.

If your baby is formula fed, make sure the bottle is made up with the right ratio of powder to water so that he gets the nutrients he needs to grow and thrive. Occasionally, slow weight gain is due to a milk intolerance or allergy, reflux, or, more rarely, a medical condition.

Q When should I try to get my baby into a routine?

In the early weeks it is a good idea to begin to teach your baby the difference between day and night, but don't worry about a routine yet.

This can be hard and you may also need to surrender yourself to your baby's world by sleeping when he sleeps, if possible. He has arrived in your world with his own around-the-clock schedule.

Newborn babies sleep for much of the time, around 14 to 18 hours in every 24, but this sleep is broken up into segments. Your baby's tiny tummy can hold only a little food, so he needs to wake every two to three hours to be fed. As your baby and his tummy grow, he will be able to go longer between being fed and a routine will emerge. A degree of flexibility is key, though—accept that sometimes your baby's needs may vary from the routine.

During these first few weeks you can subtly introduce the idea of night and day: dimming lights, reducing activity in the evening, and gradually introducing an end-of-day wind down that will evolve into a bedtime routine. Your baby will need to be fed at night for a while and it is a good idea to give these in a calm, quiet environment. If you can see past the fatigue, try to cherish these first special weeks with your new baby. This time spent cocooned with her is fleeting, and you are likely to look back on it with a sense of awe.

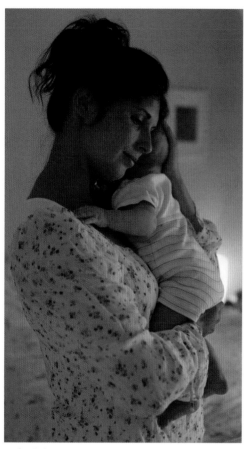

Night shift Try to help your baby understand the difference between day and night by dimming lights.

After **six weeks** your baby may begin to sleep for longer periods during the night and slightly less during the day.

Q Why is my baby often fussy when I put him down for a nap?

This happens if you miss the nap-time window, since overstimulation and overtiredness make it harder for your baby to settle down. In the first three months, your baby will start to have longer periods of alertness between naps, but he will still be doing a lot of sleeping around the clock, so it's important that he gets his daytime naps. It can be tricky to time naps since babies can move quickly from being awake and alert to being a little tired, then extremely tired. The moment to put your baby down is that period when tiredness is just starting to kick in, since this is the moment he will be best able to settle down to sleep. Tiredness cues can be as subtle as glancing away or looking a bit glazed. He may become fidgety and make jerky movements, and may clench his fists, tug his ears, or flutter his eyelids. Look for all these cues.

Q My baby often cries when he's at home with me. Is he bored?

At home, it may often be just the two of you, and the onus to keep your baby entertained and happy falls on your shoulders, which can feel like a burden. Don't try to entertain him every waking minute. He will thrive on the one-on-one attention he gets during 10 minutes of uninterrupted time with you, and he is then likely to coo happily on his play mat for 20 minutes, or be content watching you as you get on with chores.

Moving your baby around the house with you will help him feel secure and confident that you are close by, and this can make him less fretful. Newborns enjoy looking at the world around them so place him by an interesting house plant, a window, or patterned wallpaper to keep him fascinated, and keep changing the view. Remember that your baby knows that you are the one who meets his needs, and his cries are his way of communicating with you—when it's just the two of you, he may be more focused on his needs.

Q My friends and family want to visit the baby. How can I manage the visits so I am not overwhelmed?

When you return home from the hospital, you and your baby need plenty of time to adjust. Eager visitors need to understand this and their expectations should be managed. It is a good idea to invite them for a short visit and limit visits to one or two per day with space between them. Let them know when you are tired and need to rest. Close friends and famiy may want to help so try to think of a task to give them such as shopping or small household chores.

 Did you know...

As little as 5–10 minutes of deep relaxation can refresh you. Instead of doing housework, try taking a short nap while your baby sleeps. It is a good idea to learn about different relaxation techniques either online or from your local library.

Q What help is available during the early weeks if I feel that I am beginning to struggle?

Taking care of a newborn can be chaotic, tiring, and sometimes overwhelming. Depending on your personal circumstances, you may want some extra, paid help when you return home from the hospital.

There are various options available and it is important to remember that paid child care is generally not cheap. Speak to other mothers for recommendations of good nanny agencies. Magazines and newspapers are also a good source of child-care advertisements. With all forms of child care, it is vital to follow up all the references.

Maternity nurse She will help you take care of your baby in the early weeks. These are generally the most expensive form of child care since they usually live in and cover 24 hours a day, six days a week. Most people employ a maternity nurse for about six weeks. Their role is to help with daytime care as well as taking care of your baby at night, bringing them to you to be fed, and settling them down afterward.

Night nurse If you need help with nighttime duties, this can be a good option. However, the difference between this kind of help and that of a maternity nurse is that they go home during the day and simply come to help with feeding and settling your baby at night. Night nurses can be useful if your partner cannot share the night feedings. Some people choose to have them a couple of nights a week.

Doula This is an experienced woman who offers practical and emotional (nonmedical) support to a mother during and/or after childbirth. Employing a doula as a caregiver has become popular. The time they spend with you is flexible and can range from a few visits at the beginning to fixed hours for a period of eight weeks. They provide breast-feeding support, help around the house, and let you catch up on a few hours of much-needed sleep.

Q How should I plan for my baby's first trip outside?

Getting out of the house with a young baby can be nerve racking and challenging. However, with a little preparation and planning you'll be able to make your first trip easier and more enjoyable. The first thing to remember is that you'll need to be able to transport your baby reliably and safely when you are out. If you are going by car, you are legally obligated to have an age-appropriate car seat. Think about whether it would be easier to have your baby in a front pack or stroller. If you are using public transportation, it might be a good idea to find out if there are stairs to negotiate. If you are

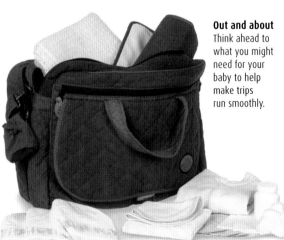

Out and about Think ahead to what you might need for your baby to help make trips run smoothly.

driving, plan the route, allowing for more stops for feeding and changing your baby. For a first trip outside, try not to be too ambitious. You will still be recovering from the birth so will need to take care of yourself as well as your baby. Whether you are going for a longer drive or walking to local stores, preparation is key.

A diaper bag is vital for any trip outside and should contain the following items:
» diapers
» wipes
» burp cloths
» change of baby clothes
» sunscreen (in the summer)
» spare clothing for yourself in case your baby regurgitates a lot on you.
» a sanitized bottle and formula if your baby is bottle-fed. (See also p.281).

Q Why do I have to take my baby to see the doctor at six weeks?

Your baby's checkup at six weeks old (though it can be up to eight weeks) is an opportune moment to check that everything is on track. This is done at your doctor's office, and you will also be given a postpartum checkup at this time (see p.259). You may have specific questions about your baby's care, feeding, and sleep patterns, or want to discuss any concerns you have. You can also learn about the

immunization program that your baby will follow into childhood.

The six-week checkup monitors your baby's progress. The doctor will examine her hips to make sure they are still positioned correctly; listen for any heart irregularities such as a heart murmur; check the alignment of her spine and that there is no dimple at its base that could indicate a nerve problem. For boys, the opening of the penis and the position of the testes will be checked, and for girls, the vaginal area.

Although these things will have already been checked at birth, they are sometimes not detectable until your baby is a bit older. For example, at this point your baby's eyes can be examined to see if she can focus on and follow a moving object. You will be asked whether your baby is smiling and socializing well, and making gurgling and cooing noises as expected. If there are any problems you will be referred to a specialist.

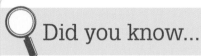 Did you know...

Many hospitals in the US make it easy for you to register your baby for her very own Social Security number. They'll provide you with the paperwork when they give you the forms to file for her birth certificate.

Q My baby is plumper than other babies the same age. Am I overfeeding her?

It's likely that you just have a plump baby on your hands. Your baby will double her body weight in the first three months. Until she is on the move, her sedentary lifestyle means that her muscles are yet to develop and she will gain a covering of fat.

Some babies are naturally bigger—much is dependent on genetics. Any differences usually iron out by toddlerhood. However, with a global rise in obesity, it's worth being aware of potential pitfalls of weight gain.

Formula-fed babies

A cohort of studies shows that breast-fed babies tend to be leaner, largely because they tend to stop drinking milk when they've had their fill. If your baby is formula fed, be careful that you are paying attention to her "full-up" cues. It may be tempting to encourage her to finish a bottle, but if she loses interest in a feeding before the end, perhaps becoming restless and turning her head, she is signaling that her tummy is full. When parents ignore these natural cues, however well intentioned, they are encouraging a habit of overeating that can continue throughout childhood and beyond.

TIPS FOR A HEALTHY BABY WEIGHT

Don't become too focused on your baby's weight, but do be aware of the following guidelines:

» Regular checkups: your pediatrician can check your baby's weight and length charts and advise you if they think there is a concern. If your baby has moved up two percentiles on her growth chart, this could flag a weight issue that needs attention.

» Sleep: getting enough sleep is linked to a healthy metabolism and weight control; at three months, your baby needs around 15 hours of sleep a day, so putting healthy sleep routines in place is important.

» Starting solids correctly: starting solids before four to six months has been shown to adversely affect weight, so don't be in a hurry to get your baby onto baby rice. When you do start solids, introduce plenty of fruit and vegetable purées among the rice and cereals.

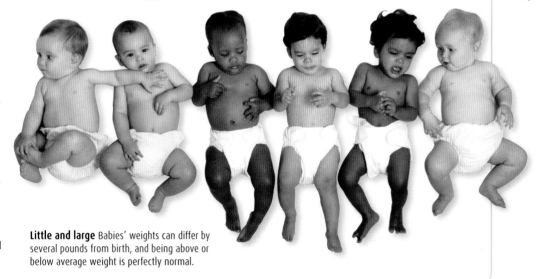

Little and large Babies' weights can differ by several pounds from birth, and being above or below average weight is perfectly normal.

Q Should I be concerned that my child is lagging behind others of the same age in our baby group?

The rate at which babies reach certain milestones can vary enormously. Socializing with parents who have babies of the same age is beneficial, but it can make you anxious as to whether your baby is doing everything she should be doing for her age and stage.

The truth is that while babies follow the same developmental progression, they do so at their own pace. Your baby develops in four areas: physically; verbally; socially; and cognitively. Learning in one area is often linked to skill acquisition in another arena. But often, a certain skill set takes a back seat while your baby spends time concentrating on something else. For example, while one baby may tirelessly swipe at objects on her play mat, another may be concentrating on the new noises she can make, fascinated by the coos and gurgles she is producing. Eventually both babies will build muscle strength and develop their communication skills.

As long as your baby has the opportunities and stimulation to learn new skills, often the actual learning of a new skill is more important than the time frame for when the skill is mastered. For example, if a developmental chart suggests your baby will walk between 12 and 15 months, and she doesn't take her first step until 17 months, this doesn't mean that there is a problem. If you are concerned about any aspect of your baby's development, always seek advice and reassurance from your baby's pediatrician.

If you have **twin babies,** try not to compare their development too closely. Remember, **they are individuals** and will each develop at their own rate.

Q When will my baby have to be immunized?

Your baby should have received his first immunization in the hopsital. His immunization program will continue through his first year and beyond, with additional vaccinations at his doctor appointments at 1, 2 4, 6, and 12 months.

IMMUNIZATION PROGRAM

In addition to newborn shots, further vaccinations are given in early childhood and in the adolescent years. A detailed breakdown of the immunization program is given in this table.

AGE	VACCINE RECEIVED	REASON
Birth	HepB	Protects against hepatitis B
1–2 months	HepB	Second dose
2 months	DtaP	Protects against diphtheria, tetanus, and pertussis (whooping cough)
	RV	Protects against rotavirus
	Hib	Protects against Haemophilus influenzae type b
	PCV13	Protects against Pneumococcal conjugate
4 months	IPV	Protects against poliovirus
	DTaP	Second dose
	RV	Second dose
	Hib	Second dose
	PCV13	Second dose
	IPV	Protects against poliovirus
6 months	DTaP	Third dose
	RV (in some cases)	Third dose (depends on the vaccine used)
	Hib (in some cases)	Third dose (depends on the vaccine used)
	PCV13	Third dose
6–18 months	HepB	Third dose
	IPV	Third dose
6–24 months	IIV	Inactivated influenza vaccine should be given annually to protect against influenza (flu); one or two doses may be required the first year. After age two, the annual vaccine can either be IIV or LAIV (live attenuated influenza vaccine).
12–15 months	Hib	Third or fourth dose
	PCV13	Fourth dose
	MMR	Protects against measles, mumps, and rubella (German measles)
	VAR	Protects against varicella (chicken pox)
15–18 months	DTaP	Fourth dose

Q What exactly do immunizations do and why are they needed?

Being immunized protects your baby from developing potentially serious illnesses. Immunity is a natural, learned process in the body; once we are exposed to an infection, our body creates antibodies to resist it in the future. A vaccine is a very diluted version of a disease, usually given by injection, designed to let your baby develop immunity to the disease without actually catching it.

All new babies have some immunity from their mother, but this effect wears off after about two months, which is why immunizations begin after this age.

Q My friend said my baby doesn't have to have immunizations. Is it true that I can refuse them?

Your consent will be asked before any of the routine vaccines offered for your baby (see chart, left) are given. If you decide against allowing your baby to have a vaccination, your pediatrician should report this in your baby's records.

Do, however, carefully weigh the benefits against potential risks before deciding not to immunize your child. Vaccination programs have successfully managed to significantly reduce or eliminate many serious and fatal diseases. If you don't vaccinate your child, you are not just increasing your child's risk of contracting a disease, but you are also affecting what's termed "herd immunity"—an effect of vaccination that makes it difficult for a disease to pass around the general populace when enough people have been immunized.

Side effects

The side effects of vaccinations tend to be mild (see opposite)—more serious side effects are rare. Some parents worry that having several vaccinations at one time could weaken their young baby's immune system. However, just a tiny fraction of the immune system is involved in creating the antibodies against live vaccines. In reality, your baby is exposed to many bacteria and viruses that are far stronger than the weakened bacteria and viruses given in vaccines, and his body handles these perfectly well.

Q How can I prepare for my baby's injections and comfort him after?

Like most new parents, you may feel ill at ease about taking your baby for his immunizations but rest assured it is a very quick and efficient procedure.

Your young baby will be unaware that he is being immunized, but he may pick up on your tension if you feel stressed. While it's a natural instinct to be concerned, try to stay as relaxed as possible and remember that being immunized is in your baby's best interests.

Try not to plan anything else for that day, before or after the immunizations, so that you don't feel rushed and have proper time to focus on your baby's needs afterward.

What happens

When you take your baby to the doctor's office for his immunization, the nurse may suggest that you sit him on your lap while the injection is given. He will be soothed by your presence, touch, and voice, so talk to him gently, and give him a reassuring hug as he is immunized. You may also want to breast-feed your baby while he is being injected, which will be comforting

for him and provide a distraction from the shot. Some babies may not even cry or have a reaction if they are nursing when they receive their vaccinations. Your baby will most likely receive his vaccinations at his regular well-visit appointments, unless you're told to make a separate appointment.

Giving pain relief

If your baby develops a fever and seems uncomfortable, you can give the recommended dose of infant acetaminophen or ibuprofen, and continue with his regular feedings to keep him well hydrated.

It's very important that you do not give a dose of pain relief before an immunization, in anticipation of your baby developing a fever, because doing this could compromise the effectiveness of the vaccine.

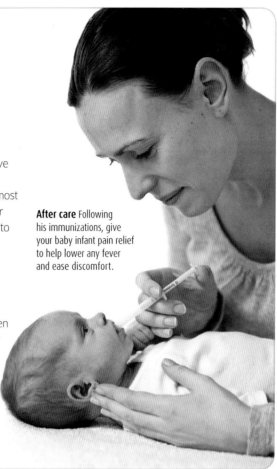

After care Following his immunizations, give your baby infant pain relief to help lower any fever and ease discomfort.

 Did you know...

Vaccination programs have been extremely effective around the world. For example, in 1914 in England and Wales there were approximately 60,000 cases of diphtheria, which caused 5,800 deaths. Following the introduction of the vaccine in 1942, there were 41,404 known cases and 1,827 deaths from the disease. By 1946, the diphtheria death rate had fallen to just 472.

In Japan in 1974, around 70 percent of Japanese children were being vaccinated against whooping cough and there were only 393 cases in all of Japan. When immunizations rates began to drop, only 10 percent of children were being vaccinated. The result was that more than 13,000 people developed whooping cough in 1979, of which 41 died. When children began to be routinely vaccinated again, the cases of whooping cough fell again.

Q Will there be any side effects from the immunizations?

It's natural to worry about possible side effects from vaccinations, but these tend to be mild and short-lived if they occur at all. There may be some local swelling and redness, and possibly a small lump at the injection site (usually the top of the thigh), all of which are harmless and disappear within a couple of days.

Occasionally babies develop a fever after an injection, in which case infant acetaminophen can be given. It's very rare for babies to have an allergic reaction to a vaccination. If it does happen, it is treatable.

Premature babies have immunizations at the same age as other babies—**their immunity** from their mother lasts the **same two months.**

Q My baby has eczema. Can he still have his immunizations?

Having an allergy, such as eczema, asthma, or any type of food intolerance, does not prevent your baby from being immunized. The only reasons for not immunizing your baby on a particular day would be if he had a fever, in which case the appointment would be rescheduled. If you are concerned that your child is not well enough on that day, seek advice from the doctor. If your child had a previous bad reaction to an immunization, (although this is rare) again, seek advice from the pediatrician

---

Q Is it true that I can't take my baby swimming until he has had his shots?

It is a common myth that babies can't go swimming before they have their injections. You can take your baby swimming at any time before or after he has been immunized.

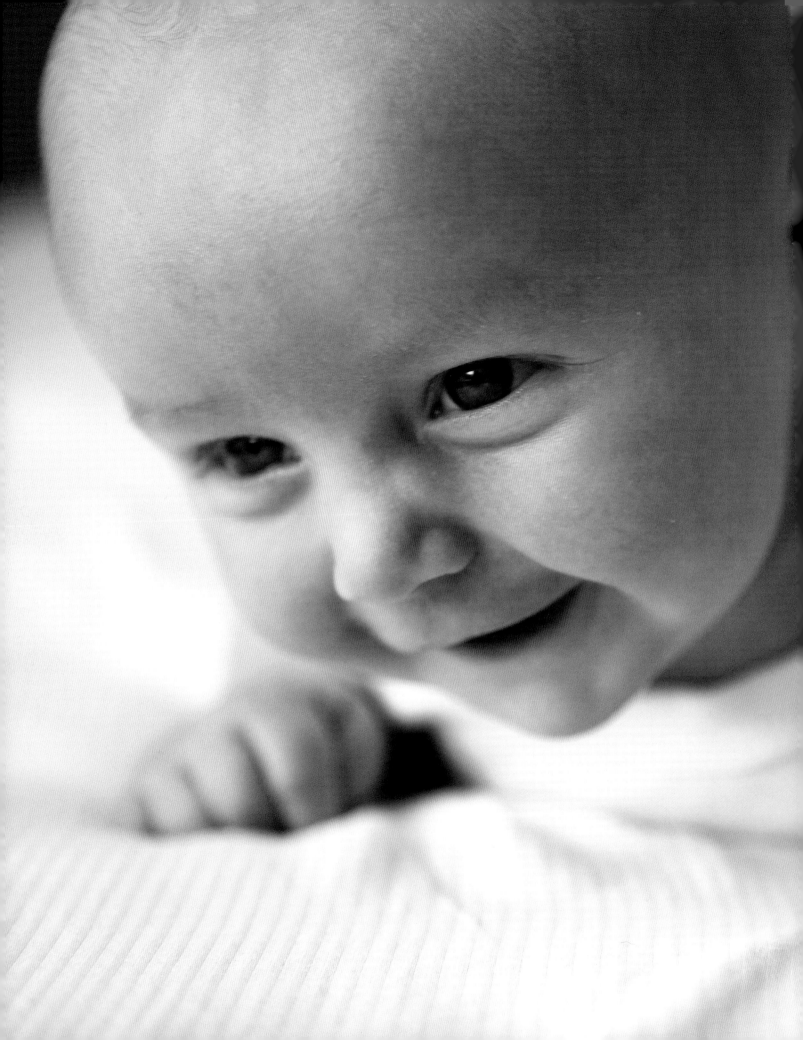

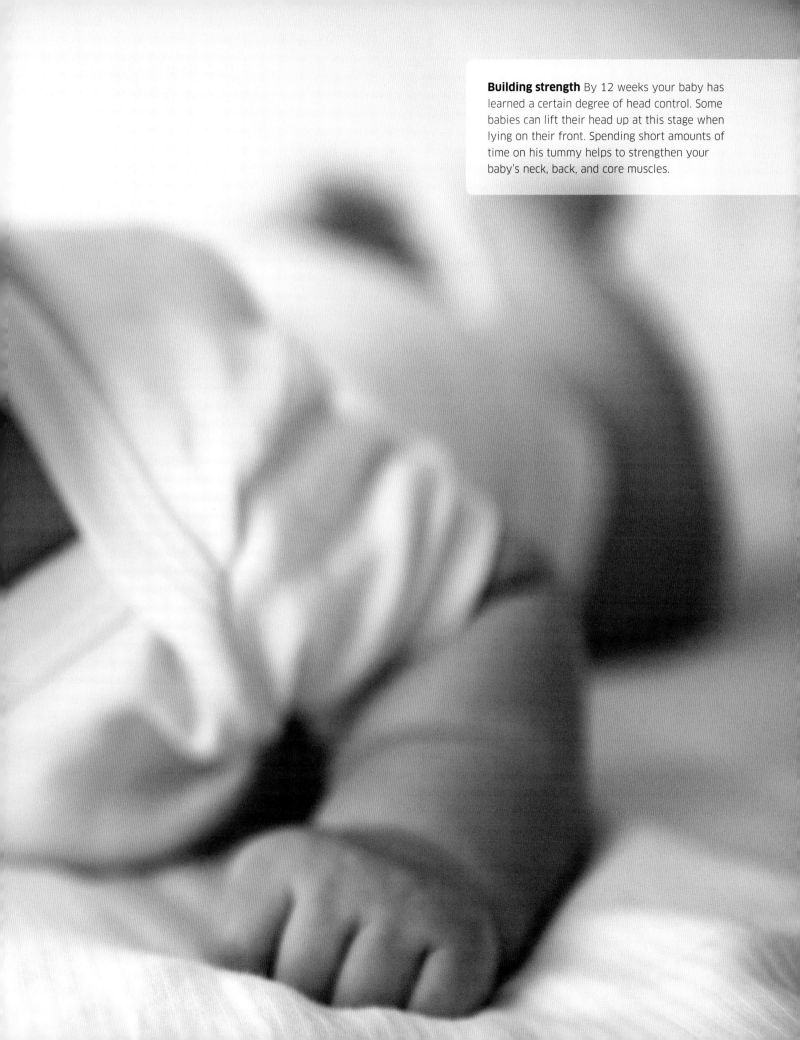

Building strength By 12 weeks your baby has learned a certain degree of head control. Some babies can lift their head up at this stage when lying on their front. Spending short amounts of time on his tummy helps to strengthen your baby's neck, back, and core muscles.

It's really important to **take care of yourself** as well as your new baby. Being in labor will leave you exhausted, or you might have had a C-section. Either way, you will need time to recover as well as adapt to your new life. Your body will also undergo an **enormous amount of change** as you return to your prepregnant state.

Birth recovery

Physical impact

Whatever type of labor and birth you had, you will be feeling the physical effects. You are likely to be exhausted, especially if you had a long labor. If you tore or had an episiotomy (a cut to the vagina and perineal area), you will be sore from the stitches, which can make sitting uncomfortable and may sting when you urinate. If you had a cesarean section, you will be recovering from major abdominal surgery, which takes several weeks. You will need to take it easy and draw on all the support you can.

Your body has done an amazing job in the past nine months, and now it will begin to return to its prepregnancy state, which will involve some dramatic hormonal changes. Your breasts will start to fill with milk to feed your baby.

Emotional roller coaster

Your emotions after birth can swing wildly: one minute you feel intensely happy, imbued with the joy of motherhood as you nestle in with your new baby, but the next moment you may feel anxious and weepy as exhaustion sets in. Hormones play havoc with your emotions, and you may feel an odd sense of emptiness since, bereft of your belly, you have lost the intimacy of carrying your baby around with you. Most women experience "the baby blues" a few days after the birth. In the middle of this physical and emotional upheaval, you are trying to deal with one of the most important tasks of your life: taking care of your new baby. This is the time to accept all the support you can get. The most significant being from your partner, who is there to hold the helm in the first few days while you recover, and give you the emotional and physical support you need.

Help from family and friends over the coming weeks will make a real and valuable contribution and each gesture will make all the difference—whether it's having meals cooked, ironing done, or simply letting someone take care of your baby for an hour or two while you sleep Be honest with those close to you about what you need.

Give yourself time

While six weeks is often talked about as the period of time it takes to recover from birth, this figure is somewhat arbitrary. A recent study found that women need a year to recover completely and get back on track after birth, so it's vital to go slowly. Give yourself time to put your feet up, and to concentrate on you: eat well, find ways to relax, and gradually regain your activity levels, eventually returning to a gentle exercise regimen. All of these things will help you to recover well.

Q I'm experiencing what feel like mild labor pains. What's happening?

Your uterus doesn't stop working right after the delivery. Having stretched ten-fold during pregnancy, it begins the job of returning to its prepregnancy size—a process known as involution.

As your uterus shrinks back down, you will experience cramping pains, like mild labor contractions, commonly called "after pains." These are generally quite manageable, especially in a first pregnancy, when the previously unstretched muscles are stronger and able to contract back down more easily.

If you do find the pains too much to bear, seek advice from your doctor. You can take acetaminophen for the pain and you can also try using the breathing techniques you used in labor. You may notice that the pains are stronger when you breast-feed; this is because the hormone oxytocin released during breast-feeding to let down your milk is the same one that encouraged uterine contractions. While you may not welcome the stronger sensation, breast-feeding helps your uterus to contract back down more quickly. It takes up to six weeks for your uterus to get back to its prepregnancy size. Pains are usually felt most strongly in the first week or so, and many women find they are barely noticeable after this time.

YOUR SHRINKING UTERUS

Within a couple of days of the birth, your uterus will be the size it was about midway through your pregnancy. It will then rapidly reduce in size, until at about six weeks after birth it is no bigger than a plum (the size it is prepregnancy).

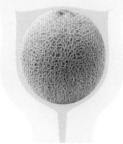 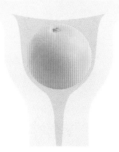 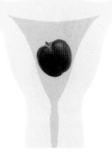

One to two days after birth
By this time, the uterus is about the size of a cantaloupe melon and weighs around 1 lb (450 g).

Seven days after birth A week after giving birth your uterus is approximately the size of grapefruit and weighs around 11 oz (300 g).

Six weeks after birth Some weeks after the birth the uterus is no bigger than a plum and weighs around 3½ oz (100 g).

Q I'm shocked by the heavy bleeding. Is this normal?

It's completely normal: as the uterus shrinks, it sheds blood and tissue called lochia. At first it's like a heavy period, but then tails off. Lochia changes from red to a watery pink color, and then becomes a yellow discharge. Wear a sanitary pad since a tampon could infect the uterus. Heavy bleeding can last up to two weeks. Seek medical help if: the bleeding becomes heavy and red again after having lightened; is so heavy that you need more than one sanitary pad an hour; you pass large clots of blood; the discharge is smelly; or you feel feverish or dizzy. Excessive bleeding anytime from 24 hours to six weeks after the birth is known as secondary postpartum hemorrhage (PPH). This may happen because part of the placenta is still attached to the lining of the uterus.

Q When is my follow-up appointment and what will the OB/GYN check?

Your "six-week checkup" can take place six to eight weeks after the birth, (your bleeding/lochia should have stopped flowing by then). The doctor will check your blood pressure and examine your abdomen to make sure that your uterus has returned to the correct size. Your doctor may examine any stitches or scars to check that everything has healed. Make an appointment sooner if you have any physical effects of breast-feeding (e.g. blocked milk ducts or mastitis) that need treatment. Your doctor will also advise you about contraception. This is a chance to talk about how you're feeling, so be honest so he or she can direct you to support.

It is possible to become pregnant while you are still breast-feeding, so don't rely on it as a form of contraception.

Q Why is my cesarean-section scar sensitive to touch and painful?

It's normal for your scar to feel tender to the touch while it's healing. You have had a major incision and your body is undergoing the complex job of knitting back together the layers of muscles and fibers to seal the wound.

As the wound site heals, it's common to experience some pain, especially if you move in an awkward way and "catch" your scar. Be careful how you move around. Gradually building up your activity levels will give the wound time to heal. It may not be glamorous, but for comfort, wear big pants (or your partner's boxer shorts). Smaller pants are likely to rub against your scar, causing discomfort.

Aside from the first couple of days after a cesarean section, when even the slightest movement can be extremely painful and you have to make careful, small steps, often with support, the pain should be fairly manageable, albeit with some soreness. If you take your analgesics regularly, you should feel quite comfortable, perhaps experiencing occasional twinges if you overdo things or are especially tired. If after the initial couple of days pain feels extreme, constant, or seems to be getting worse, and if the scar is red and inflamed, be sure to talk to your doctor.

The collagen that makes up scar tissue tends to be less elastic than the original tissue, and when the new collagen fibers form, they often do so in a haphazard fashion, which can cause hardness and restrict movement in surrounding tissues.

Adhesions can also develop, where the scar tissue sticks to surrounding tissues and other organs, which can cause discomfort. Once your scar is well healed, usually at around six weeks, some gentle fingertip massage can help to soften scar tissue, break up adhesions that may be forming, and also improve circulation, which in turn promotes good healing. Rubbing in some vitamin E oil can also help. In addition, a healthy lifestyle will help the incision heal well and reduce discomfort. Gentle walking is perfect exercise after a cesarean section.

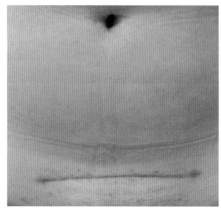

Time to heal To begin with the C-section scar, which is usually along the bikini line, will look very red. As it heals, the redness will fade. It is normal to experience some itchiness as the scar heals.

layers of muscle and skin slowly knit back together. As with any major surgery, trying to do too much too soon can set you back. At six weeks, your scar may look fairly well-healed, but there is still internal healing taking place.

If you feel a sharp twinge while attempting something strenuous, such as picking up a heavy bag, it's a sign to rest. Continue to be careful with how you move around, for example get out of bed by rolling onto your side, and avoid lifting heavy weights for two to three months after the birth.

Some women experience pain from trapped gas after a cesarean section. Eat a fiber-rich diet, drink plenty of fluids, and chew food slowly. The trapped air can irritate the diaphragm and cause shoulder-tip pain; drinking peppermint water or peppermint tea can help. While rest is essential, gentle activity is also important for improving circulation, which reduces the risk of conditions such as deep vein thrombosis and also promotes healing.

Q I feel disappointed that the birth didn't go as I'd planned. How can I come to terms with it?

All pregnant women are encouraged to write a birth plan (see p.88), but this may not come to fruition on that day. Events might have unfolded very differently from how you had hoped; you might feel that you lacked control throughout labor, and birth may not have been the joyous occasion that you envisioned it to be. However, with time you will come to terms with your feelings of disappointment.

The best way to deal with your experience and help yourself to resolve any feelings of disappointment or failure is to talk to people about what happened—to your partner, family, and, in particular, the obstetrician. If this doesn't happen before you leave the hospital, make an appointment to speak to him or her at a later date. If you become pregnant again, discuss what happened with your doctor so that you can, if possible, avoid the same experience again. You can also speak to friends about your experience or read online forums. You will soon feel that you're not alone and that it's completely normal to feel disappointed, upset, or even angry at how things went.

Try not to blame yourself or your baby for what took place and speak to your doctor if you are feeling anxious or depressed.

Q Did you know...

After a C-section, you can begin doing Kegel exercises (see pp.66–67) as soon as you feel ready. If those feel comfortable, you can go for short walks to work your lower abdominal muscles. After six weeks, you can begin light sit-ups, and gentle cycling, walking, or swimming—build your pace up slowly in periods of 10 minutes at a time. Stop if you are in pain and consult your doctor.

Q I'm still getting pains four weeks after my C-section. Is this normal?

It's very common to feel twinges as your body heals. The incisions through your abdominal wall, the underlying muscles, and your uterus understandably need time to join back together. The recovery time varies, but it is often six to eight weeks before you feel back to normal after this major surgery.

Women usually experience an improvement after a few days, but while it becomes easier to move around, there may be considerable tenderness at the incision site as the various

Q How long will it take for my body to get back to normal?

Once you've had your baby, it's understandable that you want to feel like your old self again. It may, however, take several months for your body to return to normal so be patient and don't expect too much too soon.

There is no such thing as a **miracle cream** to get rid of stretch marks, but using moisturizer will keep your skin **smooth and supple**.

BODY CHANGES

Your body has been affected by growing and carrying your baby, so some physical changes are perfectly normal.

» **Breasts:** your breasts become swollen and hard, and may be sore as your milk comes in a few days after birth. This usually eases as breast-feeding becomes established.

» **Skin:** most women are left with some stretch marks. These are caused by the collagen beneath your skin tearing as it stretches to accommodate your growing baby. They may not go completely but they will fade with time.

» **Pelvic floor muscles:** you may have temporary urinary incontinence, so find that a little bit of urine seeps out when you laugh, sneeze, or cough. Do Kegel exercises (see p.67) to strengthen the muscles.

» **Hair:** due to changes in estrogen levels, it's normal to experience some hair loss for six to 12 months after the birth.

» **Abdomen:** your abdominal and pelvic muscles will be slack. If you had a vaginal delivery, you can do gentle abdominal exercises in the first few weeks. If you had a C-section, wait until after your six-week checkup.

» **Bladder:** the trauma on the bladder can put you at risk of a urinary-tract infection. Drink plenty of water to reduce the risk of this happening.

» **Anus:** many women develop hemorrhoids, (see p.132), in late pregnancy. Eat plenty of fiber and drink lots of water to ease bowel movements. Use an over-the-counter ointment on the affected area.

Q I had stitches because I tore during the delivery. What can I do to ease the discomfort?

It's normal to feel discomfort and soreness as this area heals and there are several ways to ease the discomfort. Using analgesics will help you feel less pain. It can also help to apply towel-wrapped ice packs to your perineum, no longer than an hour at a time, in the first couple of days. Keep the perineum clean to avoid an infection, washing your hands before touching the area and bathing or showering regularly. Two or three drops of pure essential oils added to bath water can soothe perineal discomfort; lavender, geranium, and chamomile are recommended. Kegel exercises help blood flow to the perineal area, which promotes healing. Pouring a pitcher of warm water over your vulva or using a water spray can be soothing and reduce the stinging sensation when you urinate. Urinating in a warm shower has the same effect. Squatting over rather than sitting on the toilet seat, or sitting with your feet and knees raised a little, can reduce stinging. Avoid getting constipated. Drink plenty of water and eat fiber-rich foods. If you had a bad tear or are constipated, you may be prescribed a mild laxative to soften your stools. Don't hold off going to the bathroom since it increases the risk of a UTI and constipation. Talk to your doctor if the area is still sore after a few weeks.

Q I'm exhausted and can hardly get out of bed. Is this normal?

It's normal to feel exhausted in the early weeks and months. Give your body time to heal. The hormone relaxin lingers in your body after the birth. In pregnancy, it makes your ligaments more elastic to deal with labor, but after the delivery, it can exacerbate complaints such as backaches and joint pain. If getting out of bed feels like an achievement, it is because it is! Sleeping when you can, eating well, and slowly becoming more active are key to recovery.

As soon as you are able, get up and **move around** because **activity** can help with many things, including getting your digestive system working.

Q I should be happy that my baby's here, so why am I weepy and overwhelmed?

Your wonderful baby may be everything you dreamed of, and yet the challenges of new parenthood can be difficult to handle. The days following your baby's birth are intense, and emotions tend to seasaw as your hormones surge and you grapple with adjusting to your new role while feeling exhausted from the birth.

A touch of the blues

The "baby blues" are experienced by women shortly after giving birth (usually around day four). The blues tend to last a day or so. During this time women feel weepy, irrational, and generally a little overwhelmed by everything.

There are various reasons for the baby blues. After birth, your body undergoes dramatic changes as it returns to its prepregnant condition. The hormones progesterone and estrogen that helped sustain your pregnancy plummet and breast-feeding hormones rapidly rise. While these hormonal swings alone can play havoc, you are also recovering from the after effects of the birth, including exhaustion, stitches, and perhaps major surgery. If you had a difficult birth experience, you may be struggling to process this. In addition, your breasts feel tender as they fill with milk, and your sleep is disrupted. Not least, you are adapting to your new role as a parent.

Feeling depressed

If, like 1 in 10 women, you still feel low and weepy beyond the baby blues, or find that negative feelings develop around one to two months after the birth, you may have postpartum depression (PPD) and should seek medical help.

SHORT-TERM BABY BLUES

There's no need to seek treatment for the baby blues since they will pass naturally as your hormones settle down, but getting adequate rest, feeling supported, and giving yourself time can make them more bearable. All these things will help with postpartum depression, too, although you will also need medical treatment.

» Getting adequate rest: we all struggle to cope when we are overly tired and when you have a new baby to take care of this can be exacerbated. After the exertion of the birth and delivery, you need quiet, restful time, which can be hard for new mothers to come by. Being inundated with visitors, coping with a noisy hospital ward, and dealing with a crying newborn and disrupted sleep are not conducive to good rest. Don't feel that you should "do it all"—putting your feet up while your baby sleeps isn't lazy, but crucial because it allows your body to recover from the birth and builds your energy back up.

» Love and understanding: partners and loved ones play a crucial role, both practically and emotionally. They need to encourage the mother to rest as much as possible while they hold the fort; be patient; allow the mother to cry and listen to her concerns; make sure she is well-nourished; and reassure her that her feelings are natural and that she will feel better soon. In turn, be honest with those around you about what you need.

» Time to adjust: having a baby may be the most life-changing event of your life, and yet it's a role that is hard to prepare for in advance. This is a period of adjustment. You need to shift your priorities and take life at a slower pace for the moment. Give yourself time and be good to yourself.

Approximately **70 percent** of new mothers experience a form of mild depression, called the "baby blues" about four days after birth.

POSTPARTUM DEPRESSION (PPD)

Be aware of the risk factors and warning signs of PPD and don't hesitate to seek support. Speak to someone as soon as you notice any of the warning signs.

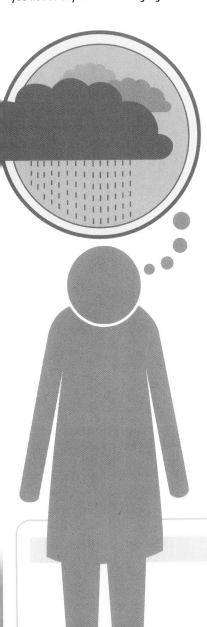

Risk factors

The risk factors listed below make it more likely you will suffer with PPD. If any of them apply to you, take steps to reduce your chances of developing the condition; it's easier to take preventative action than to motivate yourself to find help once you are depressed.

» You have been depressed before or during your pregnancy.
» You had a traumatic delivery.
» You had a recent stressful event, such as a bereavement.
» You generally have little support.

Warning signs

» You find it hard to sleep, have fitful sleep, or wake too early feeling anxious.
» You feel low-level anxiety, or perhaps feel very anxious and suffer from panic attacks.
» You feel irritable and lack concentration.
» You struggle to feel enjoyment or pleasure in life, and lack humor.
» You feel guilty and generally miserable.
» Your appetite is poor, or you overeat.
» You feel lethargic, tired, and unmotivated, and you aren't managing to take care of yourself properly.
» You feel isolated.
» You have little interest in your baby.

Support

Talk to your partner, or other loved ones, and consult your doctor if you experience any of the warning signs more than a week after the birth. Don't ignore these feelings since they are easily treatable—if left they can affect your relationship with your baby, partner, and others.

If you have suffered from depression before, the symptoms will feel familiar, although with PPD there is the added factor of how your illness impacts your baby and your relationship with him. Getting help may make all the difference in your experience of motherhood.

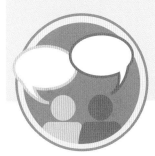

GETTING HELP

There is help available to treat PPD, so make an appointment to see your doctor as soon as possible.

Many women recover from PPD without treatment, but up to a quarter of women still have PPD after a year. In this time, their relationship with their baby will have suffered, which might affect the baby's social development.

Your doctor may refer you for talking therapy, prescribe antidepressant medication, or do both. Antidepressants may help to lift your mood to enable you to explore the root causes of your depression. There are antidepressants that are compatible with breast-feeding. Antidepressants take around two weeks to start working and need to be taken for six months to deal with the depression effectively.

Your thyroid function may be tested, since levels of the hormone thyroid can drop after pregnancy, which can cause some of the symptoms of depression.

A CLOSER LOOK
Skin to skin

Skin to skin is when you place your naked baby (except for her diaper) directly onto your bare chest. Take time to relax in each others' quiet company—time spent doing absolutely nothing other than being together is valuable bonding time, especially if you choose to do it skin to skin. Pull a sheet over you both to keep snug. Allow yourself to enjoy your baby's physical presence: her warm weight on your chest, her small hand curling around your finger, and her soft head against your cheek.

Getting acquainted The more time you spend skin to skin the quicker you will get to know each other in the early days and weeks. It's a way of communicating your love for your baby and feeling confident that you can provide for her as you have during your pregnancy.

Skin-to-skin contact This provides benefits immediately after birth. Direct contact can help you and your baby feel close throughout the first hours of her life. It's a perfect transition from the warmth and protection of your uterus to the coziness of your body.

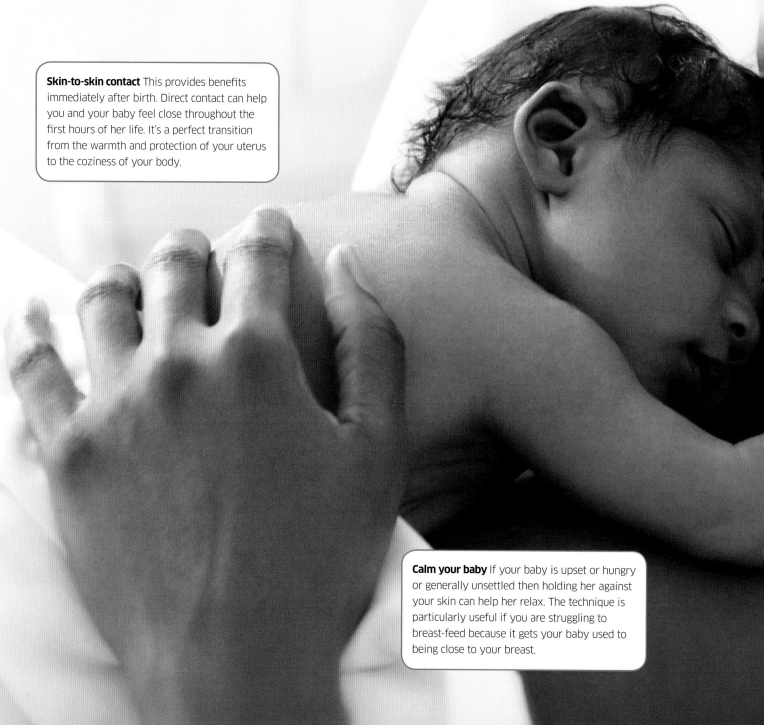

Calm your baby If your baby is upset or hungry or generally unsettled then holding her against your skin can help her relax. The technique is particularly useful if you are struggling to breast-feed because it gets your baby used to being close to your breast.

Family bonding Your partner can use skin to skin as a way to bond with your newborn. Encourage your partner to spend time alone with the baby to help build a closeness with the new addition to your family. It will give you a chance to get some sleep or rest.

FASCINATING FACTS

One hour of skin-to-skin contact immediately after birth makes a baby significantly less stressed after the trauma of the birth experience.

During skin-to-skin contact, your baby's **heartbeat and breathing** are more regular and stable.

Babies who have regular skin-to-skin contact tend to **cry less**.

Babies who have skin-to-skin contact **digest their food better**.

98.6° F (37.5° C) is the normal body temperature. During skin-to-skin contact your body helps to regulate your baby's temperature and keep it at the right level.

Skin-to-skin contact helps your baby pick up friendly bacteria from your skin, which **protect her from catching infections**.

Skin-to-skin contact **helps establish breast-feeding** because your baby can see and smell the nipple, which encourages her to feed.

Skin-to-skin contact helps **trigger your breast milk** to flow.

Skin-to-skin contact helps make you feel **more confident** that you can take care of your baby.

The milk you make for your baby is **uniquely tailored** to meet all his **nutritional needs** for about the first six months, and provide **immunity protection** at birth and beyond. The composition of this dynamic fluid constantly adapts and changes to give your baby **exactly what he needs** at each stage of his development.

Breast-feeding

Tailor-made nutrition

From the moment your baby is born, your breasts are primed to feed him, first with the pre-milk colostrum made during pregnancy and ready for your baby right away, and then, after about three days, with your breast milk. The production of breast milk is triggered by a surge in the hormone prolactin at birth.

Your milk production works on a supply-and-demand basis, so each time your baby breast-feeds, your breasts are stimulated to produce more milk for his next feeding. During growth spurts, your breasts respond to increased sucking by producing a greater quantity of milk, and in this way, your baby grows and thrives. Even if you manage only a handful of feedings in the first few days, your baby will receive concentrated nutrients and immunity-boosting antibodies that can't be obtained from formula, and that will give him the best possible start.

Benefits for you and your baby

In addition to being free and nutritionally perfect, countless breast-feeding studies point to health benefits. Breast-fed babies have fewer ear, chest, and gastrointestinal infections in the first year, and later on a lower incidence of childhood obesity and diabetes. Breast-feeding is thought to offer some protection against childhood eczema, and there are fewer incidents of Sudden Infant Death Syndrome (SIDS) in breast-fed babies. Several studies have looked at the link between breast-fed babies and higher IQs. Studies have found that breast-fed babies do better at school and beyond, regardless of wealth or class, which may be due to the high number of special fatty acids in breast milk that promote healthy neural development.

Moms also benefit from breast-feeding, often losing weight more quickly since breast-feeding burns additional calories, and the oxytocin released during breast-feeding helps the uterus contract after birth. Breast-feeding moms are also less likely to develop postpartum depression, or in the long-term, breast, ovarian, and endometrial cancers, or osteoporosis.

Getting started

Although breast-feeding is a natural process, it does not necessarily come naturally to new moms. It takes time and practice to perfect, and it can feel uncomfortable at first. Advice and support can make a real difference, so take advantage of any help provided by the hospital, and ask a breast-feeding consultant for advice when you're back home. You will soon find that you get better at reading your baby's hunger cues, which makes the feeding experience calmer and easier.

Q I've heard that "breast is best" but what exactly is in breast milk?

Your breasts won't fill with milk until three to five days after the birth. Before that time, they contain the "pre-milk" colostrum, a highly concentrated, thick, creamy-yellow substance that has countless health benefits for your baby.

Colostrum is the perfect first food, delivering vital nutrients as well as protective antibodies that give your baby an instant immune boost. Colostrum is made in very small quantities, with your baby receiving no more than a few teaspoons worth in the first few days. This amount is exactly right for your baby, whose tiny stomach is the size of a walnut.

Colostrum is protein-rich, providing amino acids for growth and development; high in carbohydrates and fat-soluble vitamins and minerals; and low in fats, which are difficult for your baby to digest at first. Key nutrients in colostrum are essential for the development of the brain, heart, and the central nervous system. Colostrum provides a high concentration of disease-fighting white blood cells, and immunoglobulins that protect against germs. It also acts as a natural laxative, triggering your baby's bowels to excrete meconimum (see p.247).

In addition to giving him colostrum, getting your newborn to nurse will stimulate your breasts to produce milk. The composition of breast milk is also highly remarkable, as outlined below.

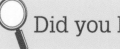

Magic milk Breast milk contains the perfect balance of nutrients, as well as protective antibodies.

WATER 88.1%

Mature breast milk is just under 90 percent water. At the beginning of a feeding, your baby receives a more watery hydrating foremilk; then, as he continues sucking, the creamier, more calorie-dense hindmilk, essential for weight gain, is released from the fat cells and makes its way more slowly up the milk ducts to the nipple. So each time your baby nurses, he receives a complete meal that both hydrates and nourishes him.

FAT 3.8%

Fats make up nearly 4 percent and are essential for growth, the development of the brain and nervous system, and easy absorption of vitamins. Breast milk is rich in long-chain polyunsaturated fatty acids, key to eye and neural development.

PROTEIN 0.9%

The main proteins in mature breast milk are whey and casein. Other specific proteins include secretory IgA, the main antibody in mature milk, which protects against ear, nose, and throat infections.

LACTOSE 7.0%

The principal carbohydrate in breast milk is lactose, which provides energy. It prevents the growth of harmful bacteria in the gut, in turn helping the absorption of essential nutrients such as calcium and phosphorus.

OTHER 0.2%

Vitamins and minerals reflect your intake. The exception is vitamin D, so it is recommended that you take a daily 10 mcg vitamin D supplement if you are breast-feeding.

Q I've been told that breast-feeding is natural, but how do I start?

f your birth is straightforward, you will be encouraged to latch your baby on right away. Hold him skin to skin, so that he can seek out your nipple. He will do this naturally if he is given uninterrupted time. Try not to rush and remember it is a new experience for him, too. Stroke his cheek to trigger his rooting reflex, talk to him, and make eye contact. If he makes mouthing and sucking movements, gently guide him to the nipple. He may suck intermittently while he gets used to the mechanics of nursing. At birth, your baby's tiny stomach holds no more than about 1 tablespoon (15ml) of milk so he needs to be fed at regular intervals.

Q Sometimes I'm breast-feeding for an hour. How long should it take?

Breast-feedings can be anything from a few minutes to an hour or more. Once feeding is more established, you will probably find it becomes more efficient and quicker. The length may be up to the baby's temperament. While some nurse enthusiastically for a short period of time, others prefer to take it more slowly, perhaps pausing for a break midway through.

It's important that you don't limit your baby's time on the breast because that could stop him from getting the fattier, nourishing hindmilk that is released from the ducts toward the end of a feeding, which satisfies his hunger and ensures healthy growth.

Did you know...

The general guideline is that newborn babies should be fed at least eight to 12 times in a 24-hour period, with feedings given evenly throughout the day and night. If your baby is very sleepy after the birth, you may need to stir him every two to three hours to offer a feeding, stroking his cheek to stimulate his rooting reflex. Feeding frequently in these first few days allows your baby to practice latching on and sucking while your breasts are relatively empty, before your milk comes in after about three days.

How can I make sure my baby is latched onto the breast correctly?

The key to successful breast-feeding—feeding that is comfortable for you and ensures your baby gets sufficient milk—is to position your baby well on the breast. There is an art to getting your little one "latched on" properly. You may not get it right until you have breast-fed a few times, but give yourself time and seek support if necessary.

Why a good latch is important

When your baby isn't latched on correctly, she will drag on your nipple rather than massage your breast tissue with her sucking. The result is sore and cracked nipples and possibly problems with milk supply, since your baby's weak sucking may not be stimulating your breasts to make enough milk. If your baby isn't emptying your breast properly, it also increases your risk of developing complications, such as mastitis (see pp.274–75), because breast milk can stagnate in the ducts and become infected.

The nurses at the hospital will help and advise you. You can also find help with breast-feeding organizations and from breast-feeding consultants.

A STEP-BY-STEP GUIDE TO LATCHING ON

Get as comfortable as possible before you begin a feeding. Choose a chair that supports your lower back, and use cushions for additional support of your back and arms if this helps. Specially designed U-shaped feeding cushions that support your baby can be helpful, especially after a cesarean section, since they bear the weight of your baby and thereby avoid putting pressure on your scar.

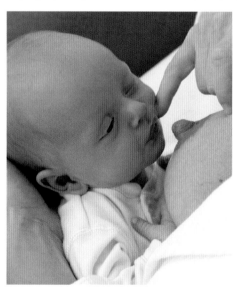

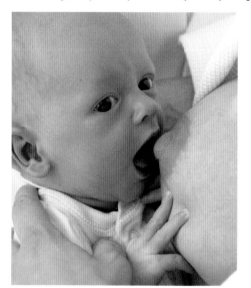

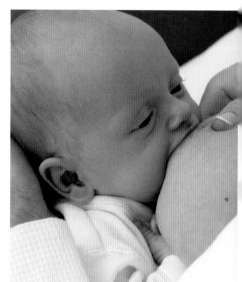

1 HOLD YOUR BABY NOSE TO NIPPLE

Position your baby facing you ("tummy to mommy") with her nose opposite your nipple. Gently support her head and shoulders with one hand. Her head and body should be in a straight line so that she doesn't have to twist to get to the nipple. Bring your baby close to your breast: her head should tilt back slightly, her chin touching your lower breast, and your nipple should be aimed toward the roof of her mouth, far closer to her top lip than the middle of her mouth. You can gently stroke her cheek with your finger or brush her nose/upper lip with your nipple, which will trigger her to open her mouth wide.

2 WAIT FOR A WIDE-OPEN MOUTH

Hold back until your baby's mouth is open very wide, as though she is yawning, before latching her on to your breast. This is crucial because she needs to suck on a good mouthful of your breast tissue. If she is sucking only on your nipple, it will be painful and cause breast-feeding problems.

3 LATCH HER ON

Once her mouth is open wide, quickly bring her onto the breast, bringing her whole body to you so she isn't craning forward. Aim your nipple toward the roof of her mouth, making sure it is well back in her mouth. If she has difficulty latching on, try using your thumb and forefinger in a U-shape to compress the nipple area a little, but don't press on the breast tissue too much.

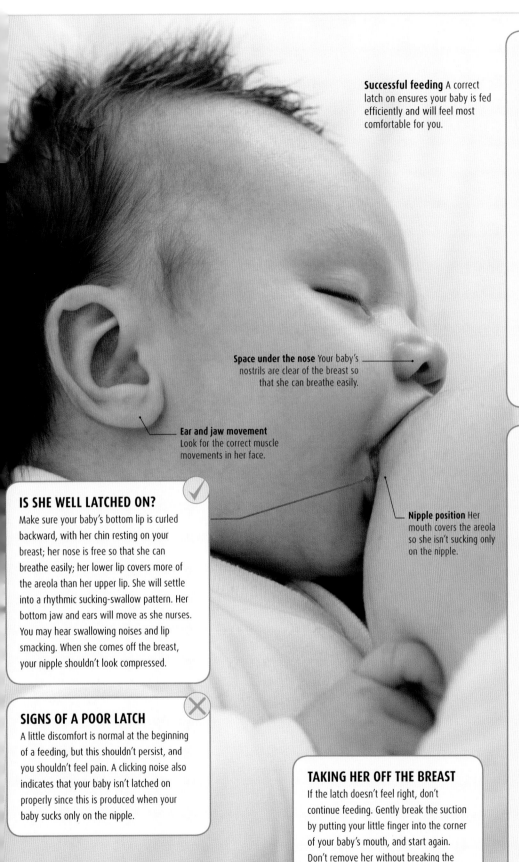

Successful feeding A correct latch on ensures your baby is fed efficiently and will feel most comfortable for you.

Space under the nose Your baby's nostrils are clear of the breast so that she can breathe easily.

Ear and jaw movement Look for the correct muscle movements in her face.

Nipple position Her mouth covers the areola so she isn't sucking only on the nipple.

IS SHE WELL LATCHED ON?

Make sure your baby's bottom lip is curled backward, with her chin resting on your breast; her nose is free so that she can breathe easily; her lower lip covers more of the areola than her upper lip. She will settle into a rhythmic sucking-swallow pattern. Her bottom jaw and ears will move as she nurses. You may hear swallowing noises and lip smacking. When she comes off the breast, your nipple shouldn't look compressed.

SIGNS OF A POOR LATCH

A little discomfort is normal at the beginning of a feeding, but this shouldn't persist, and you shouldn't feel pain. A clicking noise also indicates that your baby isn't latched on properly since this is produced when your baby sucks only on the nipple.

TAKING HER OFF THE BREAST

If the latch doesn't feel right, don't continue feeding. Gently break the suction by putting your little finger into the corner of your baby's mouth, and start again. Don't remove her without breaking the suction since this will pull on your nipple.

EARLY HUNGER SIGNS

It will be much harder to latch on a hungry baby, so learn to read her hunger cues:

» Her eyelids flutter as she stirs from sleep.
» She opens and closes her mouth and may make sucking actions and stick out her tongue.
» She puts her hand to her mouth and may suck it.
» She clenches her fist.
» She turns her head side to side and "roots" or nuzzles toward your nipple.
» She makes jerky leg and arm movements.

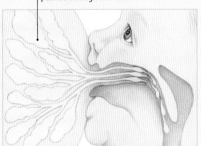

Tasty hand If your baby is sucking her hand, it is quite likely she is ready for a feeding.

THE LETDOWN REFLEX

As your baby starts sucking at your breast, nerves in your nipple are stimulated, which in turn triggers the release of hormones.

The hormone prolactin sends a signal to your breast tissues to produce more milk. The hormone oxytocin stimulates cells in your breast to release milk, which is pushed through the ducts toward the nipple, a process known as the "letdown." This can create a tingling sensation when your baby starts sucking. Some women feel a slight pain that quickly passes, or discomfort and a sensation of pressure.

Milk ducts Breast milk is pushed through the ducts

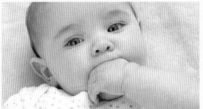

Milk flow The milk released by the letdown reflex flows toward the nipple to feed your baby.

Q How should I prepare for a feeding and what are the best positions?

Make sure you are comfortable and well supported when you settle down into a feeding session. This is key to making sure that breast-feeding goes smoothly. If it is likely to be a fairly lengthy session, make sure you have a snack and beverage on hand.

Since you will be spending a considerable amount of time sitting still while your baby nurses, you need to make sure that your upper back, shoulders, and neck aren't strained, and that your lower back and arms feel supported. If you are slouched, it can lead to back and shoulder pain and make it harder for your baby to latch on well, which in turn can result in sore nipples and other breast-feeding problems. Tension resulting from bad posture could impede your flow of milk.

Sit in a firm-backed chair, or use cushions to support your lower back so that you can hold an upright posture throughout the feeding. Try not to hunch your shoulders, which we tend to do when we are tense; instead, consciously bring them down, which is instantly relaxing.

It is possible to breast-feed twins at the same time, for example by using the football hold position (see below). Seek advice from a breast-feeding consultant about breast-feeding twins.

FEEDING POSITIONS

How you position your baby at the breast can help him nurse effectively and prevent sore nipples. If your breasts feel a bit tender or your nipples are sore, alternating positions from one feeding to another will make sure pressure is more evenly distributed around the nipple area (areola).

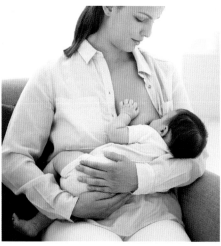

Cradle hold Sitting upright, hold your baby with his tummy facing your tummy, supporting his back and bottom. You may find it helpful to put a cushion on your lap to support your arm and your baby's weight throughout the feeding.

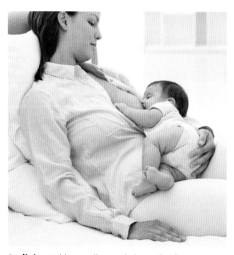

Reclining Hold or cradle your baby so that he is completely supported by you. You may find that this is a good position for night feedings. Support your back with pillows or cushions so that you are comfortable as you recline in this semi-upright position.

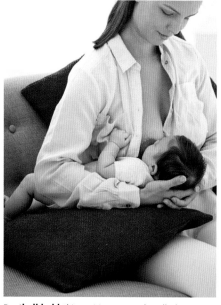

Football hold This position can work well after a C-section, since it prevents putting pressure your abdomen, or for feeding twins. Put your baby on a cushion, on the side he will nurse from, that supports his whole body. Support his head with your hand.

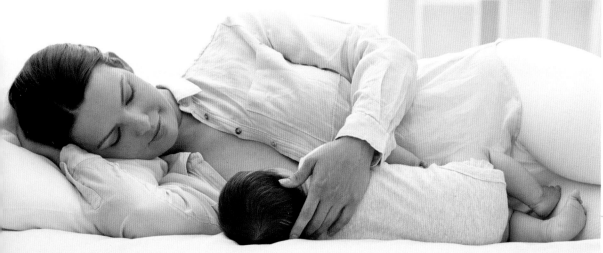

Side by side Lie on your side with your baby facing you. You may want a pillow behind you for support or to raise your body by lying on a folded blanket or towel. Prop yourself up on your elbow, or rest your head on your forearm, then use your free hand to support your baby's head and upper body and gently guide him to the breast. This relaxing position is ideal for the first feeding following a cesarean section, and while recovering from a C-section, because it avoids putting any pressure on your abdomen, and of course is perfect for nighttime feeding.

Q Should I always offer my baby both breasts at every feeding?

There are no hard and fast rules—it's best to be guided by your baby and watch out for signs that he is full. You may find that when your milk comes in, sometime during the first week, your breasts are very full and your baby may be satisfied feeding from one side only. This is fine and you just need to remember to start the next feeding session on the other side so that your

milk supply is even, and so that one nipple doesn't become sore from overuse. If you struggle to remember which side you last fed from, try switching a bracelet or hair band from one wrist to the other, or just make a note of which side you fed from.

You may find that your baby continues to be happy feeding from just one side. Or, as your milk supply settles down, your baby may want to feed from both sides in one feeding session. If he seems unsettled when you take him off the breast, try offering the second side.

It's important that your baby stays on one breast long enough to get both the watery hydrating foremilk, and the creamier hindmilk, so don't move him to the other breast too soon.

When your baby has growth spurts, which are frequent in the first weeks and months, you may find that he is dissatisfied for a day or so after just one side and needs to nurse from the second breast. If he is very hungry, you may even need to return to the first breast and nurse until he is satisfied. Your breasts will increase their supply in line with your baby's needs.

Q How do I burp my baby and is it always necessary?

It is good practice to burp your baby after a feeding because this will release any trapped air that he has swallowed along with his milk that could make him fussy, uncomfortable, and hard to settle down.

If your baby appears to be fussy midway through a feeding, perhaps squirming and coming away from the breast unsettled, he may need to be burped to release trapped air before he can continue. Bottle-fed babies (see pp.278–81) tend to take in more air.

As your baby grows, you will become accustomed to his needs, and you may find that you need to burp him routinely, or that sometimes he settles down without being burped.

Your baby may bring up, or spit up, a little of his milk when he burps—this is quite normal. Having a burp cloth ready to catch any milk spit-up can save your clothes.

If your baby suffers quite a bit with gas, try keeping him upright for around 20 minutes after a feeding since this can help to bring up trapped gas, easing his discomfort. If he's having trouble burping, try switching positions or applying a little more pressure.

BURPING POSITIONS

There are a few positions for burping. As with feeding positions, you and your baby will probably settle on the burping technique you both find most comfortable and effective.

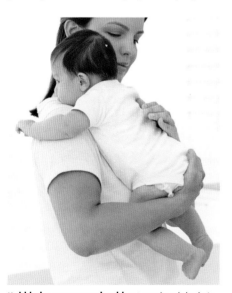

Hold baby over your shoulder A newborn's body is suited to being held upright with his head supported over your shoulder, while you gently rub or pat his back. Place a burp cloth over your shoulder to protect your clothing in case your baby spits up some milk.

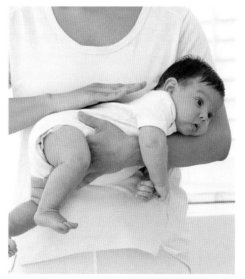

Lay baby face down Hold your baby face down across your arm or your lap, with his head a little higher than his body. Make sure his head is properly supported, then gently rub or pat his back to help release the trapped air in his tummy.

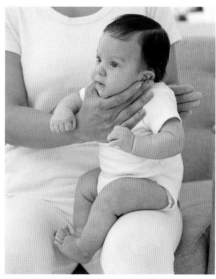

Sit baby upright, chin supported When your baby's neck muscles are a little stronger, try sitting him on your lap, your palm supporting his chest and your thumb and forefinger spread out to support his chin. Rub or pat his back.

Q What does "expressing" breast milk mean and why should I do it?

Expressing your breast milk involves extracting milk from your breasts without your baby nursing, and it is done for a whole range of reasons.

If your baby is premature or sick and unable to breast-feed, expressing means she can be fed breast milk and get the health benefits. If your breasts are full and uncomfortably engorged in the early weeks, your baby may find it tricky to latch on (see pp.268–69) to a very full breast. Expressing a little milk can reduce the fullness and make latching on easier. If your baby has a weak suck, expressing can help to stimulate your milk supply and keep this at a good level.

Expressing your breast milk also allows you to delegate feeding to someone else. Having a supply of breast milk in the freezer can be handy if you're not feeling well, or need to be away from your baby. If you are returning to work, putting in place an expressing regimen means your baby can continue enjoying your breast milk. If you are still breast-feeding at the time you start your baby on solids, you may want to express milk to mix with her baby rice or purées.

How to express

You can express breast milk with your hands or by using a pump. As you get used to expressing, you may combine methods, perhaps using your hands to stimulate the release of milk, and then a pump. Electric pumps are available to rent if you want to express for a short period, for a premature baby for example. Speak a breast-feeding organization or lactation consultant about renting one.

EXPRESSING WITH A BREAST PUMP

Before expressing, make sure that your hands are clean and that all the equipment you use has been washed and sanitized (see p.279).

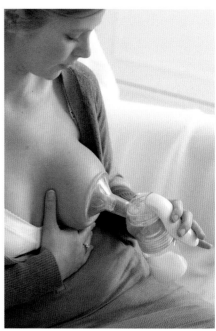

Expressing with a manual pump This is a bottle with a pump mechanism and a shield that creates a vacuum over your breast. Place the shield over your breast with the nipple area in the middle, then start pumping. Manual pumps are lightweight, but the action of pumping can be tiring.

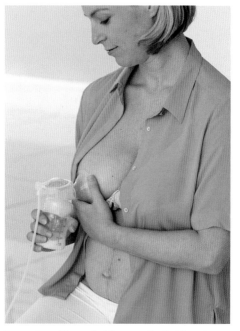

Expressing with an electric pump An electric motor does the pumping. You can usually adapt the strength of the pump to find a comfortable suction level. These pumps can be more fussy to sanitize than manual ones, but they extract milk more quickly so are a good option if you plan to do a lot of expressing.

HOW TO EXPRESS BY HAND

Have a sterilized container ready to collect your expressed milk. It can take a bit of practice to express your milk by hand, so if you manage to squeeze out only a few drops on the first attempt, try not to give up.

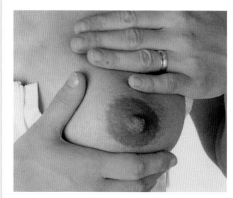

Manipulate the milk Support your breast with one hand and place the other hand above your areola to manipulate the milk toward the nipple.

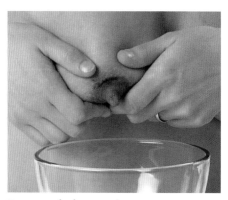

Squeeze and release Gently squeeze your breast and then release. Repeat this action, gradually building up your speed.

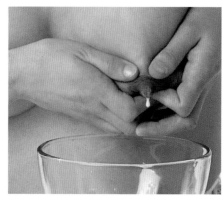

Catch the milk It can take a couple of minutes before milk appears and starts to flow. Catch the expressed milk in a sanitized container. You may need to move the position of your thumb and fingers around your breast to milk all areas.

A

Q How soon can I start expressing and giving my baby a bottle?

This can depend on your reasons for expressing. If you want breast milk for your premature baby, you can start expressing right away in the hospital. If you are breast-feeding, you might want to wait until it is well established.

Waiting a few weeks before giving your baby expressed milk in a bottle will allow her to develop her sucking technique, which for breast-feeding involves coordinating her tongue and jaw movements in a unique action. Feeding from a bottle is very different, since gravity rather than your baby's sucking brings the milk to your baby, and the milk flow tends to be faster.

Introducing a bottle (and by the same token a pacifier) in the early weeks of breast-feeding can lead to the phenomenon known as "nipple confusion," whereby your baby loses the sucking action needed for breast-feeding and, together with frustration at the slower flow of milk, shows a preference for feeding from a bottle. However, not all babies experience nipple confusion—some happily take to a bottle and are happy to switch between a breast and a bottle.

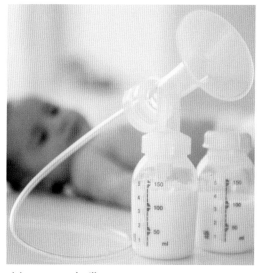

Giving expressed milk Once breast-feeding is well established, you should be able to feed your baby from the breast and give her expressed milk in bottles.

Q Should I be expressing my breast milk at a particular time of day?

There are no set rules about when you should express. Some experts recommend expressing after a feeding, so that you don't remove milk your baby would have fed on, but if you are confident that your supply is plentiful, you can express either before or after a feeding.

If you express before a feeding, do this away from your baby so that she doesn't smell your milk or see your breasts and then want to start feeding. Women often find their supply of milk is most abundant in the morning after a night's sleep, so after your baby's first feeding of the day can be a good time to express.

Once you grow more confident expressing, you can pump one breast while your baby is feeding from the other one. Your breasts will replace whatever milk is removed so you don't need to worry about your supply running out.

Did you know...

Breast milk contains substances that either relax or stimulate your baby depending on the time of day. Relaxing nucleotides are present in the evening and stimulating ones found earlier in the day.

Q I can express only a few drops of milk at a time. Does this mean I'm not producing enough breast milk?

Your breasts are almost certainly producing enough milk. Don't judge your overall supply on how much milk you manage to express. While some women fill bottles effortlessly, others don't find it as easy. Perhaps expressing works best for you by producing smaller amounts more frequently. Each woman is different.

Some women who find that expressing is unproductive have thriving, growing babies and are clearly producing enough milk. Your baby's sucking is by far the most effective way of extracting milk, so even if you aren't producing much when you express, she is almost certainly extracting more when she is feeding.

There are ways to help stimulate your letdown reflex (see p.269). Tension can hinder the letdown of your milk, so get comfortable and relaxed. Taking a warm shower or putting a warm washcloth on your breast can help. Choose a time when you are less likely to be interrupted, pick a quiet spot, have a hot beverage, and listen to some music if it helps. Massaging your breasts can help your milk to start flowing—use circular movements and then stroke downward toward your nipples. Try to think about your baby when you start to express—imagine you are feeding or cradling her—since this can trigger the letdown reflex.

It is normal for the smell, color, and consistency of **expressed breast milk** to vary depending on what you have eaten.

Q Are there any guidelines on how breast milk should be stored and how long I can keep it?

Always refrigerate or freeze your expressed milk right away. Pour breast milk into a sanitized container—a plastic bottle, specially sanitized breast milk bag, or ice-cube trays (these smaller quantities are very handy for quick defrosting). Always make a note of the date on the container.

Your milk will keep in a refrigerator kept at 39°F (4°C) or lower for three to eight days. Store it at the back since the temperature can fluctuate near the door. You can also store it in the freezer compartment of a refrigerator for two weeks, or for three to six months in the freezer attached to your refrigerator if there are separate doors and if it's kept at 0°F (-18°C). If you have a deep freezer kept at -20°C (-4°F), it can stay for six to 12 months. Defrost frozen milk overnight in the refrigerator or by running cool, then warm water over it. Do not microwave.

Q I've been breast-feeding for two weeks and my nipples are sore and cracked. What can I do?

Your breasts and nipples are not used to doing the job of breast-feeding so it is common for discomforts to occur, especially in the first few weeks.

It is important to address any physical discomforts early on, so that breast-feeding becomes a positive experience for you. If you dread any discomfort it causes, this won't be good for your well-being and it may affect how your baby nurses.

Sore and cracked nipples are a common discomfort, but should not be an ongoing problem once your baby is latching on correctly and nursing efficiently. Mostly because shorter feedings will mean your nipples get a break.

Problems such as cracked nipples can prevent your baby from nursing efficiently and lead to other discomforts. If milk isn't properly drained, it can cause blocked ducts and, in a worst-case scenario, mastitis. Both can be painful and make you feel sick so should be treated without delay.

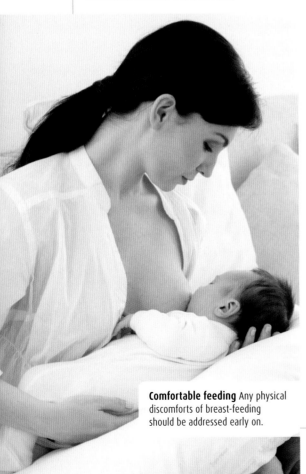

Comfortable feeding Any physical discomforts of breast-feeding should be addressed early on.

BREAST-FEEDING: COMMON CONCERNS

Understanding the causes of breast-feeding discomforts can help prevent them from becoming worse. Take action as soon as possible to resolve any problems so that efficient feeding can be established.

PROBLEM	DESCRIPTION	CAUSES
Sore, cracked, and bleeding nipples	It's normal for your nipples to feel tender since your baby's sucking stretches them, but sore nipples that last beyond the first week can indicate a problem that needs addressing. If the nipples become cracked, you may experience sharp pain for a few seconds at the beginning of a feeding. Cracked nipples may also bleed, and your baby may swallow some blood. Streaks of blood may appear in your baby's stools or when he spits up. Although alarming, this isn't harmful for your baby.	If your baby isn't latched on correctly, he may suck on your nipple, rather than your breast tissue. This makes the nipple increasingly tender, and the pressure of the sucking can cause the nipple to crack, and sometimes bleed. Since your nipples are often moist when breast-feeding, it is hard for the cracks to heal. If nipples suddenly become red and sore after a period of being fine, you may have thrush, a fungal infection that can pass between you and your baby. You will both need medical care.
Blocked milk duct	A blocked duct can result in a lump with swelling and inflammation, and the area may be tender. The swelling may be alleviated slightly after breast-feeding. If bacteria reach the blocked duct, it can lead to mastitis (see below).	Milk ducts form a series of channels that carry milk to your nipple. A milk duct can become blocked if your breast isn't drained completely, often because your baby has a poor latch or has a weak suck. In the early days, when your breasts are producing a lot of milk, they may become engorged, leading to a blocked duct. A badly fitting bra can put pressure on a part of the breast and cause a blockage. If you have redness, swelling, and lumps, contact your doctor. Early treatment can help avoid further complications, such as mastitis.
Mastitis and breast abscess	If you have hardness, swelling, and redness, and your temperature is slightly raised, you may have mastitis. If the infection worsens, it can become very painful, your temperature may escalate, and you may have flulike symptoms. Occasionally, pus forms in the area and an abscess develops, which feels like an extremely painful lump. Mastitis is most common in the early weeks of breast-feeding when your milk supply hasn't yet settled down.	Problems can stem from your baby having a poor latch or weak sucking, which leads to a blocked duct or an area where there is a build up of milk, referred to as milk stasis. If bacteria present on your skin travel to a blocked milk duct, it can cause a mastitis infection. If you are anemic, or very run down, your resistance may be lowered, making you more susceptible to infection.

Putting **cabbage leaves** on the breast helps soothe and cool down the affected area.

WHAT YOU CAN DO

» Check your latching-on technique (see p.268).

» At the end of a feeding, allow air to get to your nipples so they dry naturally. Try rubbing a couple of drops of breast milk into them, since breast milk has antibacterial properties.

» Apply a little purified lanolin cream, which is safe to use even before breast-feeding.

» Avoid breast pads since they keep moisture in.

» Nipple shields can help but only use them for a short time since they can affect your baby's latch.

» Don't stop breast-feeding from the sore breast.

» Continue to breast-feed, checking that he is latched on properly to ensure effective sucking.

» Babies often suck most strongly at the start of a feeding, so putting your baby on the affected side first may help to drain the milk.

» Warmth can help your milk flow, so placing a warm washcloth on your breast at the beginning of a feeding may be helpful, and gently massaging your breast can help to reduce swelling.

» Contact your doctor. He or she can put you in touch with a breast-feeding consultant who can help improve your baby's latch.

» Contact your doctor right away if you think you have mastitis. If infection has set in, your doctor will prescribe antibiotics that are safe to take while breast-feeding. It's important to keep breast-feeding so that milk is removed regularly and your breasts don't become engorged. You may need to nurse more often than usual, and express milk so that the breast is sufficiently drained.

» Many women find placing a cold washcloth or chilled cabbage leaf against the breast soothing since these remove heat from the breast.

» It's important to get plenty of rest.

» Mild pain relief can help. Ibuprofen also acts as an anti-inflammatory.

» An abscess that doesn't respond to antibiotics may need to be surgically drained.

Q My breasts feel as though they're about to burst. Will this last?

This feeling of fullness, or engorgement, should subside within one or two days. It's common for women to feel that their breasts have gone up a cup size or two when their milk "comes in," about three to five days after the birth.

In addition to filling with milk, blood flow to the breasts increases during breast-feeding and aside from feeling very full, breasts may feel hot, hard, lumpy, and tender. This engorgement is usually relieved when you nurse your baby and the milk supply starts to settle down.

If the engorgement is uncomfortable, or your baby is finding it hard to latch on, you can hand express or pump a small amount of milk (see p.272) to reduce the fullness just enough to make latching on easier. Be careful not to express too much, though, since you don't want your breasts to make even more milk.

Massaging your breasts a little while your baby nurses may help the milk flow. Or try putting a hot washcloth on your breast or taking a hot shower before feeding to help trigger the letdown reflex. After a feeding, a cold washcloth or compress, or a chilled cabbage leaf, can be soothing and take any heat out of the breast. A properly fitted nursing bra will support your breasts and make them more comfortable; you may want keep a bra on at night too.

Q My breasts keep leaking milk. How can I deal with this?

An overabundant milk supply can mean that breasts leak. This leaking can also happen when your letdown reflex (see p.269) is triggered unexpectedly. Leaking may occur in one breast while you're feeding your baby on the other side, or when you're in a warm environment, such as the shower, or when you hear your baby cry, or even just think about your baby.

Expressing a little milk before or after nursing may reduce leaking, and nursing frequently will ensure that milk is regularly removed and milk production falls into sync with your growing baby's needs. If you sense that you're about to leak milk, discreetly crossing your arms over your chest so that you are putting gentle pressure on your nipples may stem the flow. Putting breast pads inside your bra can contain leaks. Bring spare clothes when you go out.

Q My baby falls asleep while breast-feeing. What should I do?

If your baby nods off during a feeding you should gently wake him. Your baby may come off the breast on his own once he is full, but sometimes babies can fall asleep while on the breast, or continue comfort sucking. If his jaw is no longer moving, or his sucking has become lighter and quicker, but he doesn't appear to be swallowing, he may be full. If this happens, or he falls asleep, gently rouse him and burp him, then check if he wants to continue before ending the session.

Q My baby cries when he comes off the breast. Am I making enough milk?

If you breast-feed your baby regularly you will almost certainly be able to make enough milk for him. Your baby may need more milk for a day or two because he is going through a growth spurt. He may cry as soon as he finishes, or shortly after being fed, and you may feel like you're breast-feeding continuously.

If you meet your baby's increased demands, your supply will increase to meet his needs. Offering both breasts at each feeding will help your milk supply increase more rapidly, and you might even need to keep switching breasts until your baby seems completely satisfied.

The clearest sign that your baby is feeding well and thriving is that he is gaining weight. Being nice and alert when awake, and having more than six wet diapers a day are also sure signs that your baby is well-nourished. Talk to your pediatrician if you have any concerns.

Q I have inverted nipples. Will this prevent me from breast-feeding?

It is possible to breast-feed if your nipples are inverted, but you will need some guidance. A breast-feeding consultant can check how you are managing to feed. She may recommend using a breast pump to draw out the nipple before you begin feeding, or using a nipple shield to help the baby latch on. Pulling the breast tissue back as your baby latches on will also help the nipple to protrude. Seek advice from your doctor if you are finding it hard.

Q I'm still finding it tricky to get my baby latched on properly. Where can I get more support?

There are numerous avenues of support. In the early days, you may be able to access support from a breast-feeding consultant in your hospital or birth center. In hospital, nurses can check your technique and when you get home your pediatrician or a private lactation consultant can help.

If you need to talk to someone quickly, there are breast-feeding organizations that have help lines allowing you to talk to an experienced mother or breast-feeding consultant trained to offer advice and support. While talking on the phone can be very helpful, sometimes it isn't a substitute for sitting with someone while they watch your feeding technique. Organizations such as La Leche League and local breast-feeding support groups provide drop-in meetings where you can meet other moms and often get one-on-one help from health-care professionals such as lactation consultants and nurses. When you were discharged from the hospital, you may have been given information about local chapters of La Leche League, support groups or even Meetup groups that gather regularly. If not, you can do an online search to find a group in your area. The camaraderie and support these group meetings provide can be invaluable.

Feeling supported by your partner is important, too. Having your partner's backing can give you encouragement to overcome problems and continue breast-feeding. Don't delay seeking help if you encounter problems, since if you don't get on top of an issue, it can quickly escalate. Most problems can be resolved with the right advice and support.

Around 75% of new moms **seek help with breast-feeding.** Most work through their problems and go on to breast-feed successfully.

Q Breast-feeding is so convenient, but I feel anxious about doing it in public. How can I get confidence?

Knowing your rights and thinking ahead can help counter initial jitters about public breast-feeding. It is normal to feel self-conscious in the beginning, but in time you will grow in confidence and it will become second nature.

One of the joys of breast-feeding is that you can feed your baby any time or place as soon as she is hungry. Your breast milk is always available at the right temperature in the exact amount your baby needs, so when you start to venture out with your baby, you don't have to do preparation such as sanitizing bottles and measuring the formula you need.

Breast-feeding is simply extremely convenient. Most mothers find that it's easy to choose a spot where they can feed their baby discreetly, and that actually the majority of people barely notice, or if they do, they are entirely respectful.

Your right to breast-feed in public

Occasionally, you may get a disapproving look or comment, which makes you feel self-conscious and perhaps even a little humiliated, even though breast-feeding is the most natural thing in the world. So it's good to know that you do have rights in such a situation. In the US, 49 states (all except Idaho) and the District of Columbia have laws which allow women to breast-feed their babies at any private or public location within the state. And 29 states specifically address breast-feeding and public indecency, stating that breast-feeding is exempt from such a charge. You have rights in the workplace, too. The Affordable Care Act of 2010 requires employers to provide reasonable break time for nursing moms to express breast milk for the first year of a baby's life, in a location other than a bathroom. And 27 states have added their own laws about breast-feeding in the workplace.

Planning ahead

Think about what you are wearing: loose tops you can lift up a little to let your baby latch on help to make breast-feeding discreet. Aside from an initial flash of flesh, it's pretty hard to see anything other than your baby. Wearing a loose tank under a T-shirt means you can pull this down to hide your postpartum belly, and often, your arm cradling your baby will do this job. Practice opening your nursing bra with one hand, too.

Some women use a burp cloth or a breast-feeding scarf for a little extra cover, but others feel that this actually draws attention to you. Go with whatever feels best—if covering up feels more reassuring, that's fine, but you shouldn't ever feel you have to hide yourself when breast-feeding your baby.

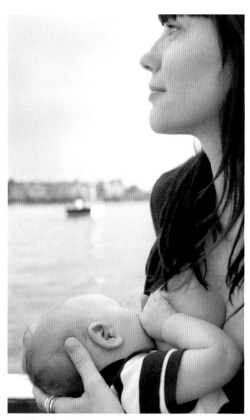

Confident feeding Breast-feeding your baby is natural and not something you should have to hide or be embarrassed about.

Q I want to continue breast-feeding, but I'm struggling. Is it really worth persevering?

Breast-feeding is time consuming, tiring, and, in some circumstances, leads to physical discomfort. For these reasons, it's not uncommon for mothers to reach a point where they are unsure if they can continue.

Like many new moms, you may be surprised at the demands of breast-feeding. After all, unless you have started to express milk, you are the only one that can feed your baby. It's natural to want to share the feeding and consider putting your baby on formula, mainly so that you can have a break and a night of undisrupted sleep while your partner bottle-feeds the baby.

Give it time

Rest assured, though, that once you have settled into breast-feeding, it becomes easier. Your baby will nurse more efficiently, meaning that feedings are likely to be shorter and less time consuming. You will also, hopefully, have overcome initial breast-feeding discomforts (see pp.274–75). Don't forget, rather than using formula you can also begin to express your milk (see p.272), which can give you a break while ensuring your baby is still getting all the benefits of breast milk.

Reaping the rewards

Most women who persevere with breast-feeding are incredibly glad they did as they reach the stage when breast-feeding becomes a real joy—convenient, easy, and a wonderful bonding experience. So yes, it is worth persevering because breast-feeding can be such a mutually rewarding experience. But if you really feel that breast-feeding isn't for you, there is no shame in giving it up.

For many women **breast-feeding becomes pleasurable,** which more than compensates for any initial difficulties.

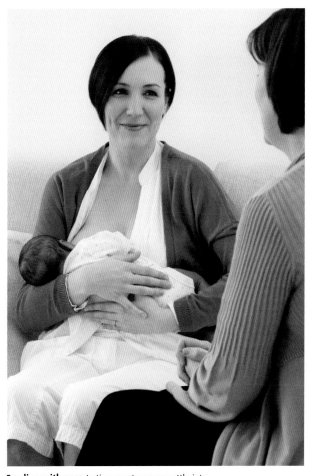

Feeding with ease In time most women settle into breast-feeding and find it mutually rewarding.

Q Will introducing a bottle of formula for one of our baby's feedings affect my milk supply?

It depends on when you decide to do this.
Giving your baby a bottle of formula allows you the occasional break and your partner a chance to feed your baby, and perhaps to help with night feeding. However, if you want to continue breast-feeding for a while, albeit on a reduced schedule, it's advisable to wait for about six to eight weeks before you introduce your baby to a bottle.

In the first few weeks, your breasts are adapting to feeding your baby and your milk supply is becoming established. If you introduce a bottle of formula, it might reduce your milk

supply, since it works on a supply and demand basis. Introducing a bottle and nipple also means that your baby has to learn a new sucking technique, which could lead to "nipple confusion" (see p.273).

After six to eight weeks, your milk supply will settle down and you can try to introduce a bottle. However, this will reduce the amount of breast milk you make, and it can be hard to reverse this decision, so be certain this is what you want to do before you introduce the formula.

It's also worthwhile to keep in mind that if you are hoping to have a break from night feedings, preparing a bottle of formula at night can be a lot more time-consuming than breast-feeding, and your partner may not be able or willing to do every nighttime feeding.

Q Did you know...

It is recommended that you breast-feed your baby exclusively until you start introducing solid food at about six months. This means only giving your baby breast milk—no other food or drink until then. Once you start solids, you can continue to breast-feed and use your breast milk to prepare foods. It is quite common for women who return to work to continue to breast-feed or combine breast-feeding with formula. Expressed milk can be given to your baby by the person taking care of her.

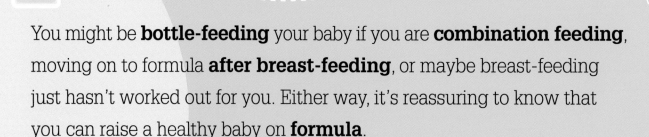

You might be **bottle-feeding** your baby if you are **combination feeding**, moving on to formula **after breast-feeding**, or maybe breast-feeding just hasn't worked out for you. Either way, it's reassuring to know that you can raise a healthy baby on **formula**.

Bottle-feeding your baby

Why bottle-feed

There is a lot of pressure put on new moms to breast-feed, but some women are uncomfortable with breast-feeding, or are unable to breast-feed. It's important that your baby gets the right amount of food to grow, so try not to worry about where her nourishment comes from; you will give her a good start in life with formula. Feeding your baby from either the breast or a bottle is a wonderful bonding experience. Some moms express breast milk from the beginning and their baby drinks it from a bottle, while others combine breast and bottle-feeding. There are some advantages to bottle-feeding. First, someone other than you can prepare and give a feeding, giving you time to rest. Second, bottle-fed babies tend to have fewer feedings. Third, they generally sleep better at night (after the first few weeks) since they're less likely to wake up for a feeding—cow's milk forms a more solid curd that takes longer to digest than breast milk. If you bottle-feed from the beginning, it will take around seven to 10 days for the milk your breasts produced after the birth to dry up, during which time your breasts may feel heavy and full.

First feeds

Your newborn needs to be fed little and often, so offer her the bottle when you notice her hunger cues (see p.269). Young babies are especially vulnerable to germs while their immunity builds up, so be meticulous about hygiene rules when preparing feedings and sanitizing bottles and nipples. Bottle-fed babies take in more air during feedings (their mouths form less of a seal around the bottle's nipple compared to your nipple) so burp your baby regularly.

Switching to bottle-feeding

If you want to go from breast to formula feedings, or to give bottles of expressed breast milk, you will need to get equipped with bottles, nipples, and a cleaning system (see p.191). Some bottles boast a similar feel to your own nipple to help a baby make the switch from breast to bottle. If you want to continue breast-feeding while trying a bottle, called combination feeding, start with one bottle a day, so that your baby gets used to the different taste and the feel of it. It can help if your partner does the first few bottle feedings until your baby gets used to the bottle.

Q What is the best way to sanitize bottles and nipples for my baby?

It's good to know that there are a few different safe methods you can use to sanitize baby feeding equipment, rather a single correct way. Before sanitizing, wash bottles, nipples, and the equipment used to make up your baby's formula thoroughly in hot, soapy water to remove all traces of milk residue. This is easier to do soon after a feeding, and using a bottle brush to clean the crevices. Rinse off the detergent. Parts from breast pumps should be washed this way after each use and then sanitized according to the manufacturer's instructions.

Washing alone does not kill harmful bacteria and viruses, so the bottles, nipples, and related equipment need to be sanitized. Cold-water sanitization involves submerging the equipment in cold water treated with a chemical agent, which comes in tablet or liquid form. Leave the equipment covered in the solution for at least 30 minutes before use, to keep it sanitized.

Steam sanitizers range from quick-to-use microwave steamers to electric sanitizers. Place the openings of bottles and nipples face down so that the insides are sanitized by rising steam.

To boil the equipment, immerse the items completely in a large, lidded pan of water. Boil for at least 10 minutes to kill germs, and keep the lid on the pan until equipment is needed.

Boiling nipples can wear them out quicker, so check for signs of damage before using them.

Q How much formula does my baby need each day? Does it depend on his appetite, or should I stick to a set amount?

In the first week or so, just like a breast-fed baby, your baby will probably manage just small amounts of formula at each feeding. After this, and until about six months of age, the rule of thumb is to give 2.5 ounces of formula a day for every pound of body weight.

Q Is there a certain way I should make up my baby's bottles?

There is a particular method that you must follow each time you make up a powdered formula bottle for your baby (see below).

Special care needs to be taken when making up formula for two reasons. One is that cartons of formula powder, although sealed, are not sterile (unlike ready-to-drink cartons of formula, which are), so could contain bacteria such as salmonella that could make your baby extremely ill. This means that meticulous hygiene is paramount when making up bottles. Secondly, the ratio of

powder to milk needs to be exactly right to make sure your baby is getting the correct balance of nutrients. Too little powder can mean that your baby isn't getting enough nourishment; and too much powder could make your baby constipated and dehydrated. Always read the manufacturer's instructions carefully before you begin and make up a bottle using the scoop provided.

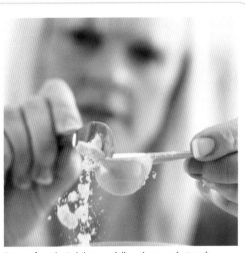

Be precise It's vital that you follow the manufacturer's instructions when making up powdered formula.

STEPS TO MAKING UP POWDERED FORMULA

Here are the steps to follow each time you make up a bottle. You'll soon get the hang of it and will be able to follow the steps effortlessly. However, you must continue to be stringent with the process.

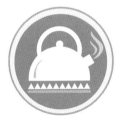 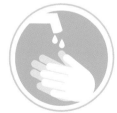 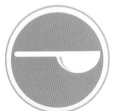 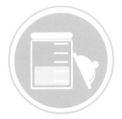 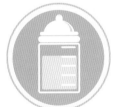 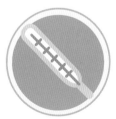

1 Start by boiling a quart (1 liter) of fresh tap water (rather than water sitting in a kettle). Let the water cool for no more than 30 minutes so that it is at least 158° F (70° C)—hot enough to kill off any bacteria present.

2 Wash your hands thoroughly and make sure the surface where you are preparing the bottle is scrupulously clean. You can spray the area with antibacterial spray and wipe it down before you start to make up a bottle.

3 Put the water in the bottle first, pouring in the exact amount recommended by the manufacturer on the packaging. Don't dilute or strengthen the formula because it can affect your baby's digestive system.

4 Using the scoop provided, loosely scoop out some formula, then level this off with a clean, dry knife, or with the leveler provided, and add the specified number of scoops to the water. Always use the scoop that came with the formula.

5 Holding the nipple by its edge, push it through the retaining ring, screw the ring onto the bottle, and cover with the cap. Shake the bottle so that all the powder dissolves. Let the formula cool before you give it to your baby.

6 Test the temperature on the inside of your wrist to help you gauge whether it's ready for your baby: it should be just warm, but not hot. To cool it down, place the bottle in a bowl of cold water or run the bottom half of the bottle under a cold faucet.

Q What's the best way to give my baby his bottle?

First, get comfortable yourself, sitting upright with your back straight and supported. Feeding can take a while, so you don't want to strain your back.

Hold your baby close to you, cradling him against your body and facing you, so you can talk and make eye contact during a feeding. It's a wonderful chance to bond with your baby. Keep him upright holding him at your chest height, since this will help him swallow at a steady pace. Allow him to pause during a feeding if he wants (as he would naturally when breast-feeding), then resume. If he squirms or seems restless midway through, remove the bottle and try burping him, then continue when he has settled. It's important that you never leave your baby with a bottle propped up in his mouth since he could suffocate or choke.

HOW TO BOTTLE-FEED STEP BY STEP

By following these simple steps you will soon become a natural at giving a bottle. It will quickly turn into a familiar routine that you and your baby both enjoy.

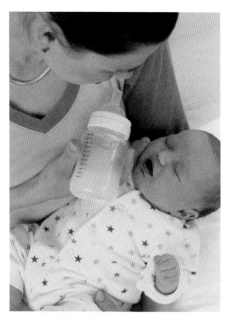

1 **Gently rub his cheek** to encourage the rooting reflex. Then place the nipple so that it is touching his top lip. Don't push the nipple into his mouth, wait for him to open his mouth to take it, or gently nuzzle it against his lips to encourage him to take it.

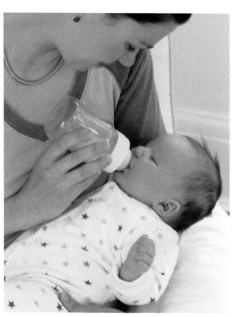

2 **Hold the bottle** slightly upright, making sure the milk covers the opening of the nipple and the neck of the bottle. This will help to make sure that your baby isn't taking in too much extra air during a feeding. Support your baby's head with the cradle of your arm.

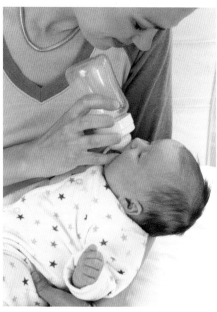

3 **Tilt the bottle** up a bit more as the bottle empties so that the milk continues to cover the nipple. At the end of a feeding you can put your little finger (make sure it's clean) into your baby's mouth to break off the suction and remove the bottle.

Q I am breast-feeding and plan to introduce a bottle. Any tips on making this switch?

While some babies switch from breast to bottle without a hitch, others go into a screaming meltdown. If your baby protests loudly whenever a bottle comes near him, there are a few tactics you can try. Getting your partner to give a bottle means that your baby can't smell your milk. Choose a time when your baby isn't very hungry, perhaps an afternoon feeding, so that he is less likely to get distressed if he isn't getting the milk he wants. If you're not in a rush to get him onto formula, you could try giving expressed milk first, since he may be more willing to try a bottle if the contents are familiar.

Keep in mind, too, that breast-fed babies need to suck harder to get their milk, so starting off with a slow-flow nipple can help ensure your baby isn't overwhelmed by a fast flow of milk. Conversely, if your baby is very hungry, a slower flow may frustrate him. Experiment to find the nipple that suits him. Let your baby play with and get used to the bottle, and don't continue trying if he refuses after about three attempts. Take a break, offer a breast-feed after about 10 minutes, then try the bottle again in a few days.

Q Should I make up each bottle of formula fresh when our baby needs it?

Yes, in recent years the guidelines on making up and storing bottles have been revised. You should always freshly make up each bottle of formula.

It used to be common practice to make up bottles for one day and keep them in the fridge until needed. However, bacteria are still able to multiply in a refrigerator (and at room temperature this can happen very quickly), so this increases the risk of harmful bacteria reaching a baby. Each bottle should be made up fresh and any remaining milk should be discarded. If you do need to make a bottle in advance, store it in the back of the refrigerator and use it within 24 hours. Unused formula that has been left at room temperature should be thrown away.

WHAT YOU NEED TO KNOW

» **Make up bottles fresh** as and when your baby needs them.

» **Make the bottle within 30 minutes** of boiling the water. Always use fresh water.

» **Put the correct amount of water** in the bottle before adding the formula powder.

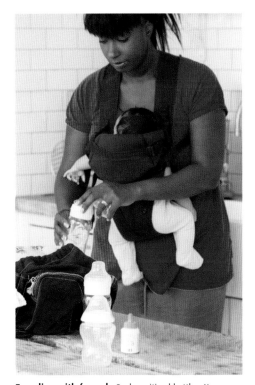

Traveling with formula Pack sanitized bottles. You can purchase travel containers with built-in dividers to keep powdered formula in premeasured quantities.

Feeding on the go

If you are away from home, there are a few options for bottle-feeding. Think about your day and how long you will be out since you don't want to get left short.

» **Take a sanitized bottle** and a carton of ready-made formula, then use this when needed. This is by far the easiest solution. You might need to bring a pair of clean scissors since opening ready-made cartons of formula isn't always that easy.

» **Put the correct amount of formula** in a clean, plastic container and pack this along with a thermos of just-boiled water and a sanitized bottle, then make up the bottle when needed, allowing the water to cool before you give the bottle to your baby.

» **If you need to make up** a bottle for someone else to give to your baby when you're not there, for example, for a babysitter or grandparent, cool it at the back of the refrigerator for an hour, then transport it in a cool bag with an ice pack and let the caregiver know it should be used within four hours.

Q Can I put my bottle-fed baby on a feeding schedule?

No, bottle-fed babies should be fed on demand just as breast-fed babies are, since your baby's small tummy means he needs to be fed more frequently at first. Although bottle-feeding can feel more structured since you make up bottles according to your baby's weight and know exactly how much milk your baby takes each day, it doesn't follow that bottle-fed babies adapt well to a schedule. Formula manufacturers suggest giving larger feedings at more spaced apart intervals, but this may not suit even your older baby, who may need smaller, more frequent feedings, especially if he spits up a lot of milk after feedings. Feedings that are too large can make your baby overly full, possibly sick, and could lead to him becoming overweight.

Q Which formula should I choose? Do I have to give my baby cow's milk formula?

Choose a formula that is appropriate for your baby's age. First infant formula is recommended from birth (and your baby can continue to enjoy it until his first birthday). First formula replicates the same of ratio of 60:40 whey to casein proteins that is in breast milk, to ensure it is digestible for your baby and provides the right balance of hydration and nutrition. "Follow-up" formulas contain a greater percentage of the thicker casein protein, but they are harder for your baby to digest and are not suitable in the first six months.

Cow's milk formula is the recommended choice for your baby. It has been formulated to strict nutritional guidelines to ensure it is a suitable food for a growing baby. Unless your doctor says otherwise, your baby should have formula derived from cow's milk in his first year. Some babies react to the proteins or the sugar lactose in cow's milk formula. In this case, your doctor can prescribe a special type of formula called "fully hydrolyzed," in which the protein is broken down and the lactose removed. Soy-based formula is rarely recommended because babies who react to proteins in cow's milk often react to proteins in soy milk too. There are also concerns that phytoestrogens in soy formula may affect the reproductive organs, and some soy products have glucose added, which could affect your baby's emerging teeth. Soy milk formula should not be given to babies under six months old, and then only if your doctor recommends it, which might be the case for vegan families, or if your baby won't drink other alternatives.

For such a little person, your **amazing new baby** requires a lot of taking care of. If this is your first time taking care of a newborn, you may feel you lack the full qualifications for the job. Rest assured that, while it's very natural for new parents to feel a little nervous, your **confidence will grow** in the coming days and weeks.

Taking care of your baby

On-the-job training

So much of parenting is about learning on the job, and you will find that your baby is naturally forgiving of any initial awkwardness. What he needs from the outset is your love, attention, and reassurance that you are there to meet his needs. The rest of your parenting skills will soon fall into place: where those early cries perplexed, before long you will be able to decipher what it is your baby is asking for, and from those first tentative holds, you'll become adept at handling and holding your baby just the way he likes while you wash, dress, and soothe him.

Taking care of your baby every day

An important part of taking care of your baby is making sure he is kept clean and comfortable and he is safe in his environment. From preventing diaper rash to ensuring good sleep hygiene—making sure his sleep environment is safe and conducive to rest—the everyday care you give your baby helps him feel content. Many of the practices you put in place in these early days will instill good habits for life. In addition to your baby's everyday practical care,

he also needs stimulation and interaction with you and his environment. At first, this may be as simple as making eye contact, copying facial expressions, and exchanging smiles. Then, increasingly, play and stimulation will involve activities, toys, and exploring other environments. All the time you spend together, both in play and with simple caring tasks, helps strengthen your bond.

Young babies are vulnerable to infection, so avoiding contact with germs is a good idea. However, your baby will inevitably be unwell at some point. Knowing what signs indicate that your baby is sick, and when to seek medical help, can reassure you that you will give your baby the care he needs.

Taking care of you

These early weeks and months taking care of your little one are amazing and all consuming. Getting the right amount of rest, being mutually supportive with your partner about your baby's care, and paying attention to your diet and lifestyle will ensure you have the energy and resources needed to give your baby your very best care.

Q I've never changed a diaper before! Where do I start?

Pick a warm, draft-free spot—babies can object to the feel of cold air on their skin—and lay your baby down on a wiped-clean diaper mat or a towel.

Changing your baby's diaper at floor level is safest for your baby, but it can be tough on your back. A purpose-made changing table is convenient and easier for you, but you need to keep an eye on your baby at all times. Have everything you need on hand: the quicker and more efficient the diaper change, the less likely it is that your baby will become distressed.

YOU WILL NEED

» **A clean diaper**, and diaper liner if you are using disposable diapers.

» **Cotton balls and warm water.** Baby wipes can be harsh on your baby's skin, so limit their use and avoid them for newborns.

» **Diaper disposal system**, for disposal

» **Diaper cream** (optional)

CHANGING YOUR BABY'S DIAPER

Remove the old diaper. If it's dirty, use the front of the diaper to wipe away feces. Fold the diaper in on itself, seal with the tabs, and dispose of it (or flush a disposable liner if using reusables). When removing a boy's diaper, hold it over his penis for a moment so you don't get sprayed by urine.

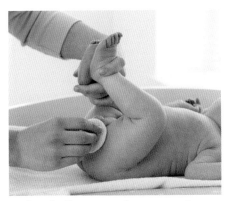

1 Clean the diaper area with wet cotton pads, a washcloth, or wipes. Wipe girls from front to back to stop bacteria from reaching the vagina. Carefully clean around a boy's testes and penis, and don't pull foreskin.

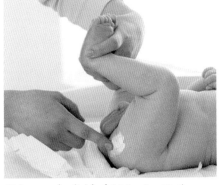

2 Once you've finished, let the air get to the diaper area for a few minutes since this can help to prevent, or soothe, sore diaper rash. If you want, you can apply a thin layer of diaper cream to the skin.

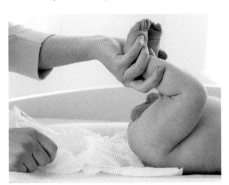

3 Gently lift up his legs by the ankles, then slip a clean diaper under his bottom, bringing the side tabs level with the waist. Check that a boy's penis is facing down before bringing up the front of the diaper.

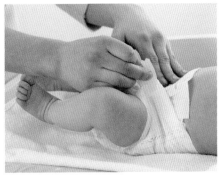

4 Bring the diaper up between the legs, and secure with the side tabs. You should be able to fit a finger between the diaper and tummy. For a reusable, put a liner inside the diaper, and add an outer wrap if using.

Q How often should I change my baby's diaper? It's hard to tell when it's wet.

It goes without saying that you should change your baby's diaper each time he has a bowel movement. With today's super absorbent disposables, it can be hard to tell if a diaper is wet. To get an idea, pour four tablespoons of water into a dry diaper—this is what a soaked one feels like. You'll change your baby's diaper at least six times a day after the first week.

Q Do I always need to change a diaper after a night feeding?

Use common sense and judgment when it comes to nighttime diaper changes. Some parents worry that the extra disruption this causes will make a sleepy, satisfied, and ready-to-settle-down baby suddenly very awake. Check the diaper. If it feels fairly dry and your baby doesn't have uncomfortable diaper rash, it's probably okay to leave it on. You may prefer, though, to be on the safe side and change his diaper so that he doesn't wake again shortly afterward feeling wet and uncomfortable.

Q What's the best way to treat my baby's sore bottom?

While diaper rash is common, when your baby's bottom becomes red, take this as a cue to check that you are practicing good diaper hygiene. Spending time in wet and dirty diapers irritates your baby's skin. Babies usually let you know when they're dirty—or you can smell it!—but they don't always complain when a diaper is wet. Keep an eye on the state of his diapers and change them frequently. Baby wipes can be irritating on your baby's delicate skin, so avoid these while your baby's bottom looks sore, and use just warm water and cotton pads for cleaning. Let your baby go diaper-free for a short while every day so that the air can get to his skin to speed up healing. Before putting a new diaper on, apply a thin layer of zinc oxide diaper cream to protect his skin. If you have reusable diapers, make sure they are rinsed thoroughly after washing so that all traces of detergent are removed.

Q What's the best way to keep my baby clean each day?

Until your baby is on the move, crawling around and picking up dirt, a daily bath isn't vital, but you do need to give her a thorough cleaning, or sponge bath, each day.

This involves washing her face, bottom, and in the skin creases where dirt and spit-up milk accumulate. Get organized first, so you don't have to root around for diapers or cloths in the middle of cleaning, and instead can give your baby your full attention so she doesn't become anxious and restless. See page 186 for the equipment you'll need for bathing your baby.

YOU WILL NEED

» **A bowl, or sink, of warm water.**

» **Some cotton pads** and a washcloth.

» **a clean diaper**, and diaper liner if you are using disposable diapers.

SPONGE BATHING YOUR BABY

Wash your hands before you start. Lay your baby down on her changing mat in a draft-free room. Put a towel on top of the mat for added comfort if you'd like. Then either undress your baby down to her undershirt and diaper, or if it's a bit chilly, keep her sleep suit on and undo the top and bottom half separately, keeping one half of her covered while you clean the other half.

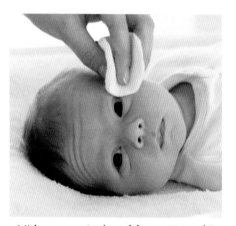

1 **Using a separate piece of damp cotton pad** for each eye, gently wipe your baby's eyes from the inner to the outer edge. Use a new piece of cotton pad to clean behind (not inside) the ears and around the neck, cleaning out milk residue from skin creases.

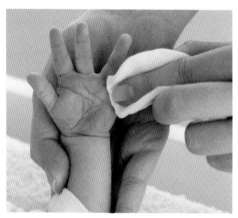

2 **Gently lift up your baby's arms** and clean in her armpits; then clean the palm of your baby's hand and uncurl her fingers to clean in between each one. Wash your baby's feet, again gently cleaning between the toes, and clean her legs, wiping the creases under the knees.

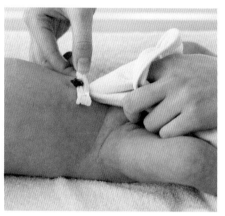

3 **Use a clean damp washcloth** to clean around the umbilical cord area. You can use plain water, or mild baby soap if the area is dirty with feces. Pat the area dry and let air get to the skin. Then clean the diaper area (see p.283) before putting on a new diaper.

Q How can I dress my baby so that she isn't too hot or too cold?

Generally, the advice is for your baby to wear one more layer of clothing than you are wearing, which may just mean adding a onesie under a sleep suit and cardigan, or putting a blanket over her in the carriage. You should regularly check, though, whether your baby seems comfortable. Young babies aren't good at regulating their body temperature, and so rely on you to make sure they are just right. By dressing your baby in several lightweight layers, you can quickly adapt her clothing when you are moving between indoors and outdoors, perhaps adding a cotton blanket, or removing a jacket, as required. It's important, too, not to leave your baby sleeping in outdoor layers when you get home, however tempting it may be not to disturb her, since she may overheat.

Gauge your baby's temperature by feeling her tummy, chest, or the nape of her neck—if these areas feel hot to touch, remove a layer, or add a layer if they feel cold. Keep in mind that babies' hands and feet are often on the cool side, so don't use these to judge temperature.

On sunny days, make sure your baby's shoulders are covered up and put a wide-brimmed sun hat on her. Your baby's skin is very delicate and can burn quickly, so in addition to keeping her covered, keep her out of direct sunshine during the part of the day when the sun is strongest. Use a sunshade on her carriage, and apply sunscreen that is specially formulated for babies, with a minimum of SPF 30.

Q What's the easiest way to put on my baby's onesie and sleep suit?

Onesies with envelope-style necks can be pulled wide, making them easy to pass over a baby's head. Lay your baby down, gently lift the back of her head, then pull the neckline over, lifting the fabric off her face. Pull each onesie arm out to pop her hands through, then smooth it over her body and close the snaps.

Lay the sleep suit out, snaps open, and place your baby on it. Gently bend her legs and place them in the sleep suit legs, then close the snaps around the legs and diaper area. Gather the fabric on an arm and pass her hand through the sleeve, putting your hand through the other end to guide it. Close the remaining snaps.

Q Why is my baby crying? Should I assume she is hungry?

Crying is a natural state for your baby, and is her first and main means of communication. Your baby may not know why she's upset, she just knows that something is wrong. Your job is to figure out what that thing is. In the first days and weeks, hunger is often the reason for her cries; you may want to feed her if it has been a couple of hours since she was fed. As your baby grows and feedings become more spaced out, you may not want to offer a feeding instantly—in fact, if you do, she may expect to be fed every time you pick her up.

As you get to know your baby, you'll notice clues as to what's wrong. If your baby is fussing, perhaps rubbing her eyes, yawning, and looking glazed, she probably needs a nap. Babies can cry when overstimulated, whether they are feeling tired or because there is too much going on. Other reasons include wanting to change position, needing a diaper change, or feeling too hot or too cold. If she's been asleep, she may cry because she needs reassurance that you are close by. If she's uncomfortable, she may simply be craving the comfort and reassurance she feels when held in your arms.

If your baby is crying intensely (three hours a day or more) and won't be soothed, often at the same time each day, and maybe looks flushed, is clenching her fists, and drawing her legs up to her tummy while crying, she may have colic—the term used when otherwise healthy babies cry excessively. You should see your pediatrician so that he or she can rule out any other cause for her crying.

Q I love carrying my baby in a front pack, but will it make her too clingy?

Carrying your baby in a front pack, or "baby wearing," is comforting for mom, or dad, and baby. This closeness makes your baby feel secure and loved, and in turn confident you're there for her, so fears about clinginess are ungrounded. The sound of your heartbeat relaxes your baby, and you'll quickly pick up on feeding cues. Make sure your baby is safe in the pack. It should be tight enough to hold her securely and support her back, her face should be clear of the carrier fabric and her head close to yours, and her chin should not rest on her chest.

Q How can I comfort my fussing baby?

Sometimes comfort and closeness to you can be enough to soothe your baby and reassure her that all is well.

When you respond to your baby's cries with soft words, a gentle touch, and by keeping her close, she learns that she can trust you to recognize her needs and that the world is a safe place for her, and in the long run she is likely to become more independent and confident. There's no right or wrong way to soothe your baby, and you and your baby will find techniques that work for you both.

SOOTHING TECHNIQUES

Experiment with different comforting methods to find the ones that work best for you and your baby.

» **Rhythm and motion** are naturally soothing to your baby, perhaps reminding her of her time in the uterus. Gently rocking or swaying your baby, or carrying her in a front pack, is reassuring, and being close to you makes her feel safe and secure. If crying is persistent, a trip around the block in the carriage or car may lull her to sleep, though you may not want her to become too dependent on these methods of soothing.

» **Sucking** is inherently comforting for your little one, so if hunger isn't the problem, she may enjoy sucking on your finger or a pacifier (though you may be avoiding pacifiers in the early weeks to avoid nipple confusion, see page 273).

» **White noise** can help your baby to switch off and zone out when she is overstimulated. The sound of the washing machine may remind your baby of swooshing noises in the uterus and be a comfort.

» **Whispering**, talking gently, singing a soothing lullaby, and smiling can all help to calm a grouchy baby, especially one who is just in need of a bit of company.

» **Rubbing your baby's back** while held upright, or while gently swaying her as she's held face down along your arm, may help if she has gas or is colicky.

» **Physical contact** is essential to your baby's well-being. Stroking her head and gently patting her back or bottom can be soothing, and if your baby has colic, a baby massage can help her to relax if she's receptive. Stroke her arms and legs, her palms, and the soles of her feet; then stroke her brow and, if comfortable for her, stroke her tummy in a clockwise motion.

If crying is persistent, occurs around the same time each day, and your baby is inconsolable, she may have colic. Talk to your pediatrician about ways to ease this.

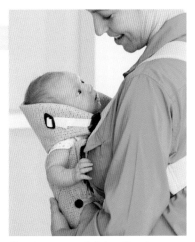

Close to you Snuggled close, listening to your heartbeat, is naturally soothing for your baby.

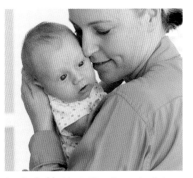

A calm hold Older babies often enjoy being held upright as you move around.

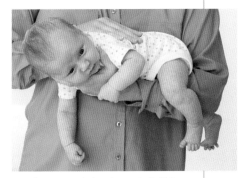

Face down Some babies love to be held face down and gently rocked back and forth.

Q How much sleep does my baby need?

On average, babies sleep 14–18 hours per day in the first few weeks. This time spent in slumber is vital for their growth and development.

Babies grow at a tremendous rate in the first few months. The time they spend asleep allows their bodies to focus on growing (growth hormone is released during sleep), and for them to process all the new information they receive each day. Newborns can manage only brief periods of sleep before their tiny tummies need to be fed again, so their sleep is spread over both night and day and they will wake as frequently at night as they do in the day. Aside from needing to wake often to be fed, your baby has short sleep cycles of 45–60 minutes, and when he stirs from a cycle, he finds it hard to drop back off naturally. All of this means that in the first six to eight weeks, you will need to feed your baby around the clock, waking every two to three hours at night to tend to him. At around two months (later for some, earlier for others), your baby will start to manage slightly longer stretches of sleep at night, and slightly shorter stretches during the day: his tummy will be bigger and his awareness of night and day is kicking in.

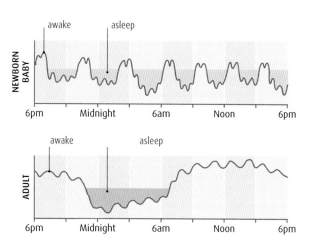

Amounts of sleep A newborn baby spends 16 hours asleep on average each day (this can range from 12 to 20 hours). The average adult requires half this amount of sleep.

AVERAGE SLEEP BY AGE

While each baby has different needs, the following is a rough guide to what you can expect for your baby's sleep over the first three months of life:

NEWBORN	ONE MONTH	TWO MONTHS	THREE MONTHS
As a new baby: he sleeps about 14-18 hours in every 24 hours, with about 7½ hours in the day, and 8½ hours at night. **During the day** sleep is divided into 3-4 periods of sleep. **At night** your baby will wake up every two to three hours to be fed.	**At one month:** your baby sleeps about 15½ hours in every 24 hours, with around 6-7 hours of sleep during the day, and 8½ hours sleep at night. **During the day** sleep is divided into about three nap times. **At night** your baby will still wake around two to three times.	**At two months** your baby will sleep about 15½ hours in every 24 hours, with around 5½ hours sleep during the day, and around 10 hours at night. **During the day** sleep is divided into about three nap times. **At night** your baby may manage slightly longer periods of sleep.	**At three months:** your baby will sleep about 15 hours in every 24 hours, with about 5 hours during the day. **During the day** sleep is divided into 3 nap times. **At night** your baby may sleep for about 10 hours, with perhaps just one or two nighttime feedings.

Q Where is the best place for my baby to sleep? Should he be in a crib?

In the first six months of life, it's recommended that the safest place for your baby to sleep is in a bassinet or crib in a room with you at night and for daytime naps. Keeping your baby nearby means you will be aware quickly of his needs, and he will feel comforted to be close to you. If you'd like, you can put your baby in a crib from the beginning. However, a full-sized crib can be too big for a newborn baby, and he may be more comfortable in a bassinet for the first few weeks. It mimics the feeling of being cocooned in the uterus, and is portable. You may find that at about two

months, your baby is looking a bit cramped in his bassinet. He should be able to sleep with his arms out to the side, or flung up by his head, without touching either the side or top of the bassinet.

Q Can I co-sleep with my newborn baby? What are the risks?

Sharing a bed with your new baby can feel like the most natural thing in the world. If you are breast-feeding, being in the same sleeping space means you can feed your baby as soon as he stirs, minimizing sleep disruption. Some studies also suggest that co-sleeping could actually help

to regulate babies' breathing, and that generally the sleep patterns of mother and baby become more synchronized. The mother may be more responsive to the baby's needs. Your baby is also likely to feel very secure being so close to you, and may settle back to sleep more easily. However, the American Academy of Pediatrics doesn't recommend co-sleeping (or bed-sharing) as a safe activity. If you choose to do it anyway, avoid doing it with infants younger than three months old, if anyone in the bed smokes, or if you smoked while pregnant or if anyone in the bed is excessively tired or taking medications or substances that make it hard to be aroused or awakened easily. Only use a firm mattress (not a soft surface) and keep all soft bedding (pillows, blankets, sheets) out of the bed.

Q How many daytime naps should my baby have? Will it prevent him from sleeping at night?

In general, you should be aiming to let your baby have three naps during the day to make sure he does not get overtired. He will probably get himself into a pattern of taking a nap in the morning shortly after he has woken up and been fed, another nap at lunchtime, and then a third nap late afternoon. The third nap should not be too close to bedtime or he might struggle to fall asleep later. It is also important to make sure he does not sleep too much during the day, since this can affect the quality of his nighttime sleep. As he grows, he will start dropping his naps, usually the late afternoon nap goes first.

Q What is a good bedtime routine for my young baby and is it too early to try to establish one?

After six weeks, as part of helping him learn the difference between day and night, it can be helpful to set up a regular bedtime routine. Following the same steps every bedtime means your baby will become familiar with the routine, and in turn associate the process with bedtime. If you follow the same pattern every night, your baby will feel safe and secure, and learn to differentiate between daytime naps and bedtime. A relaxing bath, followed by a long feeding, and a story will help your baby unwind. Even if you just point out the pictures, your baby will love hearing your voice and having your undivided attention. If your baby is really tired, a bath will revive him to allow him to have a good feeding before bed. Many parents find this a special time of day when they share quiet cuddling with their baby.

Night-lights can **trick your baby's** brain into perceiving daylight and awake time. Try using a **red lightbulb** instead (which our brains don't see as daylight) to find your way during night feedings.

Q What is SIDS and how can I prevent it? Are there any key risk factors?

There are several steps you can take to keep your baby safe while he sleeps. Most important is that you are always in the same room as your baby while he is asleep.

Very rarely, a baby dies in his sleep, known as Sudden Infant Death syndrome (SIDS), or crib death. While the causes still aren't completely understood, there are a number of factors that have been shown to increase the risk of SIDS significantly, and the greatest risk occurs in the first six months of life. Low birth weight and premature babies, as well as male infants, are also more at risk.

PRECAUTIONS AND PREVENTION

The following will help to ensure that your baby sleeps safely:

» Put your baby down to sleep on his back with his feet at the very end of is crib ("feet to foot") so that he can't wiggle down under bedding.

» For the first six months, it is safer to put your baby to sleep in a crib or bassinet in the same room as you.

» Avoid pillows, baby duvets, and soft toys in the crib for at least the first year.

» Keep the room temperature where your baby sleeps around 60–68° F (16–20° C).

» Don't smoke near your baby, or allow anyone else to. Never sleep in the same bed as your baby if you have smoked, drunk alcohol, or taken drugs or medication that makes you drowsy.

» If possible, breast-feed your baby. There is a lower incidence of SIDS in breast-fed babies.

» Never sleep on a sofa or chair with your baby.

» Using a pacifier (after one month if you're breast-feeding) may reduce the risk of SIDS.

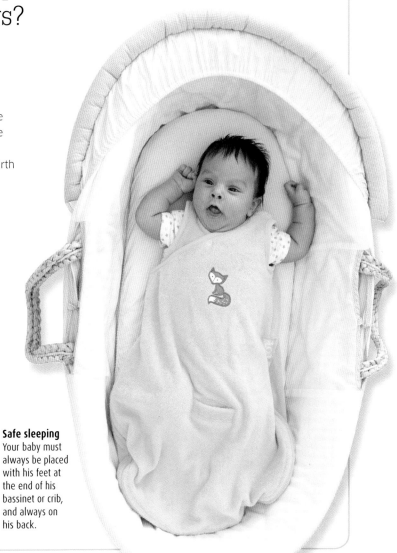

Safe sleeping
Your baby must always be placed with his feet at the end of his bassinet or crib, and always on his back.

{Q How can I interact and play with my new baby? She's too young to do very much!

Your baby may seem to do nothing but eat and sleep in the first few weeks of life—she is very busy growing after all—but she is also primed for interaction and discovery. Play and stimulation are essential for your baby's development, helping her to learn about her world, about you, and how she fits in to this new place.

Early learning

You are your baby's first playmate—your play and responses guide your baby and give her the confidence to try new things. In the early months, your baby interacts with you and her surroundings in simple ways: looking, cooing and gurgling, making facial expressions, touching, and grasping. By providing stimulation appropriate to her age and stage, you enable your baby to practice and learn new skills that will take her forward to the next stage of development. You can dedicate some one-on-one time to playing, maybe five minutes playing peekaboo, 10 minutes settling down to explore a book with fun textures, or a few moments showing her a new object or toy. Equally, much of your interaction will be woven into the fabric of your day: chatting during a diaper change, pointing out objects around the home, or spontaneously blowing a raspberry on her tummy as you dress her. Each interaction is intrinsically valuable.

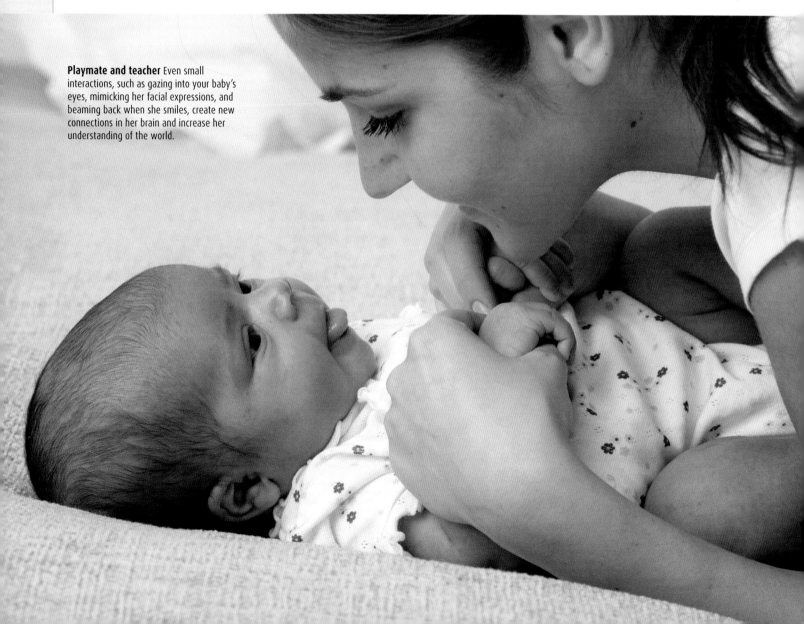

Playmate and teacher Even small interactions, such as gazing into your baby's eyes, mimicking her facial expressions, and beaming back when she smiles, create new connections in her brain and increase her understanding of the world.

HOW YOUR BABY DEVELOPS

eing aware of your baby's pattern of development in these early months can also help you to target play to nhance her development, and make sure that you aren't frustrating her with activities beyond her capabilities.

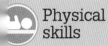 ## Physical skills

 ## Social and cognitive skills

 ## Your baby's senses

 ## Outdoor Exploration

Your baby will need some time to learn control of her limbs. Her movements are uncoordinated in the early weeks; she is slowly unfurling and stretching her limbs after being curled up in your uterus. As her muscles strengthen, however, you can provide opportunities for her to practice moving her limbs and body.

》 Place your baby on her back to allow her to get used to moving her limbs around, waving her arms, and kicking her legs. This gentle exercise will develop and strengthen her muscles.

》 Join your little one on the floor and talk to her about what she is doing, or put her under a play gym so she can swoosh and bat at the dangling objects.

》 Put your baby on her tummy, when she is a little stronger. As your baby gets older, she is likely to become increasingly excited and to kick and wave enthusiastically. A few moments of "tummy time" each day will help to strengthen her back and neck muscles, and will set her on the path to rolling and crawling.

》 Give your baby an incentive to reach out when her strength and coordination grow. Place your baby on her tummy on the floor with a colorful toy just in front of her so she can practice reaching out. Always supervise tummy time when your baby is very young, and don't leave her on her tummy if she becomes frustrated.

Reading, singing, and talking to your baby all help develop her language skills. Your first "conversations"—responding to your baby's coos and gurgles with ones of your own—enable her to watch the shapes your mouth makes, learn about sounds, and copy the noises you make. These interactions also teach important social skills: how conversations involve taking turns and listening.

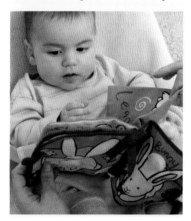

Stimulating your baby's senses is incredibly important in these early months. Your baby learns about the world around her through touch, and also derives comfort from cuddling, caresses, and skin-to-skin contact. Although she can focus her eyes only a short distance at birth, she will soon be taking in everything she sees.

》 Provide a feast for your baby's eyes with bold patterns, mirrors, and bright objects.

》 Cloth books with different textures help teach concepts such as smooth and bumpy, soft and hard, furry and crinkly.

》 Talk about and identify textures and point out contrasts in everyday objects.

》 Comment on different noises that you can hear inside the house or outside, and talk about the aromas in the kitchen.

Day trips out with your baby can keep you both feeling fresh. A walk to the store, a longer trip to the park, or just some time in the yard all provide a change of environment and new stimulation for your baby. Talk to her about the sights and sounds outside: look at the leaves blowing in the breeze, at the pattern of clouds or shadows on the ground, and at the buses, trains, and planes passing by.

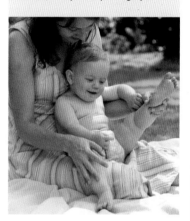

WHEN YOUR BABY HAS HAD ENOUGH

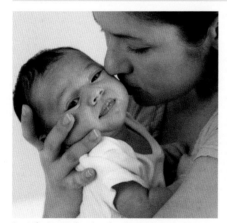

Rest time Even low-key family visits can feel intense for a baby, especially if she's passed around.

Every day your baby is absorbing and enjoying new sights, sounds, and information, but she also tires easily. If she doesn't have an opportunity for some downtime, she can feel overwhelmed by too many new noises, activities, and sensations.

Try to plan your baby's day so that there are times when activities are downscaled, and be alert to signs that your baby has had enough. Symptoms of overstimulation and fatigue include:
》 Becoming fussy and cranky.
》 Turning her head away from you and from toys and activities.
》 Appearing withdrawn.

If your young baby has been awake for about two hours, she probably needs to be put down for a nap. Or she may just benefit from some quiet time in her crib, or being cradled in your arms.

Q My baby isn't her usual self, but there's nothing specific I can put my finger on. Should I call the doctor?

As a new parent, it can be hard to judge when your baby needs medical attention, or whether you are overreacting to a harmless sniffle. Perhaps your baby hasn't been feeding well for a couple of days, or isn't quite as alert as usual. Since young babies often don't show many symptoms when they are sick, sometimes it can be hard to tell whether a baby is just a little under the weather or if there is something a bit more serious going on. For this reason, it's always best to listen to your voice of doubt and trust your instincts and get her checked over by your doctor. The chances are that there is nothing seriously wrong, but doctors are always happy to see young babies—and often prioritize them—and would rather that you erred on the side of caution. For example, a slight fever is usually nothing to worry about in an older child, but a fever is relatively unusual in a baby under three months old, and is sometimes the only sign of a more serious infection, so it's vital not to ignore it. Because a baby's immune system is still immature, they can be more susceptible to a secondary bacterial infection, and can deteriorate quite quickly. It's most likely that your doctor will be able to ease your mind but he or she will also reassure you that you did the right thing by making an appointment.

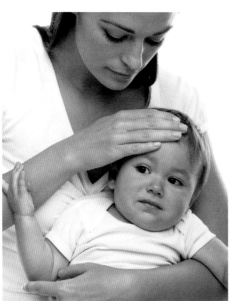

Keeping calm Try to stay calm since your baby will respond to how you are acting and will pick up on any stress.

Q Which symptoms always require medical attention?

There are certain symptoms and signs that should not be ignored and that should be dealt with quickly. Some signs (see bottom) need urgent attention.

 ## SIGNS OF A SERIOUS ILLNESS

The following signs could signal that your baby has an illness and needs to see her pediatrician. Do not hesitate to call and make an appointment if you notice:

» **Behavioral changes** are often the first sign that something isn't right. If your baby is lethargic, drowsy, hard to rouse to be fed, or persistently irritable for no reason, this may indicate that she isn't feeling well.

» **Changes in crying patterns** or sounds, for example a lack of crying or unusual high-pitched cries.

» **Changes in feeding patterns** and feeding poorly, or if your baby refuses several feedings in a row.

» **Severe vomiting or diarrhea** that lasts for longer than 12 hours (see p.295), or that is streaked with blood or mucus should be assessed.

» **Signs of an eye infection,** or a discharge from the eyes.

» **Your baby isn't responding to sounds** or has a discharge from the ears.

» **A temperature of 100.4° F** (38° C) or more if she is under three months old; or of 102. 2°F (39° C) or more if she is under six months old.

» **A sunken or bulging fontanelle,** the soft spot on your baby's head should be checked. Usually, this should be firm to the touch and may dip in a little. When your baby cries, lies down, or is sick, the fontanelle can bulge, but it should return to normal when your baby is upright and calm.

» **An unexplained rash,** especially if it accompanies a fever or diarrhea.

» **Signs of dehydration** (see p.294).

» **Signs of constipation,** such as hard, small stools, with fewer bowel movements than usual.

 ## CALL AN AMBULANCE

You should always call an ambulance if you notice that your baby is displaying any of these symptoms:

» **Stops breathing** or is struggling for breath.

» **Is unconscious** or unaware of what's going on.

» **A seizure,** even if she recovers.

» **One or more symptoms** of meningitis (see p.295).

 ## GO TO THE EMERGENCY ROOM

Go immediately to the emergency room (ER) if you spot your baby showing any of the symptoms and issues listed below:

» **Has a fever and is persistently lethargic,** despite taking medication.

» **Is having difficulty breathing,** including fast or panting breathing, or is very wheezy.

» **Has severe abdominal pain.**

» **Has a cut that won't stop bleeding** or is gaping open.

» **Has a serious fall or bump to the head.**

» **Is turning blue.**

Did you know...

When taking care of a sick baby it's important that you keep her fluids up, keep informed (know the signs and symptoms), let go of routines, don't overdress her, keep her room draft-free (but not too stuffy or warm), and remain calm so as not to alarm her.

Q What might I need to ask or tell the doctor?

To make the most out of the possibly limited time you have with your pediatrician, think about the information your doctor might need to know, and have questions ready. Taking a pad and pen means you can have questions written down so that you don't forget to ask anything, which is easily done when you're busy listening to what the doctor has to say.

Jot down any instructions or suggestions your doctor gives you for taking care of your baby at home. Be ready to give your doctor information about your baby's symptoms and when they started; about whether your baby has been feeding well and has had wet diapers; and about changes in your baby's temperature, and the time you checked her temperature. If you have given your baby any medicine, let your doctor know what you have given, how much, and when. Have your baby's immunization history ready.

Q What are the signs of a fever and how should I treat it?

If your baby looks unusually flushed, her skin is clammy and sweaty, and if her forehead, the back or her neck, or her tummy feel hot to touch, she may have a raised temperature that needs to be checked (see p.292). Your baby may also be cranky and drowsier than usual.

Most babies and infants work through a fever in a matter of days. If your doctor has seen your baby and is fine for her to be taken care of at home, continue to monitor her for as long as she isn't her normal self. Keep her fluid intake up and be on the lookout for signs of dehydration, such as fewer wet diapers than normal or a sunken fontanelle (see p.294). Once your baby starts to rally, don't launch right back into normal activities—your little one may still be tired and need a bit of time to get back to her normal self. Having said that, babies often bounce back surprisingly quickly from minor illnesses. If at any point she deteriorates, perhaps becoming drowsier or clearly dehydrated, or if she develops a rash, or you just feel concerned, listen to your instincts and go right back to the doctor, or to the hospital if you are very worried.

HOW TO TREAT A FEVER

Follow these methods to help reduce your baby's temperature. You can also talk to your baby soothingly and reassure her that you're there to help.

» **While the first port of call** is to get medical advice when your young baby has a fever, you also need to make sure that she doesn't become dehydrated. A fever makes your baby sweat more, so she loses water as it evaporates on the skin. Keep topping up her fluids with frequent breast or formula feedings, and for formula-fed babies, give top-ups of water (fresh water that has been boiled and cooled).

» **Make sure** that your baby's environment isn't too hot—it should be around 64° F (18° C).

» **If your baby is distressed** by the fever, call your pediatrician to find out what dose of baby acetaminophen you can give her. The dosage will vary based on your baby's age and weight. Don't give babies younger than 6 months baby ibuprofen. And never give aspirin to babies or children. Baby acetaminophen and baby ibuprofen are available over the counter. Both come in liquid form with a dropper to make it easy to administer.

» **There is no need** to sponge your baby with lukewarm water, or remove layers of clothes—check, though, that your baby isn't uncomfortably hot with too many layers of clothing. You can strip her down to her diaper if she is incredibly hot.

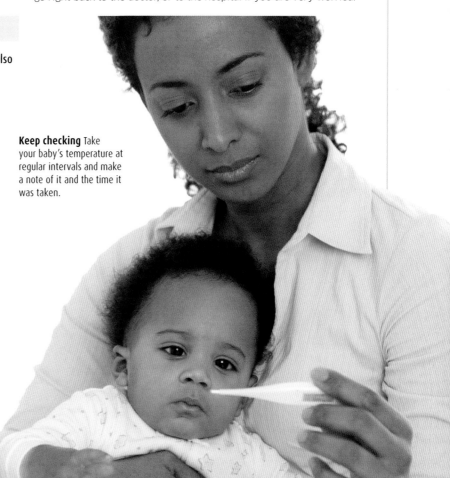

Keep checking Take your baby's temperature at regular intervals and make a note of it and the time it was taken.

Q How do I take my baby's temperature, and what is a normal reading?

A normal temperature for your baby is around 98.6°F (37°C), with slight variations being usual between children.

If your baby's temperature is higher than 99.5°F (37.5°C), then she has a fever. If your baby is under three months and her temperature reaches 100.4°F (38°C) or higher, or she is under six months with a temperature of 102.2°F (39°C) or more, consult a doctor right away.

Is a fever always a concern?
In babies over six months and toddlers and children, a fever in itself isn't such a great concern, and other signs of illness are used to gauge a child's well-being. In older infants, a raised temperature is actually a positive sign that her body is fighting off an infection, since it is harder for bacteria and viruses to survive in a hot environment.

Fevers in young babies are less common, and because with young babies it can be harder to spot other signs of illness, or to tell if there is a potentially serious underlying infection, a raised temperature should always be taken more seriously since it may be the only clear sign that something is wrong. You should therefore consult your doctor right away or go to the emergency room (ER) if your young baby has a high temperature and you can't contact your doctor.

TAKING YOUR BABY'S TEMPERATURE

While you may be able to gauge if your baby has a fever by looking at or touching her, taking her temperature lets you know exactly what her temperature is, which is important in young babies. There are several types of thermometer you can use.

THERMOMETER TYPE	DESCRIPTION	
Strip thermometer	Very convenient and easy to use, especially if your baby is fidgety, you just hold the strip on your baby's forehead. However, they are not very accurate because they measure skin, rather than body, temperature.	STRIP THERMOMETER
Digital underarm thermometer	These are cheap and fairly accurate. Place the bulb of the thermometer under your baby's arm in her armpit, then gently hold her arm alongside her body. You need to hold the thermometer in the armpit for a set amount of time—some beep when they are ready to read. Often the trickiest part of taking a baby's temperature with this type of thermometer is getting her to stay still. Hold and soothe her before you start, and talk to her calmly while you take her temperature. Never place a thermometer in the mouth of a child under five years old.	DIGITAL UNDERARM THERMOMETER
Digital ear thermometer	Although more expensive, these take a reading quickly. However, if they aren't placed correctly, they may not be that accurate.	DIGITAL EAR THERMOMETER

In the US, young children and babies with a high temperature account for around **20 percent** of the admissions to the children's emergency room (ER) at the hospital.

Q Can a high temperature increase my baby's risk of having a seizure?

Yes, febrile seizures are brought on when a baby or child has a raised temperature. However, although they can look alarming, they are usually harmless. Seizures most often occur between six months and three years old, and are fairly unusual in babies younger than six months old. During a seizure, a baby or child may become stiff, and may lose consciousness and shake her limbs. If your baby has a seizure, hold her on her side and remove anything from her mouth that she could choke on, such as a pacifier. Make sure her head is turned to the side so that she doesn't choke if she vomits. Stay with her, and time how long the seizure lasts. A baby who has had a first seizure should always be checked by a doctor at the hospital. If your baby has had a seizure before and a subsequent one lasts longer than five minutes, she should be checked by a doctor, and if a subsequent seizure lasts less than five minutes, call your doctor for advice.

Q How do I give medicine to a wiggling baby?

Getting a baby to take medicine or tolerate drops being put in her eye can be one of the most exasperating tasks for parents. As much as possible, try to stay calm.

Your baby's distress coupled with your concern about helping her get better means that it is easy for both of you to end up in a tight ball of stress. Even if you don't feel calm, try to sound reassuring and be matter of fact. Time medicine for when your baby is most receptive, perhaps after being cuddled, or before being fed, when she's a little hungry and will swallow something.

ADMINISTERING MEDICINE AND DROPS

Before you give medicine or drops, always check that they haven't passed their use-by date, and after using, store the medicine or drops as recommended by the manufacturer or pharmacist.

» Giving oral medicines: these can be given via the syringe or dosage spoon provided by the manufacturer. For a very young baby, a syringe can be the easiest way to get the medicine into her mouth since the contents are less likely to be spilled. Also, up until about four months, your baby has a thrust reflex, which means she automatically pushes things out of her mouth, so it's easier to use a syringe. Draw up the correct dosage of medicine into the syringe. Hold your baby close to you in an upright position, and, if it helps, stroke her cheek to encourage her to open her mouth, then place the syringe in your baby's mouth. Let your baby suck on the syringe if she seems willing to, or squirt the contents slowly, or a little at a time, into the side, rather than the back, of her mouth, so she doesn't choke. If you use a spoon, gently tip the medicine into the mouth, giving small amounts at a time if this works best.

» Administering eye drops: if possible, get someone else to help you do this, with one of you holding your baby while the other gives the drops. You may also find wrapping your baby in a blanket helpful, if this doesn't distress her, so that she isn't able to thrash her arms and legs around. Wash your hands. With your baby laid flat or in a reclined position, gently pull down the lower eyelid, then squeeze one drop into the lower lid, being careful not to touch any part of the eye with the dropper. Once you let go of the lid, your baby should blink, which helps to disperse the drop. If your baby won't allow you to pull down her lid, place the drop onto the side of the closed eye closest to the nose. Although not as effective, some of the fluid will hopefully make its way into the eye once open.

» Administering saline nose drops: your doctor or pharmacist may recommend these if a clogged nose is interfering with your baby's feeding or breathing. Wash your hands. As with eye drops, recruit a helper if possible. Wipe away any mucus. With your baby lying flat, place the dropper just inside the nostril and squeeze the right amount of drops into the nostril. Try to hold your baby in this position for a minute or so to help the drops spread through the nose.

» Giving ear drops: the sensation of liquid going into her ear may upset your baby and she may wiggle, so wrapping her in a blanket can help to keep her still while you give her the drops. Wash your hands. Lay your baby down and try to tilt her head to one side. Gently pull the ear lobe down to open up the ear canal, then squeeze the correct number of drops into the ear. Keep her in this position for a couple of minutes so that the drops can work their way into the ear.

Administering eye drops Do this as quickly and calmly as possible, talking to your baby constantly during the procedure to reassure her.

Q How can I help protect my baby from catching bugs?

Infections are inevitable in babies and young children as their immune system builds up its resistance over time. However, there are a few things you can do to limit the number of infections your little one picks up. Breast-feeding for as long as possible is one of the best ways to keep your baby well, since your milk passes on protective antibodies. When your baby is very young, it's also good to limit, or avoid contact with people with colds and bugs. Throughout infancy, she'll be offered many vaccinations, so keep up with her scheduled immunization program.

Q How can I best comfort and take care of my baby when she is sick?

Taking care of a sick baby is a new experience for many parents, and understandably, anxiety can take hold of you. Keep in mind that your comforting presence is an important factor in keeping her calm, which in turn helps her body fight illness. Your baby feels less secure when she is sick, so staying close by, cuddling her, and talking soothingly will all help reassure her.

While young babies can go downhill quite rapidly, with the right attention they usually recover quickly too. Knowing what to look for, when to seek medical help, or when to tend to her at home, gives you the confidence that you're equipped to give her the right care.

{Q How can I identify common illnesses and complaints?

Often it's clear when your baby is not well—he may be irritable, not feeding as usual, and lethargic. A fever is a clear sign that he is fighting infection (see p.291), and a stuffed nose and cough are easy to spot, as are stomach upsets. Other signs are less obvious: perhaps your baby is clingier than usual or isn't feeding well. Trust your instincts: if you think something isn't quite right, call your doctor.

Dehydration

» Symptoms:

Fewer wet diapers than usual, dark yellow urine, hard stools, and constipation are all signs of dehydration. Other signs include lethargy, crying without producing tears; a dry, sticky mouth; and/or a sunken fontanelle (the soft spot on his head).

» What you should do:

If your baby is suffering with vomiting, diarrhea, or has a temperature (see p.292), try to keep his fluid intake up to prevent dehydration from occurring in the first place. Offer frequent breast or formula feeding (you may need to give small feedings more often). If your baby has any of the above symptoms of dehydration, contact your doctor. He may suggest oral rehydration solution (available from pharmacies) between feeds; cooled, boiled water may be given instead if your baby refuses the solution.

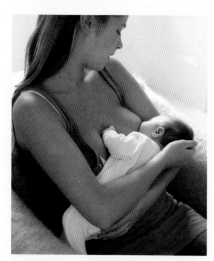

Frequent breast-feeding Feeding your baby often ensures that his fluid levels are maintained.

Cradle cap

» Symptoms:

Scaly patches on the scalp that may be thick and crusty. These may be caused by overactive sebaceous glands in the first months, which then settle down. Cradle cap is usually harmless and doesn't cause itchiness or discomfort.

» What you should do:

Cradle cap typically clears up within weeks or months, and can usually be managed at home. For mild cradle cap, wash your baby's hair regularly with a baby shampoo to prevent scales from building up, and use a baby brush to loosen flakes. Massaging a little olive oil into the head and leaving this overnight softens the scales before brushing in the morning. Don't pick the scales since this could damage skin and cause an infection. If cradle cap is persistent, ask your pharmacist about stronger shampoos to loosen cradle cap. If patches spread to the face or body, self-help measures don't work, or there's bleeding or inflammation, consult your doctor.

Eczema

» Symptoms:

Red, dry, and itchy skin on the face, and in areas where the skin creases, such as the elbows, knees, and in the neck. The condition often starts in babies between two and four months old and may be connected to an allergy to milk.

» What you should do:

Talk to your doctor about managing your baby's eczema. He or she can advise you on treatments such as emollient moisturizing creams, and may prescribe a topical corticosteroid. Scratch mittens can stop your baby from damaging his skin further, and keep your baby's nails short. Avoid bath products if your baby has a flare-up, and use nonbiological laundry detergent for your baby's clothes. If the eczema is stubborn and sore, talk to your doctor about other remedies, such as wet wraps, which can help the skin to heal.

Thrush

» Symptoms:

If your baby has oral thrush, a condition caused by the yeast fungus *Candida albicans*, he may have a white coating on his tongue and white patches around the mouth with a curdlike texture. These don't rub off easily and, if sore, can interfere with feeding. Your baby may also have a diaper rash caused by the same infection. If you are breast-feeding, the infection can be passed between you and your baby and can make your nipples sore and painful.

» What you should do:

Make an appointment with your doctor. While the condition isn't usually serious, he or she may prescribe an antifungal medicine or gel for your baby. If you're breast-feeding, your doctor may prescribe an antifungal cream for your nipples.

Conjunctivitis

» Symptoms:

This eye infection causes an inflammation of the thin membrane (conjunctiva) covering the white of the eye. The eye is red, inflamed, itchy, sticky, and watery, and there may be a discharge. The eye may be crusted over after sleep. It is caused either by an infection, or an allergy or irritant, such as cigarette smoke. In newborns, conjunctivitis may be contracted from bacteria in the birth canal.

» What you should do:

Use cotton pads soaked in cooled boiled water to remove the crust and goo from your baby's eye, using a separate cotton pad for each eye so you don't pass infection between them. Wash your hands after touching your baby and use a separate towel to stop the infection from spreading to others. If your baby is under 28 days old, or the infection is severe or doesn't clear up after a week or so, contact your doctor because your baby may have a bacterial infection that needs treatment with eye drops.

Diarrhea and vomiting

» Symptoms:

Watery, loose stools, that may be mucus stained and smelly, indicate diarrhea. Vomiting is when your baby brings up a sizeable quantity of milk (rather than a few teaspoons' worth). Causes include gastroenteritis, reflux, and allergy.

» What you should do:

Talk to your doctor. He or she may suggest replacing fluids your baby is losing to prevent dehydration by offering frequent feedings; giving oral rehydration solution in addition, or cooled, boiled water if your baby refuses the solution. Make sure to consult your doctor if your baby has had diarrhea six or more times, or has vomited three or more times, in the last 24 hours, has a rash, fever, signs of dehydration, or blood in his vomit or stool. For more advice about fluids, see Dehydration, left.

Reflux

» Symptoms:

Frequent regurgitation of milk and stomach acid. (Some spitting up is normal—the muscular valve that closes the stomach doesn't fully develop until 12–18 months.)

» What you should do:

Feed in smaller amounts more frequently, and burp often. Avoid overfeeding; for bottle-fed babies, try a nipple with a smaller hole. Hold your baby upright after feeding to ease reflux. See your doctor if your baby has frequent reflux with coughing, gagging, persistent crying, or poor weight gain.

Colds and flu

» Symptoms:

A runny nose, a cough, red eyes, and sometimes a raised temperature. Cold symptoms combined with a sudden fever of 100.4° F (38° C) or more may indicate a flu. Other signs of flu are lethargy, lack of appetite, vomiting, and diarrhea.

» What you should do:

Call your doctor who might recommend making sure your baby gets plenty of fluids (see Dehydration, left). If your baby has a stuffed nose and feeding is difficult, try raising the humidity levels to loosen his mucus: put a bowl of warm water in the room or sit in a steamy room. You can buy saline nasal drops to help thin the mucus from pharmacies. Your baby will also need to sleep more while he is recovering from a cold.

Ear infections

» Symptoms:

It can be hard to tell if a baby has an ear infection, but if he rubs or tugs on his ear, is irritable, isn't feeding normally, vomits, doesn't respond to quieter noises, and has a temperature a few days after the onset of a cold, he may have an ear infection. Pus may appear if the eardrum is damaged.

» What you should do:

Ear infections usually clear up in about three days without treatment. If your baby is under three months old and has a temperature of 100.4° F (38° C) or more, or is under six months old with a temperature of 102.2° F (39° C), consult your doctor. He or she may prescribe antibiotics if your baby is under three months old. A warm washcloth over the ear can be soothing. Repeated infections may be treated with tympanostomy tubes—tubes inserted in the ear to drain fluid.

Bronchiolitis

» Symptoms:

Symptoms are similar to a cold with a fever. They may worsen after a few days and include a dry, rasping cough, noisy or fast breathing, brief pauses between breaths, vomiting, feeding less, and having fewer wet diapers.

» What you should do:

Symptoms usually clear up in a couple of weeks. If your baby is under three months and has a temperature of 100.4° F (38° C) or more, or is under six months with a temperature of 102.2° F (39° C), consult your doctor. Keep your baby hydrated, and upright as much as possible to ease congestion. A humidifier, or bowl of warm water in a room keeps the air moist. Call your doctor (or an ambulance if you're very concerned) if your baby is having difficulty breathing, is breathing rapidly, isn't feeding well and hasn't had a wet diaper in the last 12 hours, or is unresponsive or is irritable.

Croup

» Symptoms:

Difficulty in breathing and a distinctive barking cough. Croup most commonly affects children between six months and three years old, but can occur in younger babies.

» What you should do:

Mild croup can be managed at home. Keep your baby hydrated, hold him upright to ease breathing, and comfort him, as crying worsens symptoms. Your doctor may prescribe an oral corticosteroid to reduce swelling in the throat.

Whooping cough (pertussis)

» Symptoms:

A dry, persistent cough with prolonged bouts of coughing, interspersed with gasps for air. There may be a runny nose, fever, and vomiting. Coughing may last for months.

» What you should do:

Get a vaccination against the virus between 28 and 38 weeks of pregnancy to protect your baby at birth, and have your baby vaccinated at two months old. If your baby has symptoms, consult your doctor immediately, who may give antibiotics. If he has trouble breathing, call an ambulance.

Meningitis

» Symptoms in babies:

Meningitis is a viral or bacterial infection of the membranes surrounding the brain and spinal cord. Symptoms include a bulging fontanelle; a fever with cold hands and feet (although young babies may have a normal or low temperature); sleepiness; rapid breathing; grunting; a high-pitched or moaning cry; shivering; stiffness and jerking or floppiness; irritability from muscle aches—perhaps not wanting to be picked up; diarrhea and vomiting; a stiff neck; dislike of bright lights; blotchy skin; and convulsions or seizures. A purple "pinprick" rash or purple bruises that don't disappear under a pressed glass, may indicate blood poisoning—a medical emergency. Symptoms can occur in any order.

» What you should do:

Don't wait for a rash to appear before getting help. If you suspect meningitis, call an ambulance immediately and say that you suspect meningitis.

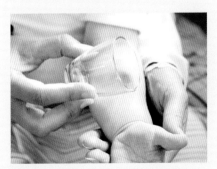

The glass test A rash that doesn't disappear under a pressed glass indicates blood poisoning.

Life with your **new baby** is full of novel experiences, intense emotions, and **positive changes**. It also brings with it many new **responsibilities** and considerations, and you will find that you need to **plan ahead** far more than you did in the past.

Planning for the future

Thinking ahead to work

One of the main considerations when taking time off with your baby is when, or if, you plan to return to work after the birth. You may have already set a date with your employer, though you might change your mind about this date when you are on leave—maybe wanting to return earlier for financial reasons, or to take an extended period of time off. Many women take three months of maternity leave. Whether or not it's paid depends on your company's policy. With the Family and Medical Leave Act, many people can get three months of unpaid leave. Individual employers may have their own terms and offers, so discuss these with yours. If you plan to return to work, arranging child care early on means you can relax and enjoy precious time with your baby.

A growing family

After a certain period of time, and once you are settled in with your new family unit, you and your partner might start to think about adding a new addition to the family, providing a sibling for your baby. There are so many reasons for and against different age gaps between siblings, and you may feel that some of these are worth considering. Essentially, though, if you and your partner feel ready emotionally, physically, and financially for this step, the time could be right to try to become pregnant again. Keep discussions open with your partner so that you are aware of each other's feelings and expectations, and any differences of opinion can be talked through.

Changes to the home

Now you are three, it's natural to reevaluate your home setup and consider how well this works for your new family unit. Perhaps you are thinking about a move to a new area where you can get a larger home for your money, which is something many parents consider in the preschool years. Or if a move isn't on the agenda, you might think about changes you can make to your existing home. Keep in mind that your child will feel happy wherever she is as long as she is surrounded by love and has good care, so don't feel you have to make changes to your home if it is likely that these are going to be stressful or financially challenging.

Q What things could I be putting in place now that will benefit my child's future?

There are a number of issues that may not have worried you too much until you had a baby and became a responsible parent. The issues discussed below are worth considering and prioritizing.

While many of these are financial, such as whether you want to start a savings account for private schooling or college, some are practical, such as leaving a will and assigning guardians to your new child if anything happens to you and your partner. You may also like to consider "legacy" issues such as family stories, letters, heirlooms, and cultural matters (particularly if there are varied nationalities in the family) you would like your child to read or know about in the future. Here is a checklist for some of the things you may want to put in place.

PLANNING FOR THE FUTURE

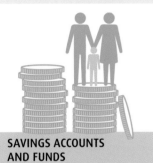

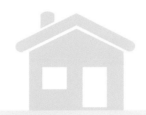

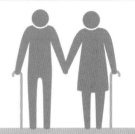

SAVINGS ACCOUNTS AND FUNDS

Whether starting to save now for her future education or first home, or a trust to safeguard your child from having large tax bills in the future, you may want to consider setting up a bank account now.

INSURANCE

Look at life and health insurance since you may want to increase your plans now that a child is in your life, so you are financially covered if something happens to you or your partner. If you have private health or dental plans, you should add the name of your baby.

WILLS AND GUARDIANSHIP

Set up a will to avoid leaving the fate of your child's guardianship and your assets in the court's hands. Assign a guardian who would be able to step in to raise your child, if the worst happened, and help her with her education, health, and keep her safe and taken care of until she is an adult.

PENSIONS AND RETIREMENT

It may seem a long way off but you will want to make sure that there is sufficient money in the pot for you later in life, so that the burden of old age and what it may bring with it doesn't fall on your child.

Q We definitely want to become pregnant again. Is there an ideal age gap between siblings?

There are pros and cons for different age gaps, and your decision on when to try again is likely to be influenced by how you both feel about managing family life. You may feel that having a second baby while your first child is still very young means that you will be able to deal with the intense baby and toddler stages all at the same time. Your children are likely to be natural playmates and develop a strong bond, and can be companions when at school. Also, if you are planning to have a big family you may not want to wait too long before you have a second child. Some suggest, though, that siblings very close in age may squabble more when competing for toys and attention. Conversely, you may want to wait until your first child is out of diapers before considering another baby, so that you

have more time to dedicate both to your first child's early years and then to the new baby. Physically, this may also be more appealing, giving your body plenty of time to recover from the birth of your first baby, so that you have more energy for the new arrival. Financially, a bigger age gap means you may not need to invest in items such as a double stroller or an additional crib, and you can spread the cost of child care out over a longer period.

Q Healthwise, is there an optimal time to wait before getting pregnant again?

Both you, and your future baby, can benefit from having some space between pregnancies. Pregnancy and breast-feeding can deplete your reserves of essential nutrients such as folate and iron, so giving your body some time to

build these reserves before you conceive again can benefit both your own and your unborn baby's health. Furthermore, recent studies have shown that women who gave birth again within 18 months of having a baby were considerably more likely to have a premature delivery than those who waited longer to get pregnant again. Waiting at least 12–18 months after having a baby before conceiving again is thought to eliminate the increased risk of premature birth.

There are **factors** other than age, such as **personality** and **gender**, that will determine how well or not your **children do.**

Q I'm undecided about whether or not to return to work. What should I consider?

For many families, one of the deciding factors about returning to work is the financial situation and balancing salaries with the cost of child care.

The most important thing is doing what is right for you and your partner. Both of you need to review your job circumstances, the long-term and short-term salary implications, and feelings about staying at home to make sure the appropriate person is the main caregiver. Whatever you decide, be prepared to be flexible. What you thought might work for you when you were pregnant might not turn out to be the case once your baby arrives. Well-thought out plans can change,

and you may feel you want to take a bit more time off than planned, or that an earlier return works better. If you adore being at home, then it's likely that you will find this a fulfilling option. Your feelings may change later on. You may find that you are missing your work environment and that you are eager to pursue your career. If parents are happy and fulfilled, and you feel completely comfortable with your child-care of choice, then the whole family is likely to thrive.

DISCUSSION POINTS

If you have a choice between staying at home and going back to work it's a good idea to communicate with your partner and ask yourself a few key questions:

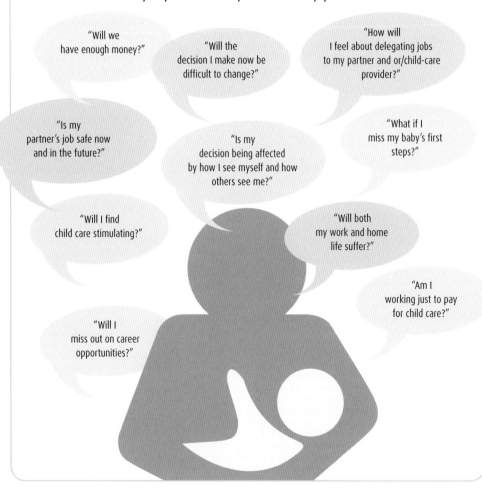

"Will we have enough money?"

"Will the decision I make now be difficult to change?"

"How will I feel about delegating jobs to my partner and or/child-care provider?"

"Is my partner's job safe now and in the future?"

"Is my decision being affected by how I see myself and how others see me?"

"What if I miss my baby's first steps?"

"Will I find child care stimulating?"

"Will both my work and home life suffer?"

"Am I working just to pay for child care?"

"Will I miss out on career opportunities?"

Q I will be returning to work when my baby is three months old. When should I think about arranging child care?

Though your return to work may seem a long way off, and handing your baby over to a caregiver is probably the last thing you want to think about at the beginning of your maternity leave, it is definitely worth looking into this now. You may have already given some thought at the end of pregnancy to the type of child care you would prefer—if not, start considering what you think would suit you as a family. What will your finances allow? Start making inquiries locally, look online, ask your pediatrician's office or your local government for lists of day-care centers or nannies in your area, ask parents you know for recommendations, and talk to friends with older children, who will have good advice.

Q My partner and I are thinking about dividing child care between us and another caregiver. Is this a good idea?

If you are all onboard and you are happy with your choice of child care, this can be a good solution. Often, fathers can feel regretful that they aren't spending enough time with their child, and many find that taking over one or two days a week can be extremely fulfilling. For yourself, returning to work part-time allows you to achieve a satisfactory work/life balance, and your baby gets quality time with both parents. It is worth checking that you are all following a similar nap-time and feeding routine, and that you agree on things like discipline and toilet training methods so that your baby doesn't become confused and unsure of what's expected of him.

72%
of two-parent families and **60 percent** of single mothers **work**, an increase of one-fifth since the mid-1990s.

Q How can I help my baby adjust to a new child-care arrangement?

Make sure that you have chosen a caregiver that you are happy with, so that you can be as relaxed as possible. Your baby will pick up on your anxieties.

Give your baby plenty of time to get used to the new person and routine and try to start the settling in process well before—preferably a few weeks—you go back to work. Babies are far more adaptable than we give them credit for and, with time and patience, can get used to any new arrangements. Initially, it is helpful for you and your baby to spend time with the new caregiver before introducing short periods of time when he is alone with the caregiver. Gradually build up the time he spends away from you with the caregiver so that by the time you go back to work you are all used to the situation and he is completely happy to be left.

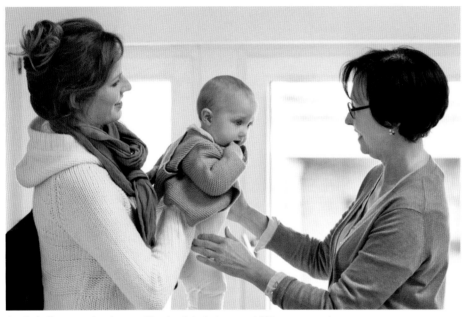

Gentle hello Be as relaxed as possible when introducing your child to a new caregiver.

SETTLING IN TIPS

Here are a few pointers to make the transition easier for you and your child:

» Keep calm: however anxious you might feel about leaving your baby, try to be as relaxed as you can; your baby will pick up on any nerves. Think positive!

» Home visit: your baby probably feels more relaxed and confident in his own surroundings so it can be useful for a babysitter, or staff member from the day-care center you are considering to visit you at home in order for you both to get to know each other better.

» Take a toy: it can be helpful for your baby to have something familiar with him, such as a favorite toy or comfort object.

» Keep it brief: try to make a clean break when you say goodbye to your baby, even if he cries. However upsetting this can be, if you go back to him repeatedly it may simply prolong his distress (and therefore yours). Most babies are easily distracted once you have gone. You could ask the caregiver to call you later to let you know that he has happily settled down.

» Communicate: while this is a challenging new experience for you and your baby, your caregiver has probably been through this many times. Share any worries and concerns that you have. Your caregiver will want to listen and talk through how best to deal with any distress that you or your baby is experiencing. Remember that you are all working toward the same goal: a happy baby.

Q I'm worried about putting my baby into child care. Will he miss me or will he love his caregiver more than me?

Rest assured that your baby will benefit from forming new relationships with different adults who he will indeed form a strong bond with and grow to love—but this doesn't mean that he will love you any less. Leaving your precious baby with a caregiver can cause a whole range of emotions from guilt to sadness, not to mention some relief that you have a little time to yourself. He will be thrilled to see you each time you pick him up and you will cherish these moments. Your baby has more than enough love for you, his family, and his caregivers.

Q The future feels unknown, but very exciting! How should I deal with not knowing what lies ahead?

Parenting constantly presents new challenges, and just when you think you've got the hang of things, your child reaches a new developmental stage, and you need to catch up. Deciding the right work/life balance and choosing child care are big decisions. At times, being a parent can seem terrifying—will you be able to do the very best for your child, and will he be happy and fulfilled? There aren't many things you can do in life that have such a profound effect on you as when you become a parent. However, the best way of managing is to try to be as organized as possible, to enjoy your child, and to be as flexible as you can. Things can and will change. Highs and lows can be intense (not helped by exhaustion in the early years), but mostly, becoming a parent is pretty exhilarating because you experience a totally new and heart-stopping kind of love, and feel a renewed sense of purpose.

> **The more people who take care of your baby,** and that he forms lasting bonds with, **the more loving he will become himself.**

{Q What do I need to think about when choosing child care?

Choosing a person or day-care center to entrust with the care of your baby is a hugely important decision, and one that you will want to consider carefully. Think about your priorities, which things you consider important and what you want for your baby, and look for child care that meets these requirements.

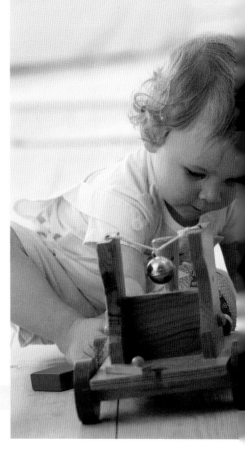

Personal choice

Talking to other parents can be useful, but keep in mind that the right child care for one family may not work for another. So while getting personal recommendations can be invaluable, you may have very different views. For example, while one family may think the social setting of a day-care center is advantageous, you may prefer your child to be in a more homey environment. Try to visit a few different types of settings rather than ruling anything out too early on. When you visit, watch how caregivers interact with your child and other children. Are they responsive and caring, is the environment clean and welcoming, are there plenty of planned activities and toys for the children, and is there dedicated down time? Do the children seem happy and relaxed, and is there outside space? Ask to see copies of any policies, procedures, or certificates—any reputable caregivers will be happy to share these. Consider speaking to some parents who currently have their child at the setting.

DIFFERENT CHILD-CARE OPTIONS

Here is some information on different settings and options for child care. The logistics and prices vary so it is a good idea to do as much research as possible so that you make the right decision.

 Day-care center

The setup: usually privately run, a day-care center offers all-day child care for young babies through to four to five years old. Staff is trained in child development, first aid, and CPR, and there are strict guidelines on ratios of staff to children. Babies and toddlers should have separate areas or rooms where the facilities are appropriate for their age.

 What to think about: your baby should get plenty of stimulation, and will have lots of other children to socialize with. One-on-one time may be rare. The cost can be high, the opening hours are set, and there may be times when it is closed. There will be an illness policy, so you will need a backup plan if your child is sick.

 Home care-center

The setup: also called licensed child-care homes, these should be licensed with the state and be background checked. Rules are different in every state, but there are limits on the number of children that can be taken care of at a time. It's usually only a handful of children under five, with only one or two children under age one or two.

What to think about: your child will be in a home environment, will have a few other children to socialize with, and will receive plenty of attention. In-home day-care staff take care of children for an extended period of time, which gives continuity, and your child is likely to form a close bond with them. If your licensed child-care worker is sick, you will need to have a backup plan.

Nanny

The setup: a qualified individual who will take care of your child in your own home.

What to think about: your child will receive one-on-one care in her own home. Nannies can become a significant part of the family and can stay in touch for years to come. They may be more flexible, occasionally being available for babysitting or weekend care. Nannying is usually the most expensive child-care option, and you are the nanny's employer so will need to pay tax, Social Security and vacation pay. Some nannies ask for extras such as the use of a car. Your child will be on her own unless your nanny meets up with other nannies and their charges.

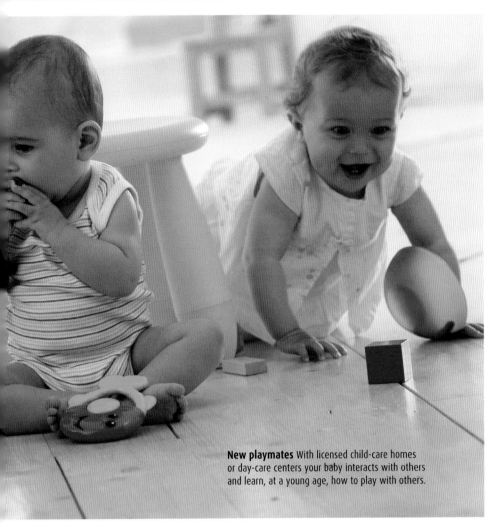

New playmates With licensed child-care homes or day-care centers your baby interacts with others and learn, at a young age, how to play with others.

QUESTIONS TO ASK

When visiting a day-care center or meeting a caregiver, it is a good idea to write down a few questions beforehand. Here are some issues you might want to ask about:

» What will my child's daily routine be? Usually a licensed child-care home will be happy to use your baby's current routine or might be able to suggest an alternative one. At a center, since there are so many babies, they may encourage her to fit in with the others.

» What will my baby be fed and where will she sleep? A day-care center will likely ask you to supply them with enough bottles filled with breast milk or baby formula to last all day. All care providers should have a quiet room for babies to nap in.

» How will you keep me informed of my child's progress? Both licensed child-care homes and other day-care centers should keep a developmental record of your child's progress. You should be able to access this at any time and it may be sent home to you so that you can review and add to it yourself.

» How do you deal with challenging behavior? All children need boundaries to keep them safe, but make sure you are happy with how the potential caregiver disciplines children and ask to see their policy document.

» What is the illness policy? Most child-care settings are happy to accept children with minor coughs and colds, but your child will need to go home and be kept home if she has a fever, sickness, or anything more serious. Ask to see the policy document regarding illness.

» What are your qualifications? It can be reassuring to know that the person taking care of your baby is fully qualified so check that day-care center staff or nannies have the relevant recognized child-care qualifications and up-to-date certificates for first aid. Always follow up on references.

 ## Family care

The setup: grandparents, uncles, and aunts take on the responsibility of caregiver. This can also take on the form of shared care between the parents.

 What to think about: depending on whether you pay your relatives, this can be one of the more cost-effective options and is particularly appropriate if the family members live nearby. Your child will be taken care of by those who love her and will be in a familiar environment. Care can also be divided between parents. In all instances of shared family care, it is vital to establish a consistent routine and rules of behavior.

Au Pair

The setup: these are generally young people who have come to the US to improve their language skills and who live with you. They have their own room and receive board and lodging, as well as some money.

What to think about: they are classified as a member of the family and as such, live in your house, have meals with you, and accompany you on outings. In return they undertake household and child-care duties, but generally for not more than 45 hours per week. Many do not have any training or previous experience of child care and you may not have the chance to meet them before they start.

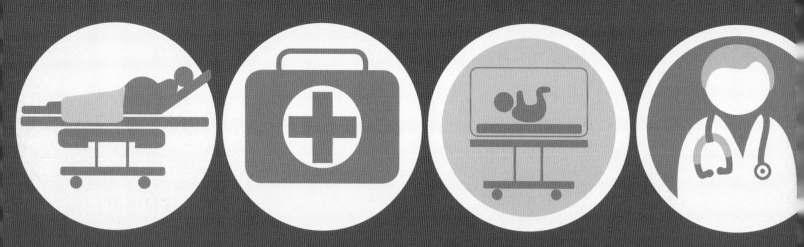

Special situations

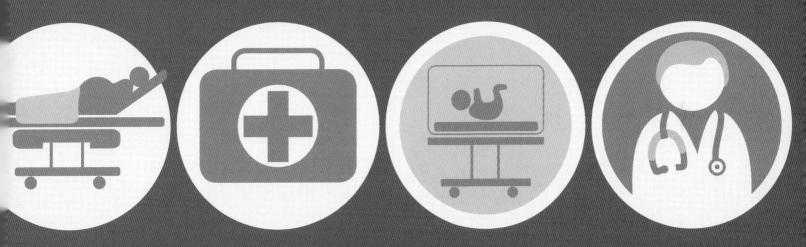

Unexpected events can take place during pregnancy and
birth, and your doctor will always advise you on your particular
circumstances. In this chapter we answer some of the questions
that commonly arise in different situations. **Support and
expert guidance** can be invaluable to help you understand
your options and enable you cope and move toward
the future with a positive outlook.

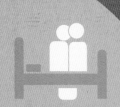

Between 15 and 20 percent of pregnancies in the US end in miscarriage, most of which occur during the first 12 weeks of pregnancy. Being **aware** of the possible causes, **symptoms**, and procedures involved in miscarriages can help you to feel more in control if this happens to you, and to enable you to make **informed choices**.

Miscarriage

What is a miscarriage?

A miscarriage is the spontaneous loss of a pregnancy during the first or second trimester, before a baby has reached 24 weeks gestation. After 24 weeks, a baby is considered "viable," which means that she is developed enough that if born this early she might be able to survive with specialized medical care. The loss of a baby after 24 weeks is known as a stillbirth (see p.309).

While some miscarriages have a specific cause, such as a structural problem with the uterus or the cervix (see opposite), most miscarriages that occur in the first trimester are thought to be due to a one-time chromosomal abnormality in the fetus. Your risk of miscarriage falls the further into your pregnancy you are, and by the beginning of the second trimester, the risk of miscarriage is around just one percent.

The symptoms of miscarriage can vary and may depend on the type of miscarriage (see box, opposite). You may have a dull ache and a bloody discharge or some spotting, or experience severe periodlike pain, which may be accompanied by heavy bleeding and clots. Sometimes a miscarriage can be symptomless and a woman may be quite unaware that there is anything wrong until a routine ultrasound scan reveals that the fetus has stopped developing in the uterus.

Investigating miscarriages

Each miscarriage is distressing, but it can be some consolation to know that, even if no cause is found, the majority of couples go on to have a healthy pregnancy in the future. About one in 100 couples experience three or more successive miscarriages, known as recurrent miscarriage. If this happens, you are likely to be given tests to try to establish a cause (see p.306). If a cause is found, there may be a treatment that can increase your chances of a successful pregnancy next time. Sometimes no cause is found, and the miscarriages are unexplained. Though upsetting, statistically you are still more likely than not to have a healthy pregnancy in the future.

Moving forward

After a miscarriage, couples need time to grieve and recover. It may take a while before you feel ready, physically and emotionally, to consider trying to become pregnant again, or you may want to try again as soon as possible. If you're undergoing tests or treatment, these can influence when you can try again. If there are no complications and the bleeding has stopped, you and your partner can try again when you feel able. It may be worthwhile to review your lifestyle to maximize your chances of a healthy future pregnancy (see p.29).

Q What are the types of miscarriage?

There are different terms for different types of miscarriage, which can be confusing at a time when you are likely to feel vulnerable and upset. Being familiar with these terms can help you to feel more informed, which in turn can help you cope better.

The two main types of miscarriage are inevitable and missed miscarriages. With an inevitable miscarriage, the cervix begins to open up before the baby is viable, and once this happens, it is unlikely that the pregnancy can be saved. This can happen during the first or second trimester. A missed miscarriage (also called a delayed or silent miscarriage) occurs when the embryo or fetus stops developing, but remains inside the uterus; this type of miscarriage is most common during the first 12 weeks of pregnancy. The developing baby dies without any clear warning signs for the mother that something has gone wrong. For a time

(sometimes days, or even weeks), the baby remains in the uterus, and the mother may continue to think that her pregnancy is progressing. Or typical early pregnancy symptoms may suddenly disappear, which may alert the mother to something being wrong. If at any time you have an instinctive sense that something is wrong, call your doctor.

A miscarriage is often a process rather than a single event. Sometimes bleeding may resolve itself (threatened miscarriage, see p.306) or bleeding may come and go and you may feel confused about what is happening. Alert your doctor to bleeding at any stage of pregnancy.

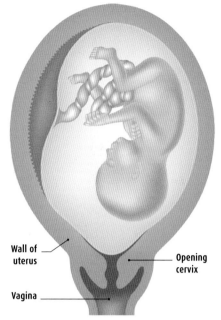

Wall of uterus

Opening cervix

Vagina

Opening cervix The most common type of miscarriage happens when the cervix opens spontaneously to stop a pregnancy that hasn't developed properly.

INEVITABLE AND MISSED MISCARRIAGES

Having an understanding of what happens in different situations can help you process events and understand your treatment options.

TYPE	WHAT HAPPENS	SYMPTOMS
Inevitable (complete or incomplete)	The cervix starts to open up before the baby is viable, and the uterus responds by contracting and starting to push out the developing fetus or embryo. This may be complete, when all of the pregnancy tissue (the embryo, sac, and placenta) is expelled, or incomplete, when some of the pregnancy tissue remains inside the uterus.	An inevitable miscarriage may be accompanied by severe periodlike pain, and is often accompanied by bleeding and clots.
Missed (also called a delayed or silent miscarriage)	The embryo or fetus stops developing, but remains inside the uterus. Eventually, the fetus dies, but with no clear warning signs, and the mother may continue to think that her pregnancy is progressing.	There may be no symptoms, or there may be a brown discharge, and pregnancy symptoms such as nausea, breast pain, and fatigue may suddenly disappear.

Q What are the causes of a miscarriage, and are there factors that increase my risk?

Around 80 percent of miscarriages that take place in the first 12 weeks of pregnancy, known as early miscarriage, occur because there is a chromosomal irregularity with the developing fetus. The baby may have too many or too few chromosomes, which means that there is incomplete chromosomal information, and as a result the baby is unable to develop properly.

A miscarriage in the second trimester, known as a late miscarriage, is more likely to have had another trigger, and is often the result of an underlying health problem or condition in the mother. There are several possible reasons for a late miscarriage, including:

» If you develop an infection.
» If you have a preexisting condition, such as thyroid disease, polycystic ovary syndrome, or diabetes, that increases the risk of miscarriage.
» If you have a weakened cervix.
» If you have a problem with your uterus,

such as a structural abnormality.
» If you have an immunological or endocrine disorder.

There are also several other factors that increase your risk of miscarriage. These include maternal age—you are at a greater risk of miscarriage over the age of 35—and lifestyle choices. For example, being obese increases your risk of miscarriage, as does smoking during pregnancy, taking recreational drugs, or drinking alcohol. Drinking caffeine is also thought to be a risk factor in whether you might have a miscarriage.

Q Is bleeding in pregnancy always a concern?

Not always. There are lots of unexplained incidences of bleeding early in pregnancies that lead to perfectly healthy, full-term babies. However, bleeding in pregnancy, at any stage, should never go unchecked.

In some cases, women experience bleeding, but the cervix remains closed, the symptoms pass, and the pregnancy continues. This is known as a "threatened miscarriage." Doctors used to prescribe bed rest for this, but there's insufficient evidence that this affects the outcome. If the cervix does go on to dilate, there is really nothing you can do to stop it and a miscarriage is inevitable. Bleeding in early pregnancy can also indicate an ectopic pregnancy (see p.308). If you have any bleeding, consult your doctor as soon as possible.

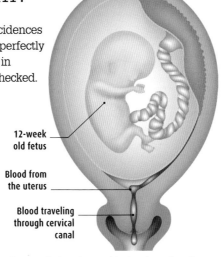

12-week old fetus

Blood from the uterus

Blood traveling through cervical canal

Threatened miscarriage In this situation, miscarriage symptoms such as bleeding can occur, but the cervix stays tightly closed, and a healthy pregnancy continues to term.

Q How is an early miscarriage in the first trimester treated?

If you have symptoms such as bleeding, you will be given an early ultrasound. If this reveals that your pregnancy isn't developing, you have a choice of letting the miscarriage happen naturally, without medical intervention, which is known as "expectant management," or of having the miscarriage medically managed, either by speeding up the process with drugs, or by surgically removing the pregnancy tissues.

Doctors often advise letting nature take its course for an early miscarriage, so unless you are at risk of a hemmorhage, your doctor will likely recommend that you have a natural, or expectant, management. This gives your body a natural hormonal response to the loss, which is thought to help you adjust physically and emotionally.

It can be hard to predict the exact course of a miscarriage, but at some point you will have bleeding, and, often, painful cramps. You may be asked to take a pregnancy test two to three weeks later to see if hormone levels indicate that the pregnancy has ended. Your doctor will support you and your partner throughout, and you will be offered counseling. If symptoms persist after this time, you will need to see your doctor again. He or she may recommend that

you take a suppository or oral medicine to dilate your cervix to encourage the expulsion of the pregnancy tissues. You will usually begin to bleed within 24 hours of taking the medication, but if you don't start to bleed, or if a pregnancy test three weeks later indicates that you are still pregnant, you may be referred for surgery.

Surgical removal of pregnancy tissues happens either under a general or (most likely) local anesthestic. In both cases, an instrument called a curette is inserted into your vagina. The curette has a plastic end that gently scrapes away pregnancy tissues, and a hollow tube provides suction to remove the tissues.

Q Is a miscarriage in the second trimester treated differently?

A late-stage miscarriage means that your doctor may suggest that you give birth to your baby. Although this may sound harrowing, studies show that going through birth can help women cope better long-term both physically and psychologically. You may go into spontaneous labor, but if this doesn't happen, you will be given a suppository to trigger labor. Your doctor may ask you if you would like to hold your baby. Don't worry if you don't want to right

away—or even at all—you must do what feels right for you and your partner. If you would like a photograph of your baby, one of the maternity staff will take one for you.

Q Will I be able to find out what caused my miscarriage?

Sometimes, but not always. It's often hard to be certain about what caused a miscarriage, and many aren't investigated. After an early miscarriage, you're most likely to have a healthy pregnancy next time. For this reason, it's only when you have had three early miscarriages in a row, known as "recurrent miscarriage," that your doctor will consider tests to try to find out the cause. You may have tests after one or two late miscarriages. Recurrent miscarriage may be caused by irregularities in the uterus or cervix, recurring genetic issues, or problems with the immune system, endocrine system, the clotting system in the blood, or with your partner's sperm. Or (most likely of all), there may be no identifiable reason.

During testing, you and your partner may be asked for blood samples to test for genetic causes, doctors will check the placenta if there is one, and for a late miscarriage, you'll be asked if you would like your baby to have a postmortem. Sometimes the examination of the placenta tells doctors all they need to know. However, it's important to prepare yourself for the fact that even after investigation, you may never know for certain what went wrong.

Q How long should we wait before trying for another pregnancy?

You should wait until bleeding has stopped before you try to get pregnant again to avoid the risk of infection. It's also advisable to have at least one period before trying again, since this makes it easier to date a pregnancy—after the uncertainty of miscarriage, it can be best to avoid confusion in a future pregnancy. Otherwise, it's up to you both. You may need more time to recover from your loss, or factors such as your age or how long you had been trying to get pregnant may mean you want to try again as soon as possible. Taking folic acid, reducing stress, eating healthily, and monitoring alcohol intake can help maximize your fertility.

Q How can we deal with my pregnancy loss and look forward to the future again?

After the devastating loss of your pregnancy, giving yourselves time to grieve can help you process what has happened and to start to look to the future. You may feel a range of emotions during this time. Finding coping strategies and seeking support can help the healing process.

There are many emotions associated with grieving, and you may feel some, or all, of these at different times. It's common to feel numb at first, and this is your body's way of dealing with the shock of the loss of your pregnancy. In time, feeling numb will pass and you may feel angry, cheated, or resentful. When those feelings also pass, you may feel deeply sad, withdrawn, or even depressed—not wanting to see friends or family, crying uncontrollably, or retreating into yourself. All these responses are perfectly normal and are symptoms of your intensely personal response to your loss. Eventually, though, you will emerge adjusted for life without your baby. Although "getting over it" isn't the right term—you will always remember your loss—you will be able to accept what has happened, and to start to move forward. There are a range of things you can do, and steps you can take, to help you to deal with your loss, and throughout your grief, the most important thing you can do is to express how you're feeling—through words and actions.

» Try writing a letter to your baby Tell her how loved she was, and what you had hoped for her. Fold the letter and put it in an envelope and keep it somewhere safe.

» Keep a daily journal of your feelings Putting your thoughts down on paper can help to formalize and organize them, which can help you feel more in control of them, if this is what you need.

» Talk it through with your partner You may not feel like doing this at first, but when you're both ready, don't shut each other out. Remember that just as you intend to parent together, you have both experienced the loss together. Try to give each other room to express your grief in your own ways, and support and comfort each other, too.

» Have a ceremony to remember your baby You might want to plant a tree in your yard or dedicate a bench in your local park so that you have somewhere to go to remember and reflect on the baby you lost.

» Join a miscarriage support group This way you can meet other couples who have experienced what you're going through. Sharing how you feel with those who truly understand provides a unique network of comfort and understanding that can reassure you that you're not alone.

While everyone deals with loss in their own way, how you respond to your miscarriage can often depend on your individual circumstances, and may be influenced by the course your miscarriage took. For example, if you had a lot of pain and bleeding, it may take longer for you to feel physically recovered. If the miscarriage played out over a relatively long period of time, you may feel particularly exhausted, though you may also feel a sense of relief that the miscarriage is behind you. Allowing yourself time to recover and to process your emotions is likely to help

you move on more completely. If, though, after a period of time you are finding it hard to shift your emotions, or you still feel below par physically, talk to your doctor, who can review your recovery and may have suggestions to help you to cope. Getting the right help and support can help you to avoid feeling isolated with your loss and give you the strength and resilience you need to look forward to the future again.

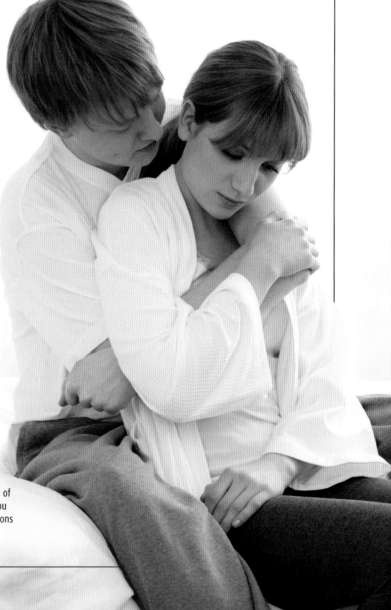

Support each other Facing the loss of your pregnancy together can help you both to cope with the difficult emotions that miscarriage brings up.

Q What is an ectopic pregnancy?

This is a pregnancy in which a fertilized egg implants outside the uterus. In about 95 percent of cases, ectopic pregnancy occurs in a fallopian tube, but it can also happen, for example, in the cervix, on an ovary, or in the abdominal wall.

Ectopic pregnancy is a serious condition that not only means that the embryo cannot survive, but can also be life threatening for the mother if a fallopian tube ruptures. However, it is also very rare–occurring in just under 2 percent of pregnancies in the US.

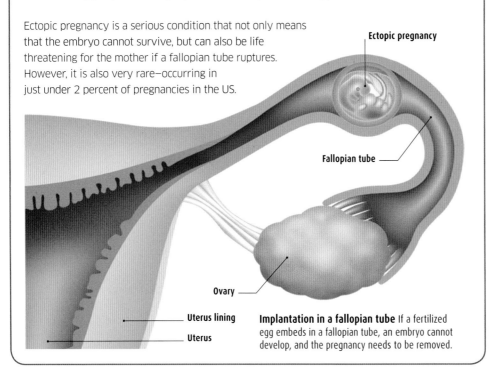

Ectopic pregnancy

Fallopian tube

Ovary

Uterus lining

Uterus

Implantation in a fallopian tube If a fertilized egg embeds in a fallopian tube, an embryo cannot develop, and the pregnancy needs to be removed.

Q How will I know if I have an ectopic pregnancy?

There is no one set of symptoms for an ectopic pregnancy. Some women may have no signs or symptoms at first, or the body may respond to the implantation of the egg as a normal pregnancy and respond accordingly. In this case, it can take up to 10 weeks for the symptoms of ectopic pregnancy to appear. Only when the ectopic pregnancy is discovered at a routine ultrasound, or the blastocyst gets so big as to cause swelling or rupture at the implantation site will you receive warning signs that something is wrong. Early symptoms can include:

» Severe cramping, similar to bad period pain.
» Pain and tenderness on one side of the abdomen.
» Vaginal bleeding.
» Stomach upset, such as diarrhea and nausea.
» Pain on defecation.
» Shoulder-tip pain.

Q Are there circumstances that increase my risk of an ectopic pregnancy?

You are at increased risk of ectopic pregnancy if you have had previous problems with your fallopian tubes, such as damage caused by an infection such as chlamydia, or a previous ectopic pregnancy; IVF treatment; patches of endometriosis that have spread to the fallopian tubes; pelvic inflammatory disease; or an appendectomy or other abdominal surgery that left scars. Some types of contraception, the IUD and progesterone-only pill, also increase the risk of ectopic pregnancy since they work by preventing implantation in the uterus, but they do not always prevent fertilization.

Q How will my ectopic pregnancy be dealt with?

An ectopic pregnancy is a medical emergency and you will need to go to the hospital. Once there, you will be given an internal ultrasound, during which a long, thin ultrasound scanner is inserted into your vagina, to check whether there are any signs of pregnancy within your uterus. A blood sample will be taken to measure your levels of the pregnancy hormone human chorionic gonadotrophin (hCG). Depending on the level of the hormone and your symptoms, one of the following will be recommended:

» **Expectant management** means that your ectopic pregnancy will be expected to resolve itself naturally without intervention. You will be closely monitored in the hospital.

» **Medical management** will be suggested if your pregnancy is in its very early stages. You will be given an injection to prevent the fertilized egg from growing any further. It will die and then be reabsorbed into your body's tissue.

» **Surgical management** will be given if there is a high chance that you will suffer a rupture in your fallopian tube. Surgery will be performed under general anesthesia to remove the fertilized egg and possibly to remove the affected tube. Although sometimes the tube can be saved, losing one tube doesn't affect your chances of becoming pregnant again. Unless your tube has already ruptured and you are not well enough to give consent, you will always be asked before you go into surgery if you agree to the affected tube being removed if necessary.

Q Will I be able to have a normal pregnancy after an ectopic one?

Yes. Although there's a slightly increased chance of suffering another ectopic pregnancy, statistically you are far more likely to go on to have a safe and healthy pregnancy next time.

65% of women have a **successful pregnancy** within **18 months** of an ectopic pregnancy. It's thought that this figure rises to **85 percent after two years.**

Q How is stillbirth dealt with?

Stillbirth occurs when a baby dies inside the uterus after 24 weeks of pregnancy. It is the term used when the baby would have been "viable," or developed enough to have potentially survived (albeit with assistance) if he had been born living. Stillbirth may occur before labor, while the baby is in the uterus, or a baby may die during labor. In the US, about three babies per 1,000 births are stillborn.

Only around one stillbirth in 10 occurs as the result of a serious congenital abnormality, that is, a birth defect that has put the baby's life at risk. In most other cases where a cause can be found, stillbirth occurs as a result of a pregnancy complication rather than from the baby's genetic makeup.

They are often picked up at routine prenatal appointments, when your doctor can't detect a heartbeat. If you are in late pregnancy, you may have alerted her to the fact that you haven't felt your baby's usual pattern of movement. If your doctor is concerned, she'll immediately send you for an ultrasound. Two sonographers will be there to confirm your diagnosis. You'll be encouraged to have someone with you for support and to listen to what the doctor tells you, since it can be hard to take in at such a sad time.

If you have a known medical condition, such as preeclampsia, you'll be encouraged to have your labor induced right away. If you are in no immediate danger, you may be able to return home for a few days to give yourself a little time to come to terms with what's happened before going through labor. After the delivery, you will be given quiet time to hold your baby if you would like to. You will be given medicine to stop your milk from coming in. You'll be asked if you want for a postmortem to be done; this will be done only with your consent. Going to all prenatal appointments and reporting any changes in your baby's pattern or strength of movement reduces the risk of stillbirth.

POSSIBLE CAUSES OF STILLBIRTH

The chart below gives some of the possible causes of stillbirth, though in some cases a definite reason for the stillbirth is never established.

WHAT HAS GONE WRONG	WHAT DOES IT MEAN?
Preexisting conditions	Conditions such as kidney failure, high blood pressure, diabetes (prior to becoming pregnant), and other chronic illness can cause pregnancy complications, so you will be monitored closely during your pregnancy.
Maternal age	Mothers over 40 years old are more likely to have a stillbirth than women who are in their 20s. This is because becoming pregnant when you're older increases your likelihood of having other risk factors for stillbirth—including congenital or chromosomal abnormalities in the developing baby, gestational diabetes, and high blood pressure.
Lifestyle factors	Heavy drinking, smoking, and recreational drug use are all risk factors for stillbirth, because they restrict the baby's access to oxygen and nutrients. Obesity can also increase the risk.
Multiples births	Possible complications with multiples may result in stillbirths, but your babies will be monitored throughout your pregnancy to ensure their well-being.
Preeclampsia	This condition causes high blood pressure in the mother, which in turn reduces blood flow to the baby, starving him of oxygen.
Problems with the placenta (including abruption)	Your placenta is your baby's life-support system in the uterus. Your doctor will check the growth of your baby at your appointments. If your baby is smaller than expected it may be due to the poor function of the placenta. If it stops working for any reason, your baby is starved of the oxygen and essential nutrients he needs for life. Placental abruption (when the placenta comes away from the uterine lining) can be why the placenta might stop working. Over 50 percent of unexplained stillbirths are thought to be because of placental problems, but all the causes are not yet fully understood.
Hemorrhaging (including abruption)	Losing blood during pregnancy has the automatic consequence that your baby receives a restricted blood supply, increasing the risks of stillbirth.
Obstetric cholestasis	This is a rare liver condition that's been linked with stillbirth, although it's unclear why the two are related. Your doctor may suggest delivering your baby at 37 weeks if you suffer from obstetric cholestasis.
Maternal infection	Although the placenta and amniotic sac provide a barrier against many infections, in some cases bacteria and viruses can make their way into your baby's system. The most common culprits are infections that travel from the vagina into the uterus such as Group B streptoccocus, E.coli, and enterococcus, but this rarely happens before your water breaks—contact your doctor at this point and he or she will monitor you. Many sexually transmitted infections, such as chlamydia and mycoplasma can also increase the risk of stillbirth.
Problems with the umbilical cord	If your baby becomes entangled in his umbilical cord during labor, or lies on it in such a way that the vein and arteries within it become compressed, he can restrict his oxygen supply. A prolapsed cord, which protrudes into the birth canal, is another possible cause of stillbirth.

Your newborn may need **extra care** or medical attention before he can go home if he was born prematurely, or needs to be **monitored or treated** because of occurences during his development, or the birth itself. This section looks at some **situations and conditions** that require special care, and the type of care your baby will receive.

Special-care babies

After the birth

If you had complications during pregnancy, or a problem with your baby was identified during prenatal screening, you may have been prepared for your baby to be taken care of by a medical team immediately after the birth. Your doctor should have explained what he or she will need to do before the birth, so you will know what to expect. You may also have had a chance to visit the neonatal intensive care unit (NICU) in the hospital and will be familiar with the facilities. If a problem wasn't anticipated, it can be a shock and extremely worrying if your baby needs medical attention at birth. The maternity staff may not have time to fully explain what is happening, because their priority will be your baby's health and well-being. As soon as possible, though, they will inform you about your baby's condition, and explain to you why your baby needs medical care.

Your role in the care of your special-care baby

Seeing your baby carried off and into the care of nurses feels totally counterintuitive for most parents—since the important first moments of parenthood are literally taken from your hands. However, even though your baby needs extra medical help, his emotional and psychological well-being relies upon you. He has been listening to your voice from within your uterus, so talking to him, as well as caressing him and holding him whenever you can, make sure that his recovery is as rapid as it possibly can be.

Where special-care babies are taken care of

Many hospitals have a neonatal intensive care unit (NICU) where babies are taken when they need help after birth. Usually this unit has four divisions, each one providing a different level of care appropriate to the seriousness of a baby's condition. Occasionally, a hospital may be unable to provide the level of specialized care your baby requires, and in this case your baby may need to be transferred to a hospital with the right facilities.

» **Level I units** treat babies who were born between 35–37 weeks and need a little bit of extra care.

» **Level II units** treat babies older than 32 weeks who have breathing problems or other issues that are expected to resolve fairly quickly.

» **Level III units** provide life-sustaining care for newborns younger than 32 weeks and/or low-birthweight babies, and these units have pediatric specialists on hand in addition to neonatal specialists.

» **Level IIII units** can do all of these things, plus babies who need intensive surgery can get it here.

Q Why would my baby need medical care?

There are many reasons why a newborn might need medical care. Some relate to premature births and others may occur in full-term babies. The following is a list of the most common reasons:

>> **Respiratory disorders:** your baby may need extra oxygen or help with breathing in the short term if his respiratory system hasn't fully formed yet, or because he has an infection or meconium in his lungs.

>> **Temperature control:** even full-term babies are very bad at regulating their temperatures after birth. Your baby may need to go into an incubator until his body systems are better developed.

>> **Hypoglycemia:** this describes a condition when your baby's glucose levels

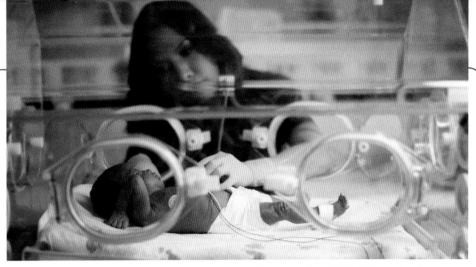

fall too low. This can be the case in babies of mothers with diabetes, or in premature babies. Your baby's brain and body need glucose to function, so if he's unable to raise his sugar levels through feeding, he may have to go onto a nasogastric feeding tube to correct the imbalance.

>> **Jaundice (see p.322):** this is a relatively common newborn condition in which a baby's liver doesn't break down bilirubin (a by-product of red blood cells) in his blood. It occurs in around 60 percent of full-term babies, and approximately 80 percent of premature babies. Most cases are harmless. Your baby may need

Your reassuring presence Staying close by, talking to, and stroking your baby will help him to feel calm, and is a comfort for you, too.

treatment if he's premature, or has particularly high levels of bilirubin in his blood. Exposure to light or phototherapy might be recommended.

>> **Patent ductus arteriosus:** when your baby is born, the vessel that keeps blood-flow away from the lungs during pregnancy should close off. If this doesn't happen—your baby's lungs and heart can be strained (patent ductus arteriosus). See p.323.

Q When is a baby considered premature and why do some babies arrive early?

A premature (or "preterm") baby is a baby **born before 37 weeks of pregnancy. In the US, approximately 11 percent of births (almost eight percent in the UK) are premature.** It's unusual for there to be a single, clear reason why a baby arrives early; usually preterm labor is the result of a combination of factors. For up to 30 percent of premature births, the cause doesn't ever become clear. In another 25 percent of premature births, labor is medically induced before the baby reaches full term because a problem has been detected. This means that an early delivery is the safest option for the mother and/or baby. The following list sets out some of the reasons why babies are born prematurely:

>> **If you have a pregnancy condition** such as preeclampsia (see p.144), where your baby's growth may be restricted, or gestational diabetes (see p.145), where your baby can grow very large, you may be induced early on.

>> **Placental problems**, including placenta previa (see p.147) and placental bleeding, can mean that labor needs to be induced early.

>> **You may have a weak cervix**, which cannot support the baby and membranes to full term.

>> **If amniotic fluid begins to leak** from the sac around the baby, known as premature prolonged rupture of membranes, your baby is at risk of infection, and labor may need to be induced.

>> **Having had a premature baby** in a previous pregnancy or having had a previous late miscarriage increases your risk of premature labor.

>> **Carrying twins or more** adds to pressure on the uterine muscles. Similarly, excess amniotic fluid can distend the uterus and trigger labor.

>> **Preexisting maternal conditions**, such as high blood pressure, diabetes, or kidney disease, and irregularities in the shape or structure of the uterus, can mean labor is induced earlier.

>> **Being younger than 25 or older than 35** increases the risk of premature labor.

>> **Lifestyle factors,** such as smoking, drinking alcohol, taking drugs, or poor nutrition in pregnancy make premature labor more likely.

Q What will my premature baby look like?

This depends upon how close to your due date you were when you went into labor. A baby born at 36 weeks will look as you might expect a newborn to look, except smaller. A more premature baby might have very pink or reddish skin, because the fat layer under the skin hasn't formed, and he may be covered in lanugo, the soft, downy hair that protects the skin in the uterus and is shed toward the end of pregnancy. His head may seem large for his body, and, if very premature, his eyelids may be fused. The top of his skull will be soft (and his fontanelle large), since the flat bones haven't fully formed over the sides and top of his head. His limbs may seem fragile, and since his muscle tone is still quite weak, he may not be curled up as term newborns often are since he can't hold his knees to his chest. His facial features will be fully formed and he may have hair on his head.

A CLOSER LOOK
The power of touch

When a baby cries, our instinct is to pick him up and cuddle with him. However, taking care of a special-care baby can make soothing touch a little more complicated. When your baby goes into the neonatal intensive care unit (NICU), he may be in an incubator or in a special crib and attached to machines and IVs that mean you can't always pick him up when you want to. However, simply touching your baby can be hugely beneficial for him.

Contact with your baby Studies show that caressing your baby through the holes in the sides of the neonatal crib, and, once he is strong enough to be picked up, holding him whenever you can and nestling him against your bare skin as much as possible, can help with bonding and trigger the release of hormones that aid milk production.

Less stressed Being close to you and hearing your familiar voice help to reduce the amount of the stress hormone cortisol in your baby's body. Babies getting special care are more tolerant of medical care, becoming less distressed during examinations, general procedures, and administration of medication, if they've felt the power of your touch.

A sense of calm When you touch or stroke your baby, you stimulate the release of oxytocin–the calming and bonding hormone– in your body and in your baby's body, promoting the bond between you and helping your baby to feel calm and secure. The release of this hormone especially helps you feel closer to your baby if he is too tiny to be held.

Help your baby sleep Your loving touch, whether caressing him or holding him, also helps to soothe your baby and promotes sound sleep. During sleep, energy is diverted away from taking in the sights, smells, and sounds of his surroundings, and from trying to keep warm, to the growth and development of his organs, limbs, and brain.

Close contact As your baby grows stronger, and with advice from your neonatal nurses, he can spend longer amounts of time being held by you outside of his incubator. Holding your baby skin-to-skin is beneficial, and even babies who are very premature can benefit from brief periods outside the incubator being held next to their mother's skin.

FASCINATING FACTS

Touch has many benefits for both special-care baby and parents, also helping to promote a strong bond.

Boost immunity When held skin-to-skin, bacteria from the mother's skin colonize the baby, protecting him from germs.

Avoid PPD Mothers of special-care babies are more likely to suffer from postpartum depression. Oxytocin, released when you touch your baby, can help you avoid PPD.

Home early Premature babies held skin to skin are likely to need less time in the hospital. Studies also show better neurological-development scores at six and 12 months for premature babies who received kangaroo care.

Skin-to-skin contact Babies who receive kangaroo care (see below) are better able to regulate temperature, have improved oxygen levels, and breast-feed more easily.

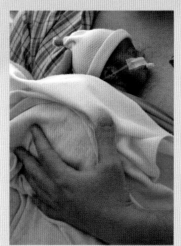

Kangaroo care This is the practice of holding your naked baby against the skin of your chest, wrapped in a sling or cloth, snuggled upright between your breasts. The technique was first used in Colombia in the 1980s when hospitals had no incubators to keep premature babies warm. With his face turned to one side, your baby can breathe easily and, crucially, maintain a warm body temperature.

Q What can I expect in the neonatal intensive unit?

As a parent, it's natural to feel anxious and scared when you see your baby in an incubator, with tubes attached and hooked up to lots of machines. However, all of the equipment in the neonatal intensive care unit (NICU) is there to help your baby breathe and keep him nourished to ensure he develops and grows so that in time he can manage on his own.

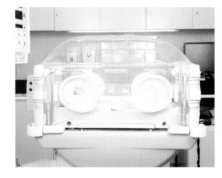

Support Babies who are born prematurely may spend time in an incubator. These are similar to usual hospital cribs, but have a lid to keep your baby warm. Holes in the sides allow you to reach in to touch and caress your baby.

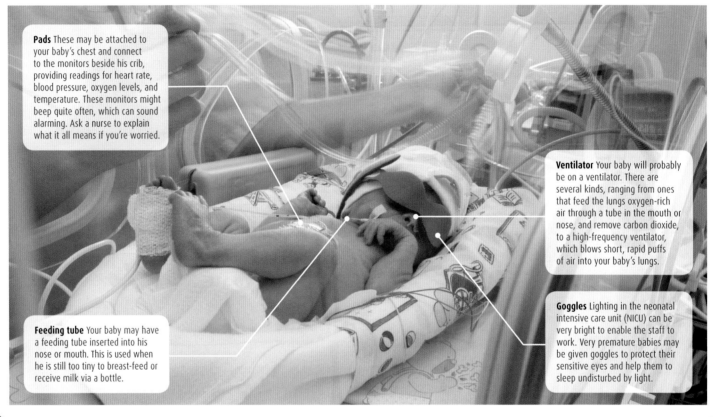

Pads These may be attached to your baby's chest and connect to the monitors beside his crib, providing readings for heart rate, blood pressure, oxygen levels, and temperature. These monitors might beep quite often, which can sound alarming. Ask a nurse to explain what it all means if you're worried.

Feeding tube Your baby may have a feeding tube inserted into his nose or mouth. This is used when he is still too tiny to breast-feed or receive milk via a bottle.

Ventilator Your baby will probably be on a ventilator. There are several kinds, ranging from ones that feed the lungs oxygen-rich air through a tube in the mouth or nose, and remove carbon dioxide, to a high-frequency ventilator, which blows short, rapid puffs of air into your baby's lungs.

Goggles Lighting in the neonatal intensive care unit (NICU) can be very bright to enable the staff to work. Very premature babies may be given goggles to protect their sensitive eyes and help them to sleep undisturbed by light.

Q How will my baby be taken care of in the NICU?

Your baby will receive around-the-clock care, specially tailored for his specific circumstances. NICU nurses will take care of your baby every minute of the day and night, with one nurse specially assigned to your baby's care. In addition to the nurses, pediatricians with expertise not just in premature babies, but also in the specific issues relating to your baby, will take care of him. For example, if your baby is showing signs of neurological damage, a neurologist will take care of this aspect of his care. Your baby will also be assigned to a neonatologist (a doctor specializing in the complex needs of special-care babies) and to a social worker, who will support you through your baby's time in the NICU. Other relevant specialists and nurses will also all be on hand to make sure that your baby receives the best care possible.

Q Can I talk to the staff at any time about my baby's progress, and can I help with his care?

The NICU nurses are always on hand to talk to, and they will encourage you to ask questions and, when possible, to help with tasks such as washing and changing your baby. If you have any questions that the nurses can't answer, they will ensure that the appropriate doctor or other clinician contacts you as soon as possible to talk to you. You should find that the doctors taking care of your baby are happy to have an open and supportive dialogue about his care, and you should feel involved in all the decisions that need to be made about his care. If you're worried or confused about anything and want a layperson's view, ask your social worker to put you in touch with other parents who have been through similar experiences. One of the best ways to get involved in your baby's care, and to get to know the medical staff who take care of him, is to be there when the doctors visit him—the nurses can tell you at what time each day this is likely to be.

Q Will I be able to stay with my baby all the time?

You will need to check the policy in your hospital, but most hospitals allow parents to stay with their baby as long as they want throughout the day and night. Being close to you, hearing you, and being caressed by you are all ways in which you can help your baby gain strength. Keep in mind, though, that you and your partner need to rest, and that your body needs to recover from birth. You may have been faced with difficult decisions and have had to deal with the unexpected circumstances of your baby's arrival in the world; though you may feel guilt if you're not with your baby the whole time, some time away from the NICU, both together and separately, is important for your well-being.

Q Can other family members and friends visit my premature baby?

Most neonatal intensive care units will allow a few visitors at a time, and siblings in particular are encouraged to come and bond with their new brother or sister. The ward will, though, have specific visiting times for visitors, whereas parents usually can stay around the clock. Keep in mind that too many people at one time can be overwhelming, so try to keep visitor numbers small at any one time. Don't feel obligated to run an open house; you have a lot to contend with so if you prefer just immediate family to visit for the time being, this is fine. Premature babies have low immunity, so anyone who has an infection, such as a cold, will be encouraged to stay away until they are completely recovered.

Q When will we be able to take our baby home?

The circumstances of every baby's special-care needs are different, and so how long your baby remains in the NICU entirely depends on his health at birth and his reasons for needing special care. In general, hospitals will recommend that premature babies stay in the NICU at least until they have reached "full term." At this stage, your baby's organs should be well developed enough that he can manage the demands of life outside the incubator.

In general, before your baby is ready to be go home, the NICU will want to ensure that he fulfills a number of criteria. First, staff needs to be confident that your baby can breathe independently, which happens in stages. As he grows stronger, the nurses will take him off the ventilation equipment for short periods of time so that he can practice breathing for himself. Gradually, the amount of time your baby spends getting help with his breathing will decrease, until he can breathe fully on his own.

In addition to being able to breathe independently, the staff wants to see that your baby is feeding well—whether breast- or formula feeding—and gaining weight, and that he is urinating and passing stools regularly and without difficulty.

When you do leave, you may be given a follow-up appointment at the hospital in a few weeks time to check your baby's progress.

Q How can I prepare to take over the care of my baby?

Before you take your baby home, the nursing staff will make sure you are confident about administering his medication (see box, below) and that you have support systems in place to ensure you get all the help (personal and professional) you need to take care of your baby. Some hospitals ask you to stay overnight with your baby just before you take him home so you can follow his 24-hour pattern of care with help on hand if you need it. It's natural to be nervous when your baby has been so closely monitored in the hospital, but remind yourself that the hospital is happy for him to leave since they are confident that you will be able to take care of him independently now, and that home is the best place for him to grow and thrive.

Q I'm worried about administering my baby's medicines. Are there any tips or techniques I should know?

The neonatal nurses in the NICU will try to make sure you're confident about administering your baby's medicines while your baby is in the NICU so that you can continue when at home. However, inevitably when you get home, without their watchful guidance, giving medicine can feel overwhelming. The following tips, techniques, and guidance can increase your confidence:

» **First and foremost** try to stay calm, because your baby will pick up on your stress and in turn will be less relaxed himself. Eye drops, nose drops, vitamins, minerals, and medicines all come in easy-to-administer liquid form for babies.

» **Most importantly, always wash your hands** before giving your baby any medicine. Shake any medicines before you give them, and have everything you might need, such as antibacterial wipes or cotton pads, within easy reach.

» **Swaddle your baby** so that his arms and legs stay still, then place him on his back on the floor or cradle him in one arm, depending upon whether you need one or two hands to give the medicine (for eye drops, you'll need two hands, for example).

» **Try to avoid** any part of the medicine bottle, for example the eye drop pipette, or the tip of a bottle of nasal drops, touching your baby's skin. If you do, don't worry—just wipe the tip with an antibacterial wipe before you use it again.

» **If your baby becomes distressed**, stop what you're doing and calm him before trying again. Never miss a dose of medicine, though, unless your doctor says that it's okay to.

» **Make a wall chart** to remind you when to give which medicines, and check them off each day so that you don't have to rely upon your memory.

» **Keep in mind that at home** you will follow the same medication routine that your baby had during his stay in the hospital, which at first can provide a helpful pattern for your day.

Q How will my premature baby be fed on the neonatal intensive care unit?

This depends on how premature your baby is. The coordinated movement of sucking, breathing, and swallowing doesn't kick in until around 34 weeks' gestation, so your baby may need to be fed through an IV or tube at first.

Babies born before 34 weeks' gestation need to be fed either directly into their blood stream (an IV), or via a tube into their stomachs.

There are two ways that premature babies can be fed if they're too small to be breast- or bottle-fed. One way is through a vein, with an IV. Babies who are a bit older may have breast milk (or a suitable alternative) fed to them through a tube that goes to the stomach through the nose or mouth. Babies can are able to feed by breast or bottle, but need extra calories and nutrition of supplemental feedings.

If your baby needs to stay on a ventilator or doesn't yet have a coordinated sucking, breathing, and swallowing movement, she will receive milk through the tube The milk feedings will be small, but frequent—once every two to three hours—and you may be able to hold your baby while she is being fed, and perhaps help to administer the milk. You can express your breast milk for your baby, or she can receive donor breast milk from a bottle bank, or enriched low-birthweight formula.

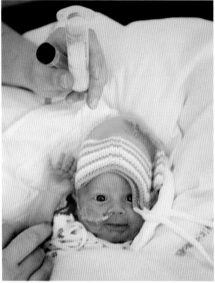

Feeding via a syringe Your baby can be fed tiny quantities of milk this way. Your expressed breast milk is nutritionally best for your baby, since your body makes it specifically for her, and it contains important antibodies that boost your baby's immature immunity.

Moving to a bottle If you want to bottle-feed, when your baby is strong enough to suck, you can use a smaller sized nipple that holds just a little milk at a time, which is easier for your tiny baby to manage.

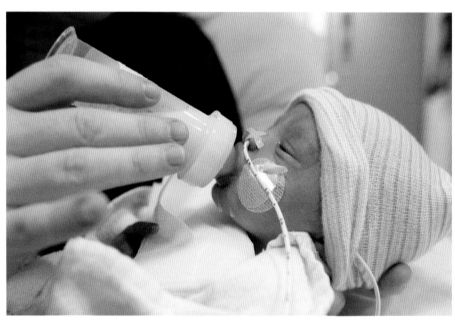

Q When can I start expressing milk for my baby?

You can begin expressing milk as soon as you feel ready, the sooner the better. Even tiny amounts of breast milk from you contain important antibodies and nutrients specially formulated for your baby's needs. The sooner you start to express, the sooner you will establish a good milk supply, and the more likely you are to breast-feed successfully once your baby can coordinate sucking, breathing, and swallowing. While your baby is too small still to latch on to the breast, your milk can be fed to her via a tube.

Q When can I start to breast-feed my baby?

As your baby becomes stronger and gradually learns to coordinate sucking, breathing, and swallowing, you can start trying to bring her to the breast. A premature baby can take time to get the hang of breast-feeding, and even when she has developed her sucking technique, she may find it hard to latch on with her tiny mouth. At first, just give your baby short periods of time to practice latching on and sucking. She may not take much milk initially, and supplements may be needed. Be guided by the NICU nurses or doctors, who can help you ease your baby into breast-feeding. They will encourage you to hold her skin to skin so she is stimulated to breast-feed, and help her to build up her time on the breast slowly.

Q My baby spits up lot of milk. Why is this?

It's common for babies to bring up some milk after being fed, known as reflux, and it is especially common in premature babies. This is because the muscles that control the valve at the bottom of the esophagus, which stops food from coming back out of the stomach and up to the throat again, are less likely to be well developed. Keeping your baby upright during and after a feeding, spending time burping her, and, if you're bottle-feeding, switching to a slower-flow nipple to avoid her guzzling down milk too quickly, can all help to minimize the problem (see p.295 for more information and advice on dealing with reflux).

Q Can my baby have normal formula?

If you want to give your premature baby formula, she will need to have special type of formula that contains additional amounts of nutrients, calories, and essential fats. Your hospital will provide this for you while you are there. When your baby has reached the due date, and is ready to go home, the hospital will probably prescribe this special high-calorie formula and recommend that she continues on this until she has reached a certain weight and is well enough to go onto ordinary formula. Don't switch formula without consulting your doctor first.

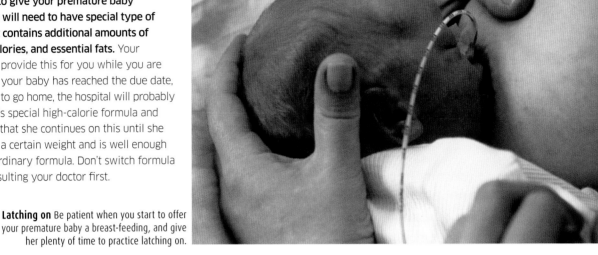

Latching on Be patient when you start to offer your premature baby a breast-feeding, and give her plenty of time to practice latching on.

Q How can I help support my baby's development and growth once she's home?

It's reassuring to know that most premature babies will usually catch up to be at least almost as tall, strong, and heavy as their classmates by the time they are four years old. This is because premature babies have two "catch-up" growth spurts (see below) that bring them in line with their peers. For your part, making sure your baby is well nourished is essential for triggering these growth spurts.

The first months

Your medical team will discharge your baby from the hospital once they are confident that she is gaining weight. If you are breast-feeding, continue to do so on demand. If you are formula-feeding, follow the advice your doctor gives you about pacing feedings. Breast-fed babies (and some formula-fed ones) need vitamin and mineral supplements to ensure they receive extra dosages of all the nutrients they need for development. Your baby may need to continue taking these until she is a year old.

Catch-up growth spurts

Between the ages of one and two years, your child may have catch-up growth spurts—this will be apparent first from an increase in her head circumference recorded on her growth chart, followed by a sharp rise in her length and weight—she may quickly start to grow out of her clothes! She may have another small catch-up growth spurt at about three years old. After this time, she will be roughly the same height and weight as all the other children her age.

Starting solid food

Although advice is that babies should start solids at around six months, for premature babies this means six months from their due date rather than their actual age. So, if your baby was four weeks premature, you would wait until she is seven months old before starting solids, when her digestive system will be mature enough to digest solid food. If your baby was very premature or you are in any doubt about when to start her on solids, the doctors who take care of your baby can guide you.

Other ways to help

» Encouraging good sleeping patterns—and, over time, teaching your baby to soothe herself to sleep—will help your baby to grow and develop. Studies show that premature babies who sleep deeply in kangaroo care (see p.313) grow and develop faster than those who don't have this experience.
» As your baby grows, periods of activity every day will help improve her muscle tone and skeletal strength, which in turn will help to maximize her growth.

While arriving home with your special-care baby is a joyful occasion, you may feel nervous about being in charge alone. Parents often find that it's only when they're home that the full force of what they've been through sinks in. Working through emotions and seeking support will help you manage.

Managing emotionally

It's very normal to begin a period of grief when you arrive home with your baby after his prolonged hospital stay—for your expectations of your first days, weeks, or months of your life as a family. You may feel anxious about the responsibility of taking care of your baby without constant medical support, and angry that life hasn't been as simple as it was supposed to be. Along

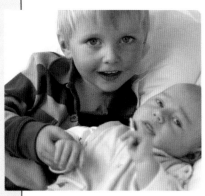

with frustration, guilt, confusion, irritability, and helplessness, these are perfectly normal reactions to your situation. The five-step plan, below, can help you work through complex feelings.

A close bond The time your older child spends with the new arrival, talking to and touching him, will help them form an enduring bond.

Your growing family

Welcoming a new baby into the family presents challenges, and when that baby needs extra care, challenges magnify. Be careful not to shut out older children. Involve them in the baby's care if you can: maybe they can help with sponge bathing or finding a diaper bag. You are bound to feel anxious about a two-year-old "cuddling" a premature infant, so set boundaries you're happy with. Be honest, but kind, and explain that the baby is tiny and has been sick, so only grown-ups can hold the baby for now, but he loves to have his head stroked or his hand held. Sing songs to the baby together, and tell your toddler how the baby loves to hear his voice and how this helps to make him better. Older children may feel confused if you are sad or irritable, and think the baby is sick because of something they've done. Reassure them that nothing that's happening is their fault. Say sorry if you're snappy, and explain that you're tired. Praise your children for any help they give you and try to spend dedicated time with them every day, even if this is just at bath- or bedtime.

FIVE-STEP PLAN

This simple five-step plan can help you work through the emotions you may feel about your baby needing special care. This isn't a cure-all, but one, some, or all of them may help you start to accept events and move forward.

 1 Acknowledge your grief

If you knew before the birth that your baby would need extra care, you may be grieving for the loss of an easy-going pregnancy. If your baby was premature, you may grieve for the loss of those last weeks of pregnancy. Or you may grieve for the loss of those first moments after birth when you could be alone with your baby. Acknowledging that events represent a loss of the experiences you might have wished for is the first step to coping.

 2 Express your emotions

The hospital can put you in touch with a therapist who has been trained to advise and help parents of special-care babies. Talking to someone who isn't emotionally involved can help you to rationalize how you feel. You can go with your partner, on your own, or a mixture of both. Keeping a journal of your baby's progress and how you feel provides a positive reminder of how far you've come.

 3 Celebrate the successes

Successes don't have to be big things. The first time you manage a walk with your baby in the carriage, to give eye drops without forgetting to keep tissues beside you, to sit down with a slice of toast in the morning, to write a thank you card or two, are all steps towards "normal" life, which makes them successes worth celebrating. They will help to remind you that every day you can achieve something.

 4 Ask for help

You don't need to be strong all the time. When possible, ask for help with the practical matters of being at home, so that you can focus on your baby and yourself. Ideally, someone else can do the cleaning, shopping, and cooking. Don't be shy about taking advantage of the resources of well-meaning friends and family, and accept all offers of practical help willingly.

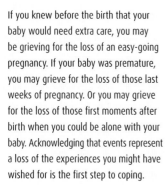

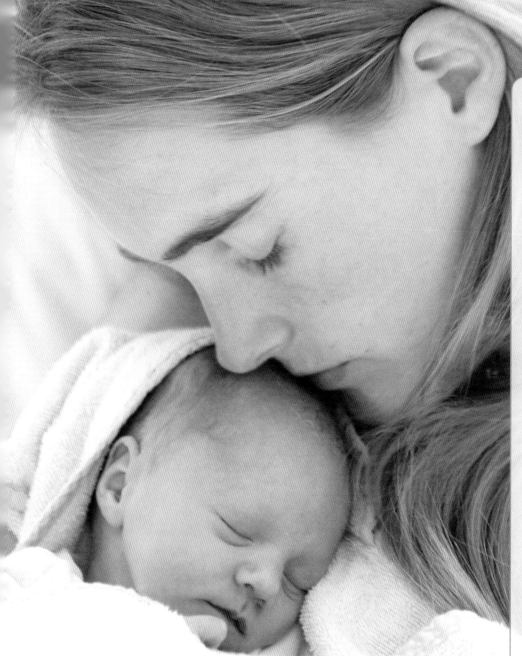

WHERE CAN I GO FOR HELP AND SUPPORT?

There are plenty of avenues of support that you can explore to help you manage when taking care of your special-care baby.

» **Your partner:** sometimes asking for help from your partner can be a trigger for him to feel more involved and positive himself.

» **Your pediatrician:** when you're home, your pediatrician will want to see his new patient within a few days. Ask him or her anything you need to know about your baby or how to best take care of him.

» **Friends and family:** ask for practical help whenever you can. Close family and good friends will want to do all they can to ease your load.

» **Other parents:** the social worker assigned to your baby in the neonatal intensive care unit can put you in touch with other parents who have been through a similar situation. Many hospitals run support groups for the parents of their special-care babies.

» **A counselor:** ask your doctor about seeing a counselor, or, if you had a neonatal counselor in the hospital, arrange to speak to him or her. Talking things through with an impassive observer can help you unload without fear of judgment.

» **The Internet:** Organizations like the nonprofit March of Dimes, which are designed to help parents of preemie babies, have online chat rooms, local chapters and e-newsletters.

 5 Take one day at a time

Making plans or giving yourself deadlines will only add to your load. Instead, try to enjoy every moment and every day for what it is, and to relish the stage that your baby has reached. Give yourself permission to roll with the punches.

Supporting each other

Though you and your partner will react in your own ways to the pressures of taking care of your baby, it's best to try to work as a team. Assign roles so you both feel valued and included, and that you're contributing your individual strengths. Your partner may also to be worried about you. Suggest practical ways for him to help, such as making you a "packed lunch" before he goes to work, or taking responsibility for the dishes. Encourage him, too, to have some skin-to-skin time with the baby to help them bond.

Mothers of babies who have spent time in intensive care have a higher risk of postpartum depression (PPD), so be aware of the symptoms (see p.263). Sharing how you feel each day will help to keep you connected, and for you to feel supported.

Time together Once home with your baby, you can enjoy a new sense of closeness.

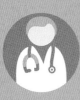

Many doctors report that one of the most common questions when a baby is born is, understandably, **"Is everything alright?"** Here, we look at some concerns parents might face. These might be conditions that you've heard others talk about, or that you' had experience of, either in a previous pregnancy or through a family member or friend

Issues at birth

Assessing your baby

As soon as your baby is born, her immediate well-being will be assessed. Then, over the following 48 hours, a staff pediatrician will do a series of checkups on your baby for complications or problems. Many of the conditions in this section, including ones such as cleft lip, tongue-tie, and hernia, will be picked up during these checkups (see p.246)—or may even have been picked up during pregnancy—and, if necessary, treatment can begin immediately. Regularly scheduled office visits to the pediatrician over the next weeks and months provide a means of ensuring that all continues to be well, that your baby is growing, and that you are recovering well, too. As the weeks and months progress, you should begin to feel more secure about your role as parent, and you'll see the proof that you're doing a good job as your baby gains weight over time. If you have any questions as time passes, always ask the doctor. While some problems are picked up on quickly, others may become apparent only after a period of time, which is why your baby's development is followed closely in these early months.

Trust your instincts

You are the person most closely attuned to your baby's well-being, so if you think something might be wrong, even if you're worried you might be imagining things, raise it with the doctor. Concerns about newborns are always taken seriously, and no one will think you are overly anxious or overly cautious.

When a problem is found

Finding out that your baby has a problem is naturally upsetting. If a concern was identified during pregnancy, you will have had some time to adjust and find out about possible treatment. If a problem is discovered after the birth, you will have questions and concerns. Many minor concerns are easily remedied. Some do require longer-term treatment and sometimes your baby may need surgery, but most problems can be either eliminated or improved. Finding out about a condition early on means that treatment is prompt and outcomes improve.

This section looks at a range of conditions that can affect newborns, some of which may be identified or suspected during pregnancy through ultrasounds or because of concerns about a baby's growth, and many of which are detected in the days and weeks following the birth. The conditions range from those that are relatively common, such as jaundice and umbilical hernias, to those that are rare. In each case the implications for your baby are explained as well as the treatment and help available.

{ Q What problems or conditions could my newborn encounter?

When you consider the myriad cell divisions and biological processes that are involved in making a baby, it is little wonder that sometimes things go wrong and babies are born with conditions that need treatment in their first months of life, or that require ongoing care. The earlier a problem is identified, the sooner treatment or attention can be given, and often this lessens any long-term repercussions for your baby.

Respiratory Distress Syndrome (RDS)

» What is this?

In order to inflate properly, a newborn baby's lungs need sufficient amounts of surfactant—a fluid that keeps the lungs inflated and prevents the air sacs within them from collapsing when your baby starts to breathe on her own at birth. The air sacs begin to produce surfactant at around 27 weeks of pregnancy. Babies born before 31 weeks don't have sufficient surfactant to enable the lungs to take in air properly, which leads to RDS. Your baby will show signs of breathing difficulties at birth, which will vary in severity depending upon how prematurely she was born, and symptoms worsen in the following days if left untreated. Some babies will need to go on to a ventilator immediately to begin breathing, while others may show signs of rasping or grunting as they try to fill their lungs.

» What can be done?

If there's time, you may be given steroids as soon as you go into premature labor to speed up the development of your baby's lungs. Once your baby is born, she may need to go into an incubator, where she can be given surfactant through a tube that goes into her mouth and directly into her tiny lungs. When she is stable, she will be put on a ventilator, which mechanically fills her lungs with air, breathing for her; or a continuous positive airways pressure machine, which allows her to breathe on her own, but prevents her lungs from collapsing between breaths.

» What does this mean for my baby?

The potential effects of RDS depend upon your baby's gestational age at birth. With quick treatment, and gentle but steady progress, your baby is likely to make a full recovery. Some babies will need help with breathing for just a few days, but if your baby was very premature, she may need assistance for weeks; sometimes it can take many months for a premature baby's lungs to work properly. Many very premature babies have RDS that develops into chronic lung disease.

Congenital infections

Viral or bacterial infections present at birth are called congenital infections, passed to the baby from the mother via the placenta in pregnancy, or during birth. The table here shows some common infections. Others include toxoplasmosis, hepatitis, HIV, and CMV.

INFECTION	WHAT IS IT?	WHAT CAN BE DONE?
Group B streptococcus (GBS infection)	A baby may contract group B streptococcus infection during birth from a mother carrying the bacteria. The baby develops blood poisoning, which can cause serious complications. Premature infants are at greater risk.	Fast treatment with antibiotics leads to no long-term effects. If the mother is a known carrier, the baby will receive antibiotics as soon as she is born to prevent the spread of infection. When the infection isn't known about, the baby may have signs such as unresponsiveness, breathing difficulties, convulsions, poor temperature control, and pale skin.
Herpes	The herpes simplex virus comes in two forms—HSV1, which causes cold sores; and HSV2, which causes genital herpes. HSV2 is most common in newborns, who catch the virus during birth. It is a potentially serious infection that can cause severe conditions, or even neonatal death.	If you know or suspect you have genital herpes, your doctor may advise a cesarean section to prevent the spread of the virus to your baby. If not, and your baby contracts the infection, she may have no symptoms at first, and may go on to be perfectly healthy. If the virus activates, babies may be unresponsive, have difficulty feeding, and have a fever. Your baby will need intravenous antiviral medication for up to three weeks to control the infection.
Rubella	Also known as German measles, this is a viral infection that can cause serious complications for premature infants (see p.139). Congenital rubella occurs when the baby contracts the virus in the uterus in the first trimester. It can cause developmental problems, which can affect the heart, and the nervous and musculoskeletal systems.	There is no way to treat the rubella infection itself, so treatment involves minimizing its effects. Some babies will be able to have heart surgery to correct defects. Sadly, any damage to brain tissues is permanent.

Jaundice

» What causes jaundice in babies?

Jaundice in newborns, known as neonatal jaundice, is a usually harmless condition caused by high levels in the blood of the substance bilirubin. Bilirubin is a yellow pigment that is produced when old red blood cells are broken down and metabolized by the liver, then excreted in the urine and feces. In the uterus, your baby needed extra red blood cells to carry oxygen to her own body and the placenta. However, for life outside the uterus she needs fewer red blood cells, and has to break down the excess. At birth, the extra red blood cells mean an extra load on your baby's immature liver; the liver can't keep up and therefore bilirubin is reabsorbed back into your baby's blood stream, causing yellowing in the skin and the whites of the eyes. The condition is very common in newborn babies, affecting 6 out of 10 babies born at term, and 8 out of 10 born prematurely. Premature babies are slightly more likely to be jaundiced since their immature liver and gut are even less well equipped to deal with an overload of red blood cells. Jaundice usually arises in the first two to three days of life, and in most babies resolves itself without treatment within a week or so. In a few babies, jaundice becomes severe, and the babies require treatment to avoid serious, but rare, complications affecting the brain.

» How will I know if my baby has jaundice?

If you notice a yellow tinge to your baby's skin, press the middle of her forehead with your finger (the skin yellowing progresses from top to toe): if your baby has jaundice, the color of the depressed skin will be yellow when you remove your finger. You may also notice a yellowing on the palms of the hands or soles of her feet. Stools may be pale (rather than brown), and urine very yellow (rather than pale). The whites of your baby's eyes may appear yellow, too.

» Can jaundice be missed?

You may not notice mild jaundice, but the pediatricians and nurses at the hospital will check your baby regularly for jaundice, and when you go home, your pediatrician will check her again within a couple of days, so it's unlikely that it will go unnoticed. Your doctor will also take into account risk factors for jaundice, such as whether or not your baby is premature, if you have other children who had neonatal jaundice, whether your baby is feeding well, whether you're breast- or bottle feeding (it is more common in breast-fed babies), and whether your baby seems alert and responsive. Poor feeding and an uninterested baby can make a case for likely jaundice. Call your doctor immediately if yellowing skin is accompanied by extreme lethargy, irritability, unwillingness to feed, or a fever.

» Will my baby have to have any tests to confirm suspected jaundice?

If the hospital is concerned about the level of your baby's jaundice, they will use a special light that shines through the skin to show bilirubin. Your doctor may also take a small blood sample to test for bilirubin levels in your baby's blood, and he or she may take a urine sample to check for an underlying condition. If jaundice is confirmed, doctors will do further tests on your baby's blood to try to establish the cause and severity.

» Will my baby need to be treated?

If jaundice is mild, your baby will usually be left alone to allow the liver to mature and resolve the jaundice naturally—usually the liver is able to metabolize excess bilirubin by two weeks after birth. If your baby is premature, or she has very high levels of bilirubin, she will be treated with a form of light therapy called phototherapy. Treatment is usually completely successful within a few days and, assuming all else is well, your baby will be able to go home. If bilirubin levels remain high, a blood transfusion may be given in a neonatal intensive care unit. Small amounts of your baby's blood are replaced with matching donor blood until the levels of bilirubin are low enough that the jaundice dissipates.

» Is there anything I can do to prevent my newborn getting jaundice?

Make sure that your baby feeds well so she doesn't become dehydrated. If you're breast-feeding, encourage her to feed every two hours. If you're bottle-feeding, try for a 30 to 60 ml feed every three hours. If you're breast-feeding, but your baby isn't taking in enough milk and begins to show early signs of jaundice, your doctor may suggest you use a breast pump to express your milk for a day or so (which will also encourage your milk-flow), feeding it to your baby in a bottle.

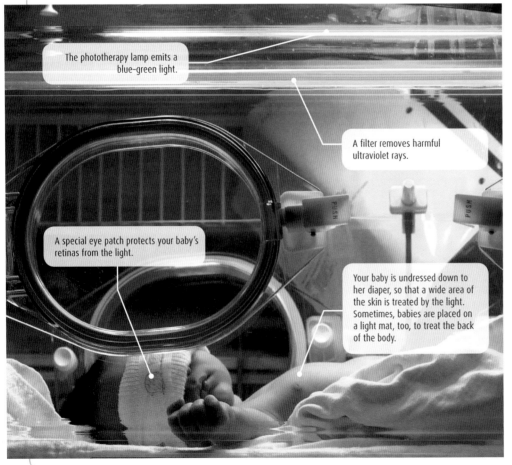

The phototherapy lamp emits a blue–green light.

A filter removes harmful ultraviolet rays.

A special eye patch protects your baby's retinas from the light.

Your baby is undressed down to her diaper, so that a wide area of the skin is treated by the light. Sometimes, babies are placed on a light mat, too, to treat the back of the body.

Phototherapy treatment Your baby is placed under a special light that changes the chemical makeup of bilirubin to make it easier to break down.

Cleft lip and palate

» What is this?
Parts of your baby's face develop independently in the uterus and then grow together. However, if they don't join successfully, a cleft lip and/or palate is the result—these are gaps in the top lip and in the roof of the mouth. A baby may have a cleft lip or a cleft palate, or both. The conditions are often inherited and can hamper your baby's ability to feed successfully, and eventually to talk. They affect more than 7,000 babies in the US each year.

» What can be done?
Your baby will need surgery to bring the two sides of the mouth together, both for the upper lip and the palate. This is usually done by your baby's first birthday; the correction of a cleft lip may be done as early as three months and is followed by a procedure to correct the palate. A few babies may go on to have slight difficulties forming some words or to have a nasal tone to their voice, most recover to have perfectly normal speech. More surgeries may be needed.

Umbilical hernia

» What is this?
This occurs when the baby's intestine pushes out through the hole in her abdominal wall where the umbilical cord was attached, and when this hole fails to close up spontaneously after birth. It is painless, and you may notice the protrusion only when your baby cries or strains. Umbilical hernia is a common conditions in newborns, affecting around 3–5 percent of healthy term babies. Premature babies are at slightly increased risk.

» What can be done?
Unless your baby's hernia is large or has become infected, it will probably be left to clear up on its own. Eventually the hole closes and the protruding portion of the intestine goes back into position. Large or infected hernias may need to be treated, possibly with surgery. As long as any infection is treated before it affects the intestine wall, there are no long-term implications.

Inguinal hernia

» What is this?
In around one in six premature babies, part of the small intestine protrudes through a hole in the abdominal wall near the groin, in the space called the inguinal canal. You may notice this hernia only when you see a swelling under the skin near the groin when she cries or strains.

» What can be done?
Your baby will need surgery to push the hernia back into position and close over the hole into the inguinal canal in order to prevent a reoccurrence. This will usually be done as soon as possible after the hernia has been diagnosed.

Congenital heart problems

» What kinds of defects can occur?
About 40,000 babies born in the US each year (about 1 percent) have a congenital heart defect, so heart problems in newborns are rare. Among the most common is one relating to a special blood vessel—the ductus arteriosus—that enables blood to bypass the baby's lungs while in the uterus. This vessel should close within 24 hours of the birth, but occasionally this doesn't happen, overloading the lungs and heart with blood (see p.311). Other congenital heart problems include:

Atrial septal defect (ASD) and ventricular septal defect (VSD). Commonly referred to as "a hole in the heart," this is when the two sides of a baby's heart fail to become distinct from one another, causing oxygenated and deoxygenated blood to mix. This is often easily resolved with surgery, and small holes may close up on their own.

Coarctation of the aorta occurs when the aorta (the heart's main artery) is narrowed, limiting blood flow. It can become a serious condition, but is treatable with the insertion of a stent (a small tube that opens the artery), or with surgery to remove the affected part of the aorta.

Stenosis of the valves occurs when the arterial or ventricular valves are narrowed, hampering blood flow between the chambers of the heart and causing a heart murmur. The condition usually requires surgery to correct.

Some babies may have more serious problems such as failure of one side of the heart to develop fully, or the arteries and veins of the heart "transposing"—developing the wrong way around.

» When will heart problems be spotted?
Some heart defects are picked up by the sonographer at your pretnatal ultrasounds, others develop at birth. If a problem is spotted, a cardiac specialist will explain the implications of the condition and what treatment, if any, your baby will need when she is born. Ask as many questions as you need to. Your doctor will be able to give you details of support groups, and other parents who have been in a similar situation.

KEY
→ Oxygen-rich blood
→ Oxygen-poor blood
→ Mixed blood

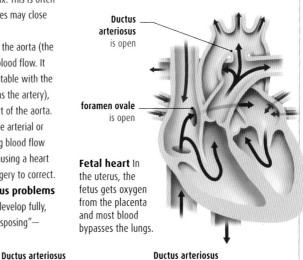

Ductus arteriosus is open

foramen ovale is open

Fetal heart In the uterus, the fetus gets oxygen from the placenta and most blood bypasses the lungs.

Ductus arteriosus has closed

Ductus arteriosus has closed

Ductus arteriosus remains open

foramen ovale has closed

foramen ovale has remained open

foramen ovale has closed

Healthy newborn heart At birth, a hole (foramen ovale) between the chambers and another at the ductus arteriosus closes—normal circulation begins.

Open foramen ovale If the hole between the chambers remains open at birth, oxygenated blood returns to the lungs, making circulation less efficient.

Open blood vessel If the ductus arteriosus fails to shut at birth, oxygenated blood meant for the body is diverted back to the lungs again.

Hip dysplasia

» What is this?
The long bone of the thigh (the femur) connects to the pelvis in a ball-and-socket joint at the hip, which gives us full range of circular movement in our legs. In about 2 percent of births, babies are born with femur joints (one or both) that completely or partially malform outside the socket. Your baby's hips will be tested for this condition within three days of birth—a doctor or doctor will manipulate her upper thighs in the hip sockets to check for freedom of movement. The condition tends to run in families and is more common in baby girls than in boys.

» What can be done?
Sometimes it's just a matter of ligaments tightening up around the joint to hold the femur bone in place, which can happen naturally. If your baby has hip dysplasia caused by malformation in the bone, however, she may need to wear a special harness to hold her legs in position so that as the bones of the pelvis harden, the socket forms properly around the top of the femur bone. If hip dysplasia isn't picked up until after your baby is six months old, or if treatment with the harness

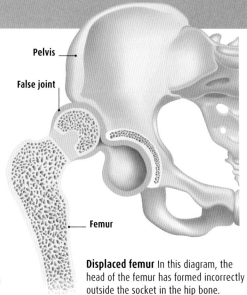

Pelvis

False joint

Femur

Displaced femur In this diagram, the head of the femur has formed incorrectly outside the socket in the hip bone.

hasn't worked, your baby will need surgery to position the femur correctly within the socket. After surgery, your baby will need to wear a cast until the bones have reformed around the corrected femur, a process that usually takes about three months.

Undescended testes

» What is this?
During the third trimester of pregnancy, a baby boy's testes should descend into the scrotal sac. However, in up to 4 percent of baby boys, the testes fail to descend and the baby is born with an empty scrotum. This doesn't cause any pain.

» What can be done?
Most of the time, the testes will descend without any intervention before the baby is six months old. If they don't, your baby will need to have surgery to move them into the correct position. The surgery usually takes place before he reaches the age of five.

Talipes

» What is this?
More commonly known as club foot, this occurs when the tendons on the inside of a baby's lower leg are tighter and shorter than those on the outside. The result is that the foot (or feet—about half of all cases of talipes show up in both feet) turns inward. Usually, the bones of the ankle are also poorly formed. It's more common in boys, and occurs in about one in 1,000 babies. The condition runs in families. There are several types of club foot, ranging from isolated conditions

that can be easily corrected to types that are an indication of other, chromosomal abnormalities.

» What can be done?
Soon after birth, your baby will begin a weekly program of manipulation and casting to coax the foot into the correct position as the bones grow. Once this process is over, he may need a simple surgery to release the tension in his Achilles tendon. To prevent retightening in the tendon, he will probably have to wear special harnesses on his feet continually, and then only nightly, until he is four or five years old. After this, children usually recover fully.

Syndactyly

» What is this?
Your baby's hands and feet form in the early weeks of pregnancy. At about five weeks, they look like paddles, with fingers or toes joined together. They begin to separate about two to three weeks later. Syndactyly occurs when two or more of the digits of the hands or feet fail to separate properly, leading to a webbed appearance. The effect may be superficial, in just the skin, or the bones may have fused. It affects about one in 2,000–3,000 babies, and can run in families.

» What can be done?
Your baby will need surgery to separate the bones and/or

skin of the fingers or toes that are joined together. If she has more than two conjoined digits, she will need more than one surgery, because only one side of each digit can be operated on at a time in order to preserve the blood flow to the whole hand or foot.

Tongue-tie

» What is this?
Tongue-tie occurs when the frenulum, the small piece of tissue that lies beneath the tongue, connecting it to the bottom of the mouth, is too far forward, so the tongue can't move forward or from side to side effectively. This can make breast-feeding especially difficult and can sometimes cause sore and ulcerated nipples for the mother if the baby is unable to achieve a good latch. If your baby is feeding well, you may never notice that she is tongue-tied. However, if you are having problems feeding, perhaps finding that your baby doesn't latch on to your nipple properly, tongue-tie could be the cause. Tongue-tie affects 4–10 percent of newborn babies and is more common in boys than girls.

» What can be done?
If your baby is having problems with feeding and it's thought that tongue-tie is the problem, doctors may perform a tongue-tie division, a procedure that involves a painless snip in the tightened frenulum to enable the free movement of the baby's mouth and tongue.

Retinopathy of prematurity (ROP)

» What is this?
Images are formed on the back of the eye, at the retina. Babies born before 31 weeks are at risk of developing abnormal blood vessels leading to the retina, impairing its ability to receive information and so distorting vision. It occurs in about 20 percent of premature births. There are no outward signs of the condition and diagnosis relies upon assessment by an ophthalmologist at birth.

» What can be done?
After birth, an eye doctor will shine a flashlight into your baby's eyes to assess the health of her retinas. Your baby may have drops put into her eyes to give the doctors a better picture of what's going on. Laser surgery may prevent the advancement of the condition and save sight.

» What does it mean for my baby?
Mild forms of ROP, which are the most common, will correct themselves in time, as the blood capillaries feeding the retinas settle down. More severe forms may lead to the retina detaching from the layers beneath it; laser surgery may correct this but it isn't always successful, and often babies will have at least some form of visual impairment, particularly in their peripheral vision.

Hypospadias

» What is this?
This condition occurs in about one in 300 baby boys when the urethra exits the penis along the shaft, rather than at the tip of the penis. Depending upon where the hypospadias occurs, the penis may not be able to straighten properly, and the foreskin may not develop normally on the underside.

» What can be done?
If the urethra appears close to the tip of the penis, the condition is considered mild and often it is left as it is. However, in more severe forms of the condition, which can cause pain when urinating and later difficulties with erectile function, are usually treated with surgery before the baby reaches 18 months old.

Pyloric stenosis

» What is this?
Around one in 500 babies are born with this condition. The pylorus is a muscular tube that connects the stomach to the bowel. Sometimes a baby may be born with a section of overdeveloped pylorus muscle and this means that milk can't pass beyond the stomach. This causes the baby to vomit back up her feedings (sometimes violently) and in turn she becomes dehydrated and undernourished. It can sometimes be a hereditary condition, and tends to affect more boys than girls. It usually develops at about six weeks after birth.

» What can be done?
Your baby will need to have surgery (often keyhole surgery) under general anesthesia to cut through the muscle and create a passage for milk to pass into the bowel from the stomach. There tend to be no long-term side effects, and babies make a full recovery, going on to feed perfectly normally throughout life.

Imperforate anus

» What is this?
This is a rare condition affecting about just one in every 5,000 babies. In the uterus, the entirety of your baby's digestive system begins, essentially, as one long tube, separated by thin membranes that gradually break down as necessary as the different sections of the gastrointestinal tract form. Sometimes, the sections that form the large intestine, anus, and rectum don't form properly, making it impossible for your baby to pass a stool. This is an imperforate anus.

» What can be done?
Imperforate anus is corrected using surgery, usually as soon as the problem is discovered (or at birth—since often it shows up on an ultrasound). Your baby will need to wear a colostomy bag until the bowel has healed. Most children go on to have a perfectly healthy and well-functioning bowel, but occasionally a child may need to go on to a special diet to relieve constipation.

Fetal alcohol syndrome

» What is this?
Fetal alcohol syndrome (FAS) occurs when the levels of alcohol a mother drinks during pregnancy affect the development of the baby. A newborn with FAS often has a small head with distinctive facial features, including droopy eyelids with skin folds in the upper inner corners, and small eyes. Ears may be set low down and the mouth may have an underdeveloped jaw, a thin upper lip, and only a shallow or indistinct groove above the lip (called the philtrum). The bridge of the baby's nose will seem low when compared with the position of the eyes, and the nose itself may seem short and upturned. In addition, FAS can cause heart problems and learning difficulties. It is estimated that about one in 1,000 children are affected by FAS.

» What can be done?
There is no treatment for FAS itself, although any heart abnormalities may be operable, and your baby will need support throughout childhood for any learning or behavioral difficulties.

Cerebral palsy

» What is this?
Cerebral palsy is the result of lack of oxygen to the brain, which can occur before a baby is born (causing damage directly to the neurons in the brain as the brain forms), during birth (as a result of hemorrhage), or as a consequence of an illness such as meningitis after birth. It affects areas of the brain that control muscle movement (including those for speech and swallowing), hearing, vision, and learning.

» What can be done?
There is no cure for the condition, but it is not progressive—that is, it doesn't get worse over time. This means that management can be uniquely tailored to each individual child. Once your child has been diagnosed with cerebral palsy, you will have a team of health professionals involved in her care. You will also have one key worker, who may be your point of contact and will help to coordinate the management of your child's condition. There is a wide range of therapies for cerebral palsy that help deal with different aspects of the condition, with the goal of relieving symptoms and maximizing your child's independence. Physical therapy is one of the main treatments, which is important to prevent muscles from weakening further and movement from becoming more restricted. Occupational therapy may be given to help your child manage everyday

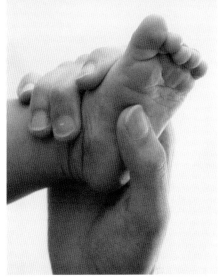

Massage therapy Complementary therapies such as massage gently manipulate soft body tissues, helping to relax and relieve muscle stiffness.

activities and tasks. Speech therapy provides exercises to help your child communicate more clearly if needed. Speech and language therapists can also help children reduce drooling. If the muscles are very stiff, your child may need medication to relax them. Occasionally surgery is needed to treat bone and joint problems.

Cerebral palsy occurs in about **3 in 1,000** births in the US, and it is more common in **boys** than girls. More than half the cases each year occur as a result of **premature births**.

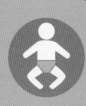

Occasionally, a baby is born with or develops a condition that requires **lifelong support**. It may be caused by a faulty **chromosome or gene**, or may have no known cause. You may have found out in pregnancy that your baby had a problem, or it may become evident only **after the birth**, or in the first months of your baby's life.

Special needs

What is meant by "special needs"?

Special needs refers to any condition that means a child, or an adult, needs extra support to reach their potential. If your baby has special needs, she may need help to maximize her opportunities to develop not just physically, but emotionally, socially, and mentally, too. Some conditions present physical or neurological challenges, others require a special diet, or a particular medication to control the condition. Essentially, special needs is an umbrella term for myriad conditions, from those that affect a baby physically, such as chronic illness or malformations in limbs or organs, to those that affect psychological or mental well-being, such as memory disorders or learning difficulties. Chromosomal conditions such as Down syndrome fall under this umbrella term, too, as do some inherited illnesses, such as cystic fibrosis. This section looks at some of the most common special-needs situations, as well as some more rare conditions that are tested for with the heel prick blood test in your baby's first week of life (see p.250).

Readjusting your outlook

In many cases, babies born with special needs aren't "suffering from" anything, but are living with and often overcoming the challenges of conditions that carve their

and your lives into a different kind of normality. Understanding your baby's condition, and knowing about its causes, features, symptoms, and prognosis, can help you to come to terms with it so that you can nurture your baby in the most positive and fulfilling ways possible.

Your role

If your baby has a condition that requires ongoing care, it can be easy to feel marginalized against the whirling backdrop of medical care, especially in the early years. However, you lie at the heart of your baby's life, and your understanding of her needs is instructive. While doctors can discuss and treat her physical condition, you know best how to ensure her emotional and social well-being. This means that doctors will look to you to take charge of your baby's care, following their advice so that it works for your family. Never underestimate the importance of your opinion, or be afraid to share it, and never be afraid to ask as many questions as you need to.

As your baby grows and gains an understanding of her situation, talk to her about her treatment or the challenges that she faces in age-appropriate terms. Involve siblings and other family members, too, making sure no subject, appropriately discussed, is off-limits, and having open discussions, which will bring you together.

Q How can we build up an effective support network?

Having a baby with a life-limiting or special-needs condition can be overwhelming for a parent. It's important that throughout your baby's diagnosis and treatment, you accept all offers of help and support available to you.

Taking care of your special-needs baby presents new challenges, and the early years are likely to be a steep learning curve. Not only are you adjusting to being a new parent, with the lifestyle changes this comes with, but you are also finding out about and dealing with the additional special needs of your baby. The right help and support can be crucial.

HELP AND SUPPORT

Accessing all the help and support that is available to you and your baby can provide you with essential practical and emotional backup, making it easier to deal with your baby's particular needs and enabling you to provide the best possible care for her.

» Communicate with your partner Although at times you may respond to challenges differently, no one knows what's going on as intimately as your partner. Don't judge each other and listen to each other's point of view. Set aside some time for just the two of you, and know when to give each other space.

» Call on your family frequently—they have a vested interest in you and your baby, and making sure a grandparent, aunt, or uncle is fully involved in the details of your baby's special upbringing will give you a babysitter you can completely trust, so that you can have a break when you need it.

» Having friends to talk to can provide welcome relief and a sense of normality. If a friend offers to grab some groceries, bring a meal over, or pick up your dry cleaning, take up the offer willingly and gratefully.

» Support groups can provide a new perspective from someone with experience of the situation you're in and provide solutions to challenges that seem hard to fathom when you're trying to cope. Even if there are no solutions, talking to someone who has been through similar events and knowing you're not alone is often enough to keep you positive.

» Counselors are trained in helping you to explore and rationalize your emotions. Taking care of a sick or special-needs baby comes with a whole range of emotions, and talking to a counselor can help you channel these for positive effect. Talk to your pediatrician about finding a counselor or therapist with an approach that will suit you.

» Your pediatrician is there to support you and your baby. He or she can give advice, a referral to a specialist if you feel you need one, and will also know about organizations in your area that offer respite care to give you a break every now and then. He or she can also advise on your entitlement to Social Security disability income or Medicaid.

» Try to have someone with you who can act as an extra pair of ears when you go to doctor appointments and meetings with therapists. This might be your partner, or a close family member or friend. Taking notes will help too, giving you something to refer to that will help you formulate questions for next time, or even for a follow-up call.

Q What causes Down syndrome?

Down syndrome, also known as Trisomy 21, is a chromosomal abnormality. Healthy babies are born with 23 pairs of chromosomes, with one chromosome in each pair received from each parent. Down syndrome occurs when a baby has an extra version of chromosome 21 thereby creating a group of three chromosomes. In the US, Down syndrome occurs in just about one in 700 births, and the chances of having a baby with Down syndrome rise with increasing maternal age (see p.97).

Q What are the signs of Down syndrome?

A person with Down syndrome has distinctive facial and anatomical characteristics, and will have some degree of learning difficulties. Some babies may be born with heart problems and a closed section in the small bowel (known as a duodenal atresia), as well as problems with hearing and vision. Characteristics include:

» Rounded face with a broad brow.
» Folds at the inner corners of the upper eyelids.
» Slanted appearance in the openings for the eyes.
» Low-set ears.
» Weakened muscles in the legs and arms.
» Flattened bridge of the nose, set low down compared with the position of the eyes.
» Single crease across the palms of the hands.
» Short little finger that may curve inward.
» Protruding tongue and overly arched palate.
» Gap between the big toe and the toe next to it.
» Short neck with loose skin.

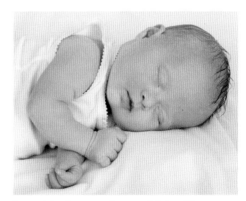

Recognizing Down syndrome Each baby with Down syndrome has an individual appearance, but there are a number of physical characteristics that are common to the condition. They are not always immediately evident at birth.

Q Will my baby with Down syndrome need to stay in the hospital longer?

Most likely, yes. Even if you were given a strong indication during pregnancy that your baby was likely to have the condition, Down syndrome won't be officially diagnosed until after the birth, when tests and checkups will be done in the hospital to confirm it. Firstly, a pediatrician will examine your baby to look for anatomical features that suggest Down syndrome is present. Then, he or she will do a blood test to see if your baby has an extra chomosome 21. Only once you have this chromosomal analysis—which may take up to 48 hours to come back, although timings vary from hospital to hospital—is the diagnosis given. Furthermore, babies with Down syndrome may have trouble feeding since a lack of muscle tone in the tongue can make sucking difficult. Like any mother of a newborn baby, you will be encouraged to stay in the hospital until you and your doctor are confident that your baby is feeding well.

Once you have the final diagnosis, your baby will need more tests to try to establish the degree to which she is affected by the condition. Effects can range from mild to severe—in the former case you may be allowed to go home soon after diagnosis, in the latter, your hospital stay may be longer.

Q What are the likely long-term challenges for babies with Down syndrome?

Although life expectancy for people with Down syndrome was once limited to middle age, men and women are now expected to live well into their 50s, and sometimes 60s. Increasingly, individuals with Down syndrome can live full lives, even leaving home as an adult to live independently. Nonetheless, the condition does pose certain challenges.

» Weakened immunity: your baby may be more susceptible to everyday infections, such as coughs, colds, and respiratory illnesses, although no one is really sure why this should be the case. Your baby is also more susceptible to serious conditions, such as leukemia.

» Thyroid problems: your baby is more likely than children without the condition to have to take medication for hypothyroidism (an underactive thyroid). Even though this is relatively straightforward to control, this will be something that your baby will have to have monitored throughout her life.

» Learning difficulties: all babies with Down syndrome grow up to have some level of learning difficulties. Obviously, the more severe your baby's learning difficulties, the greater social and behavioral challenges she will then face. Problems such as impaired hearing and vision can exacerbate issues with cognitive function, since these can further delay several developmental stages, such as learning to talk, read, and write. Difficulty sleeping is also a trait of the condition, and this too can further impede learning.

» Dementia: studies indicate that people with Down syndrome are more likely to suffer from dementia after the age of 40, which can lead to the need for long-term residential care.

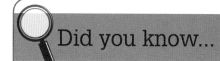

Did you know...

Down syndrome is named after the 19th-century English doctor John Haydon Down, who first registered the condition in 1862.

Q What can I do to help my baby in the future?

Like any parent, your job is to help your baby reach her potential, not just in terms of learning, but also by helping her develop confidence in herself and to become as independent as possible.

Try to avoid comparisons with other babies without Down syndrome born at the same time, and instead celebrate your baby's successes as they happen. Tailor your parenting methods to her own unique learning styles—if she is creative, get creative with her; if she finds it hard to form words, teach her sign language; if she loves music, take her to music groups and as she gets older even learn to play an instrument together. Show her that she has unique talents, just like any other child, and in this way watch her grow in confidence and independence. Give her lots of opportunity to meet and play with other children, both with and without Down syndrome. Teach her social skills, such as manners and sharing, and offer her plenty of opportunities to socialize.

Finally, it's essential that throughout your parenting you work in partnership with the medical staff who are taking care your baby—not just for her physical well-being, but also because this can help you to allay her fears or anxieties about any tests or procedures she may need to have.

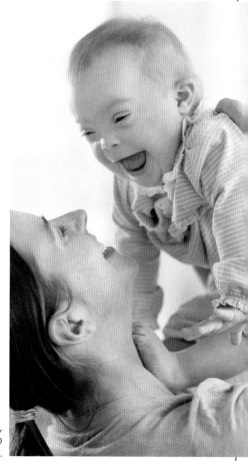

Loving support With your constant support and love, your baby will grow in confidence and flouish, ready to take on challenges, knowing that you are there for her.

Q Will I know right away if my baby has cystic fibrosis (CF)?

About one in 10 babies with CF have a condition called meconium ileus at, or shortly after, birth, which causes a bowel blockage and requires surgery. Other symptoms of CF usually emerge in the first year of life, so it may not be obvious immediately that your baby has CF. However, most cases of CF are now diagnosed shortly after birth since CF is one of the conditions screened for with the heel prick test (see p.250), done within the first few days of life. Signs of CF include difficulty breathing, a raspy, hacking cough that doesn't go away, and coughing up a lot of phlegm. If the condition affects your baby's pancreas, she'll be unable to produce the right level of enzymes to break down her food sufficiently, and her digestive juices will be too thick to absorb nutrients properly. As a result, she may show signs of malnutrition, such as having pale skin, a thin and small frame, and a distended tummy, and may pass fatty-looking stools. Her skin may taste salty, because your baby's sweat has a high concentration of salt.

Q Can cystic fibrosis (CF) be treated?

There is no cure for CF. However, although it is a life-limiting condition, advances in medicine over recent decades mean that life expectancy has dramatically improved, and now more than 80 percent of babies born with CF will live into their 50s. Treatment involves relieving symptoms, and is tailored to the individual's needs. Physical therapy, oxygen therapy, and inhalers can be used to ease breathing, while vitamin and mineral supplements, replacement digestive enzymes, and a high-calorie diet can help to improve nutrition and growth. Your baby will be more vulnerable to infections, so may also be prescribed prophylactic (preventative) antibiotics. In more serious cases, a heart and lung transplant may be needed.

There are certain characteristic effects of CF on the sufferer's body, including, most significantly, impairment of the function of the lungs and pancreas.

≫ **Damage to the pancreas** can not only cause problems with digestion, but also lead to diabetes since the pancreas is responsible for making insulin, which controls sugar levels.

Q What is cystic fibrosis, and how does it affect babies?

Cystic fibrosis (CF) is a condition caused by a faulty gene, called CFTR. The gene needs to be inherited from both parents for someone to suffer from CF. The faulty gene causes a buildup of mucus that in turn affects breathing and feeding.

The condition primarily affects the lungs and digestive system, causing a buildup of mucus in these organs. The faulty gene affects the way in which salt and water move in and out of cells in the body; an excess of salt enters the cells of certain organs, causing an imbalance of salt and water. Eventually too little water remains in the fluid surrounding the affected organ's cells, resulting in a buildup of thick mucus that impairs the organ's function. The condition affects one in 3,700 babies born in the US every year. About 10 million Americans unknowingly carry the faulty gene.

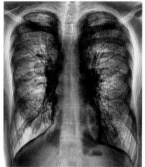

Mucus buildup Here, mucus (in green) can be seen clearly in a CF sufferer's lung, blocking airways and causing difficulty breathing.

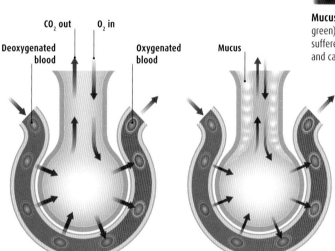

CO$_2$ out   O$_2$ in

Deoxygenated blood   Oxygenated blood   Mucus

HEALTHY AIR SAC   **INFECTED AIR SAC**

Air sacs This illustration shows how the buildup of mucus seen in the lungs of a cystic fibrosis sufferer clogs up the multitude of air sacs (alveoli). This affects the flow of oxygen in the lungs and causes difficulty with breathing.

≫ **The intestine** can't absorb nutrients properly from food.

≫ **Increased likelihood of infertility,** particularly for men.

≫ **Poor nutrition** can lead to osteoporosis later on, especially in women.

≫ **Sinus infections** are common, as well as polyps (small growths) inside the nose.

≫ **The lungs fill with mucus,** which leads to breathing difficulties, repeated chest infections, and increased coughing.

≫ **Risk of liver damage.**

Q Will cystic fibrosis affect my baby's growth?

This partly depends upon how severely she has the condition. Mutations in the gene that causes cystic fibrosis mean that it varies in its effects. Mild forms of the disease may affect only the lungs, and her pancreas may remain relatively stable. This will mean that she won't suffer from the nutritional deficiencies associated with more severe forms of the disease and is more likely to grow normally. Even in more severe cases, most sufferers are able to take supplementary pancreatic enzymes that help do the job that the pancreas is failing to do. This can help with the breakdown of food and has been shown to greatly improve growth in those with CF.

Q What can I do to help ease the symptoms of cystic fibrosis?

First and foremost make sure you get all the information and support that's available to you. Then, follow the guidelines from your specialist carefully. These will be tailored to your child's individual requirements and can help you to manage her condition. Importantly, give your baby all her medicines, including any that help her to digest her food properly, since this is essential for growth and development. In consultation with your doctor, make sure she gets all her immunizations at the correct times, since she is especially susceptible to illness.

You will also have a physical therapist involved in your baby's care. He or she will teach you age-appropriate techniques that help clear the lungs, so that you can give your child essential care at home. Ask plenty of questions while you learn the techniques until you're fully confident about using the methods on your own. Try not to panic when your baby experiences breathing difficulties since she is more likely to be anxious if she senses that you are panicking, which can worsen her symptoms. Be reassuring and matter of fact while you carefully administer the procedures you've been taught. However, if at any point you are very concerned about your baby's breathing, call the hospital—or an ambulance.

It's a good idea to extend your trusted network of friends or relatives who can use CF techniques so that you have support to call on when you need it.

Q I've been told CF may affect my baby's growth. How can I help her growth?

In addition to giving your baby supplements to assist her digestion (see p.329) to make sure she absorbs essential nutrients, you'll probably need to start her on solid foods slightly earlier than is usually recommended—perhaps as early as three months old—to make sure she gets the calories she needs to grow properly. As she gets older, keep plenty of high-calorie snacks in the home and encourage her to eat them regularly, as well as her usual meals. Also encourage your older child to take part in sports and other physical activities to help strengthen her lungs. It can seem counterintuitive, but exercise is an important part of her therapy. Not only that, but running, playing, and competing at sports with friends is essential for giving her as normal a life as possible.

Q I've been told my baby has phenylketonuria. What is this?

This rare genetic condition, referred to as PKU, occurs when the body lacks or is unable to make an enzyme called phenylalanine hydroxylase (PAH).

The enzyme PAH is needed to convert the amino acid (the building blocks of protein) phenylalanine into another amino acid, tyrosine. Tyrosine helps regulate moods, aid concentration and memory, and maintain energy levels. A buildup of phenylalanine can lead to severe neurological damage. Although potentially serious, once detected, PKU is completely treatable with a special diet (including special infant milk), which needs to be maintained throughout life. The heel prick blood test (see p.250) done in the first week of life screens for PKU, and if your baby is found to have it, early treatment is given. The condition affects only one baby in every 15,000 born in the US each year.

Inherited genes For a baby to have PKU, she must inherit the affected gene from both parents. Inheriting the gene from only one parent will make her a carrier of PKU, but she won't show the effects herself, as shown in this diagram.

FATHER (CARRIER)

MOTHER (CARRIER)

Both genes A child who inherits both

NORMAL CHILD

CARRIER CHILD

CARRIER CHILD

AFFECTED CHILD

Q How does phenylketonuria (PKU) affect babies?

A baby who inherits PKU may begin to show symptoms in the first few months of life if the condition goes undetected. Symptoms include convulsions, a musty odor on her skin or in her urine, a pale complexion and eye color, slow growth rate, a small head, and eczema. In time, if PKU goes untreated, children may develop severe learning and behavioral problems, and hyperactivity.

Q Will my baby develop healthily, even though she has PKU?

As long as you adhere to her dietary regimen (and she continues to follow it when she's older), evidence suggests that PKU has no obvious effects on growth, emotional and social development, or mental agility. A PKU diet is low in protein and includes some carbohydrates, as well as supplements of the amino acid tyrosine that supports certain brain functions (see box, left). Your baby will have regular blood tests during childhood to monitor the levels of phenylalanine in her blood to ensure they are within safe limits.

Q What are the characteristics of Turner's syndrome, and can it be treated?

This rare chromosomal condition affects only girls and occurs when there is one X chromosome missing from the pair that determines her gender. It affects about one in 2,000 baby girls born in the US every year and is named after the American doctor Henry Turner, who first described it in 1938. One of the main characteristics of the condition is short stature, and most girls with Turner's syndrome are also infertile. The condition results in several other distinctive physical features, including a broad neck, ears that are set low on the sides of the head, nipples that appear far apart, a low hairline, and swelling in the hands and feet. Other problems may include hearing problems, short fingers, thyroid problems, and diabetes.

Although there is no specific treatment for Turner's syndrome, growth-hormone supplements and supplements of estrogen can help to stimulate growth and bring on puberty, though most girls still remain infertile. The side effects of the condition are treated on a case-by-case basis.

Q What causes the condition congenital hypothyroidism?

Congenital hypothyroidism (CH) is a rare condition, occurring in only one in every 2,370 births in the US each year and is slightly more common in girls than in boys. It is thought to be caused by malformations in the thyroid gland during development in the uterus (usually because the gland doesn't move into a forward position in the throat), or perhaps the absence of the thyroid gland altogether. Occasionally, an inherited gene mutation may be the cause. The condition means that babies are born without the ability to make thyroxine, an important growth hormone, and if left untreated, hypothyroidism can lead to long-term growth problems and neurological damage.

Your baby will be tested for levels of thyroxine as part of the standard heel-prick test given at five days old. If your baby has CH, she will be given thyroxine supplements that she will need to continue throughout life. As long as the dosage remains accurate, the condition has no long-term consequences for your baby.

Q What is neurofibromatosis?

This rare genetic condition affects the nervous system, causing noncancerous tumors to grow on and along the nerves. The condition has a range of symptoms, (and is also associated with learning difficulties).

Babies may have clusters of freckles around the groin and armpits, and flat, light-brown pigmented patches of skin elsewhere on the body. Sometimes freckles appear on the whites of the eyes, and benign tumors may occur on the optic nerve. All over the skin, along nerve pathways, small lumps—as a result of the neurofibromas growing on the nerves—may appear, which can be significantly disfiguring. Children with the condition may have an unusually large head, and may develop convulsions, learning or behavioral problems, and hearing and sight may be affected. There is no treatment for this progressive disorder, although doctors may use chemotherapy or surgery to remove tumors that become cancerous, as well as surgery to remove benign tumors if these start to affect bodily function. Sufferers are offered counseling to try to come to terms with their appearance, especially if the neurofibromas are too numerous to consider removing for cosmetic reasons.

Neurofibromatosis This "dominant" gene disorder means a baby needs to inherit the gene from one parent only to develop the condition, as shown below.

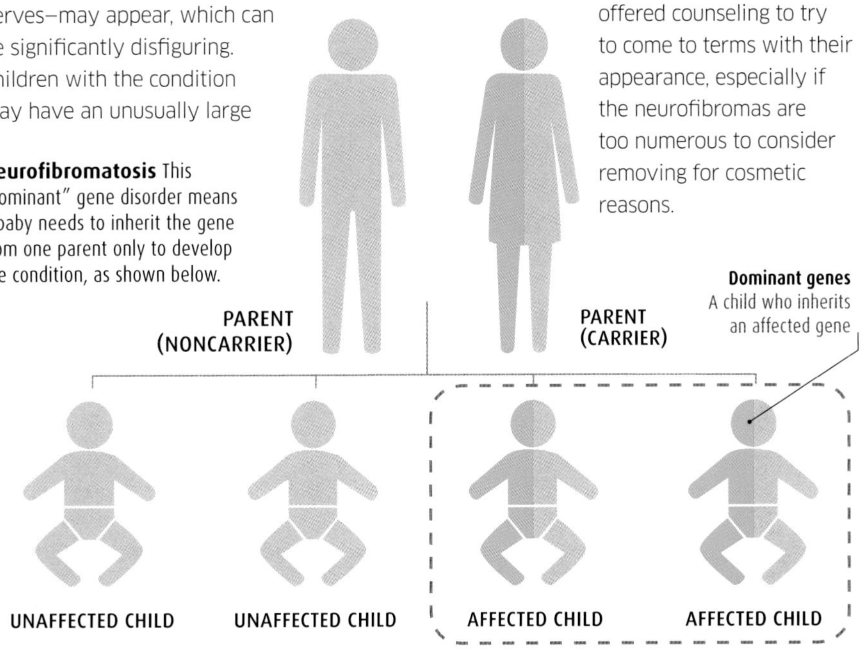

Dominant genes A child who inherits an affected gene

PARENT (NONCARRIER)

PARENT (CARRIER)

UNAFFECTED CHILD

UNAFFECTED CHILD

AFFECTED CHILD

AFFECTED CHILD

Q Is sickle-cell disease the same as sickle-cell anemia?

Sickle-cell disease is the umbrella term for a group of conditions that includes sickle-cell anemia. It is an inherited blood disorder in which red blood cells are shaped like a crescent moon—or a sickle. Healthy red blood cells are disc-shaped and bendy, enabling them to pass freely through the body's network of veins and arteries. Conversely, sickle cells are rigid and sticky, which means they become trapped in the junctions between blood vessels. This causes blockages in the circulation, starving bones, muscles, and organs of the oxygen and nutrients they need to grow and develop. In turn, organ damage, low growth rate, and pain in the joints and muscles occurs. A person with sickle-cell disease will go on to develop sickle-cell anemia, because sickle cells have a short life span and they die off faster than bone marrow can manufacture new cells to replace them. The result is anemia, which is characterized by a pale complexion and causes extreme fatigue.

Your baby is screened for sickle-cell anemia as part of the heel-prick test at five days old. There is no certain cure for sickle-cell disease, though occasionally bone marrow and stem cell transplants can work. Nonetheless, there have been major advances in the understanding of how to treat the symptoms and to minimize its effects, including prolonging life expectancy.

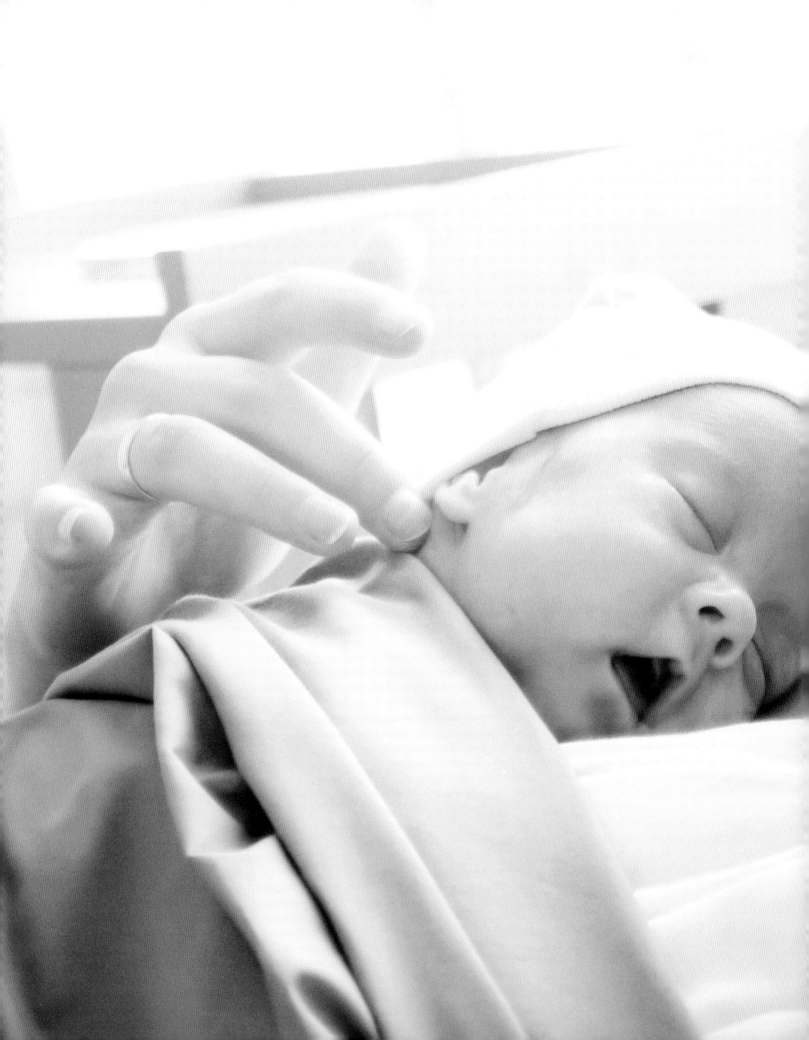

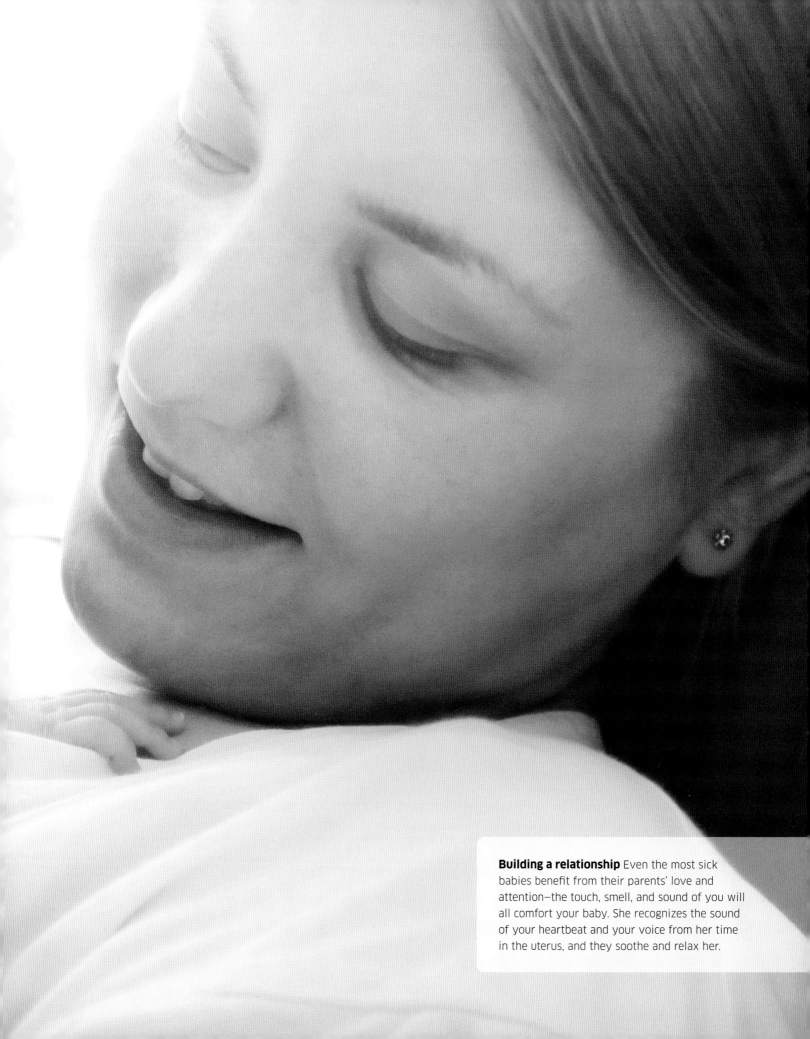

Building a relationship Even the most sick babies benefit from their parents' love and attention—the touch, smell, and sound of you will all comfort your baby. She recognizes the sound of your heartbeat and your voice from her time in the uterus, and they soothe and relax her.

Glossary

Abruption Premature separation of the placenta from the wall of the uterus.

Active positions An approach to childbirth that involves upright positions and movements during labor.

Active labor The point during labor in which the cervix begins to dilate more rapidly and contractions are stronger, last longer, and are closer together.

Alveoli Milk glands in the breasts, which produce a flow of milk when they are stimulated by prolactin and the baby's sucking.

Amniocentesis The surgical extraction of a small amount of amniotic fluid through the pregnant woman's abdomen. This procedure is usually performed as a test for fetal abnormalities.

Amnion The thin inner membrane surrounding the fetus and the amniotic fluid. It's also known as the amniotic sac.

Amniotic fluid The fluid that surrounds the fetus in the uterus. Ultrasounds may be done in late pregnancy to ensure that enough fluid is present.

Amniotomy The surgical rupture of the amniotic sac, often done to speed up labor. This is referred to as ARM (artificial rupture of the membranes).

Anemia A condition in which there is an abnormally low percentage of hemoglobin in the red blood cells. It is treated by taking iron supplements.

Anesthetic Medication that produces partial or complete insensibility to pain.

Anesthesia, general Anesthetic that affects the whole body, with temporary loss of consciousness.

Antibiotics Substances capable of destroying or limiting the growth of microorganisms, especially bacteria.

Antibodies Protein produced naturally by the body to combat any foreign bodies, germs, or bacteria.

Apgar score A general test of the baby's well-being performed at 1, 5, and 10 minutes after the birth to assess the baby's heart rate and tone, respiration, blood circulation, and nerve responses.

Areola The pigmented circle of skin surrounding the nipple.

Bilirubin Broken-down hemoglobin, normally converted to nontoxic substances by the liver. Some newborn babies have levels of bilirubin too high for their livers to deal with (neonatal jaundice).

Blastocyst An early stage of the developing egg after fertilization, when it has divided and subdivided into a group of cells.

Bloody show A vaginal discharge of bloodstained mucus occurring before labor, resulting from the onset of cervical dilatation. A sign that labor is starting.

Braxton-Hicks contractions Practice contractions of the uterus that occur throughout pregnancy, but which may not be noticed until toward the end of pregnancy.

Breast pump A device for drawing milk from the breasts.

Breech presentation When the position of the baby in the uterus is bottom down rather than head down.

Carpal tunnel syndrome Numbness and tingling of the hands arising from pressure on the nerves of the wrist. In pregnancy, it is caused by the body's accumulation of fluids.

Cephalic presentation The position of a baby who is head down in the uterus. The most common presentation.

Cephalopelvic disproportion A state in which the head of the fetus is larger than the cavity of the mother's pelvis. Delivery of the baby must therefore be by C-section.

Cervical dilation See *Dilation*.

Cervical insufficiency A disorder of the cervix, usually arising after a previous midpregnancy termination or damage to the cervix during a previous labor, in which the cervix opened up too soon, resulting in repeated midpregnancy miscarriages. It is sometimes treated by stitching to hold the cervix closed during pregnancy.

Cervix The lower entrance to the uterus, or neck of the uterus.

Cesarean section (C-section) The delivery of the baby through an incision in the abdominal and uterine walls.

Chorion The outer membrane tissue that envelops the fetus and placenta.

Chloasma Pigmentation of the skin that causes darker patches, often on the face. Also known as melasma.

Chorionic gonadotrophin See *Human chorionic gonadotrophin (hCG)*.

Chorionic villus sampling A method of screening for genetic disease by analyzing tissue from the small protrusions on the outer membrane enveloping the embryo (chorion), which later forms the placenta.

Chromosomes Rodlike structures containing genes. They occur in pairs within the nucleus of every cell. Human cells each contain 23 pairs.

Cleft palate A congenital abnormality of the roof of the mouth and upper lip. It is often treated with reconstruction surgery.

Colostrum A kind of milk, rich in proteins, formed and secreted by the breasts in late pregnancy and gradually changing to mature milk some days after the birth.

Conception The fertilization of the ripened egg by the sperm and its implantation in the uterine wall.

Contractions The regular tightening of the uterine muscles in labor as they work to dilate the cervix and press the baby down the birth canal.

Cordocentesis Fetal blood sampling or umbilical vein sampling. A diagnostic test to detect fetal abnormalities.

Crowning The moment when the baby's head appears at the entrance of the vagina during labor and does not slip back again.

Cystitis Infection of the bladder.

Diabetes Failure to metabolize glucose, indicated by excess sugar in blood and urine.

Dilation The progressive opening of the cervix caused by uterine contractions during labor.

Dizygotic See *Twins*.

Doppler A method of using ultrasound vibrations to listen to the fetal heart.

Doula A paid helper who provides support before, during, and after childbirth.

Ectopic pregnancy A pregnancy that develops outside the uterus.

Edema Swelling caused by water retention and blood pooling in the lower body. In rare cases this can be a sign of preeclampsia.

EDD The estimated date of delivery.

Electroencephalogram (EEG) A test where electrodes are placed on the scalp to record the electrical activity of the brain.

Embryo The earliest form of the baby in the uterus, from 4 weeks of pregnancy until around 10 weeks of pregnancy, after which it is termed a fetus.

Endometrium The lining of the uterus.

Engaged When the baby descends into the pelvis and three-fifths of his head have moved below pelvic bone. Usually a sign that labor is imminent.

Engorgement Congestion of the breasts with milk. If long periods are left between feedings, or the baby is not latched on well, painful engorgement can occur. This can be relieved by putting the baby to the breast or expressing the excess milk.

Epidural anesthesia A method of numbing the nerves of the lower spinal cord to ensure pain-free labor.

Episiotomy A surgical cut in the perineum to enlarge the entrance to the vagina.

Estrogen Hormone, levels of which rise rapidly in the first weeks of pregnancy, thickening the lining of the uterus, swelling breasts, and keeping hair and nails in a growth phase.

External cephalic version (ECV) The manipulation of the fetus by gentle pressure into the cephalic (head down) position. This may be done by an obstetrician or midwife at the end of pregnancy if the baby is in a breech or transverse position.

Fallopian tubes Two tubular structures (one on each side of the uterus) leading from the ovaries to the uterus.

Fertilization The meeting of the sperm with the egg to form a new life. See also *Conception*.

Fetus The developing baby in the uterus, known by this name around 10 weeks of pregnancy until birth.

Fibroids A benign (noncancerous) growth of muscle in the uterus, usually spherically shaped.

Flavonoids A group of compounds with antioxidant properties (also known as bioflavonoids).

Fontanelle The soft spot on top of a baby's head, which closes after about one and a half year's of age.

Forceps A tonglike instrument that fits on either side of the baby's head and is used to help deliver the baby.

Fundal height The distance from the pubis to the top of the uterus. It's measured regularly throughout pregnancy and is used as a marker of fetal growth.

Fundus The top of the uterus.

Hepatitis Viruses (named A, B, C, E, and others) that infect the liver, causing jaundice and generalized illness.

Hormone A chemical messenger in the blood that stimulates various organs to carry out specific actions.

Human chorionic gonadotrophin (hCG) A hormone released into the woman's bloodstream by the developing blastocyst after implantation. Its presence in the urine means that she is pregnant.

Hypnobirthing A type of self-hypnosis using visualization and breathing techniques to achieve a deep state of relaxation during labor.

Hyperemesis gravidarum Unrelenting, excessive nausea and vomiting preventing intake of adequate amounts of food and fluids. It can lead to dehydration.

Hypertension High blood pressure. During pregnancy this can reduce the fetal blood supply.

Hypotension Low blood pressure.

Implantation The embedding of the fertilized egg within the wall of the uterus.

Induction The process of artificially starting labor and keeping it going.

Intravenous (IV) The infusion of fluids directly into the bloodstream by means of a fine catheter introduced into a vein.

In vitro fertilization (IVF) A type of assisted conception where fertilization occurs outside the body and embryos are transferred back into the uterus.

Jaundice, neonatal The yellow color noticed in the eyes and skin due to an increased level of bilirubin (a substance produced when the liver breaks down red blood cells).

Kangaroo care A technique, adopted especially with premature babies, where baby and parent have prolonged skin-to-skin contact. This is thought to provide warmth, stimulation, and to encourage the baby to breast-feed.

Lanugo The fine soft hair that grows on the body of the fetus.

Letdown reflex The flow of breast milk into the nipple.

Lie The position in which the baby is lying within the uterus.

Linea nigra A line of dark pigmentation that appears on the skin of the abdomen in some women during pregnancy. It runs down the center of the abdomen over the rectus muscle.

Lochia Postpartum vaginal discharge.

Longitudinal lie The position of the fetus in the uterus in which the spines of the fetus and the mother are parallel.

Low-birth weight baby A baby who weighs below 5 lb (2.5 kg) at birth.

Meconium The first contents of the bowel, present in the fetus before birth and passed during the first few days after birth. The presence of meconium in the amniotic fluid before delivery is usually taken as a sign of fetal distress.

Melasma Dark, uneven patches of skin on the cheeks, forehead, nose, and chin during pregnancy. Exposure to the sun makes it worse. See also *Chloasma*.

Membranes Two layers of protective sacs enclosing the fetus, called the amnion and the chorion.

Meningitis A serious infection of the meninges, layers of tissue covering the brain.

Miscarriage The spontaneous loss of a baby before 20 weeks of pregnancy.

Monozygotic See *Twins*.

Morula A stage in the development of the fertilized egg, 3–4 days after fertilization, when it has grown into around 16 cells.

Multigravida A woman in her second or subsequent pregnancy.

Neonatal A baby less than 28 days old.

Nuchal scan A special ultrasound that can check for risk of Down syndrome.

Nucleus The central part or core of a cell, containing genetic information.

Occipital anterior The position of the baby in the uterus when the back of its head (the crown or occiput) is toward the mother's front (anterior).

Occipital posterior The position of the baby in the uterus when the back of its head (the crown or occiput) is toward the mother's back (posterior).

Opioids (Narcotics) Painkilling drugs that induce drowsiness and stupor.

Ovary One of the two female glands, set at the entrance of the fallopian tubes, which regularly produce eggs until menopause.

Ovulation The release of a ripe egg by the ovary.

Oxytocin Hormone that triggers the uterus to start contracting in the first stage of labor. If you are very overdue, you may be given an extra dose of synthetic oxytocin via an IV.

Palpation Feeling the parts of the fetus through the mother's abdominal wall.

Pelvic floor The springy muscular structure set within the pelvis that supports the bladder and the uterus, and through which the baby descends during labor.

Perinatal The period from the 24th week of gestation to one week following delivery.

Perineum The area of soft tissues surrounding the vagina and between the vagina and the rectum.

Placenta A flat, thick disc-shaped organ that supplies the fetus with oxygen and nutrients.

Placenta previa A placenta situated over, or close to, the entrance to the cervix. This makes a vaginal delivery unlikely.

Postpartum After delivery.

Postpartum hemorrhage (PPH) Excessive bleeding following delivery.

Preeclampsia A condition that features high blood pressure and excess proteins in the urine. May be mild or serious.

Premature A baby born before the 37th week of pregnancy.

Prenatal Before birth.

Presentation The positon of the baby according to the part of the fetus that is closest to the cervix before and during labor.

Preterm See *Premature*.

Primigravida A woman in her first pregnancy.

Progesterone A hormone produced in the ovaries and then by the placenta.

Prolactin Hormone that stimulates milk production.

Prostaglandins Natural substances that stimulate the onset of labor contractions. Prostaglandin gel may be used to soften the cervix and induce labor.

Quickening The first sensations of your baby moving. Generally felt for the first time at around 20 weeks.

Rhesus (Rh) factor A distinguishing characteristic of the red blood corpuscles. All human beings have either rhesus positive or rhesus negative blood. If the mother is rhesus negative and the fetus is rhesus positive, rhesus disease (the destruction of the red corpuscles by antibodies) may occur; usually in a subsequent pregnancy unless prevented by an injection of Rh immunoglobulin.

Rh immunoglobulin injection An injection of antibodies given to women who have a rhesus negative blood group if they may have been exposed to rhesus positive fetal blood cells.

Rooting The baby's instinctive searching for the breast in order to feed.

Rubella (German measles) A mild virus that may cause congenital abnormalities in the fetus if it is contracted by a woman during the first 12 weeks of pregnancy.

Sonographer Medical professional who operates ultrasonic imaging devices.

Spider nevi Tiny new veins noticeable on your cheeks, breasts, and legs, required to help your body disperse the extra heat generated in pregnancy.

Spinal anesthesia An injection of anesthetic into the spine for pain relief.

Startle reflex Also known as the Moro reflex. Newborns are tested for this reflex to check the nervous system is working.

Stillbirth The delivery of a deceased baby after the 24th week of pregnancy.

Stretch marks Shiny lines that sometimes appear on the skin after it has been stretched during pregnancy.

Surfactant A creamy fluid that reduces the surface tension of the lungs so that they do not stick together when deflated. Premature babies may have breathing difficulties if surfactant has not developed sufficiently.

Suture The stitching together of a tear or a surgical incision.

Thrombosis A blood clot, commonly occurring in the calf; most dangerous if in the lungs (pulmonary embolus).

Thrush A yeast infection that can form in the mucus membranes of the mouth, genitals, or nipples.

Toxoplasmosis A parasite infection that can be caught from cats or other pets. It's also found in soil and it can be present on fruit and vegetables. If it crosses the placenta during pregnancy, it can cause eye or central nervous system damage in the baby.

Transcutaneous electronic nerve stimulation (TENS) A method of pain relief that uses electrical impulses to block pain messages to the brain.

Transducer An instrument that translates echoes of high-frequency sound waves, bounced off the developing fetus in the uterus, to build an ultrasound image on a monitor. See also *Ultrasound*.

Transition A phase between the first and second stages of labor when the cervix is dilating to between 2¾–4 in (7–10 cm).

Transverse lie A sideways position of the fetus in the uterus.

Trial of labor A situation in which, although a cesarean section may be necessary, the mother labors in order to see if a vaginal delivery is possible.

Twins The simultaneous development of two babies in the uterus. If two eggs are fertilized independently by two sperm, dizygotic or fraternal twins result; more rarely, one fertilized egg divides to produce monozygotic or identical twins.

Ultrasound A way of building up a picture of an object by bouncing high-frequency soundwaves off it. Ultrasounds are used during pregnancy to show the development of the fetus in the uterus. See also *Transducer*.

Umbilical cord The cord connecting the fetus to the placenta.

Urinary tract infection (UTI) Infection affecting the kidneys and/or bladder.

Uterus (or womb) The hollow muscular organ in which the fertilized egg becomes embedded. Once implanted the egg develops into an embryo and then a fetus.

Vacuum extractor An instrument, used as an alternative to forceps, which adheres to the baby's scalp by suction and helps guide the baby out of the vagina.

Vagina The channel between the uterus and the external genitals. It receives the penis during intercourse and is the passage through which the baby is delivered (also called the birth canal).

Varicose veins Swollen veins in the legs that occur late in pregnancy.

VBAC Vaginal birth after cesarean section.

Vernix A thick, greasy substance that covers and protects the fetus's skin in the uterus.

Vertex presentation When the top of the fetus's head is the part closest to the cervix.

Vulva The external part of the female reproductive organs.

Water birth Birth of a baby under water.

Yolk sac The first source of nutrients for an embryo until the placenta takes over at around 12 weeks.

Zygote The single cell, formed by the merging of the egg and sperm.

Useful resources

WEBSITES

Here are contact details for organizations that offer support, advice, and guidance for conception, pregnancy, and life as a new parent.

Fertility

Resolve The National Infertility Association
resolve.org

Path2Parenthood (Formerly the American Fertility Association)
path2parenthood.org

American Society for Reproductive Medicine
reproductivefacts.org

Society for Assisted Reproductive Technology
sart.org

North American Surrogacy Center
northamericansurrogacycenter.com

Pregnancy

American College of Obstetricians and Gynecologists
acog.org

American Pregnancy Association
americanpregnancy.org

BabyCenter
BabyCenter.com

The Bump
thebump.com

ChooseMyPlate.gov for Pregnancy & Breastfeeding
choosemyplate.gov/moms-pregnancy-breastfeeding

March of Dimes
marchofdimes.com

Midwives Alliance of North America
mana.org

National Healthy Mothers, Healthy Babies Coalition
hmhb.org

National Women's Health Information Center
www.womenshealth.gov/pregnancy/index

Preeclampsia Foundation
preeclampsia.org

Labor and birth

American Association of Birth Centers
birthcenters.org

Bradley Method of Husband-Coached Natural Childbirth
bradleybirth.com

Childbirth Connection
childbirthconnection.org

DONA International (doulas)
dona.org

HypnoBirthing
www.hypnobirthing.com

International Cesarean Awareness Network
ican-online.org

Lamaze International
lamaze.org

Midwives Alliance of North America
mana.org

National Association of Certified Professional Midwives
nacpm.org

Breast-feeding

Baby-Friendly Hospital Initiative
babyfriendlyusa.org

Human Milk Banking Association of North America
hmbana.org

La Leche League
llli.org

National Alliance for Breastfeeding Advocacy
naba-breastfeeding.org

Support for Breastfeeding Mothers
lowmilksupply.org

United States Lactation Consultant Association
uslcaonline.org

Support groups

American Diabetes Association
diabetes.org

American SIDS Institute
sids.org

Asthma and Allergy Foundation of America
aafa.org

Birth Defect Research for Children
birthdefects.org

Cystic Fibrosis Foundation
cff.org

Epilepsy Foundation
epilepsyfoundation.org

Infants Remembered In Silence
irisremembers.com

Mental Health America: Portpartum Disorders
mentalhealthamerica.net/conditions/postpartum-disorders

National Down Syndrome Society
ndss.org

National Eczema Association
nationaleczema.org

NICU Parent Support Site
nicuparentsupport.org

Postpartum Support International
postpartum.net

Preeclampsia Foundation
preeclampsia.org

Sickle Cell Disease Association of America
sicklecelldisease.org

Spina Bifida Association
spinabifidaassociation.org

Star Legacy Foundation (stillbirth research and education)
starlegacyfoundation.org

Trisomy 18 Foundation
trisomy18.org

United Cerebral Palsy
ucp.org

Parent groups

CafeMom
cafemom.com

Mom-mentum
mom-mentum.org

Moms Meetup Group
moms.meetup.com

National Responsible Fatherhood
Clearinghouse
fatherhood.gov

National Single Parent Resource Center
nationalsingleparent.org

National Organization of Mothers
of Twins Clubs/Multiples of America
National Organization of Mothers of Twins
Clubs/Multiples of Americanomotc.org

Parents Without Partners
parentswithoutpartners.org

Rights and benefits

Family and Medical Leave Act
dol.gov/whd/fmla/

National Partnership for Women &
Families
nationalpartnership.org

General

American Academy of Pediatrics
healthychildren.org
aap.org

American Association of Acupuncture &
Oriental Medicine
aaaomonline.org

American Chiropractic Association
acatoday.org

American Red Cross
redcross.org

Centers for Disease Control and
Prevention
cdc.gov

Child Care Aware (information about
child care providers)
cpsc.gov

Infant Massage USA
infantmassageusa.org

National Assoc. for Family Child Care
nafcc.org

National Center for Complementary and
Alternative Medicine
nccam.nih.gov

National Highway Traffic Safety
Adminstration (car seat safety)
nhtsa.gov

National Institute of Child Health and
Human Development
nichd.nih.gov

Nemours Foundation
kidshealth.org

Safe Kids Worldwide
safekids.org

Smokefree (quitting smoking)
smokefree.gov

APPS

There are a multitude of apps available to download that can help with your pregnancy, labor, and taking care of your newborn. However, remember that while apps are fun and useful, never rely on them for medical advice and always consult your pediatrician first.

Pregnancy Plenty of apps are on available to assist you throughout your pregnancy journey. Certain ones contain personal journals with space to upload photos of your growing belly and images from your ultrasounds. Others have integrated communities with forums where you can connect with fellow moms-to-be.

There are apps that send you alerts for prenatal appointments, give you daily and weekly digests, monitor your baby's movements, track your weight gain, chart your pregnancy milestones, and prompt you with daily reminders to do your Kegal exercises.

Labor and birth There are a variety of apps that prepare you and your partner for the big day. They encourage you to think about what will happen from start to finish. Most labor apps have a contraction timer and a place to write out your birth plan. Some apps include suggestions on how to have a natural birth, birthing positions to try out, and videos showing various laboring techniques. These apps often list the pros and cons of different birthing methods, helping you consider all the available options. Many apps help prepare you mentally for delivering your baby—they demonstrate how to utilize meditation, relaxation, and visualization.

There are also lots of handy apps with checklists of what to pack in your hospital bag that you can check off as you pack the items in your bag. There are several apps with a birth announcement tool to help you share your happy news and upload photos of your new arrival.

Life with your baby Once you have your baby, there are apps with a range of tools to assist you with life as a new parent. Some give daily guidance during the first 6 months. You can communicate with other new moms and dads in your area through certain apps that include forums. If you're feeling tired and forgetful, there are apps to help track your baby's feedings, diaper changes, and sleeping patterns.

There are specific apps devoted to calming and soothing your baby through white noise, lullabies, or nursery rhymes. There are a few apps that find the closest diaper changing facility when you're out and about. Users can rate their experiences of cleanliness, accessibility, and location.

As your baby grows, there are apps for starting your baby on solid food available to download with tips, trackers, and recipes. There are even some that demonstrate baby signing, so you can teach your baby the basic signs for milk, sleep, eat, play, and teddy bear.

Index

Acknowledgments

Publisher's acknowledgments

Creative Publishing Manager Anna Davidson
Proofreaders Jemima Dunne, Claire Cross, and Jamie Ambrose
Indexer Hilary Bird
Art Direction for Photography Isabel de Cordova, Peggy Sadler
Models Adam Dicuru, Raquel Dicuru, Abby Dorrian, Indiana Dorrian, Myles Dorrian, Justyna Duggan, and Adele Roche
Location Agency www.1st-Option.com

Picture credits

Most of the images and photographs of the developing baby in this book are of the embryo and fetus live in utero, using endoscopic and ultrasound technology. When this has not been possible, images have been taken by reputable medical professionals as part of research or to promote educational awareness.

The publisher would like to thank the following for their kind permission to reproduce their photographs:

(Key: a-above; b-below/bottom; c-center; f-far; l-left; r-right; t-top)

4 Photolibrary: Digital Vision. **12 Maxine Pedliham:** (tr). **Science Photo Library:** P. Saada / Eurelios (br). **37 Corbis:** MedicalRF.com (tr). **49 Science Photo Library:** Anatomical Travelogue (ca). **82 Dreamstime.com:** Monkey Business Images / Monkeybusinessimages (bl). **93 iStockphoto.com:** M_a_y_a. **94 Dreamstime.com:** Ngo Thye Aun / Ngothyeaun. **95 Dreamstime.com:** Monkey Business Images / Monkeybusinessimages (bl). **Getty Images:** R. J. Sangosti / The Denver Post (cl). **96 Science Photo Library:** Dr. G. Moscoso (tr); Sovereign, ISM (bl, br). **99 Wellcome Images**. **100-101 LOGIQlibrary. 100 Science Photo Library:** Living Art Enterprises, LLC. (bc, br). **101 Getty Images:** LM Photo / The Image Bank (tl). **102 Dreamstime.com:** Natasnow. **103 Science Photo Library:** Dr. Najeeb Layyous (cra, bl, bc, br). **107 Corbis:** Tomas Rodriguez. **110 Alamy Images:** View Stock. **111 Alamy Images:** Jose Luis Pelaez Inc. / Blend Images. **113 Alamy Images:** Jose Luis Pelaez Inc. / Blend Images. **121 Corbis:** B2M Productions / Ocean (bl). **127 Alamy Images:** OJO Images Ltd. (l). **130 Dreamstime.com:** Ana Blazic Pavlovic (c). **134 Corbis:** Tomas Rodriguez (tl). **136 iStockphoto.com:** momcilog (b). **140 Corbis:** JGI / Tom Grill / Blend Images (crb). **141 Getty Images:** Westend61 (br). **142 Getty Images:** Caroline Purser (cl). **143 Science Photo Library:** (br). **145 Corbis:** B. Boissonnet / BSIP (tr). **146 Science Photo Library:** Gustoimages (cb). **158-159 Science Photo Library:** Edelmann. **163 Science Photo Library:** Neil Bromhall (t). **164-165 Science Photo Library:** Neil Bromhall. **167 Corbis:** Bernd Vogel (cr). **Getty Images:** Marc Romanelli (ca). **iStockphoto.com:** PonyWang (cra). **193 Dreamstime.com:** Indigolotos (br). **209 Mother & Baby Picture Library:** Ian Hooton (l). **218-219 Alamy Images:** Lionel Wotton. **220 Corbis:** Juergen Effner / dpa (cr). **221 Corbis:** Rune Hellestad (br). **223 Alamy Images:** Chloe Johnson (br). **225 Science Photo Library:** David Parker (r). **228 Science Photo Library:** Ian Hooton (l). **229 Science Photo Library:** Ian Hooton (cb). **230 Alamy Images:** Phanie (cra). **234 Alamy Images:** Martin Valigursky (b). **237 Alamy Images:** philipus (tr). **243 Alamy Images:** Purestock (crb). **245 Getty Images:** Layland Masuda (cl). **246 Alamy Images:** Phanie (bl). **247 Getty Images:** Siri Stafford (cra). **248-249 Dreamstime.com:** Aynur Shauerman (b). **249 Alamy Images:** Family (tl). **Science Photo Library:** Dr. P. Marazzi (cra, cra/strawberry, cr, cr/skin spot); (crb, crb/mole). **253 Getty Images:** Comstock (cr). **255 Alamy Images:** Phanie (tr). **258-259 Getty Images:** Alistair Berg. **264-265 Getty Images:** LWA. **272 Dorling Kindersley:** Antonia Deutsch (br, cr, tr). **273 Getty Images:** Jamie Grill (tr). **276 Getty Images:** Mecky (br). **290 Getty Images:** Science Photo Library (bl). **291 Getty Images:** Tetra Images (br). **293 Getty Images:** Frederic Cirou (bl). **295 Science Photo Library:** Gustoimages (br). **299 Getty Images:** ONOKY - Eric Audras (cl). **300-301 Getty Images:** Marina Raith. **311 Corbis:** ERproductions Ltd. / Blend Images (tr). **312-313 Getty Images:** Science Photo Library. **313 Getty Images:** Guillermo Legaria / AFP. **314 Corbis:** Glowimages (tr). **Getty Images:** BSIP / UIG (c). **315 Corbis:** JGI / Tom Grill / Blend Images. **316 Getty Images:** Todd Bates / E+ (bl); Cultura Science / Marc Fluri (ca). **317 Science Photo Library:** Antonia Reeve. **319 Getty Images:** Focus_on_Nature / E+. **322 Getty Images:** Fertnig / Vetta. **327 Getty Images:** Leanne Temme / Stockbyte. **328 Corbis:** JGI / Tom Grill / Blend Images. **329 Science Photo Library:** Photostock-Israel. **332-333 iStockphoto.com:** IvanJekic.

All other images © Dorling Kindersley
For further information see: **www.dkimages.com**

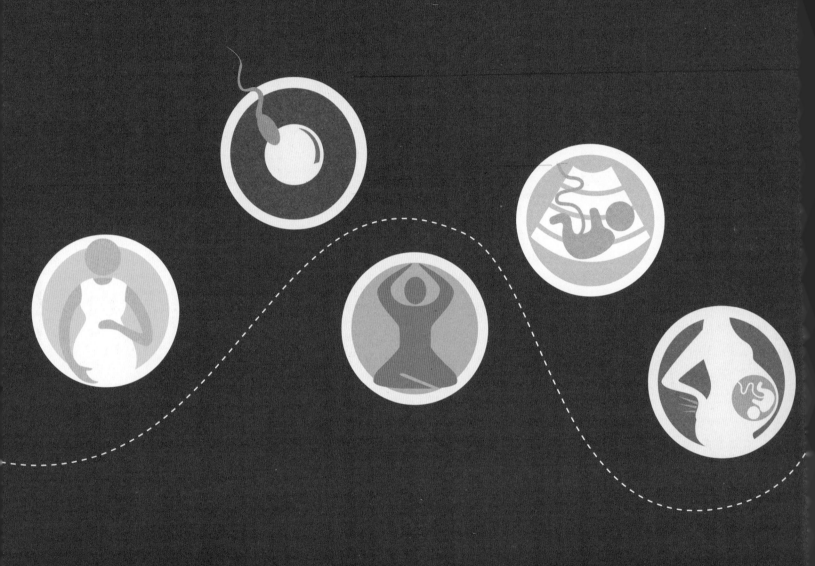